Minimizing Incisions and Maximizing Outcomes in Cataract Surgery

Jorge L. Alió
I. Howard Fine (Eds.)

Minimizing Incisions and Maximizing Outcomes in Cataract Surgery

Springer

Jorge L. Alió, MD, PhD
Professor and Chairman of Ophthalmology
Vissum
Instituto Oftalmológico de Alicante
Miguel Hernández University
Department of Ophthalmology
Av. de Denia, s/n
03016 Alicante
Spain
jlalio@vissum.com

I. Howard Fine, MD
Oregon Health & Science University
Drs. Fine, Hoffman and Packer
1550 Oak Street, Suite 5, Eugene
OR 97401, USA
hfine@finemd.com

ISBN: 978-3-662-50184-9 ISBN: 978-3-642-02862-5 (eBook)

DOI: 10.1007/978-3-642-02862-5

Springer Heidelberg Dordrecht London New York

Cover design: eStudio Calamar, Figueres/Berlin

Printed on acid-free paper

Springer is part of Springer Science+Business Media (www.springer.com)

This book is dedicated to the privilege of working with I. Howard Fine, an excellent professional model and a most highly esteemed friend and mentor, dedicated to his talent in creating progress in cataract surgery, teaching others, working hard and meticulously, being precise, and always behaving like a really good person. It has been an honour to work with Howard on this book, immediately prior to his retirement and sabbatical. I do not know anyone who really deserves it more.

Jorge Alió

Preface

This book appears at a moment in which cataract surgery is probably making the last evolution in technology and surgical practice, according to the postulates that Charles Kelman started in the early 70s. The progressive transition from the initial concept of small inicision cataract surgery, the development of more and more sophisticated technology to support the surgeon's practice of the procedure, the development of intraocular lenses capable of correcting virtually all types of refractive errors, and the scientific knowledge available today on fluidics, micromechanics, biomaterials, viscomaterials, and surgical instrument technology has made cataract surgery experience one of the greatest progressions and advances of a surgical technique throughout the history of medicine and surgery.

Cataract surgery at the moment is transforming into a practice in which minimal agressiveness and optimized outcomes are targeted and tried to achieve by surgeons. Better diagnostic technology, sophistication in calculation formulas for IOL implantation, better instruments for incisions, and deeper knowledge into the structure of the cornea and corneal optics, greater knowledge into issues related intraocular lens performance, the approach to solve pseudophakic presbyopia by multifocal or accommodative lenses are, among many others, issues that have been recently advancing cataract surgery toward its next stage.

Throughout this process, the history of cataract surgery has been related to the decrease in incision size. This is why an important part of this book is targeting biaxial microincisional surgery, which seems to be mandatory in the future evolution of cataract removal. Simplification of the procedure and separation of irrigation and aspiration seems to be related to better outcomes supported by current scientific evidence. This is possible, thanks to a better knowledge of the instrumentation, fluidics, use of ultrasound power, and indeed surgical knowledge and training. The development of new lenses capable of fitting through smaller incisions than those currently available seems to be a limit to the development of the technology. Today, we can precisely limit our capabilities for cataract removal to 1.6 mm and to 1.8 mm with IOL implantation. Throughout this book, the reader will be able to learn about the methods to achieve this benchmark of cataract surgery at this moment.

As we have already mentioned in our opinion, this book appears during the final stage of the evolution of cataract surgery as conceived today. We anticipate that sub 1 mm surgery will require new technologies, and especially, new IOL technology and biomaterials. Most probably, we are at the end of the revolution that was started by Charlie Kelman in the early 70s and in the next decade we shall start a new evolution toward new issues such as lens replacement through new biomaterials, new accommodating lenses, regenerating surgery, and new technologies to soften the cataract and to eliminate it through punctures rather than through incisions.

We both, as co-authors, think that the readers will enjoy going through this book to discover the real cutting edge but practical image offered today by high-quality cataract surgery practice. We thank all the co-authors of this book, all of them most relevant professionals and surgical scientists, for their contribution to this book and to the progress of cataract surgery. Thanks to them and to the support of our families, this book appears ready to go to your operating room as an advisor for your progression toward the last transition that cataract surgery will experience with the technology available today.

Alicante, Spain — Jorge L. Alió
Eugene, Oregon, USA — I. Howard Fine

Contents

Contributors

Amar Agarwal Eye Research Centre & Dr. Agarwal´s Group of Eye Hospitals, 19 Cathedral Road, Chennai 600 086, India
dragarwal@vsnl.com

Jorge L. Alió Vissum Instituto Oftalmológico de Alicante, Miguel Hernández University, Medical School, Alicante, Spain
Department of Ophthalmology, Miguel Hernández University, Alicante, Spain
jlalio@vissum.com

T. Amzallag Ophthalmic Institute of Somain, 28 rue Anatole France, 59490, Somain, France
thierry.amzallag@institut-ophtalmique.fr

Steve A. Arshinoff Humber River Regional Hospital, 2115 Finch Avenue, Toronto, ON, Canada M3N 2V6
The University of Toronto, Toronto, ON, Canada
ifix2is@sympatico.ca

Gerd U. Auffarth University Eye Hospital Heidelberg, International Vision Correction Research Centre (IVCRC), Ruprechts-Karls-University of Heidelberg, Im Neuenheimer Feld 400, 69120 Heidelberg, Germany
ga@uni-hd.de

George H.H. Beiko McMaster University, University of Toronto, Hamilton, ON, Canada
george.beiko@sympatico.ca

Jerome Bovet Clinique de l'oeil, 15 bois de la chapelle, 1213 Onex/Geneva, Switzerland
jbovet@vision.tv

Rosa Braga-Mele University of Toronto, Toronto, ON, Canada
Mount Sinai Hospital, Toronto, ON, Canada
Kensington Eye Institute, Toronto, ON, Canada

Miriam Casper University Eye Hospital Heidelberg, International Vision Correction Research Centre (IVCRC), Ruprechts-Karls-University of Heidelberg, Im Neuenheimer Feld 400, 69120 Heidelberg, Germany

David F. Chang 762 Altos Oaks Drive, 1 Los Altos, CA 94024

Robert J. Cionni The Eye Institute, 755 East 3900 South, Salt Lake City, UT 84107, USA
rcionni@theeyeinstitute.com

H. Burkhard Dick Center for Vision Science, Ruhr–University Eye Hospital, In der Schornau 23-25, 44892 Bochum, Germany
burkhard.dick@kk-bochum.de

I. Howard Fine Oregon Health & Science University, Drs. Fine, Hoffman and Packer, 1550 Oak Street, Suite 5, Eugene, OR 97401, USA

William J. Fishkind Fishking & Bakewell Eye Care and Surgical Center, Tucson, Arizona, USA
University of Utah, Salt Lake City, Utah, USA
University of Arizona, Tucson, Arizona, USA

Alessandro Franchini Eye Institute, University of Florence, Italy
oculist@unifi.it

Iacopo Franchini Medicine and Surgery School, University of Florence, Italy

David Hair The Eye Institute, 755 East 3900 South, Salt Lake City, UT 84107, USA

Richard S. Hoffman Oregon Health & Science University, Drs. Fine, Hoffman and Packer, 1550 Oak Street, Suite 5, Eugene, OR 97401, USA

Bassam El Kady Ain Shams University, Cairo, Egypt
Vissum-Instituto Oftalmologico de Alicante, Department of Research and Development, Alicante, Spain
bisoelkadi@yahoo.com

Hakan Kaymak Department of Ophthalmology, Knappschafts–Hospital, Sulzbach/Germany
sek-augen@kksulzbach.de

Pawel Klonowski Vissum-Instituto Oftalmologico de Alicante, Department of Research and Development, Alicante, Spain

Peter Allan Karth Medical College of Wisconsin, Department of Ophthalmology, Milwgukee, WI, USA

Stephen S. Lane University of Minnesota, 2950 Curve Crest Boulevard, Stillwater, MN 55082, USA
sslane@associatedeyecare.com

Ulrich Mester Department of Ophthalmology, Knappschafts Hospital, Sulzbach/Germany

Rupert Menapace Department of Ophthalmology, Vienna General Hospital & Medical University Vienna, Waehringer Guertel 18–20 A 1090 Vienna, Australia

Ayman Naseri Department of Ophthalmology, University of California, San Francisco, San Francisco, CA
San Francisco VA Medical Center, San Francisco, CA, USA

Silvio Di Nardo Oertli Instruments AG, Hefnerwisenstrasse 4, CH 9442 Berneck, Switzerland

Randall J. Olson Department of Ophthalmology and Visual Sciences, Moran Eye Center, University of Utah School of Medicine, 65 N Medical Drive, Salt Lake City, UT 84132, USA
randall.olson@hsc.utah.edu

James M. Osher Department of Ophthalmology, University of Cincinnati, Cincinnati, OH, USA

Robert H. Osher Department of Ophthalmology, University of Cincinnati, Cincinnati, OH, USA

Mark Packer Oregon Health & Science University, Drs. Fine, Hoffman and Packer, 1550 Oak Street, Suite 5, Eugene, OR 97401, USA

Richard Packard Prince Charles Eye Unit, Windsor, UK

Arturo Pèrez-Arteaga Centro Oftalmològico Tlalnepantla, Vallarta 42, Tlalnepantla, Mèxico, 54000, Mèxico
drarturo@prodigy.net.mx

Tanja M. Rabsilber University Eye Hospital Heidelberg, International Vision Correction Research Centre (IVCRC), Ruprechts-Karls-University of Heidelberg, Im Neuenheimer Feld 400, 69120 Heidelberg, Germany

Jose L. Rodriguez-Prats Vissum-Instituto Oftalmologico de Alicante, Department of Research and Development, Alicante, Spain

Jennifer H. Smith Department of Ophthalmology, Northwestern University, 2238 Pinehurst Drive, Glenview, IL 60025, USA

Daniele Tognetto Eye Institute, University of Trieste, Italy

L. Felipe Vejarano Fundación Oftalmológica Vejarano, Popayán, Colombia
Department of Ophthalmology, Universidad del Cauca, Popayán, Colombia

Introduction

Minimizing: A Continuous Trend in Cataract Surgery

I. Howard Fine, Jorge Alio, Mark Packer,
Richard S. Hoffman, and Peter Allan Karth

Literature Review

There is a growing body of investigation focused on minimally invasive bimanual microincision cataract surgery (MICS). The first reports of this technique published in peer-reviewed journals appeared in the mid-1970s and 1980s [1–4]. Agarwal is generally recognized as having created a renewed interest in this technique [5].

A series of cases of bimanual MICS was published in January 2002 which consisted of a noncomparative study of this procedure in 637 eyes [6]. The volume of publications on this subject has seen a considerable increase in the last 18 months. From 1995 through 2006, over 50 papers have featured bimanual, or biaxial, MICS. In 2007 and the first half of 2008, an additional 30 peer-reviewed papers have been published, addressing various topics.

Major Issues

The issues surrounding the debate between traditional, or microcoaxial, phacoemulsification and bimanual, or biaxial, microincision phacoemulsification are many. Within the published literature, these issues can be broken down into the following major groups:

1. Visual outcome: postsurgical best corrected visual acuity (BCVA), and change in astigmatism
2. Corneal/anterior chamber factors: corneal endothelial cell loss, postsurgical corneal swelling, and anterior chamber cell and flare
3. Incision-specific factors: thermal burn and incision leakage
4. Technical factors: effective phacoemulsification time (EPT) and total surgical time

Nearly all of the published studies examine one or more of these factors, either in a directly comparative setting or simply to determine the rates of these factors in biaxial MICS for comparison with historical levels in coaxial phacoemulsification. Some studies do provide data on other metrics specific to the particular aspect being studied, but these are widely variable and difficult or impossible to compare between studies [7]. We will focus on the above major issues in this review.

Major Studies

Many of the published papers on this subject use animal or cadaver eyes, are noncomparative, have significant confounding variables, or are simply opinion pieces or case reports. This leaves only a handful of studies which are considered seminal, high-quality papers. These are randomized, prospective, comparative studies conducted on human subjects by surgeons competent in the techniques being compared. Most have large sample sizes and minimal confounding variables. All were published in highly respected peer-reviewed journals. These studies are discussed individually and only statistically significant results are analyzed.

In January 2002, Tsuneoka et al. [6] published a paper evaluating thermal burn, astigmatism, and endothelial cell loss as a result of bimanual phacoemulsification using a 1.4 mm incision and a sleeveless phaco tip. This was the first large series studying bimanual phacoemulsification; 637 eyes were included.

I. H. Fine (✉)
Oregon Health & Science University, Drs. Fine, Hoffman and Packer, 1550 Oak Street, Suite 5, Eugene, OR 97401, USA
e-mail:hfine@finemd.com

J. L. Alió, I. H. Fine (eds.), *Minimizing Incisions and Maximizing Outcomes in Cataract Surgery*,
DOI: 10.1007/978-3-642-02862-5, © Springer-Verlag Berlin Heidelberg 2010

Although noncomparative, it remains an important study. Approximately 5% of the cataracts had grade 4 or 5 nuclear density. The results showed a mean operating time of 8 min and 42 s. Not one case of thermal burn was reported. Three-month postsurgical follow-up was done in 312 eyes. Measured corneal endothelial cell density had decreased by 4.6% in eyes with a nuclear hardness of grade 1, 6.9% in eyes with grade 2, 10.8% in eyes with grade 3, and 15.6% in eyes with grade 4 and above. The authors considered these levels to be similar to cell loss with traditional, coaxial, phacoemulsification methods. Corneal astigmatism was 0.35D at postoperative week 1 and 0.18D at postoperative month 3, which was deemed to be far lower than postoperative astigmatism induced by standard phacoemulsification, despite enlargement of an incision up to 4 mm for IOL insertion. The authors concluded bimanual MICS to be at least as safe and effective as traditional methods, especially considering superior astigmatic results.

Jorge Alió, a pioneering surgeon with biaxial phacoemulsification, published the first large prospective randomized landmark study in November 2005, comparing bimanual MICS with regular coaxial phacoemulsification [8]. A total of 100 eyes with cataracts graded 2–4 were randomized to two groups, one receiving biaxial phaco from 1.5 mm incisions, and the other receiving coaxial phaco via a 2.8 mm incision. All other aspects of the surgeries were designed to be identical, including equipment settings, minimizing confounding variables. Key statistically significant results showed dramatic differences in estimated phaco time (EPT = total phacoemulsification time in seconds × average power percent used): 2.19 for biaxial and 9.3 for coaxial. Postsurgical astigmatic changes were significantly lower in bimanual MICS (0.433 vs. 1.20D in the coaxial group). Postoperative corneal endothelial cell loss, anterior chamber cell/flare, and visual acuity were statistically equal in both groups. As in the Tsuneoka et al. study, no signs of thermal burns were seen with either technique. The authors understandably concluded bimanual MICS to be safe, effective, and in many ways superior to coaxial techniques.

In 2006, Kurz et al. compared biaxial microincision (1.5 mm) and coaxial small-incision (2.75 mm) cataract surgery in a well-designed study of 70 randomized eyes [9]. A multitude of outcomes were measured. BCVA on postoperative day 1 showed a mean of 20/25 in the biaxial group and 20/33 in the coaxial group. Eight weeks after surgery, BCVA in the biaxial group was 20/20 versus 20/25 in the coaxial group, showing notably better visual acuity outcomes in bimanual MICS. EPT times were measured to be greater than 3 s in 34% of bimanual patients and 68% of coaxial patients. Astigmatic changes were statistically similar (0.15 vs. 0.31D). Corneal endothelial cell losses were statistically equivalent in both groups (14–15%). Overall, using these and other metrics, the authors concluded bimanual phacoemulsification to be as efficacious as coaxial, and, in fact, superior in two aspects.

Cavallini et al. prospectively randomized 100 eyes in 50 patients to compare bimanual and coaxial phacoemulsification in a paper published in 2007 [10]. All cataracts were graded 2–4. Particularly interesting was that all 100 procedures were done using the same machine and by the same surgeon, who was quite capable at both methods. Multiple key metrics were recorded. The authors reported all metrics to be statistically equal, including EPT (3–5 s), corneal endothelial cell loss (10–12 cells/mm), and postsurgical astigmatism (<1D). Shorter surgical time was reported in the biaxial group (637 vs. 736 s). Less BSS was used in the biaxial technique. The authors concluded both methods to be safe and effective.

One must keep in mind that these studies did not address the primary benefits of biaxial technique (ability to interchange instruments by switching hands, iris management, separation of aspiration from irrigation, etc.). These studies and nearly all the published papers address measurable outcome metrics. Therefore, if biaxial phaco was deemed only equal to coaxial phaco by these measurements, it would still have tremendous benefit because of the fluidic advantages of separating aspiration from irrigation and eliminating competing fluid currents at the tip. Smaller incisions are also inherently less invasive.

Kahraman et al. published a well-designed prospective study with masked investigators to compare metrics of phacoemulsification outcomes 1 day and 3 months after surgery [11]. Thirty-three patients underwent cataract surgery, with bimanual phaco being performed in one eye and micro-coaxial (3.2 mm) in the other eye of each patient on the same day. The standard metrics for evaluating cataract surgery were recorded. The data showed no statistical differences between the two techniques, except that corneal thickness was increased on the first postoperative day in the biaxial group by 14 ∝m, ostensibly due to corneal swelling. This difference resolved at the second time point. The authors correctly concluded that bimanual MICS is safe and reproducible.

In June 2007, Cerma et al. performed standard coaxial in one eye and bimanual MICS in the fellow eye of 30 patients with 1 year follow-up in 26 patients [12]. In this study, EPT was significantly higher in the biaxial group (8.2 vs. 5.0 s). Corneal endothelial cell loss was also greater in the biaxial MICS group (8.82 vs. 6.00% cells/mm). BCVA was similar in both groups. The authors stated that the endothelial cell loss was well within safe limits and concluded that biaxial was a safe and effective method for cataract removal.

Yao et al. randomized 60 eyes to biaxial phaco with a 1.7 mm incision and coaxial phaco with 3.2 mm incisions [13]. This study was specifically designed to focus on surgically induced astigmatism and showed biaxial phaco to be equal or superior to coaxial phaco 1-month postoperatively with less astigmatic changes (0.78 vs. 1.29D). Mencucci et al. compared biaxial MICS with standard phacoemulsification in 80 eyes, using stop-and-chop in both groups [14]. Among several other metrics, there was no statistically significant difference in central corneal endothelial cell counts.

Again, these studies do not compare the overall superiority of either technique and do not address any surgical benefits of one technique over the other. All studies concluded BCVA and astigmatic changes to be equal or superior in biaxial phaco, but corneal endothelial cell loss was inconclusive or contradictory. All the major studies cited conclude that bimanual MICS is at least as safe and effective as coaxial methods. We believe that biaxial techniques are superior and that is especially true in challenging and complicated cases (see Chap. 3), many of which would be impossible to perform with coaxial procedures.

Negative Studies

As of mid-2008, the peer-reviewed literature contained less than ten papers which suggest that biaxial MICS may be an inferior technique, with their major finding being a negative outcome for biaxial phaco.

The Kahraman study showed increased corneal thickness due to swelling in the first postoperative day, but showed no other statistical differences [11]. The Cerma study reported that EPT and corneal endothelial cell loss was higher in the biaxial group [12]. It also reported similar BAVA at 1 year between the two groups.

In a comparative study in 2008, Praveen et al. compared 180 eyes randomized into three phacoemulsification groups: standard coaxial, micro-coaxial, and biaxial [15]. The ingress of trypan blue dye into the eye was measured immediately after cortex removal and again at the end of surgery after stromal hydration. The study concluded that biaxial wounds allowed increased ingress intrasurgically immediately after cortex removal when compared to other groups. However, after stromal hydration, no statistical difference was found between the three groups.

The two rabbit studies compared wound damage and bacterial ingress and concluded coaxial and micro-coaxial to be superior to biaxial in these areas [16, 17]. Two cadaver studies used small sample sizes (15 eyes and 6 eyes) to look at wound damage and temperature and concluded coaxial and micro-coaxial to be superior to biaxial in these areas [18, 19].

We have inadequate knowledge of construction and architecture of the biaxial incisions in these studies, but, as Fine has demonstrated utilizing optical coherence tomography (OCT), properly constructed micro-biaxial incisions creates architecture that is self-sealable and stable [20, 21]. Finally, all of these investigators are novices at biaxial phaco and their initial experiences cannot be compared to other techniques that they have mastered over a period of decades.

References

1. Shock JP. Removal of cataracts with ultrasonic fragmentation and continuous irrigation. Trans Pac Coast Otoophthalmol Soc Annu Meet 1972; 53:139–144.
2. Girard LJ. Ultrasonic fragmentation for cataract extraction and cataract complications. Adv Ophthalmol 1978; 37: 127–135.
3. Shearing SP, Relyea RL, Loaiza A, Shearing RL. Routine phacoemulsification through a one-millimeter non-sutured incision. Cataract 1985; 2:6–10.
4. Hara T, Hara T. Endocapsular phacoemulsification and aspiration (ECPEA) – recent surgical technique and clinical results. Ophthalmic Surg 1989; 20(7):469–475.
5. Agarwal A, Agarwal S. No anesthesia cataract surgery. In: Agarwal S (ed.) Phacoemulsification, Laser Cataract Surgery, and Foldable IOLs. New Dehli, India: Jaypee Brothers, 1998, 144–154.
6. Tsuneoka H, Shiba T, Takahashi Y. Ultrasonic phacoemulsification using a 1.4 mm incision: clinical results. J Cataract Refract Surg 2002; 28(1):81–86.
7. Olson RJ, Jin Y, Kefalopoulos G, et al. Legacy AdvanTec and Sovereign WhiteStar: a wound temperature study. J Cataract Refract Surg 2004; 30:1109–1113.
8. Alio J, Rodriguez-Prats JL, Galal A, Ramzy M. Outcomes of microincision cataract surgery versus coaxial phacoemulsification. Ophthalmology 2005; 112(11):1997–2003.

9. Kurz S, Krummenauer F, Gabriel P, Pfeiffer N, Dick HB. Biaxial microincision versus coaxial small-incision clear cornea cataract surgery. Ophthalmology 2006; 113(10): 1818–1826.
10. Cavallini GM, Campi L, Masini C, Pelloni S, Pupino A. Bimanual microphacoemulsification versus coaxial miniphacoemulsification: prospective study. J Cataract Refract Surg 2007; 33(3):387–392.
11. Kahraman G, Amon M, Franz C, Prinz A, Abela-Formanek C. Intra-individual comparison of surgical trauma after bimanual microincision and conventional small-incision coaxial phacoemulsification. J Cataract Refract Surg 2007; 33(4):618–622.
12. Crema AS, Walsh A, Yamane Y, Nosé W. Comparative study of coaxial phacoemulsification and microincision cataract surgery. One-year follow-up. J Cataract Refract Surg 2007; 33(6):1014–1018.
13. Yao K, Tang X, Ye P. Corneal astigmatism, high order aberrations, and optical quality after cataract surgery: microincision versus small incision. J Refract Surg 2006; 22(9 Suppl):S1079–S1082.
14. Mencucci R, Ponchietti C, Virgili G, Giansanti F, Menchini U. Corneal endothelial damage after cataract surgery: microincision versus standard technique. J Cataract Refract Surg 2006; 32(8):1351–1354.
15. Praveen MR, Vasavada AR, Gajjar D, Pandita D, Vasavada VA, Vasavada VA, Raj SM. Comparative quantification of ingress of trypan blue into the anterior chamber after microcoaxial, standard coaxial, and bimanual phacoemulsification: randomized clinical trial. J Cataract Refract Surg 2008; 34(6):1007–1012.
16. Johar SR, Vasavada AR, Praveen MR, Pandita D, Nihalani B, Patel U, Vemuganti G. Histomorphological and immunofluorescence evaluation of bimanual and coaxial phacoemulsification incisions in rabbits. J Cataract Refract Surg 2008; 34(4):670–676.
17. Gajjar D, Praveen MR, Vasavada AR, Pandita D, Vasavada VA, Patel DB, Johar K, Raj S. Ingress of bacterial inoculum into the anterior chamber after bimanual and microcoaxial phacoemulsification in rabbits. J Cataract Refract Surg 2007; 33(12):2129–2134.
18. Berdahl JP, DeStafeno JJ, Kim T. Corneal wound architecture and integrity after phacoemulsification evaluation of coaxial, microincision coaxial, and microincision bimanual techniques. J Cataract Refract Surg 2007; 33(3): 510–515.
19. Osher RH, Injev VP. Microcoaxial phacoemulsification Part 1: laboratory studies. J Cataract Refract Surg 2007; 33(3): 401–407.
20. Fine IH, Hoffman RS, Packer M. Profile of clear corneal cataract incisions demonstrated by ocular (optical) coherence tomography. J Cataract Refract Surg 2007; 33(1): 94–97.
21. Fine IH, Hoffman RS, Packer M. Architecture of clear corneal incisions demonstrated by ocular coherence tomography. Highlights Ophthalmol 2007; 35(4):2–4; 6–9.

1 The Transition Towards Smaller and Smaller Incisions

James M. Osher and Robert H. Osher

1.1 Micro-Coaxial Phacoemulsification with Torsional Ultrasound

James M. Osher and Robert H. Osher

Core Message

- Micro-coaxial phacoemulsification with torsional ultrasound is an exciting new technology that allows the surgeon to remove the cataract through a smaller incision with enhanced safety and efficiency.

1.1.1 Introduction

Cataract surgeons continue to explore new technologies that improve safety, efficiency and patient outcomes. Two approaches, bimanual microphacoemulsification (B-MICS) and micro-coaxial phacoemulsification (C-MICS), have allowed surgeons to operate through smaller incisions. Bimanual MICS utilizes a sleeveless tip and requires two small incisions approximately 1.0–1.5 mm in length, one for irrigation and chopping and the other for ultrasound and aspiration. Micro-coaxial phacoemulsification is a sleeved procedure allowing ultrasound, irrigation, and aspiration to be performed through a single incision approximately 2 mm in length.

R. H. Osher (✉)
Department of Ophthalmology, University of Cincinnati and the Cincinnati Eye Institute Cincinnati, Ohio USA
e-mail: RHOsher@CincinnatiEye.com

Another recent innovation in phaco technology is torsional ultrasound. Instead of the traditional jackhammer movement of longitudinal ultrasound, the torsional needle creates a side-to-side oscillatory movement, which has been proven to be more efficient with less chatter and repulsion of nuclear fragments. This chapter will review the benefits of combining micro-coaxial phacoemulsification with torsional ultrasound.

1.1.2 Micro-Coaxial Phacoemulsification

Micro-coaxial phacoemulsification was developed by Alcon in 2003 for the purpose of providing several advantages over the conventional coaxial and bimanual techniques. By introducing the smaller Ultra sleeve designed to be used with the Infiniti Vision System, it became possible to remove the cataract and implant a full-size intraocular lens (IOL) through an unenlarged 2.2 mm incision. Conventional coaxial phacoemulsification uses a 2.75–3.0 mm incision. By decreasing incision size to 2.2 mm, surgeons observed less induced astigmatism. One study found that a 3.0 mm incision induces a third to a half diopter of astigmatism, while a 2.2 mm incision approaches toric neutrality [1]. Decreasing surgically induced astigmatism has become essential as presbyopia-correcting lenses and toric lenses have gained widespread acceptance, while patient expectations for uncorrected vision have never been higher. When compared to bimanual microphacoemulsification, micro-coaxial technique has been reported to provide superior fluidics and less incisional leakage, leading to better chamber stability [2]. While the smaller sleeve used in the micro-coaxial procedure results in a 25% decrease in infusion when compared

J. L. Alió, I. H. Fine (eds.), *Minimizing Incisions and Maximizing Outcomes in Cataract Surgery*,
DOI: 10.1007/978-3-642-02862-5_1, © Springer-Verlag Berlin Heidelberg 2010

to the standard sleeve, the irrigation flow is considerably higher when compared to the volume available using 19, 20, and 21 gauge irrigating choppers. In fact, the Ultra sleeve provides as much as 60% more flow than a variety of 20-gauge irrigating choppers used in bimanual phaco [2]. The micro-coaxial surgeon has the option to access higher fluidic settings since there is no need to compensate for the limited irrigation inherent in the B-MICS procedure.

Another advantage of micro-coaxial phaco is enhanced thermal protection. Micro-coaxial phaco uses an insulating sleeve between the vibrating needle and the tissue bordering the incision. C-MICS also takes advantage of the aspiration bypass system (ABS) which is not possible with the bare needle of bimanual phaco. Several studies have suggested that the thermal profile of micro-coaxial phaco has a greater margin of safety [2–5]. When coupled with torsional ultrasound, which creates even less friction in the incision, the potential for thermal damage is substantially reduced.

A third advantage of micro-coaxial phaco involves the architectural integrity of the incision. As a general rule, a smaller incision size reduces the possibility of leakage and improves wound sealability. However, while B-MICS incisions are smaller, laboratory and clinical evidence has been published which shows a greater disruption in wound architecture when compared to micro-coaxial incisions [6–8]. Spontaneous wound leakage and India ink penetration was present in all eyes that underwent the bimanual technique but was not seen in the micro-coaxial group [6]. These authors also found more qualitative trauma to Descemet's membrane and to the corneal endothelium as demonstrated by scanning electron microscopy (SEM). A randomized clinical trial was designed to compare the ocular surface fluid ingress into the anterior chamber after cortical removal and at the end of the procedure using trypan blue as the quantifying tracer. At both points, trypan blue ingress was statistically significantly higher in the bimanual group than in the micro-coaxial group [9]. A histomorphological and immunofluorescence study in rabbits comparing bimanual and coaxial phaco demonstrated that B-MICS resulted in more disorganized collagen fibrils, excessive shrinking of stromal fibers, and more ragged tunnel margins [10, 11].

Integrity of the incision is not only important in preventing aqueous from exiting the eye, but it is also crucial in preventing bacteria from entering the eye [12]. Studies have shown that the short length and single plane of the incision in bimanual phaco may allow an increased ingress of bacteria [13, 14]. Another study based on finite analysis concluded that less incision stress is created with the micro-coaxial incision [15]. A clinical study evaluating 2.2 mm incisions using a square configuration popularized by Paul Ernst et al. [16] found no evidence of either hypotony or wound leakage [17]. One of the authors (RHO) of this chapter has not seen a postoperative complication related to the 2.2 mm incision since beginning micro-coaxial phacoemulsification in 2003.

Another advantage of micro-coaxial phaco is related to the smaller dimensions of the actual instrumentation. Better visualization when the pupil is small has been reported [18] and we have found that the emulsification is easier to perform in small eyes with shallow anterior chambers.

In the United States, where a micro-incisional IOL is not yet approved, the 2.2 mm incision of micro-coaxial phaco permits implantation of a full size, high quality optic without either an enlarged or separate incision. Several injectors requiring either a one hand or a bimanual insertion technique are able to consistently and gently deposit the IOL into the capsular bag regardless of whether the surgeon selects an AcrySof IQ, Toric, or ReStor IOL. Either the C cartridge or the smaller D cartridge manufactured by Alcon is available at the present time.

It has been surprisingly easy to transition to micro-coaxial phacoemulsification with minimal change in instrumentation and technique. Leading American educators like Richard Lindstrom, have also found that it is an easier operation to teach than B-MICS. The cataract surgeon who authored the peer-reviewed pilot study on micro-coaxial phacoemulsification found that the actual lens removal was no more difficult than performing traditional phaco. However, he did conclude that a learning curve was necessary for the IOL insertion, but with experience, this surgeon was able to achieve safe and reproducible IOL implantation [19]. The same study demonstrated a low incidence of intraoperative and postoperative complications with excellent clinical outcomes.

1.1.3 Torsional Ultrasound

Traditional longitudinal phacoemulsification was developed by Charles Kelman more than four decades ago and has remained relatively unchanged. Certainly, there have been improvements in techniques, instrumentation, and hand-piece design, as well as machine engineering. However, the basic principle of emulsifying the nucleus with longitudinal ultrasound has not undergone any major modification. At the annual meeting of the European Society of Cataract and Refractive Surgery in 2005, Alcon introduced OZil, a new platform providing torsional ultrasound on the Infiniti Vision System. While longitudinal phaco produces a jackhammer motion in which emulsification is only taking place 50% of the time, the side-to-side oscillatory movement of torsional ultrasound results in shearing and cutting 100% of the time. Because the entire stroke is utilized, torsional ultrasound is significantly more efficient than conventional ultrasound. Moreover, surgeons have the option of lowering fluidic parameters to safer levels without compromising efficiency.

The advantages of torsional phaco have been well documented. Torsional ultrasound causes less repulsion of nuclear material [20], and is best illustrated by the high-speed cinematography in a video produced by Teruyuki Miyoshi and Hironori Yoshida which won the Grand Prize at the 2007 ASCRS and ESCRS film festivals [21]. Another study found reduced turbulence with torsional vs. longitudinal phaco [22]. In a cadaver study comparing torsional ultrasound to conventional ultrasound, a high-speed camera was used to follow implanted micro-carrier beads [23]. Because there was little or no repulsion of the beads when using torsional fluidics, the removal time was 50% less with torsional ultrasound. The significance of less repulsion was implied in another award winning video from the 2008 ASCRS Film Festival by Osher and Osher, demonstrating that nuclear fragments were more easily displaced posteriorly through a tear in the posterior capsule with longitudinal rather than torsional ultrasound [24].

Torsional ultrasound has also been shown to increase the efficiency of the phacoemulsification. Simulated cataracts using a hard polymer were emulsified comparing cutting efficiency. While conventional phaco required 1.63 oz of force to cut through the cataract model, torsional ultrasound required 0.86 oz of force [25]. One investigator found a 23% reduction in BSS with torsional phaco compared to longitudinal, and lower vacuum levels appeared to achieve similar efficiency [26]. Less BSS fluid was required using torsional ultrasound in another series [27]. A European study compared fluid use during different stages of the emulsification. During quadrant removal the longitudinal ultrasound group required 55% more irrigation fluid than the torsional group [28]. The author concluded that torsional ultrasound was more efficient for dense nuclei and provided greater safety to the corneal epithelium. A Chinese study compared torsional vs. traditional ultrasound in a randomized comparative clinical study [29]. Both ultrasound time and cumulative dissipated energy proved less in the torsional group for all grades of cataract. Corneal edema, Descemet's striae, and a higher endothelial cell loss were found in the traditional ultrasound group. Best corrected visual acuity was better in the torsional group at days one and seven, although there was no difference between groups at the 1 month postoperative visit. Another European study showed faster removal times and lower energy exposure at the incision with torsional ultrasound [30]. Tip travel was investigated and found to be less with torsional ultrasound [31]. The author concluded that a shorter cumulative tip travel and less procedure time indicated improved efficiency and safety.

Torsional ultrasound generates less heat than longitudinal ultrasound due to several factors. One reason is that the frequency of OZil has been reduced from 40 to 32 kHz. In one study, torsional ultrasound was associated with a 60% reduction in temperature rise within the incision compared to longitudinal ultrasound [32]. Since longitudinal ultrasound at 100% power generates a linear stroke of 90 μm, the lateral movement of the tip is also about 90 μm. However, the angled tip used with torsional ultrasound creates a rotational movement of the shaft measuring only 40 μm. Therefore, movement of the tip within the incision with torsional ultrasound is less than half the movement characteristic of traditional phaco. When combined with the fact that the tip oscillates at a lower frequency, the heat reduction due to less frictional movement against the tissue adjacent to the incision, is approximately one-third that of longitudinal phaco [33].

One of the few perceived disadvantages of this new technology is that the surgeon is required to use a curved tip to realize the full benefits of torsional ultrasound. While it is possible to emulsify a nucleus using a straight tip with torsional ultrasound, bursts of longitudinal energy are necessary to prevent "apple-coring" of the nucleus. The 22° curvature of the Kelman tip has appealed to some, but not to all surgeons. Since the majority of cataract surgeons around the world prefer a straight phaco tip, Dr. Takayuki Akahoshi from Japan and Dr. Robert Osher independently designed a modified tip with a 12° curvature that shares high efficiency and thermal benefits similar to the Kelman tip. In addition, this new 12° tip has the opening on the same side as the curve, allowing the surgeon to embed the tip in

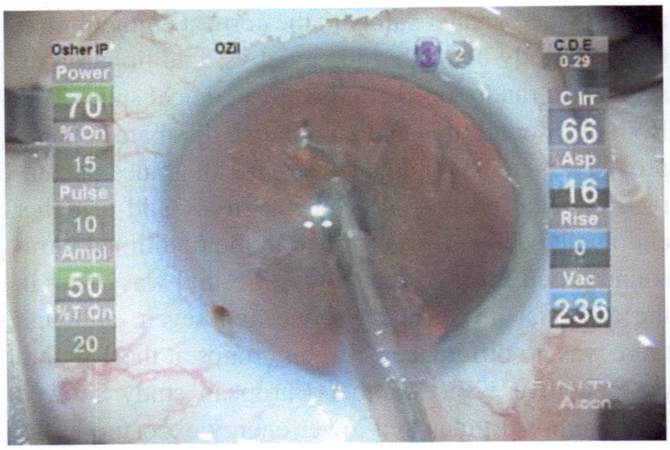

Fig. 1.1 Divot is made in lens with bevel down OZil 12

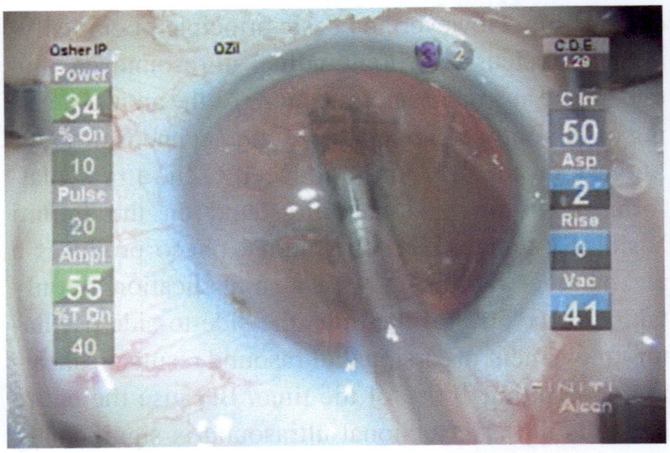

Fig. 1.2 Bevel up sculpting with low parameters

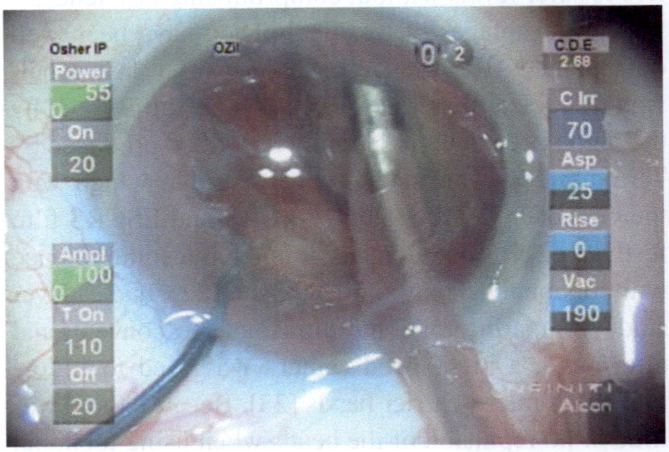

Fig. 1.3 Nucleus is divided into hemispheres

the lens without disturbing the overlying OVD, sculpt more safely, and chop more efficiently. One investigator found that the OZil 12 tip geometry translates to 50% reduction of stroke within the incision compared to traditional phaco, and a two-thirds reduction in thermal energy compared to longitudinal ultrasound [34]. In a study comparing the OZil 12 to the Kelman tip, the authors found that the clinical performance was equally effective [35]. Alcon has developed a complete line of tips to allow the surgeon to choose the size and configuration of the tip that he or she prefers.

While comments in this chapter reflect the author's experience with the Alcon technology, other companies are introducing microincisional technology such as Bausch & Lomb's Stellaris. Alternatives to traditional longitudinal phaco such as AMO's elliptical transverse ultrasound are also being introduced by industry.

1.1.4 Our Procedure for Emulsifying the Nucleus

After the capsulorhexis has been performed, the nucleus is loosened by hydrodelineation and the cortex is loosened by hydrodissection. The anterior chamber is filled with Healon5. The bevel-down OZil 12° tip is placed into the central anterior cortex where, a divot is removed to assure fluid exchange at the tip (Fig. 1.1). The tip is rotated 180° until bevel up and the parameters are reduced (slow motion phaco [36]) during the sculpting of the troth (Fig. 1.2). A nuclear chopper is introduced through the stab incision and the nucleus is divided into hemispheres (Fig. 1.3). The tip is rotated placing the bevel on its side, burying the opening in the nuclear hemisphere to facilitate chopping (Fig. 1.4) and removal of the nuclear quadrants, apex up working near the center of the capsular bag. Next, the cortex is removed with a silicone I & A tip and the posterior capsule is gently vacuumed. The capsular bag is inflated with OVD and a micro-hook is introduced through the stab incision for counter-traction during the lens implantation.

A single piece acrylic IOL (ReStor, Toric, or IQ) with a full size 6 mm optic has been loaded into the C cartridge similar to the picture on the cartridge. An Osher one-handed injector (Crestpoint and B&L) is introduced into the incision bevel down and the IOL is advanced by depressing the plunger until the lens emerges. It is inserted into the capsular bag (Fig. 1.5) where it is rotated and decentered away from the incision. The incision is hydrated (Fig. 1.6) before the OVD is removed, first from within the bag behind the lens (Fig. 1.7), and then from in front of the IOL. After the lens is centered with a silicone tip, the water-tightness of the incision is confirmed (Fig. 1.8). On the first postoperative day, the cornea is almost always clear (Fig. 1.9) and the square incision appears sealed (Fig. 1.10).

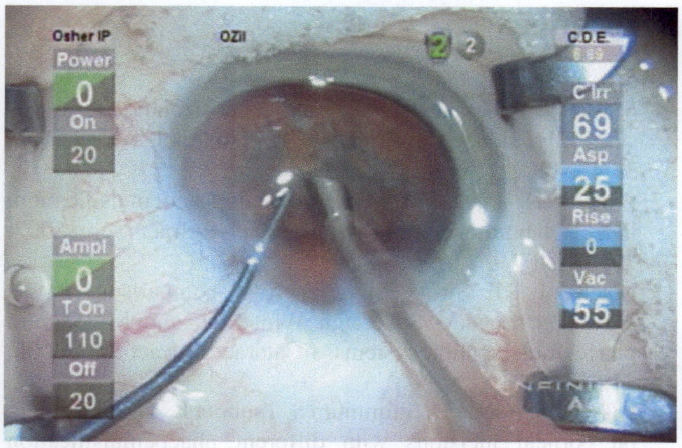

Fig. 1.4 Bevel on side for chopping of quadrants

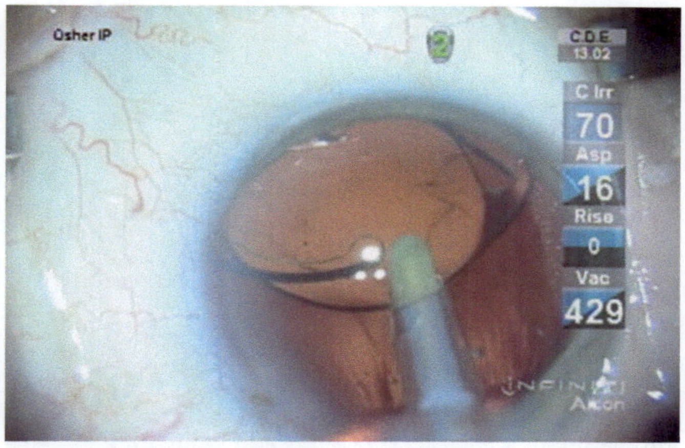

Fig. 1.7 OVD evacuated from capsular bag

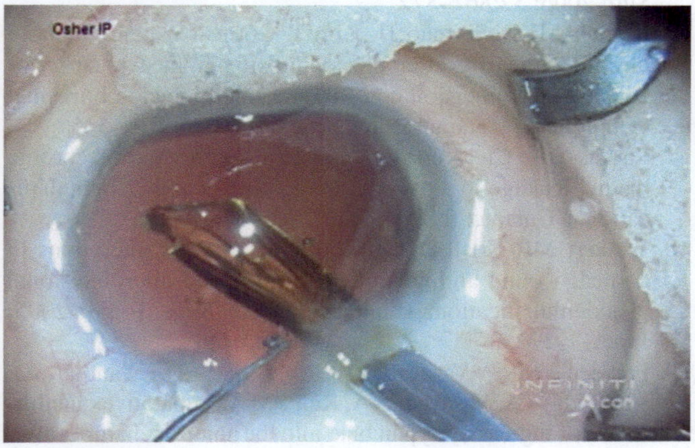

Fig. 1.5 IOL injected through 2.2 mm incision with bevel down cartridge using counter-traction technique

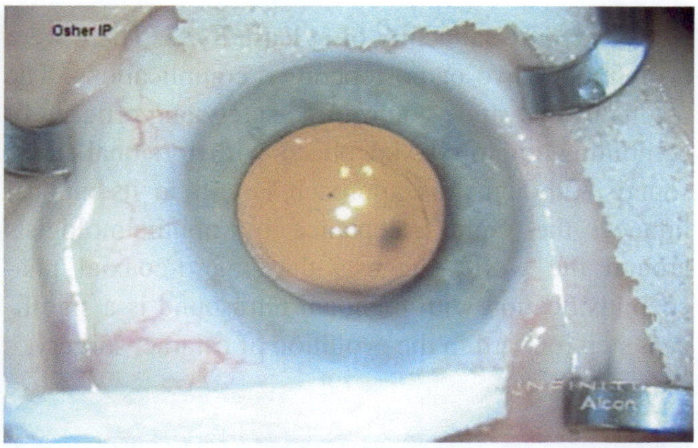

Fig. 1.8 Water-tightness of incision confirmed

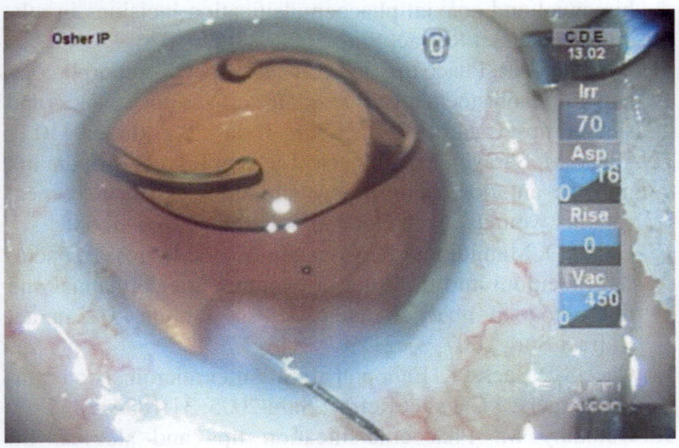

Fig. 1.6 Incision hydration precedes removal of OVD

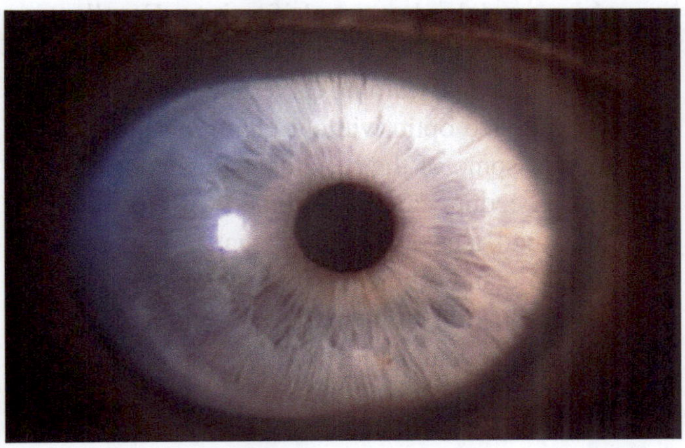

Fig. 1.9 Clear cornea on post-op day 1

1.1.5 Combining Micro-Coaxial Phacoemulsification with Torsional Ultrasound

At the 2007 annual meeting of the American Society of Cataract and Refractive Surgery, a study was presented in which an Ophthalmology Fellow independently examined 100 consecutive routine procedures using micro-coaxial phaco with torsional ultrasound and the 12° OZil tip [37]. Ninety-eight percent of the patients attained an uncorrected visual acuity of 20/40 or better on the first postoperative day and 62% attained an

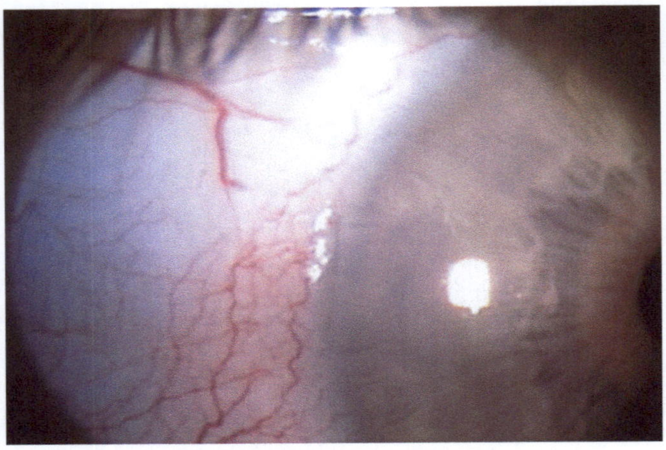

Fig. 1.10 Appearance of incision on post-op day 1

uncorrected visual acuity of at least 20/25. There were no intraoperative or postoperative complications. The results of this study confirm the safety and efficacy of combining micro-coaxial phaco with torsional ultrasound. Although this approach is still in its clinical infancy, the rapid acceptance by ophthalmologists around the world suggests that micro-coaxial phacoemulsification with torsional ultrasound is a significant step forward in the evolution of cataract surgery.

Take Home Pearls

- Smaller incisions in the 2 mm range, which offer astigmatic neutrality, can be achieved with micro-coaxial phacoemulsification. Excellent fluidics, thermal protection, competent incisions, a minimal learning curve, and implantation of a full size optic without enlarging the incision are some of the benefits of this approach. This procedure can be combined with torsional ultrasound, a new technology that appears to be more safe and efficient with less repulsion and heat production, compared to traditional longitudinal phacoemulsification.

References

1. Masket S. Coaxial 2.2 mm microphaco technique reduces surgically induced astigmatism. Ophthalmol Times 2006; 31:41–42
2. Osher RH, Injev VP. Micro-coaxial phacoemulsification. Part 1: laboratory studies. J Cataract Refract Surg 2007; 33:401–407
3. MacKool RJ, Sirota MA. Thermal comparison of the AdvanTec Legacy, Sovereign WhiteStar, and Millennium phacoemulsification systems. J Cataract Refract Surg 2005; 31:812–817
4 Bissen-Miyajima H, Shimmura S, Tsubota K. Thermal effect on corneal incisions with different phacoemulsification ultrasonic tips. J Cataract Refract Surg 1999; 25:60–64
5. Osher RH, Injev VP. Thermal study of bare tips with various system parameters and incision sizes. J Cataract Refract Surg 2006; 32:867–872
6. Berdahl JP, DeStafeno JJ, Kim T. Corneal wound architecture and integrity after phacoemulsification; evaluation of coaxial, microincision coaxial, and microincision bimanual techniques. J Cataract Refract Surg 2007; 33:510–515
7. Stratas BA. Clear corneal paracentesis: a case of chronic wound leakage in a patient having bimanual phacoemulsification. J Cataract Refract Surg 2005; 31:1075
8. Weikert MP, Koch DD. Phaco wound study: alterations in corneal wound architecture with bimanual microincisional phacoemulsification. Cataract Refract Surg Today 2005; June:11–13
9. Praveen MR, Vasavada, AR, Gajjar D, Pandita D, Vasavada VA, Vasavada VA, Raj, SM. Comparative quantification of ingress of trypan blue into the anterior chamber after micro-coaxial, standard coaxial, and bimanual phacoemulsification. J Cataract Refrac Surg 2008; 34:1007–1012
10. Kaid Johar SR, Vasavada AR, Mamidipudi R, et al Histomorphological and immunofluorescence evaluation of bimanual and coaxial phacoemulsification incisions in rabbits. J Cataract Refract Surg 2008; 34:670–676
11. Vasavada AR. Phaco tips and corneal tissue: histomorphology and immunohistochemistry reveal the effects of sleeveless and sleeved tips. Cataract Refract Surg Today 2005; June:9–10
12. Taban M, Sarayba MA, Ignacio TS, et al Ingress of India ink into the anterior chamber through sutureless clear corneal cataract wounds. Arch Ophthalmol 2005; 123:643–648
13. Gajjar D, Mamidipudi R, Vasavada A, et al Ingress of bacterial inoculum into the anterior chamber after bimanual and micro-coaxial phacoemulsification in rabbits. J Cataract Refract Surg 2007; 33:2129–2134
14. Chee S-P, Bacsal K. Endophthalmitis after microincision cataract surgery. J Cataract Refract Surg 2005; 31:1834–1835
15. Boukhny M. Phacoemulsification tips and sleeves. In: Buratto L, Werner L, Zanini M, Apple D, eds, Phacoemulsification Principles and Techniques, 2nd edn. Thorofare, NJ, Slack, 2003; 247–254
16 Ernest PH, Fenzl R, Lavery KT, Sensoli A. Relative stability of clear corneal incisions in a cadaver eye model. J Cataract Refract Surg 1995; 21:39–42
17. Masket S, Belani S. Proper wound construction to prevent short-term ocular hypotony after clear corneal incision cataract surgery. J Cataract Refract Surg 2007; 33:383–386

18. Dosso AA, Cottet L, Burgener ND, Di Nardo S. Outcomes of coaxial microincision cataract surgery versus conventional coaxial cataract surgery. J Cataract Refract Surg 2008; 34:284–288
19. Osher RH. Micro-coaxial phacoemulsification. Part 2: clinical study. J Cataract Refract Surg 2007; 33:408–412
20. Cionni RJ. Torsional to longitudinal phacoemulsification comparison. In: American Society of Cataract and Refractive Surgery Annual Meeting, San Francisco, 2006
21. Miyoshi T, Yoshida H. From phaco-cutting to true phacoemulsification. VJCRS 2007; XXIII(4)
22. Fernandez de Castro LE, Sandoval HP, Vroman DT, Solomon KD. Fluid dynamics during phacoemulsification; fluid dispersion check model. In: American Society of Cataract and Refractive Surgery Annual Meeting, San Diego, 2007
23. Solomon K. Alcon CME Program, American Academy of Ophthalmology, San Fransisco, 2006
24. Osher J, Osher R. Understanding the dropped nucleus. Video J Cataract Refract Surg 2008; XXIV(4)
25. Boukhny M. Laboratory performance comparison of torsional and conventional longitudinal phacoemulsification. In: Annual Meeting of American Society of Cataract and Refractive Surgery, San Francisco, 17–22 March 2006
26. Allen D. Efficient surgery with a new torsional phaco mode. In: Annual Meeting of the American Society of Cataract and Refractive Surgery, San Francisco, 17–22 March 2006
27. Yoo S. Transitioning to torsional phaco emulsification. Cataract Refract Surg Today 2006; (supplement):7–8
28. Tjia KF. Efficiency of torsional versus longitudinal ultrasound. Cataract Refract Surg Today Europe 2008; May:33–34
29. Liu Y, Zeng M, Liu X, et al. Torsional mode versus conventional ultrasound mode phacoemulsification: randomized comparative clinical study. J Cataract Refract Surg 2007; 33:287–292
30. Johansson C. Quantitative comparison of longitudinal versus torsional phacoemulsification. In: European Society of Cataract and Refractive Surgeons Annual Meeting, London, 9–13 September 2006
31. Davison JA. Cumulative tip travel and implied followability of longitudinal and torsional phacoemulsification. J Cataract Refract Surg May 2008; 34:986–990
32. MacKool RJ. Lens removal/torsional phacoemulsification: advantages of nonlinear ultrasound. In: Annual ASCRS Symposium on Cataract, IOL, and Refractive Surgery, San Francisco, CA, 17–22 March 2006
33. Allen D. Cataract surgery evolves: new IOL implantation and fluidics technologies make transitioning to a micro-coaxial technique easier and safer. Cataract Refract Surg Today 2007; (Supplement):3–5
34. Davison JA. Beginning micro-coaxial surgery. Eyeworld Supplement May 2008
35. Henderson B, Grimes K. Comparison of surgical efficiency using different ultrasound modulation on dense lenses and using varied angled phacoemulsification tips. ASCRS, San Diego, 2007
36. Osher RH, Marques FF, Marques D.M.V, Osher JM. Slow motion phacoemulsification technique. Tech Ophthalmol 1(2):73
37. Vaz F, Osher RH. Early uncorrected visual acuity with micro-coaxial phacoemulsification and torsional ultrasound: an independent study. In: Annual Meeting of the ASCRS, San Diego, 2007.

1.2 Transitioning to Bimanual MICS

Rosa Braga-Mele

Core Messages

- Tackle an easy case first and remember you can always default back to standard phacoemulsification.
- A clear cornea trapezoidal incision is preferred so as to allow maneuverability within the wound without stretching.
- The capsulorhexis forceps are advantageous as they create very little, if any, pressure on the incision, but require a slight change in technique.
- There are multiple irrigating second instruments available. Try a few before committing to any one.
- Most of the currently available phaco platforms will support bimanual MICS without the need to change current techniques.

1.2.1 Introduction

Microsurgery for phacoemulsification represents the next evolution in techniques for cataract surgery. When bimanual microsurgery was first introduced, the rally behind the push was that surgeons needed to learn smaller incision technique because IOLs that could be inserted into sub-2-mm incisions were on the horizon. Today, many small incision IOL's are available around the world and the procedure is a reality. The procedure uses separate irrigation instruments and a sleeveless phaco tip to remove cataracts. Irrigation during phacoemulsification is provided through an irrigating chopper or manipulator instead of through the phacoemulsification handpiece. The surgery can be performed through incisions less than 1 mm and is associated with improved maneuverability, visualization, and less refractive error after surgery. Over the

R. Braga-Mele
University of Toronto, Toronto, ON, Canada
e-mail: RHOsher@CincinnatiEye.com

last few years, a number of advancements in phacoemulsification power modulations, understanding of fluid dynamics involved in bimanual phacoemulsification, and lenses that may be inserted through smaller incisions have brought renewed interest to bimanual phacoemulsification. Since those IOLs are now available, microphaco has caught on, mainly because a smaller incision for phaco induces less trauma in the eye, and the final incision, even when enlarged to insert the IOL, seems to seal better after the surgery is complete.

This chapter will focus on techniques and pearls to utilize during the transition from standard or coaxial microincisional surgery to bimanual microincisional cataract surgery (MICS).

1.2.2 Technique

Corneal incision: Two clear corneal trapezoidal incisions of 1.4–1.6 mm width or less are created in the inferotemporal and superotemporal quadrants using a metal or diamond blade, from a temporal approach. The external width of the incision is made slightly larger than both the phaco needle and the irrigating chopper to avoid tension on the incision and allow maneuverability within the wound, and thus have the advantage of a trapezoidal wound. The smaller internal wound minimizes egress of fluid around the instruments. It is important to know the gauge size of the phaco needle so that one can match the incision size and the irrigating chopper gauge.

Capsulorhexis: The capsulorhexis can be made using a 25 gauge bent cystotome needle or 23 gauge forceps that are specifically made for the procedure. This is one of the learning curves of the procedure. To use the capsulorhexis forceps, one must slightly modify the current technique. These forceps require more of a fine finger motion as opposed to a wrist motion. Also, it is a cross-action technique for opening and closing the forceps. However, in many ways the forceps are advantageous: they create very little pressure on the wound and control is superior.

Hydrodissection: It is important to get a good, complete hydrodissection. Because the wounds are small and tight, it is best to release some of the viscoelastic from the anterior chamber by burping the wound first.

Irrigating choppers: Multiple irrigating choppers or manipulators are currently available: those with a single-ended open-irrigating port; those with two side-irrigating ports; and those with an inferior irrigating port. Each has its advantages. With the single-ended instrument, one can inflate the chamber immediately upon entering the eye, and one can direct the fluid stream where one wants it to go. However, it can be difficult to learn to utilize. With the two side-irrigating ports, the fluidics remain relatively similar to coaxial phaco, but by positioning the chopper in certain directions, one can direct nuclear segment or inflate the capsular bag. The inferior port directs the fluid toward the posterior chamber keeping the capsule away from the phaco tip. There are many different types of irrigating handpieces available and today most deliver over 55–65 mL of fluid. My suggestion is to try different types and see which are best suited to your technique and comfort level.

Bimanual phacoemulsification: A 19 or 20 gauge irrigating chopper or manipulator is inserted into the inferotemporal stab incision using the left hand, and the phaco needle is inserted through the superotemporal incision with the right hand (or vice versa depending on the dominant hand). Note that this is counterintuitive to standard phaco where the phaco needle enters the eye first followed by the chopper. This is because the chopper now carries the fluid that helps maintain the chamber. Most of the currently available phaco units can be used to perform MICS because of the development of new phacoemulsification technologies and power modulations which allow the emulsification and fragmentation of nuclear material without the generation of significant thermal energy. Power modulations such as hyperpulse or microburst (with longer off than on times) are best utilized for this procedure. Techniques such as chop (horizontal or vertical), flip, or even divide and conquer can be utilized. One must either slightly lower the vacuum below settings used in conventional coaxial phacoemulsification, raise the bottle height, or pressurize the infusion. One can also use stable chamber tubing, which is more compliant with a small area of cylindrical filter mesh that increases resistance within the tubing and stabilizes the anterior chamber by essentially lowering the effective vacuum. The irrigating handpiece and phaco handpiece are used to engage the nucleus and fragment and emulsify it. The irrigating handpiece can be used to direct lens material to the phaco needle.

Irrigation and aspiration of cortex: This is perhaps an area where bimanual MICS is truly advantageous. Twenty gauge bimanual irrigating and aspirating instruments are each inserted into the eye. The aspirating probe is used to remove the cortex and if there is difficulty removing the subincisional cortex, the probes may be switched to reach the subincisional cortex.

IOL insertion: There are two methods commonly used for insertion of the IOL: either a 2.8 mm incision may be created between the two stab incisions or one of the stab incisions may be enlarged. Following the injection of the IOL into the capsular bag, residual viscoelastic is removed and all wounds are stromally hydrated. However, more recently, newer generation IOLs have become available that can easily go through a sub-2.0 mm incision.

1.2.3 Summary

Biaxial microincisional cataract surgery has its advantages. Irrigation through the side-port can help direct pieces of nuclear material towards the phaco tip. It minimizes the opposing forces of coaxial irrigation at pushing the nuclear material away. Slightly lower infusion pressure and the split of irrigation with the ability to control the fluid stream direction away from areas of zonular instability make it more beneficial in challenging cases. Also, if needed, nuclear material can be approached from both incision sites. With the availability of microincision IOLs, the procedure is more tightly controlled, the eye is more stable and less astigmatism is induced. This is the procedure of today and the future.

Take-Home Pearls

- Microsurgery for phacoemulsification represents the next evolution in techniques for cataract surgery.
- Do not change your technique or change too many parameters at one time.
- Start slowly and pick the right case and patient.
- Bimanual MICS is safe and effective.

1.3 0.7 mm Microincision Cataract Surgery

Jorge L. Alió, Amar Agarwal, and Pawel Klonowski

Core Messages

- To perform 0.7 mm MICS (microincision cataract surgery) you need new 21 gauge instruments
- To achieve stable fluidics in the anterior chamber it is necessary to use pressurized infusion
- 0.7 mm MICS is the new limit of cataract surgery in terms of incision size
- 0.7 mm MICS is possible in all cataract cases with today's improvements in phaco technology

1.3.1 Sub 1 mm MICS: Why?

The natural trend of modern surgery is to minimize the physical aspects of intervention in the human body. During the last 40 years, cataract surgery has made the huge step from the 10–12 mm incision to the 0.7 mm incision. Not only the incision, but even the energy delivered, the surgical trauma and the time of the surgery have decreased. Nowadays, with millions of cataract surgeries performed annually around the world, the technique and outcome of surgery have become more efficient and predictable. Only minimal invasive surgery can improve the refractive result [1–3]. Many papers have confirmed the dependence between incision size and postoperative astigmatism, or corneal aberrations [4, 5]. This makes the surgery more efficient and faster. Reduction of incision size seems to be the trend in the normal evolution of surgery, and it will continue to be a challenge even in the future.

A. Agarwal (✉)
Eye Research Centre & Dr. Agarwal's Group of Eye Hospitals, 19 Cathedral Road, Chennai 600 086, India
email: dragarwal@vsnl.com

On 15 August 1998, Amar Agarwal performed 1 mm cataract surgery by a technique he called Phaconit (phaco being done with a needle incision technology) [6–11]. One of the authors, Jorge Alió, coined the term MICS – microincision cataract surgery – for all sub-2 mm surgeries [12]. On 21 May 2005, for the first time, a 0.7 mm phaco needle tip with a 0.7 mm irrigating chopper was used by one of the authors to remove cataracts through the smallest incision possible so far (Microphaconit – 0.7 mm MICS).

The MICS concept was put into practice following the MICS principles:

1. New MICS instruments
2. Increased use of vacuum and improved fluidics
3. Closed and stable anterior chamber
4. Less use of power settings, reduced use of ultrasound energy
5. Adequate MICS IOL

These conditions allow applying MICS surgery and making surgery much more:

1. Predictable
   a. Diminishing surgically induced astigmatism
2. Controllable
   a. Stable anterior chamber
   b. Stable position of the posterior capsule
   c. Higher effectiveness of the phaco fragmentation and aspiration
3. Uncomplicated
   a. Bimanual access
   b. Small tools maneuvers
   c. Stable conditions

The appropriate combination of these conditions and the proper application of the instruments and machine setting make sub-1 mm surgery possible. Now MICS and 0.7 mm MICS are the standard procedures performed by authors. The right use of the tools and the adequate setup of the machine fluidics help to operate all grades of cataracts, including complicated cataracts. The surgery is more controllable if properly performed.

By choosing the right instruments and fluidics, it is possible to get all types of cataracts, even complicated ones, through sub-1 mm incision.

The main purpose of this chapter is to describe the approaches and techniques used by the authors to make a transition towards 0.7 mm MICS.

1.3.2 Potential Drawbacks of a Sub-1 m Incision

The transition towards performing 0.7 mm MICS requires more attention to the incision and fluidics. The inadequate settings of machine parameters (US power, vacuum and pressured infusion) may result in incision burn, corneal trauma and anterior chamber instability.

The principles of application for 0.7 mm instrumentation are the same as in MICS. The most important change is the diameter of instruments and the use of high vacuum and pressured fluidics. The instruments have to be compatible with these parameters.

New micro MICS instrumentation should allow better fluidics and should

- Fit through minimal new incisions
- Be ergonomic
- Allow multiple functions
- Be safe
- Be easy to use

The main problem in 0.7 mm MICS is the destabilization of the anterior chamber during surgery. Smaller dimension of the instruments needs to be achieved by increasing the potential of the fluidics. Now with a 22 gauge (0.7 mm) irrigating chopper it is essential that pressured infusion be used in the surgery. Some of the new phaco machines are equipped with internal air pumps: Accurus (Alcon Laboratories) and the Millennium (Bausch & Lomb). This technique is called internal gas forced infusion (IFI). The filtered air is pressed into the BSS bottle. The anterior chamber is filled with the salt solution under stable conditions. This type of GFI is well verified in MICS surgery. The surgeon has perfect control of this parameter at the machine platform during different stages of the surgery. These machines maintain the infusion at a stable level.

The second option is to connect the external air pump to the infusion bottle. This option is inexpensive but gives less control of the infusion (Fig. 1.11).

The advantages of pressured infusion are listed below:

1. The surgeon can control all the parameters (forced infusion rate, ultrasonic power modulations and vacuum settings) in the same panel of the surgical system.

Fig. 1.11 Air pump

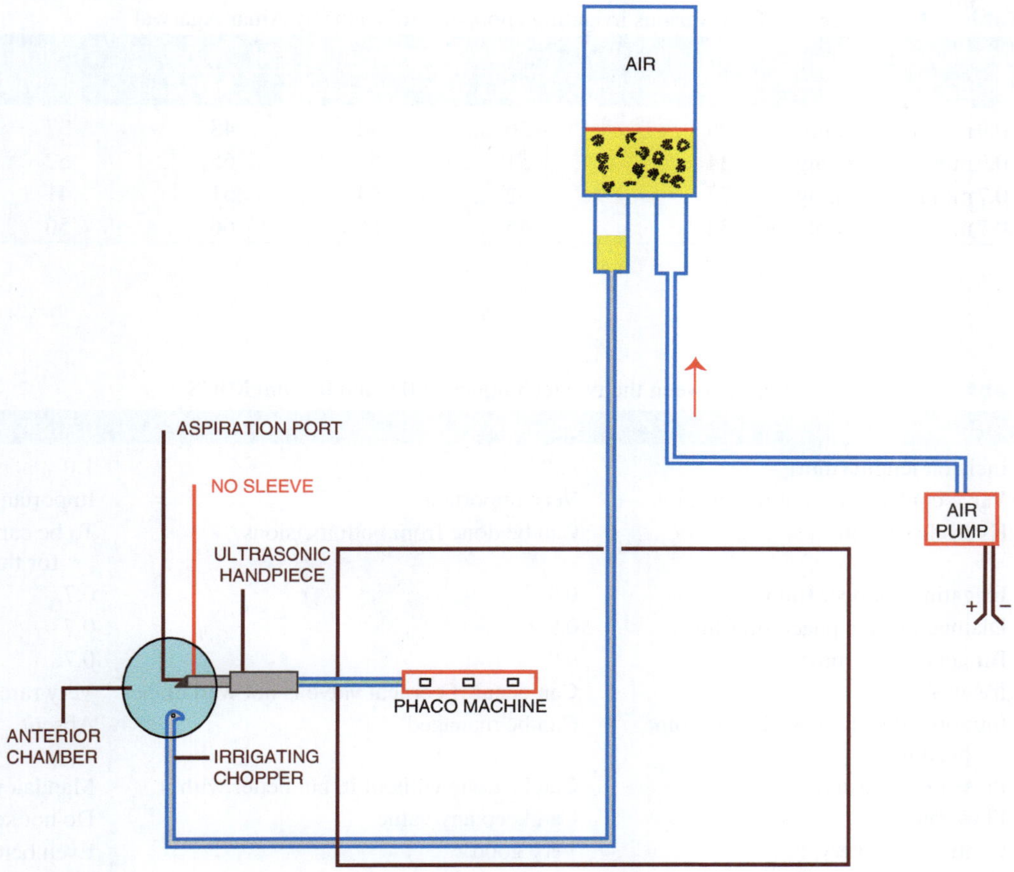

2. The forced infusion rate can be actively and digitally controlled during the surgery, adjusting the parameters to the conditions and/or the surgical steps of each individual case and balancing the inflow and outflow by internal intraocular pressure (IOP) control in modern cataract machines.
3. Bottle height becomes irrelevant as a key factor in surgical control with the consequent advantages for OR design.

Other advantages of ressured infusion are:

1. Continuous and active infusion
2. Stable amount of fluid delivered into the eye
3. Maintaining stability of the anterior chamber
4. Continuous rapid cooling of the phaco tip
5. Posterior capsule is situated in the secure position
6. Gives opportunity for safe maneuverings in the anterior chamber

One of the authors (Amar Agarwal) has mainly worked with anterior vented gas forced infusion system (AVGFI) of the Accurus surgical machine that helps in the performance of MICS/Phakonit [13–15]. This was started by Dr. Arturo Pérez-Arteaga from Mexico. The AVGFI is a system incorporated into the Accurus machine that creates a positive infusion pressure inside the eye. It consists of an air pump and a regulator which are inside the machine; the air is pushed inside the bottle of intraocular solution, and so the fluid is actively pushed inside the eye without raising or lowering the bottle. The control of the air pump is digitally integrated in the Accurus panel.

Table 1.1 presents the outflow of fluid from various types of irrigating choppers when the Accurus infusion pump is set at 100 mmHg or when the external pump is connected (Table 1.1) The external air pump has two modes of action. Mode high is equal to using the Accurus machine at about 100 mmHg pressure. Mode low of the air pump is equal to using the Accurus machine at 50 mmHg pressure. The use of the millipore filter is mandatory to protect against and prevent any infection. We measured the amount of fluid coming out of the various irrigating choppers with and without an air pump. We measured the values using the simple external air pump (external gas forced infusion) and the Accurus machine with IFI.

Table 1.1 Fluid exiting from various irrigating choppers (mL/min) by Amar Agarwal

Irrigating chopper	Without gas forced infusion	With gas forced infusion at			Air pump with regulator at low	Air pump with regulator at high
		50 mmHg	75 mmHg	100 mmHg		
0.9 mm Side opening	25	36	42	48	37	51
0.9 mm End opening	34	51	57	65	52	68
0.7 mm End opening	27	39	44	51	41	54
0.7 mm Inferior opening	32	45	55	66	50	66

Table 1.2 The differences between the two techniques of 0.9 and 0.7 mm MICS

Features	0.9 mm MICS	0.7 mm MICS
Incision length (mm)	1.2	1.0
Valve configuration of the incision	Very important	Important as incision is much smaller
Hydrodissection	Can be done from both incisions	To be careful as there is very little space for fluid to exit the eye
Irrigating chopper (mm)	0.9	0.7
Diameter of the phaco tip (mm)	0.9	0.7
Bimanual I/A (mm)	0.9	0.7
Iris prolapse	Can occur if corneal valve is not well done	Very rare
Intraoperative floppy iris syndrome prevention	Can be managed	Absent
Pressured infusion	Can be done without it, but better with it	Mandatory
Flow rate	Can keep any value	Do not keep it very high. 20–24 mL/min
Control in surgery	Very good	Even better
Closing incision	Hydration is mandatory	Hydration is not necessary

The difference between 0.9 and 0.7 mm surgery is not only the diameter of the instruments, but also the quality of the surgery. The smaller width of the tools gives us the opportunity to control more precisely the surgery and the maneuvers in the anterior chamber. The use of the pressured infusion and high vacuum MICS instruments provides control over anterior chamber stability. The problem with iris prolapse practically does not exist. Smaller incisions prevent leakage. The main features in 0.9 and 0.7 mm MICS are shown in Table 1.2.

The second parameter that should be maintained is the vacuum. One of the authors (Jorge Alió) started work with the Bausch & Lomb Stellaris platform. As the 0.7 mm MICS requires higher parameters for sufficient flow, this can be hazardous for anterior chamber stability. The lack of inflow compensation after the occlusion can cause anterior chamber collapse. To prevent the surge during occlusion breaks at higher vacuum levels, the flow restrictor can be installed between the phacoemulsification handpiece and the aspiration tubing. Stable Chamber System® (Bausch & Lomb Company Rochester, NY) and Cruise Control™ (STAAR Surgical Company Monrovia, CA) are devices specially designed to restrict outflow for increased safety in MICS at high vacuum settings. They have disposable flow restrictor and mesh filter against blocking. The lens masses remain on the filter. The restrictor limits the flow. At the vacuum level of 500 mmHg, the anterior chamber does not become shallow, especially when working with pressured infusion. Pressured infusion with IOP control allows fine-tuning and matches the fluidics in 0.7 mm MICS [16].

1.3.3 Instrumentation

1.3.3.1 Phaco Tip (0.7 mm)

The main challenges in 0.7 mm MICS are to project the phaco tip, which can transmit ultrasound energy, and have liquid flow efficiency as well as standard MICS tools.

The problem in the minimization of the phaco tip is not only the tip diameter, but also the fluid flow and energy transmission. If the diameter of the phaco tip becomes smaller, from a 0.9 mm phaco needle to a 0.7 mm phaco needle, the expected speed of the surgery would decrease. Flow rate aspiration would also decrease. The inner diameter of the tip regulates the flow rate. To obtain flow rate aspiration on the standard MICS level, the wall of 0.7 mm MICS phaco tip must be thinner and thus the internal diameter of the tip can be increased. The 0.7 mm MICS needle was designed for a 22 gauge (0.7 mm) chopper. The 30° tip end makes it even better. The special 0.7 mm phaco needle is currently produced by MST (cat. numb. PT-29130 MST, Redmond, Washington) (Fig. 1.12).

1.3.3.2 0.7 mm Irrigating Instruments

There are many designs of irrigating instruments. The construction of irrigating instruments can have an end-opening, lateral-opening or inferior-opening hole. The rules of the fluidics flow are the same as in the aspiration tip. The previous set used was the 0.9 mm set. Now with the 0.7 mm MICS set, the new 0.7 mm bimanual irrigation-aspiration cannulas can be positioned in the anterior chamber without enlarging the incision after the nucleus removal.

All these instruments of the 0.7 mm set fit onto the handles of the Duet System. These instruments are designed by MST. So, if a surgeon already has the handles and is using it for phakonit, the same handles can be used for microphakonit, and only the tips are needed.

The end-opening chopper has an advantage of more fluid coming out of the chopper, but greater turbulence of the fluid can occur in the anterior chamber. MST in their irrigating chopper increased the flow by removing the flow restrictions incorporated in other irrigating choppers. They have also developed control on incisional outflow by making all the instruments of one size and creating a matching knife of the proper size and geometry.

The first irrigating chopper for a 0.7 mm surgery was an end-opening irrigating chopper (Fig. 1.13). The idea was to diminish the diameter of the tool and to increase the infusion. The amount of fluid coming out of it would be less, so an end-opening chopper would maintain the fluidics better. With gas forced infusion, we thought we would be able to balance the entry and exit of the fluid into the anterior chamber and we succeeded in doing so.

Two different instruments are preferred by the authors:

The Agarwal Micro Phaconit 0.7 mm irrigating chopper (Cat. No. Du-02353 MST) is basically a sharp chopper which has a sharp cutting edge and helps in karate chopping or quick chopping. It can chop any type of cataract.

The Alio Stinger irrigating chopper Duet System (Cat. No. Du-02362 MST) is a 22 gauge inferior-opening instrument. It has one hole on the inferior side of the cannula and provides the infusion stream directly backward, forcing cataract fragments to levitate towards the phaco tip pointed towards masses and the posterior capsule. This allows maintaining the anterior chamber at

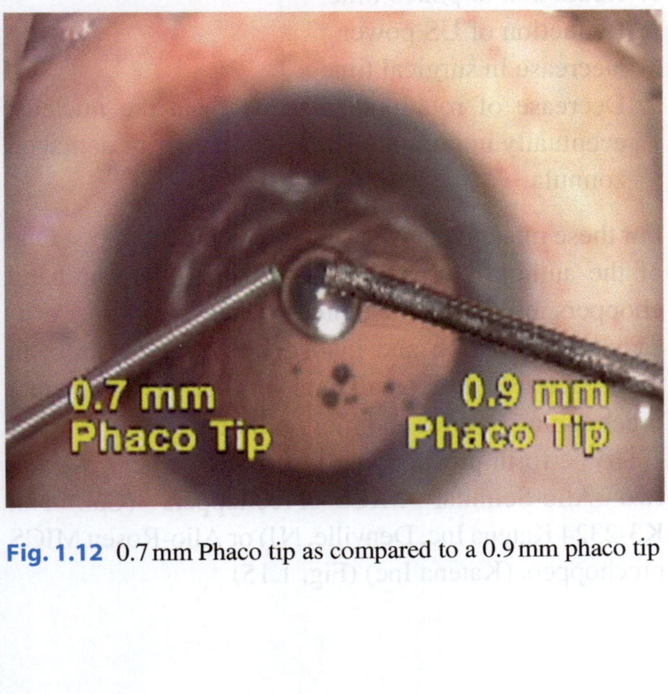

Fig. 1.12 0.7 mm Phaco tip as compared to a 0.9 mm phaco tip

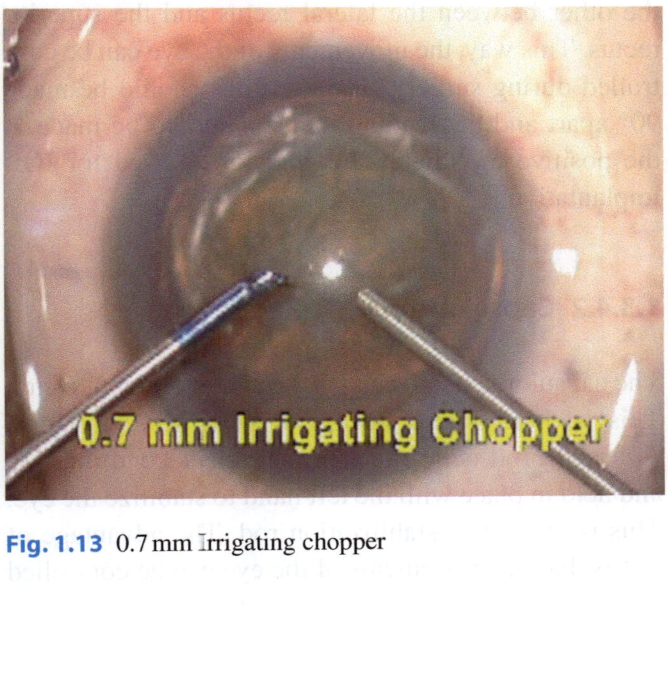

Fig. 1.13 0.7 mm Irrigating chopper

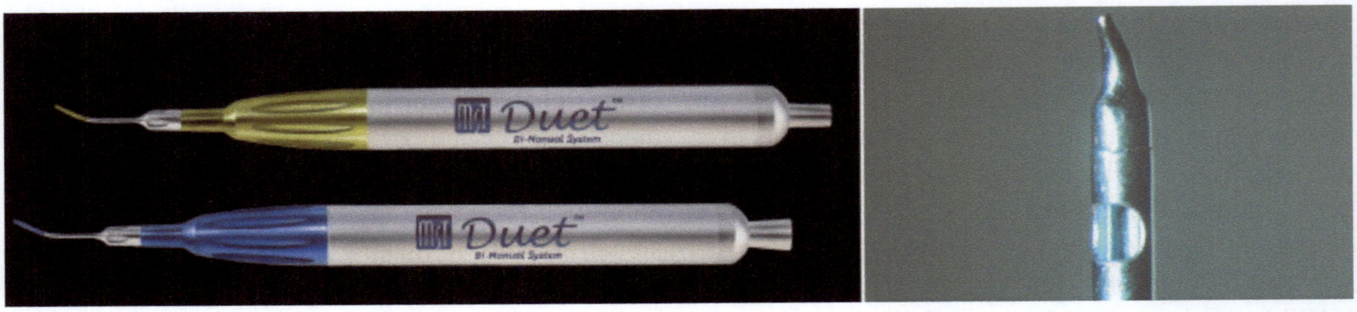

Fig. 1.14 The 0.7 mm (22 gauge) Duet® System Alio Stinger irrigating chopper

the required depth and holding the capsule far from the phaco tip. The fluid infusion due to pressured infusion is sufficient for 0.7 mm MICS. The end of the Stinger is equipped with a pointed tip which is angled downwards. It enables breaking masses with ease and guides them to the aspiration hole (Fig. 1.14).

1.3.4 Surgery

1.3.4.1 Incision

A biplanar valved incision is made with a 1 mm keratome. The preference of one of the authors (Amar Agarwal) is a sapphire knife or a stainless-steel knife. A tight incision is mandatory in 0.7 mm MICS. Ill-fitted incisions would not seal the anterior chamber when gas forced infusion is used in 0.7 mm MICS. The viscoelastic is then injected inside the eye. This will distend the eye so that a clear corneal incision can be made easily. One clear corneal incision will be made between the lateral rectus and the inferior rectus and the other between the lateral rectus and the superior rectus. This way, the movements of the eye can be controlled during surgery. The incisions should be made 90° apart and the leading incision should be made at the positive meridian. This incision is used for IOL implantation.

1.3.4.2 Capsulorhexis

The capsulorhexis is then performed of about 5–6 mm. This is done with a needle or with MICS forceps. A straight rod is inserted through the second incision and held in place with the left hand to stabilize the eye. This is the Globe stabilization rod. The advantage of this is that the movements of the eye can be controlled while working, without any anesthesia or under topical anesthesia.

1.3.4.3 Hydrodissection

Hydrodissection is performed after removing the small amount of viscoelastic from the anterior chamber. The fluid wave should pass under the nucleus. Both incisions are suitable for the purpose of hydrodissection and even the subincisional areas can get easily hydrodissected. The problem is that there is not much space for fluid escape through the 1 mm incision. Careful hydrodissection and fluid control during these maneuvers can avoid complications.

1.3.4.4 Prechopping

Prechopping is a maneuver that can decrease ultrasound surgery time and power use. The advantages of bimanual prechopping are the following:

1. Reduction of phaco time
2. Reduction of US power
3. Decrease in surgical time
4. Decrease of rotational maneuvers at the nucleus, eventually important in cases with poor or damaged zonnula

For these maneuvers we need tools – prechoppers. One of the authors (Jorge Alio) concludes that one-hand choppers are not recommended because of lesser efficacy of this action and inadequate zonullar stress in hard cataracts. For small incision surgery, bimanual prechopping is safer and more efficient.

To perform prechopping in 0.7 mm surgery, we use two Alio-Scimitar MICS Prechoppers (Cat. No. K3-2324 Katena Inc, Denville, NJ) or Alio-Rosen MICS prechoppers (Katena Inc) (Fig. 1.15)

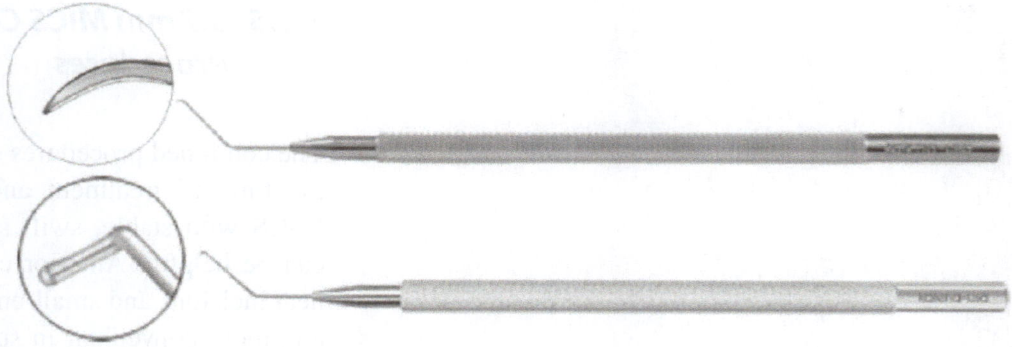

Fig. 1.15 Alio Scimitar prechopper and Alio-Rosen Phaco prechopper for microincision cataract surgery (Katena Inc)

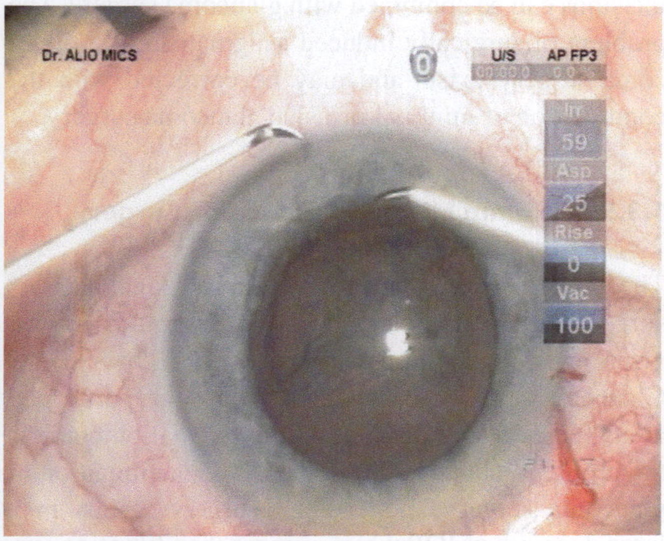

Fig. 1.16 Bimanual use of Alio's Scimitar prechoppers

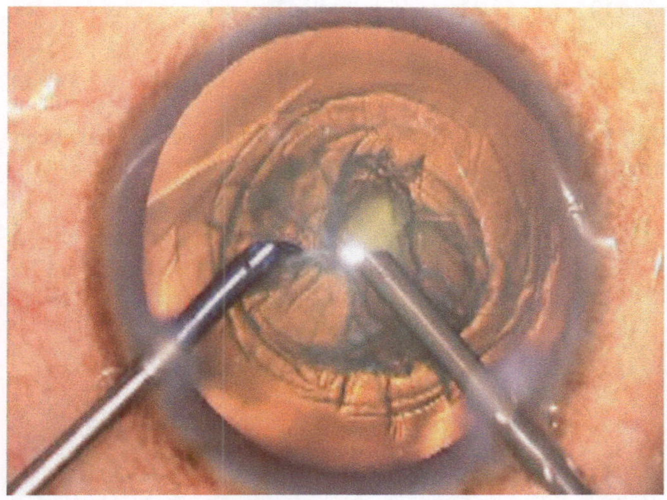

Fig. 1.17 0.7 mm MICS started, 0.7 mm irrigating chopper and 0.7 mm phaco tip without the sleeve inside the eye. (Instruments are made by MST)

The shape of the Scimitar Prechopper is designed to perform and facilitate 700 µm surgery. The Scimitar Prechopper has a curved tip with a blunt end and a sharp inferior edge. The choppers are crossed by situating them symmetrically opposite each other (Fig. 1.16). Then the cuts are made by gently crossing the prechoppers. The cuts are made from the perimeter to the center of the nuclei. The internal edge is sharp and this facilitates incisions of lens masses. The mass is cut into two dividing hemispheres. The nucleus is then rotated 90° and then prechopping is repeated for the second time as described earlier.

1.3.4.5 Phacoemulsification

The 22 (0.7 mm) gauge irrigating chopper connected to the infusion line of the phaco machine is introduced with a foot pedal on position 1. The phaco probe is connected to the aspiration line, and the 0.7 mm phaco tip without an infusion sleeve is introduced through the clear corneal incision (Fig. 1.17).

Using the phaco tip with moderate ultrasound power, the center of the nucleus is directly embedded, starting from the superior edge of the rhexis, with the phaco probe directed obliquely downwards towards the vitreous according to one of the authors (Amar Agarwal). The settings at this stage are 50% phaco power, 20 mL/min flow rate and 100–200 mmHg vacuum. Using the karate chop technique the nucleus is chopped [17]. Thus the whole nucleus is removed (Fig. 1.18).

The other method is to aspirate the nuclear fragment with the phaco tip after successful prechopping. The nuclear fragment lifted by the phaco tip and aspiration is broken with the help of the Alio Stinger Irrigating Chopper. The Stinger cannula is equipped with the hook at its end, which facilitates fragmentation of the nucleus. Small fragments of the nuclei are aspirated by high vacuum, practically without using U/S power.

Cortical wash-up is then done with the bimanual irrigation aspiration (0.7 mm set) technique (Figs. 1.19 and 1.20). During this whole procedure gas forced infusion is used.

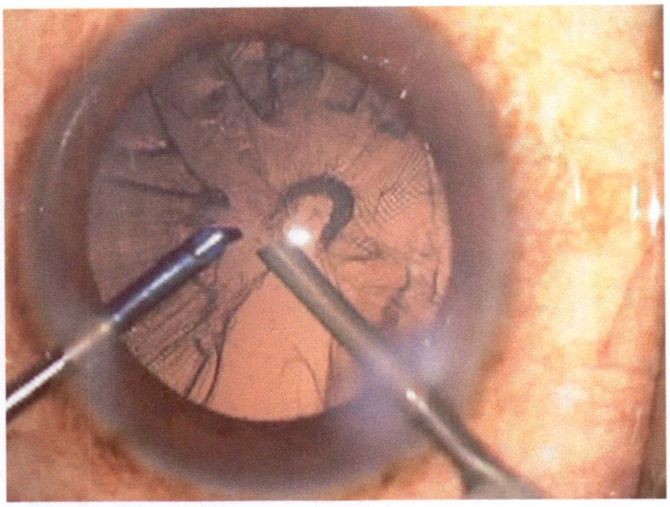

Fig. 1.18 0.7 mm MICS completed, the nucleus has been removed

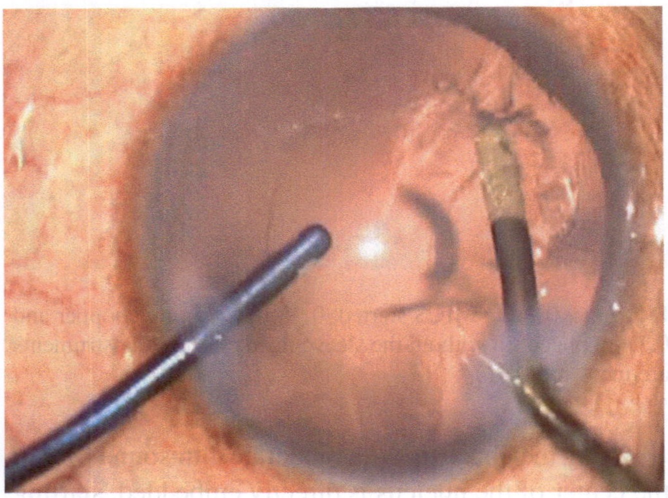

Fig. 1.19 Bimanual irrigation aspiration started with the 0.7 mm set

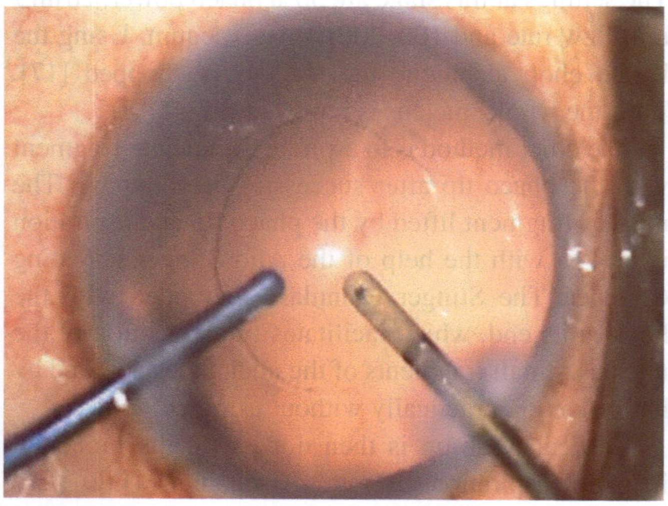

Fig. 1.20 Bimanual irrigation aspiration completed

1.3.5 0.7 mm MICS Combined Procedures

The combined procedures of eye surgery can diminish the time of treatment and complement each other. MICS with stable, swift surgery and small incisions can be helpful. Anterior chamber stability, tight corneal incisions and small-energy surgery can be helpful and more convenient in surgeries combined with vitrectomy. The characteristic astigmatic neutral MICS incisions can be combined with glaucoma surgery. The problem of surgically induced astigmatism after glaucoma surgery exists and may be corrected with the combination of minimal invasive glaucoma surgery.

1.3.5.1 0.7 mm MICS and Glaucoma Surgery

The combination of glaucoma surgery and cataract surgery with IOL implantation ideally should improve visual acuity and diminish visual patient recovery time. Glaucoma surgery and the cataract surgery are performed at all stages of the diseases. So the visual outcome is the problem that has to be solved. The combination of glaucoma surgery and cataract surgery results in a large decrease of IOP which is more than filtration surgery alone. But the standard trabeculectomy can increase corneal astigmatism. The conjunctival bleb, the scleral flap incisions, and the lack of tissue at the site of trabeculectomy can increase astigmatism. The use of minimal invasive surgery has become more important. Standard MICS surgery with MICS lenses can diminish corneal astigmatism and improve visual outcome of the operated eye [18, 19]. The use of micro filtration valves can decrease the IOP value by 50%. The mini shunt ExPress Corneal Surgery does not require the removal of the scleral and trabecular tissues. This nonvalved device was originally designed to provide a direct conduit from the anterior chamber to the sub-conjunctival space. The results of this procedure are very promising. The combination of MICS surgery and filtration surgery with mini shunt ExPress can diminish postoperative refractive error and be very useful in diminishing the postoperative IOP values in glaucomatous and cataract eyes [20] (Fig. 1.21).

Our first results of combined surgery of MICS and mini shunt ExPress after 3 months of follow-up on 5 patients indicated that BCVA and IOP had statistically improved. Before surgery, BCVA was 0.36 and was

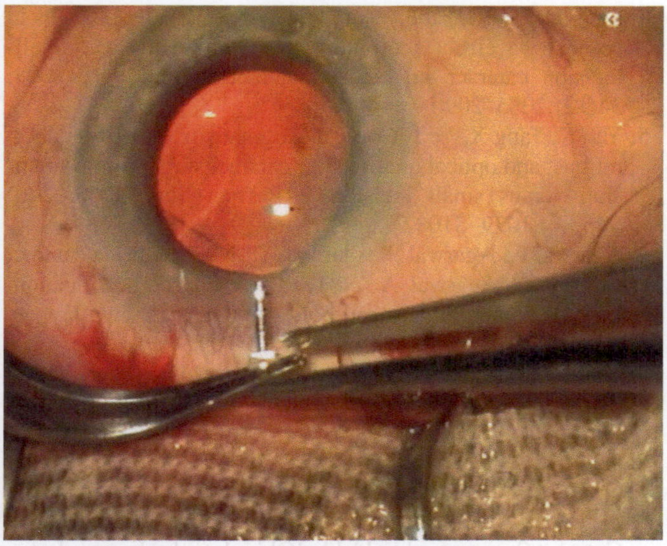

Fig. 1.21 Combined procedure of MICS and filtration surgery. The ExPress shunt implantation

improved to 0.85 after surgery. The media IOP before surgery was 23 mmHg and was reduced to 12.5 mmHg 3 months after surgery. The 46% of IOP reduction in glaucoma eyes is an excellent outcome. Further follow-up is necessary to confirm and evaluate this result. But these preliminary results are very promising (Tables 1.3 and 1.4). Other authors confirm usefulness, biocompatibility and beneficial effects of mini shunt ExPress [21, 22].

1.3.5.2 0.7 mm MICS and 25-Gauge Transconjunctival Sutureless Vitrectomy

It is very difficult to obtain stable conditions during combined surgery of the anterior and posterior segments of the eye. The problems with incisions and IOP may still occur. In earlier cataract and vitrectomy surgery techniques, the vitrectomy infusion cannula was inserted before phacoemulsification. The need to reduce complications leads to the application of less traumatic small incision surgery. One of the authors (Amar Agarwal) was the first to apply the combination of two surgical techniques: Transconjunctival Sutureless Vitrectomy (TSV25) and 0.7 mm MICS [23, 24]. The 0.7 mm MICS incisions are small, stable and self-sealing. They are able to withstand high intravitreal pressure during vitrectomy without leakage, chamber shallowing or iris prolapse (Fig. 1.22). The

Table 1.3 Results in BCVA and UCVA changes during 3 months after MICS and mini ExPress shunt surgery

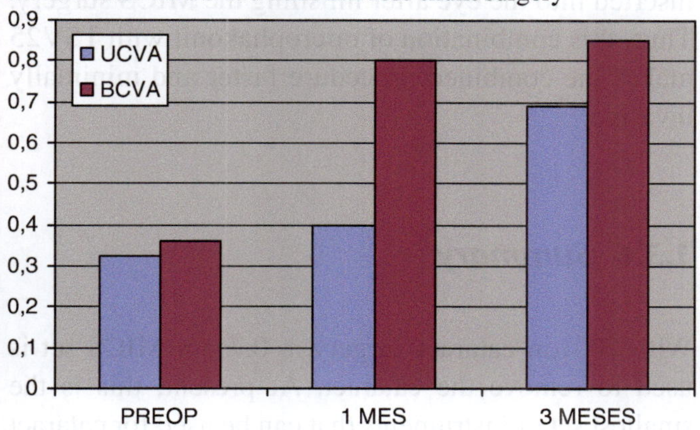

Table 1.4 Results in IOP changes during 3 months follow up after MICS and mini ExPress shunt surgery

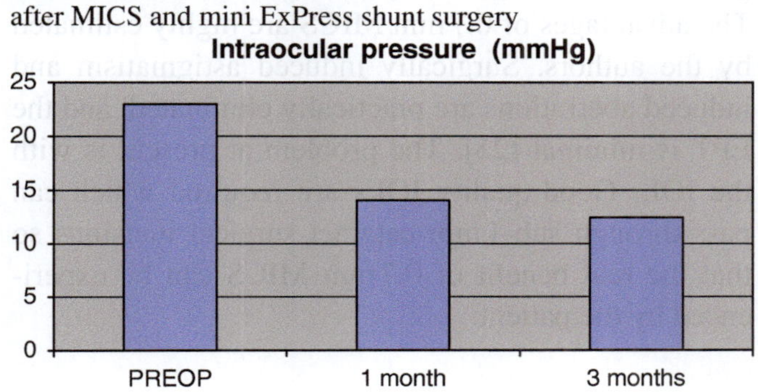

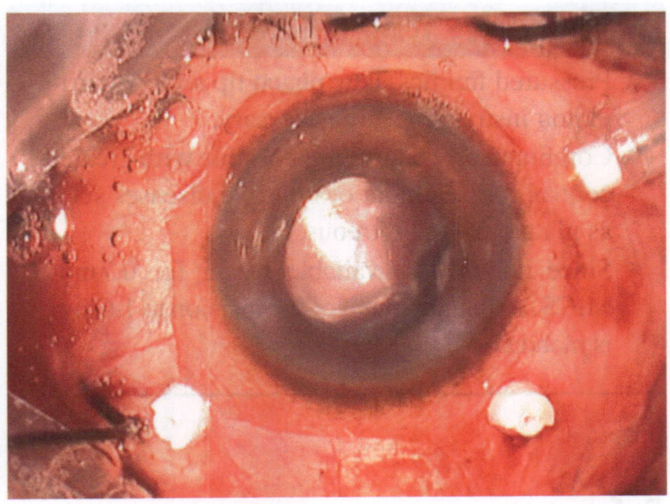

Fig. 1.22 Combined 0.7 mm MICS and 25-gauge transconjunctival sutureless vitrectomy. Self-sealing 0.7 mm MICS cataract incisions withstand high intravitreal pressure during vitrectomy without leakage, chamber shallowing, or iris prolapse [23]

problems of reduced resistance of the eye globe and the instability of the incisions during the infusion cannula insertion are not encountered with the 0.7 mm MICS technique at the first stage of vitrectomy.

Nowadays, the vitrectomy TSV25 infusion cannula is inserted into the eye after finishing the MICS surgery. Thus, this combination of microphakonit with TSV25 makes the combined procedure faster and minimally invasive.

1.3.6 Summary

With 700 μm cataract surgery, a 0.7 mm MICS set is used to remove the cataract. At present, this is the smallest set of instruments that can be used for cataract surgery. With time, surgery will be able to be performed with smaller and better instruments and devices. The advantages of 0.7 mm MICS are highly estimated by the authors. Surgically induced astigmatism and induced aberrations are practically eliminated, and the EPT is minimal [25]. The problem at present is with the IOL. Good-quality IOLs are required which can pass through sub-1 mm cataract surgical incisions so that the real benefit of 0.7 mm MICS can be experienced by the patient.

Take Home Pearls

- Pressured fluidics, new phaco tip and new irrigation instruments are necessary.
- Combined procedures are possible with greater control for treatment of multiple diseases such as glaucoma and vitreous.
- Since no IOL is available so far for 0.7 mm MICS, the enlargement of the incision to 1.6 mm is mandatory.

References

1. Agarwal A, Agarwal C, Agarwal AT. The Phakonit Thinoptx IOL. In Agarwals A (ed) Textbook Presbyopia. Slack, USA, 2002; pp 187–194
2. Pandey S, Wener L, Agarwal A, Agarwal S, Agarwal At, Hoyos J. Phakonit: cataract removal through a sub 1.0 mm incision with implantation of the Thinoptx rollable IOL. J Cataract Refract Surg 2002; 28:1710
3. Agarwal A, Agarwal S, Agarwal AT. Phakonit with an acritec IOL. J Cataract Refract Surg 2003; 29:854–855
4. Tong N, He JC, Lu F, Wang Q, Qu J, Zhao YE. Changes in corneal wavefront aberrations in microincision and small-incision cataract surgery. J Cataract Refract Surg 2008; 34(12):2085–2090
5. Yao K, Tang X, Ye P. Corneal astigmatism, high order aberrations, and optical quality after cataract surgery: microincision versus small incision. J Refract Surg 2006; 22(9 Suppl):S1079–S1082
6. Agarwal A, Agarwal S, Agarwal AT. No anesthesia cataract surgery. In Agarwal A (ed)Textbook Phacoemulsification, Laser Cataract Surgery and Foldable IOL's, 1st edn. Jaypee, India, 1998; pp 144–154
7. Pandey S, Wener L, Agarwal A, Agarwal S, Agarwal AT. Apple D: no anesthesia cataract surgery. J Cataract Refract Surg 2001; 28:1710
8. Agarwal A, Agarwal S, Agarwal AT. Phakonit: a new technique of removing cataracts through a 0.9 mm incision. In Agarwal A (ed) Textbook Phacoemulsification, Laser Cataract Surgery and Foldable IOL's, 1st edn. Jaypee, India, 1998; pp 139–143
9. Agarwal A, Agarwal S, Agarwal AT. Phakonit and laser phakonit: lens surgery through a 0.9 mm incision. In Agarwal (ed) Textbook Phacoemulsification, Laser Cataract Surgery and Foldable IOL's, 2nd edn. Jaypee, India, 2000; pp 204–216
10. Agarwal A, Agarwal S, Agarwal AT. Phakonit: phacoemulsification through a 0.9 mm incision. J Cataract Refract Surg 2001; 27:1548–1552
11. Agarwal S, Agarwal A, Agarwal AT. Phakonit with Acritec IOL. Highlights of ophthalmology, Panama, 2000
12. Alio J. What Does MICS Require in Alio´s Textbook MICS. Highlights of Ophthalmology, Panama 2004; pp 1–4
13. Agarwal A, Agarwal S, Agarwal AT. Phakonit. In Agarwal (ed) Textbook Phacoemulsification, Laser Cataract Surgery and Foldable IOL's, 3rd edn. Jaypee, India, 2003; pp 317–329
14. Agarwal A, Agarwal S, Agarwal AT. Phakonit and laser phakonit. In Boyd B, Agarwal A, et al (eds) Textbook Lasik and Beyond Lasik. Higlights of Ophthalmology, Panama, 2000; pp 463–468
15. Agarwal A, Agarwal S, Agarwal AT. Phakonit and laser phakonit-cataract surgery through a 0.9 mm incision. In Boyd B, Agarwal A, et al. (eds) Textbook Phako, Phakonit and Laser Phako. Higlights of Ophthalmology, Panama, 2000; pp 327–334
16. Agarwal A, Agarwal S, Agarwal AT. Antichamber collapser. J Cataract Refrac Surg 2002; 28:1085
17. Agarwal A. Air pump. In Agarwal A (ed) Bimanual Phaco: Mastering the Phakonit/MICS Technique. Slack, USA, 2005
18. Alio J, Rodriguez-Prats JL, Galal A. Advances in microincision cataract surgery intraocular lenses. Curr Opin Ophthalmol 2006; 17:80–93
19. Alió JL, Schimchak P, Montés-Micó R, Galal A. Retinal image quality after microincision intraocular lens implantation. J Cataract Refract Surg 2005; 31:1557–1560
20. Alio J. MICS in complicated cases (including management of complications in MICS). In XXX Seminar in Microincision Cataract Surgery, Riyadh, Saudi Arabia, 13–14 October 2008
21. Maris PJ, Smith ME, Netland PA. Clinical outcomes with the ExPress miniature glaucoma implant. Invest Ophthalmol Vis Sci 2005; 46:E-Abstract 71

22. Nyska A, Glovinsky Y, Belkin M, Epstein Y. Biocompatibility of the Ex-PRESS miniature glaucoma drainage implant. J Glaucoma 2003; 12(3):275–280
23. Agarwal A, Trivedi RH, Jacob S, et al. Microphakonit: 700 micron cataract surgery. Clin Ophthalmol 2007; 1(3): 323–325
24. Agarwal A, Jacob S, Agarwal AT. Combined microphakonit and 25-gauge transconjunctival sutureless vitrectomy. J Cataract Refract Surg 2007; 33:1839–1840
25. Alio J.L, Rodriguez-Prats JL, Galal A, Ramzy M. Outcomes of microincision cataract surgery versus coaxial phacoemulsification. Ophthalmology 2005; 112:1997–2003

2 MICS Instrumentation

Jorge L. Alió, Pawel Klonowski, and Jose L. Rodriguez-Prats

Core messages

- Specific instruments should be used to start the microincisional cataract surgery (MICS) transition.
- The most important instruments are the irrigating chopper (or stinger) and an adequately calibrated corneal knife to match the right incision size.
- The adequate use of irrigation device converts the inflow into operation advantage for MICS surgery.
- Nowadays, caliper surgical irrigation, aspiration instruments are 19 gauge.

2.1 MICS Instrument Choice: The First Step in the Transition

Minimization technology provides an opportunity to progress with new surgical techniques. The surgical tools have become slimmer and better designed. The lenses have advanced optics and have become thinner. Therefore, the evolution of the lens surgery is due to the minimization of the surgical trauma and incision, and maximization of the visual outcome. Returning to a 3–4 mm incision is impossible [1–3]. The Kelman concept of cataract surgery has been improved [4]. Now surgeons aspire to do phacoemulsification almost without ultrasound energy. The concept of MICS (Microincisional Cataract Surgery) and 0.7 mm MICS may be the way to merge the idea of the small incision corneal surgery with the new lens technology. MICS has catalyzed the design of a new set of instruments which can be used in minimized incisions.

In 2003, Jorge Alió registered MICS as a name of the new operating method. The definition of the MICS is the surgery performed through incisions of 2.0 mm or less [T.M. 2.534.071, March 2003, Spain] (Fig. 2.1).

Understanding this global concept implies that it is not only about achieving a smaller incision size but also about making a global transformation of the surgical procedure towards minimal aggressiveness [5].

The idea of separating infusion and aspiration is not new. Shearing did a cataract surgery using bimanual irrigation – aspiration tools 20 years ago [6]. Nevertheless, the concept was based on awider incision and different flow of the fluidics.

The basic concept of MICS is to diminish the energy required for disassembling the cataract lens and implantating the artificial lens with less corneal damage. To achieve this goal, many different authors have been looking for new instruments or they made the existing instruments more efficient [7]. Thus the idea of bimanual prechopping or irrigating choppers came into being.

The premises of MICS tools are that they should:

- Allow better fluidics
- Fit through minimal new incisions
- Be ergonomic
- Allow multiple functions
- Be safe
- Be easy to use

J. L. Alió (✉)
Vissum/Instituto Oftalmológico de Alicante, Avda de Denia s/n, Edificio Vissum, 03016 Alicante, Spain
email: jlalio@vissum.com

J. L. Alió, I. H. Fine (eds.), *Minimizing Incisions and Maximizing Outcomes in Cataract Surgery*,
DOI: 10.1007/978-3-642-02862-5_2, © Springer-Verlag Berlin Heidelberg 2010

MINISTERIO DE CIENCIA Y TECNOLOGÍA

Oficina Española de Patentes y Marcas

TÍTULO DE REGISTRO DE MARCA

Cumplidas las disposiciones establecidas en la vigente Ley 17/2001, de 7 de diciembre, de Marcas, se expide el presente título de registro de la marca que más abajo se identifica.

Conforme a la citada Ley de Marcas, el registro de la marca, confiere a su titular el derecho exclusivo a utilizarla en el tráfico económico. El registro ha quedado otorgado, sin perjuicio de tercero, por diez años, contados desde la fecha de presentación de la solicitud, y podrá renovarse indefinidamente por periodos ulteriores de diez años. De no efectuarse la renovación en la forma y plazos previstos legalmente, el registro de la marca será caducado.

Marca Nº. 2.534.071

TITULAR DE LA MARCA: *INSTITUTO OFTALMOLOGICO DE ALICANTE, S.L.*

DISTINTIVO MICS MICROINCISION CATARAT SURGERY	TIPO DISTINTIVO: **DENOMINATIVO** COLORES REIVINDICADOS DESCRIPCIÓN Y/O INDICACIÓN DE ELEMENTOS NO REIVINDICADOS EN EXCLUSIVA: *NO SE REIVINDICAN A TITULO PRIVATIVO LOS VOCABLOS MICROINCISION CATARAT SURGERY.*

FECHA PRESENTACIÓN SOLICITUD 18 de marzo de 2.003	FECHA CONCESIÓN REGISTRO: 13 de octubre de 2.003	PRIORIDADES REIVINDICADAS: PAÍS, NÚMERO, SOLICITUD, FECHA
MARCA ESPAÑOLA POR TRANSFORMACIÓN		
FECHA PRESENTACIÓN EN OFICINA DE ORIGEN	MODALIDAD MARCA DE ORIGEN Y NÚMERO:	
FECHA ANTIGUEDAD REIVINDICADA:	ANTIGÜEDAD DE LA MARCA ESPAÑOLA Nº:	

Fig. 2.1 Trade Mark 2.534.071, March 2003

By using surgical instruments to disassemble the cataract using prechoppers, one can diminish the use the phaco energy and decrease EPT. Bimanuality and separation of irrigation-aspiration functions help in using the tools parallelly in both hands and they can act together to improve the efficiency of the maneuvers. Therefore, many surgeons are creating new instruments in the search for new techniques of operation.

MICS instruments can be divided into the following sections:

- Incision instruments
- Capsulorhexis instruments
- Prechopping instruments
- Irrigation/aspiration instruments
- Auxiliary instruments

Converting the standard phacoemulsification mode to the MICS surgery would not be a problem for the ophthalmologist surgeon because the principle idea of manipulation inside the eye remains unchanged. The main aim of MICS is to understand the principles and to use proper tools. In this chapter, we present the instruments that are presented in various papers about MICS surgery and the instruments recommended by tool manufacturers that conform to the requirements of MICS.

2.2 MICS Incision

The surgery starts with two corneal equal incisions with a distance of 90–110° angle steps. The shape of the wound is very important. The basic conditions of the incision are that it has to be watertight and allow correct tool manipulation. The MICS incision should have a trapezoidal shape with two different size of incisions; one with a small measurement of 1.2 mm breadth inside the wound near the Descemet membrane, and the other with a wider measurement of 1.4 mm, outside near the epithelium. This is essential as the structure of the wound will allow us to insert the tools easily, it will protect against leakage, and at the same time, it will provide an opportunity to work with minimal anxiety and tissue injury. The lateral manipulations are very easy and safe in this type of wound. The mechanical injury of the tissues can suppress and extend the time of healing, and lead to leakage and hypotony. If the incision is too small, it will prevent us from correctly manipulating inside the anterior chamber and if the incision is too big it will lead to an unchecked leakage from the wound. The watertightness of the wound guarantees holding stability and the right depth of the anterior chamber, and it also reduces the possibility of exchanging liquids between the anterior chamber and the conjunctiva sack. It is essential for the minimization of the risk of endophthalmitis [8–10]. The great advantage of this incision is the optical result. The clinical data of MICS incision and surgically induced astigmatism suggest that three months after the MICS surgery, there is no statistically important change in the corneal astigmatism. The MICS incision is a neutral incision and this means that the size and shape of the incision do not affect on the postoperative corneal shape and astigmatism. It is important to say that no changes in astigmatism are caused by MICS incisions. To assure the reduction of the existing astigmatism, relaxing incisions can be made on the corneal periphery [1, 11, 12].

To carry out 1.5 mm MICS, we use trapezoidal knives, which have a changeable gauged breadth of the incision from 1.2 mm on the peak to 1.4 mm by the base (Katena Inc, Denville, NJ). To achieve this target, two kinds of knives can be used: Alio's MICS Knife (Cat. No. K20-2360, Katena Inc) and MICS Diamond Knife (Cat. No. K2-6660. Katena Inc) with trapezoid shape 1.25/1.4/2.0 mm angled, double bevel (Figs. 2.2 and 2.3).

This size of the wound is adapted to phacoemulsification tip with 0.9 mm breadth. For smaller phacoemulsification tips the breadth of the incision should be appropriately smaller. Through this incision, we can inject anesthetics and ophthalmic viscoelastic devices (OVD) without any problem, using standard infusion cannulas.

Sharpoint ClearTrap trapezoidal angled knife has different breadth of edge (1.2–1.4 mm) width indicator.

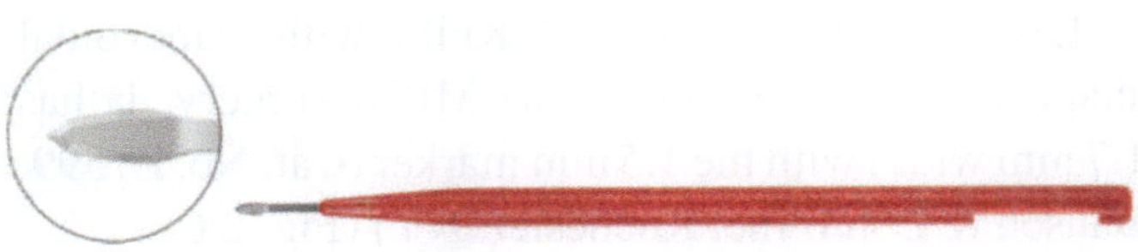

Fig. 2.2 Alio's MICS metal knife (Katena Inc)

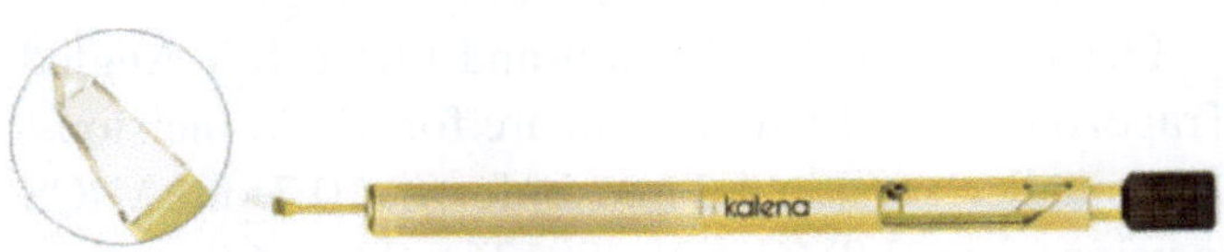

Fig. 2.3 Alio's MICS diamond knife (Katena Inc)

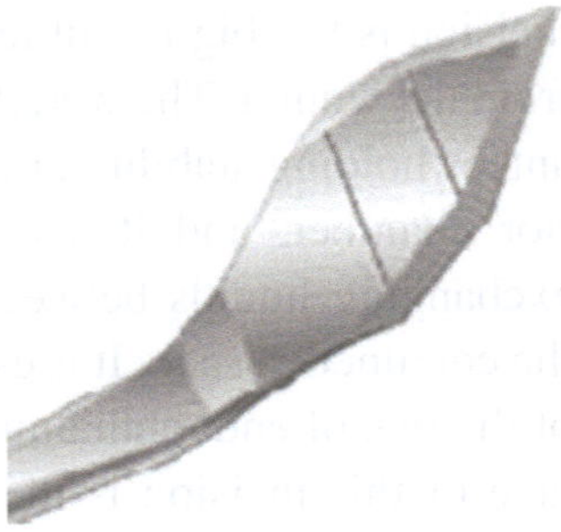

Fig. 2.4 Sharpoint ClearTrap trapezoidal knife (Angiotech)

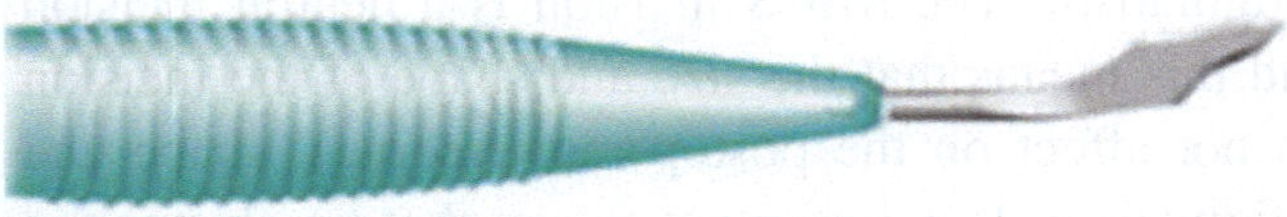

Fig. 2.5 Oasis MICS Medical PremierEdge knife (Oasis Medical)

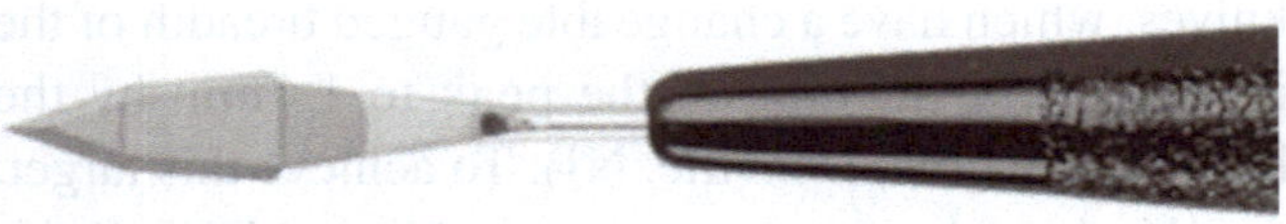

Fig. 2.6 Laseredge® clear corneal knife, trapezoidal (Bausch & Lomb Inc)

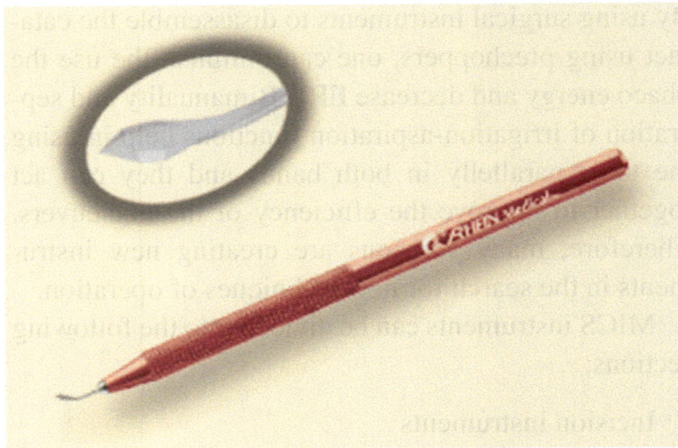

Fig. 2.7 3D Bi-Manual phaco blade (Rhein Medical Inc)

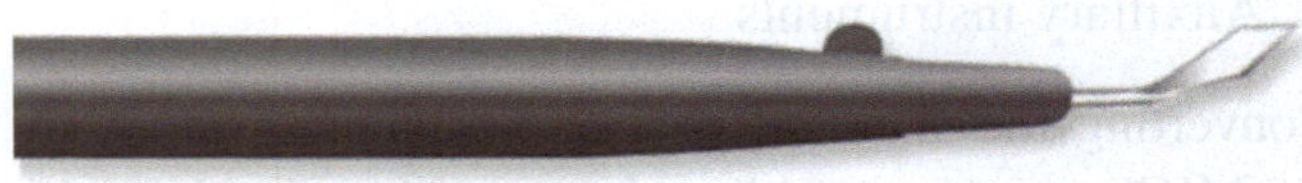

Fig. 2.8 Phaco slit angled 1.3 mm knife (Surgistar Inc)

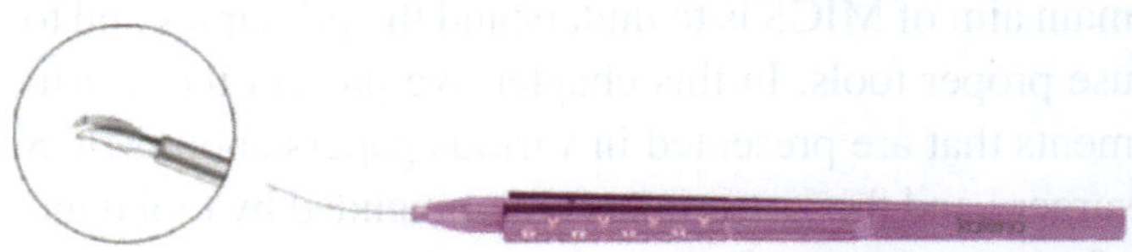

Fig. 2.9 Alio's MICS capsulorhexis forceps (Katena Inc)

This knife can make the intended shape of the incision (Cat. No. 75-1214, Angiotech, Reading, PA) (Fig. 2.4).

Oasis Medical PremierEdge knife (Cat. No. PE3915, Oasis Medical, Glendora, CA) is a blade with incremental widths of 1.0, 1.5, and 3.0 mm. The new Oasis MICS knife is angled with a single bevel up blade and has incremental widths of 1.0, 1.3, and 1.5 mm (Fig. 2.5).

A Microcut is a trapezoidal knife with widths 1.2 and 1.4 mm, and satisfies the conditions of MICS incision (PhysIOL, Toulouse, France).

Laseredge Clear Corneal Knife with trapezoidal shape can be also adapted to MICS surgery. It has 1.7 mm width with the 1.5 mm marker (Cat. No. E7599, Bausch & Lomb Inc, Rochester, NY) (Fig. 2.6).

3D Bi-Manual Phaco Blade, made by Rhien, is a knife with progressive width from 1.2 to 1.4 mm (Cat. No. 03-3011, Rhein Medical Inc, CA) (Fig. 2.7).

Phaco Slit Angled 1.3 mm and Phaco Slit Angled Trapezoid 1.4 × 1.6 mm knife are for MICS incisions. The smaller version 1.1 mm is for the 0.7 mm MICS incisions (Fig. 2.8) (Cat. No. 901361, 971416 Surgistar, Inc. Knoxville, TN).

2.3 MICS Capsulorhexis

The MICS incision is too tight for standard capsulorhexis forceps. The capsulorhexis can be made by cystotome or by MICS capsulorhexis forceps. The use of special forceps is thought to be much more adequate. The MICS capsulorhexis forceps allows for more flexible and precise surgery, with better control of the capsular bag and it should be the preferred technique in MICS. We use Alio's MICS Capsulorhexis Forceps (Cat. No. K5-7651, Katena Inc). This 23 guage diameter tool can easily be inserted in the wound of the cornea without stretching it. At the end of the forceps, a pointed catch is found. It enables a controlled puncturing of the anterior bag of the lens. Pressure is applied on the bag and then with a little movement, the slice is made in the anterior bag. The forceps enables a free manipulation of the torn capsular bag. The size of the surgical wound and the diameter of the forceps prevent the possibility of OVD leakage and flattening of the anterior chamber, stabilize the cataract lens and the bag and reduce the probability of bad tearing (Fig. 2.9).

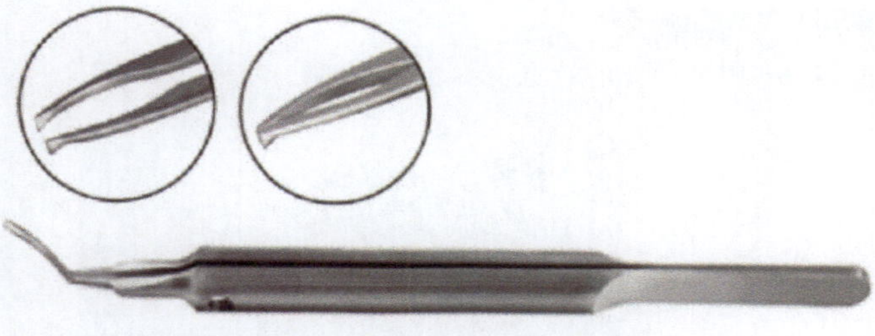

Fig. 2.10 Giannetti MICS capsulorrhexis forceps (Katena Inc)

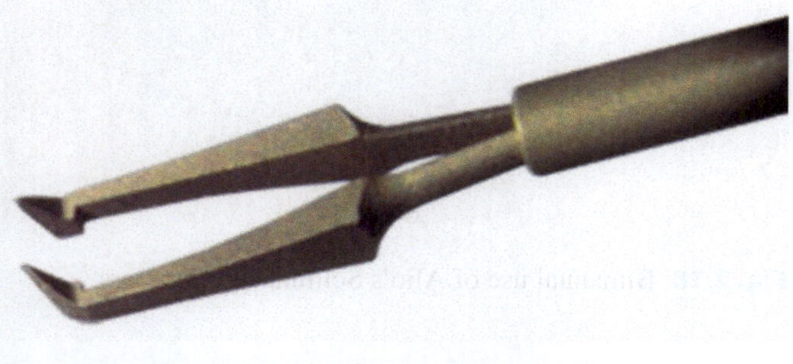

Fig. 2.11 Kelman capsulorhexis forceps 23G (Synergetics Inc.)

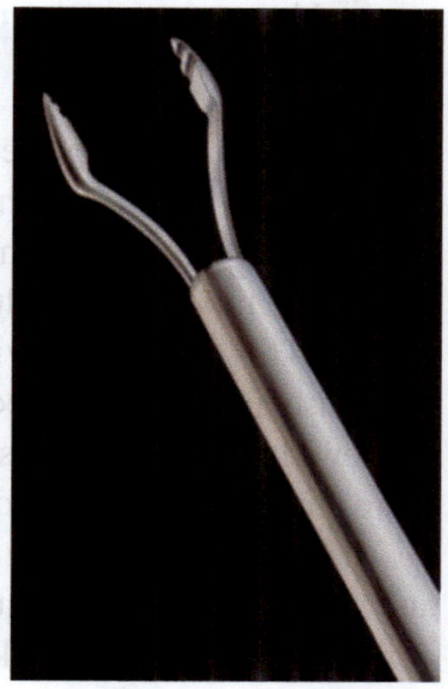

Fig. 2.12 Fine–Hoffman capsulorhexis forceps (MST Redmond)

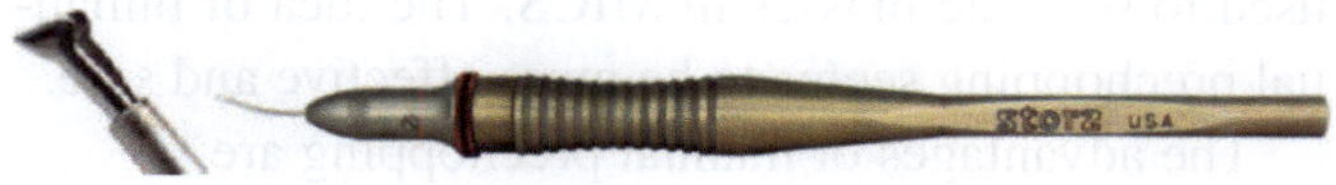

Fig. 2.13 Storz MICS capsulorhexis forceps (Storz, Bausch & Lomb)

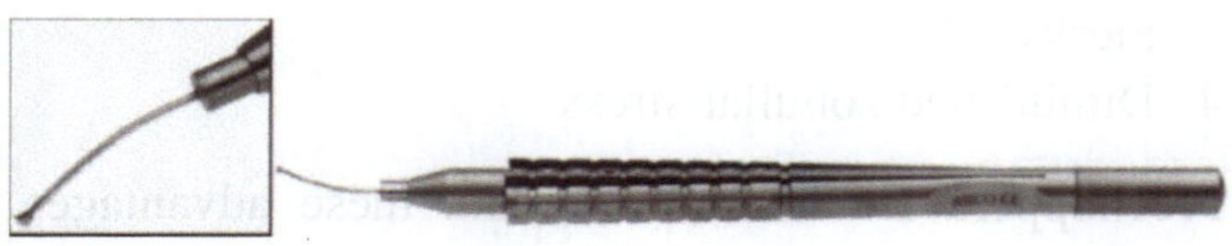

Fig. 2.14 Fine/Ikeda super micro capsulororhexis forceps 23G (ASICO LLC)

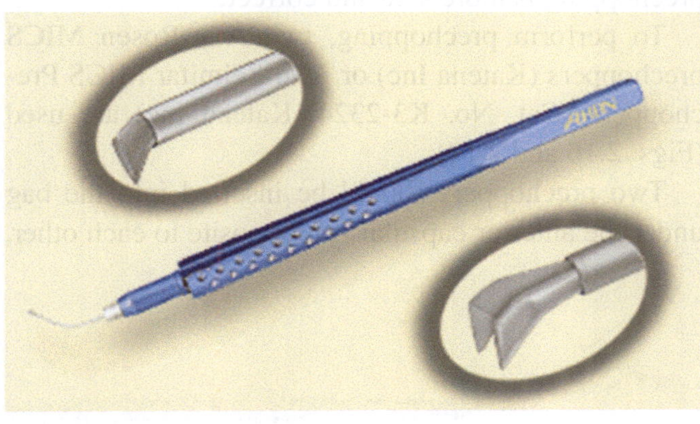

Fig. 2.15 Rhein tubular 23g capsulorhexis forceps (Rhein Medical Inc)

The forceps can be helpful to manipulate and release small adhesions with ease.

The other type of capsulorhexis forceps is the Giannetti MICS Capsulorhexis Forceps (Cat. No. K5-5090, Katena Inc). The construction of this forceps is based on the standard forceps structure. The 1 mm shanks allows for manipulation in the wound with minimal stretch of the corneal tissue (Fig. 2.10).

The Kelman Capsulorhexis Forceps has a very thin and curved shaft and facilitates maneuvers with the capsule. The forceps has a diameter of 23 guage (Cat. No. D100.23 Synergetics Inc. O'Fallon, MO) (Fig. 2.11).

Fine–Hoffman Capsulorhexis Forceps 23G was also designed for MICS surgery (Cay. No. DFH-0020, MST Redmond, Washington). The construction of this instrument is based on the structure of the micro forceps. This type of construction is ideal for wound protection and for maneuvring into the anterior chamber (Fig. 2.12).

Capsulorhexis Tip is designed to perform capsulorhexis through a 1.4 mm phaco incision. A nonrotating squeeze handle is used for control during MICS procedures (Cat. No. ET8190 H Storz, Bausch & Lomb, CA) (Fig. 2.13).

Fine Ikeda Super Micro Capsulororhexis Forceps 23G has a tip length of 0.95 mm. Tapered tips allow for easy maneuverability through the paracentesis incision. The 13 mm shaft from tip to handle, gives adequate access within the anterior chamber. It features a 90° tip that can be used as a cystotome. Proximity of the tip allows for easy working in the subincisional area without snagging the Descemet membrane. Compressible handle allows for maximum tactile feedback (Cat. No. AE-4389S ASICO LLC, IL) (Fig. 2.14).

Rhein Tubular 23g Capsulorhexis Forceps is adapted to 1.0 mm incision (Cat. No. 05-2362, Rhein Medical Inc) (Fig. 2.15).

2.4 MICS Prechopping

The ultrasound energy delivered into the eye during surgery is always too high. Prechopping is one of the saving elements here. This maneuver will diminish ultrasound time surgery, ultrasound energy and thermal energy. This type of activity is much better and does not cause any adverse effect when performed in accordancewith the rules. This is an upcoming trend now and more surgeons have started to perform this procedure.

The idea of prechopping led to development bimanual and monomanual techniques. Frequently used choppers like Fukasaku and Akahoshi choppers are monomanual choppers. However, two equal incisions can be used to separate masses in MICS. The idea of bimanual prechopping seems to be more effective and safe.

The advantages of manual prechopping are:

1. Reduction of phaco time
2. Lower amount of liberated ultrasound energy
3. Diminished damage to endothelium and trabecular meshwork
4. Diminished zonullar stress

Prechoppers are needed to attain these advantages. One-hand chopper maneuvers are not recommended because of the lesser efficacy of this action and huge zonullar stress. For small incision surgery bimanual prechopping is more safe and correct.

To perform prechopping, two Alio-Rosen MICS prechoppers (Katena Inc) or Alio-Scimitar MICS Prechoppers (Cat. No. K3-2324, Katena Inc) are used (Figs. 2.16 and 2.17).

Two prechoppers should be inserted into the bag under the anterior capsular rim opposite to each other.

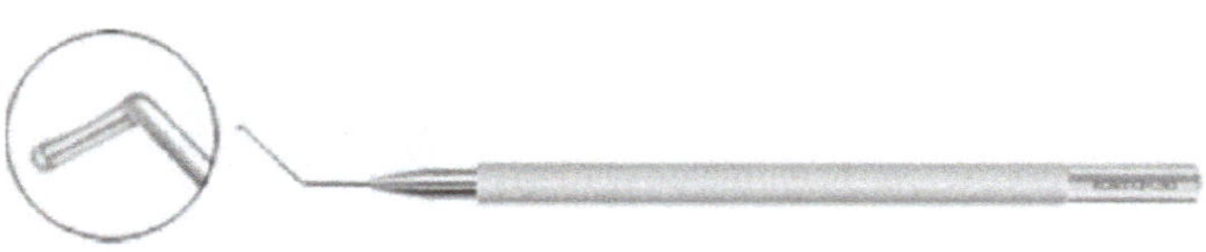

Fig. 2.16 Alio-Rosen phaco prechopper for micro incision cataract surgery (Katena Inc)

Fig. 2.17 Alio Scimitar prechopper for micro incision cataract surgery (Katena Inc)

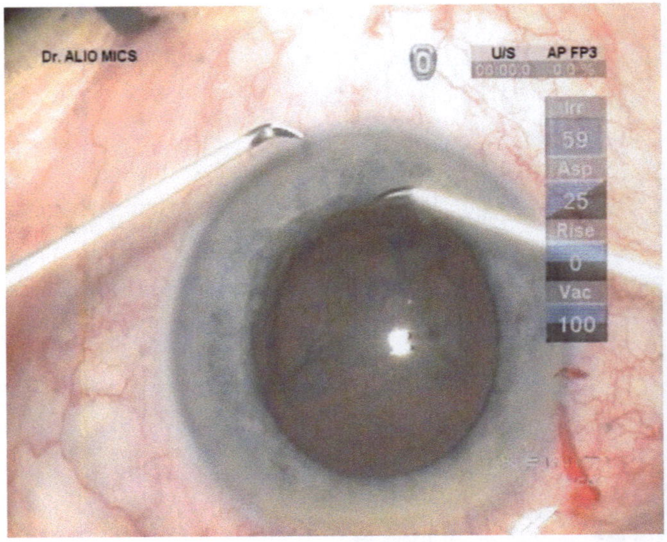

Fig. 2.18 Bimanual use of Alio's Scimitar prechoppers

The hooks of the choppers should be parallel to the anterior capsule bag. Next, the choppers should be gently rotated along the axis of the tool. The choppers should now be situated behind the masses of the lens under the bag on the perimeter. Both the hands should symmetrically carry out this activity. The choppers are crossed by symmetrically situating them opposite oneself. Now, cutting movements are made by gently crossing the prechoppers (Fig. 2.18).

The cut will be made from the perimeter to the center of the nuclei. Internal edge prechoppers have sharp edges that facilitate the incisions of the lens masses. This ambidextrous activity is important to prevent zonullar stress. It can also be carried out in the case of subluxated cataracts. When the cut is made, two dividing hemispheres are formed. The nucleus is then rotated about 90° and then for the second time, prechopping is repeated as described. After carrying out prechopping, we have four lens quadrants in the bag. Fast and effective division of the nuclei reduce the duration of operation. The new Alio Scimitar Prechoppers are made for the same type of maneuvers, but they have different endings. Scimitar Prechopper has a curved tip with a blunt end and a sharp inferior edge. This makes the cortical and the nuclear cut easier and can diminish zonullar stress at all stages of prechopping. The shape of the Scimitar Prechopper is prepared to perform and facilitate the 0.7 mm MICS surgery.

Nichamin triple choppers are ambidextrous choppers and can be used in MICS (Cat. No. 8-14506V, Rhein Medical Inc) (Fig. 2.19).

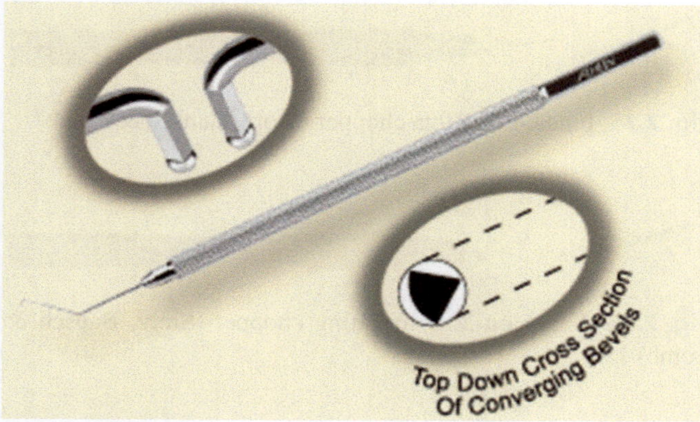

Fig. 2.19 Nichamin triple choppers (Rhein Medical Inc)

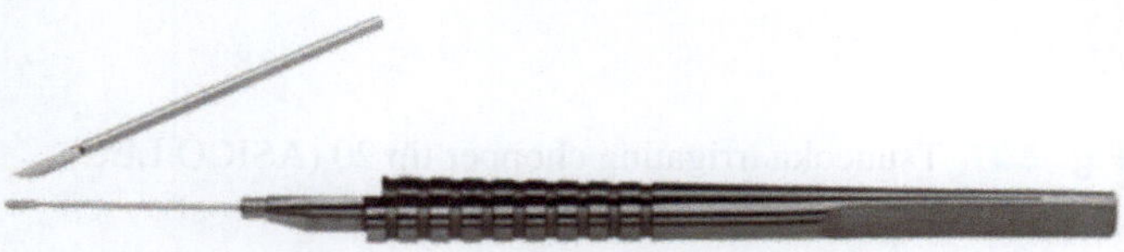

Fig. 2.20 Akahoshi super micro combo prechopper (Asico LLC).

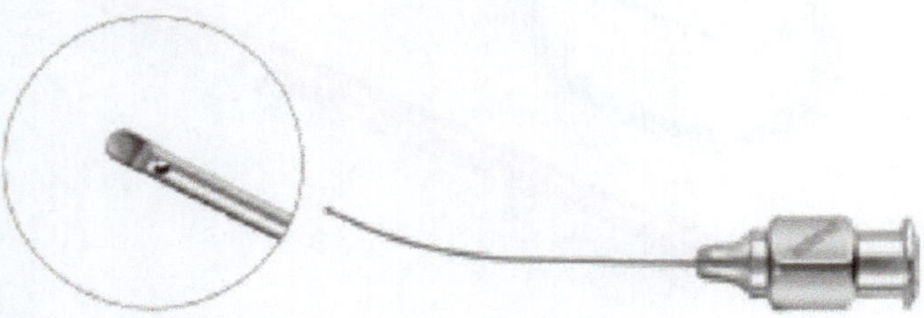

Fig. 2.21 Fukasaku hydrochop canula (Katena Inc)

Akahoshi Super Micro Combo prechopper can also be useful to make MICS nucleotomy. This 20 gauge combo prechopper is able to fit through a 1.2 mm incision (Cat. No. AE-4287 Asico LLC). The cataract lens can divide before phacoemulsification and without nuclear grooving (Fig. 2.20).

The Fukasaku hydrochop canula (Cat. No. K7-5462, Katena Inc) is also useful in dividing the nucleus. Thin cannula with liquid irrigation can divide the nucleus into parts (Fig. 2.21).

2.5 MICS Irrigation/Aspiration Instruments

Other ideas of fluidics management and ultrasound power management have led to the development of newer types of irrigating choppers. The most important factor was to connect the irrigating performance of the cannula with the mechanical properties of the chopper. The small diameter of the instrument was a challenge. Olson, Fine, Nagahara, and Tsuneoka made the first infusion cannulas with a high flow. Their cannulas had liquid flow up to 60 mL/min. Nevertheless, the first MICS cannula with a liquid flow of more than than 70 mL/min was the Alio's MICS Irrigating Stinger. This chopper has a high liquid infusion efficiency. All these infusion cannulas satisfy the requirements of MICS fluidics.

2.5.1 19 G Instruments

Irrigation Cannulas. The phacoemulsification can start when the quadrants are divided. In bimanual surgery, both incisions are involved in fluid transport. Use of irrigation cannula is obligatory. Infusion cannula has an additional application in MICS. It functions as both, chopper and manipulator. The end of the instrument, which is provided with a special hook, facilitates tearing and crumbling large fragments of the masses. It is very useful in the first part of nuclei phacoemulsification. The plane end is very practical to manipulate the masses and translocate them to the phaco tip or the aspiration cannula, when small fragments or soft cortical masses circulate in the anterior chamber.

The irrigation hole of the MICS irrigation tool should be on the bottom of the lower side. The diameter of the hole is 1 mm. Very thin walls and increased internal diameter of the instrument allows achieving irrigation in borders 72 cm^3/min. The stability of the anterior chamber is the result of irrigation, and direction of the liquid to the lens masses at the bag back (Fig. 2.22).

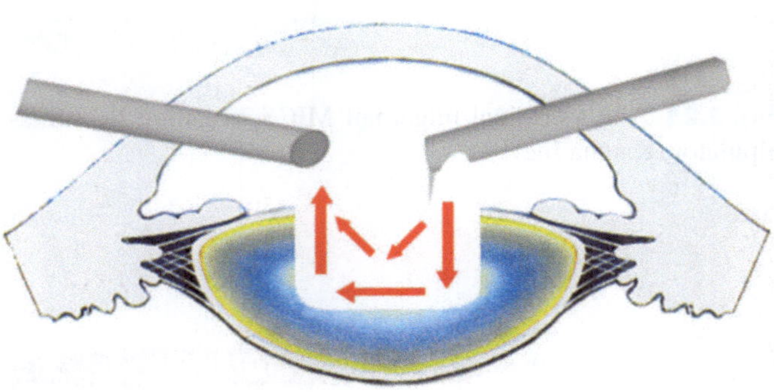

Fig. 2.22 Posterior irrigation in the irrigating cannula

The strength of the stream permits the bag to be held at a safe distance from the phacoemulsification tip and at the same time, enables convenient manipulations of the tools and lens masses. Additionally, this stream can clean the back bag from remaining cortical cells. A stream to the back bag is provided for the preservation of corneal endothelial cells before mechanical and thermal damage, instead of the cannulas with lateral holes. The posterior- directed stream gives the masses from the posterior chamber, the opportunity to circulate directly to the phaco tip. This helps the surgeon to avoid putting the phaco tip inside the capsular bag.

While starting phacoemulsification, vacuum levels should be set at 500–550 mmHg as the process involves pressured infusion. In most cases, when the cataract is not very hard, Alio's MICS hydromanipulator irrigating fingernail can be used. This makes it possible to divide and aspirate fragment masses of the lens without using ultrasound or torsional energy or to use them in the minimum way. In the case of hard cataracts, when total occlusion of the tip makes aspiration impossible, the Stinger Alio's MICS Irrigating Chopper would be more useful. This tool has a narrow edge at the end, which divides the masses and allows easy aspiration of the phacoemulsification tip. The fragmented elements of the hard cataracts are now easily aspirated, using the high under pressure and, at times, using ultrasound energy.

The Alio's MICS hydromanipulator irrigating fingernail (Cat. No. K7-5860 Katena Inc) is the first tool inserted in the anterior chamber during this stage of operation (Fig. 2.23).

This tool's end is shaped like a fingernail. It helps to remove rather soft cataracts. The tool that allows the removal of harder cataracts is Alio's MICS Irrigating Stinger (Cat. No. K7-5861, Katena Inc) (Fig. 2.24).

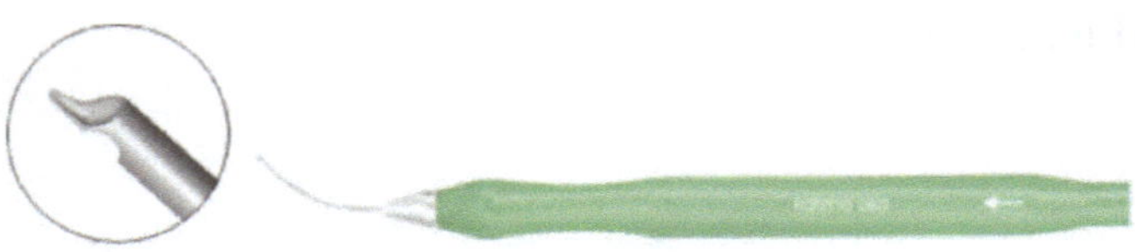

Fig. 2.23 Alio's original fingernail MICS irrigating hydromanipulator (Katena Inc)

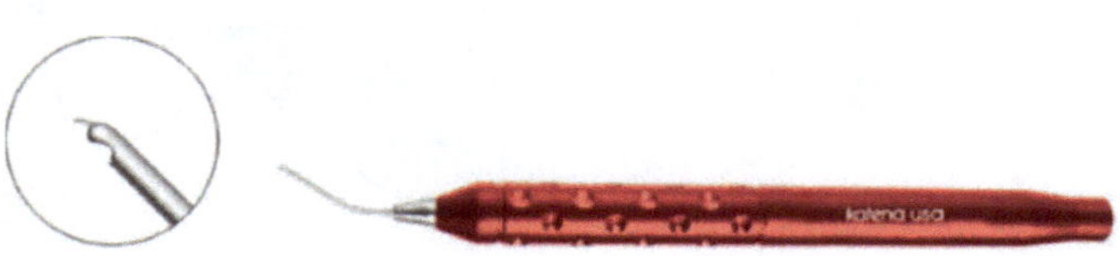

Fig. 2.24 Alio's MICS irrigating stinger (Katena Inc)

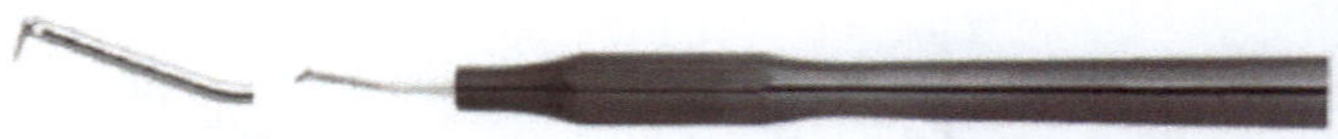

Fig. 2.25 Fine Olson 19ga chopper (Storz, Bausch & Lomb)

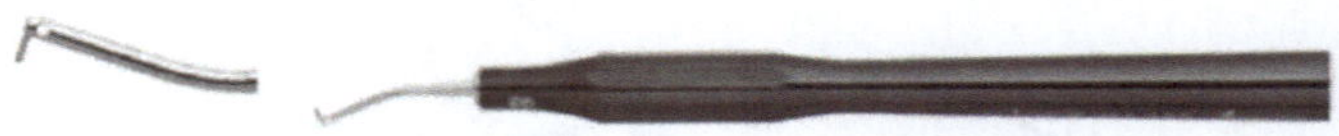

Fig. 2.26 Nagahara 20G irrigating chopper (Storz, Bausch & Lomb)

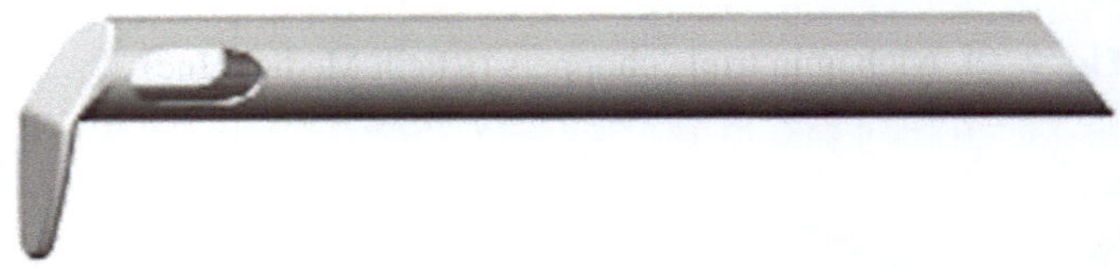

Fig. 2.27 Tsuneoka irrigating chopper tip 20 (ASICO LLC)

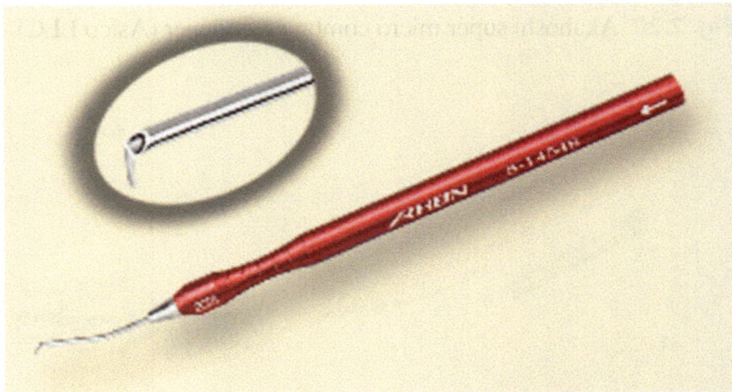

Fig. 2.28 Olson 20g irrigating chopper (Rhein Medical Inc)

Fine Olson 19ga chopper is a bimanual irrigating chopping instrument with an angled chopping tip. The irrigating hole is on the lateral side of the instrument (Cat. No. MVS1099 Storz, Bausch & Lomb) (Fig. 2.25).

Nagahara 20G chopper is for bimanual irrigation chopping The irrigating hole is on the lateral side of the instrument (Cat. No. MVS1095 Storz, Bausch & Lomb) (Fig. 2.26).

Duo Max Tsuneoka irrigating chopper tip 20 guage has large dual oval ports at the distal end for maximum irrigation. The side port configuration avoids pushing away the nucleus being chopped (Cat. No. AE7-3028 ASICO LLC) (Fig. 2.27).

Olson 20g Irrigating Chopper is the instrument with open- end irrigation. It can be used in 1.4 mm incision surgery (Cat. No. 8-14548, Rhein Medical Inc) (Fig. 2.28).

Aspiration cannula. The aspiration cannula has a smaller internal diameter than the irrigation cannula.

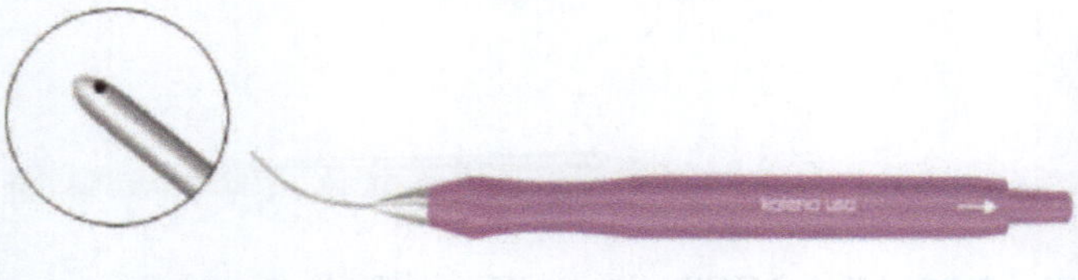

Fig. 2.29 Alio's MICS aspiration handpiece (Katena Inc)

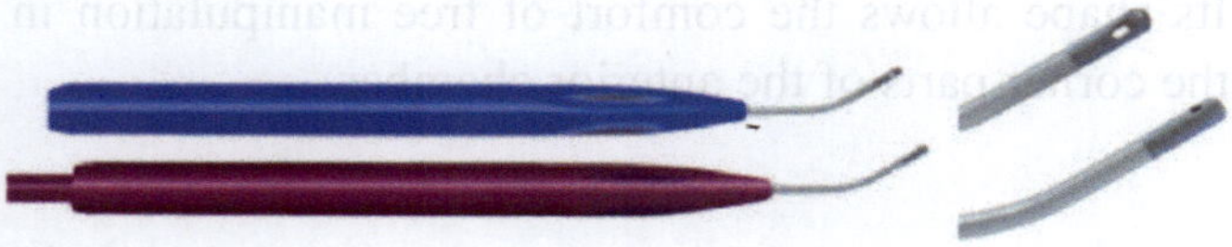

Fig. 2.30 Oasis bimanual microincisional kit (Oasis Medical)

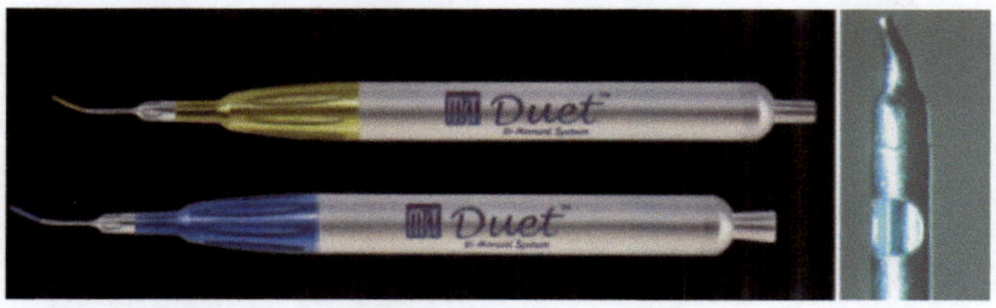

Fig. 2.31 MST Duet® BiManual system (MST, Redmond)

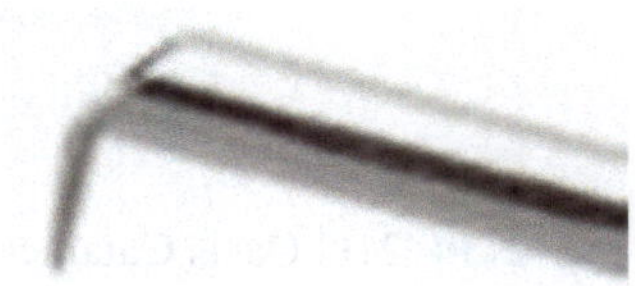

Fig. 2.32 Fine/Olsen irrigating chopper 20G (Storz, Bausch & Lomb)

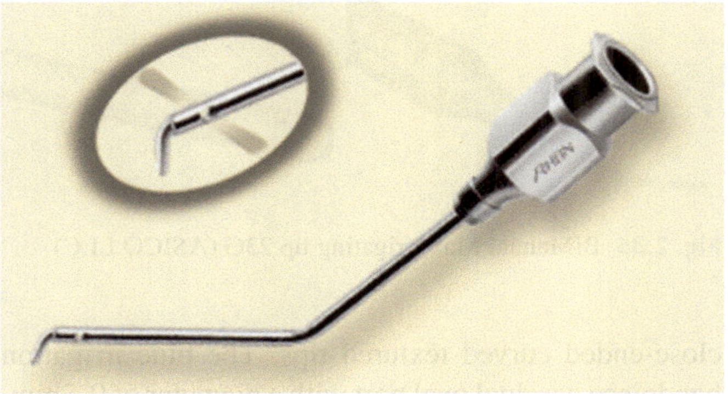

Fig. 2.33 Olson Cannula irrigating chopper 21G (Rhein Medical Inc)

This will cause disproportion in the resistance of flow between infusion and aspiration and will guarantee the anterior chamber stability. The increase in the depth of the anterior chamber causes the movement of the lens diaphragm. This can cause the lens masses movement into the space behind the iris. Masses can be placed between the iris and the anterior bag in the space surrounding the sulcus which does not allow the masses to be seen. However, the masses can be seen in the anterior chamber after few hours of the operation. Rinsing out and cleaning this space is extremely important.

The stability of the anterior chamber, in case of MICS, is definitely higher than in coaxial phacoemulsification. MICS does not cause frequent and considerable changes in the proportion anatomy of the eyeball and there is no traction during the operation. It is possible to maintain the anterior chamber stable from the capsulorhexis to the OVD injection before lens implantation during the MICS surgery [11].

Alio's MICS Aspiration Handpiece (Cat. No. K7-5820, Katena Inc) also serves to remove the remains of cortical masses. It has a port diameter of 0.3 mm (Fig. 2.29).

Oasis bimanual kit for 19 and 21 guage surgeries have instruments with open or closed ended curved textured tips. This is the singe use tip. The blue irrigation handpiece has dual oval port with a diameter of 0.5 mm. The purple aspiration handpiece has one round port of 0.3 mm (Cat. No. 1719, Oasis Medical) (Fig. 2.30).

2.5.2 21 G Instruments

The minimization of MICS tools surgery allows us to carry out phaco through 0.7 mm. Part of the standard MICS tools can be adapted to 0.7 mm MICS, but irrigation and aspiration cannulas are not fitted. The 22G Alio Stinger irrigating chopper Duet System (MST, Redmond, WA) allows to perform the 0.7 mm MICS through 1 mm incision (Fig. 2.31).

The decreased thickness of the walls and the appropriate internal profile gives an opportunity to achieve the required inflow of the fluid into the anterior chamber. Stinger irrigating chopper 22G also has a narrow edge at the end, this allows to divide and conduct the masses into the aspiration cannula.

Fine/Olsen irrigating chopper is an open- ended 20 guage instrument, especially designed forMICS. This instrument has external diameter of 0.89 mm. It allows easy insertion into MICS incision (Fig. 2.32) (Cat. No. MVS2000 20 Storz, Bausch & Lomb).

Olson Cannula irrigating chopper 21G is the instrument with horizontal infusion holes (Cat. No. 91-7146-L, Rhein Medical Inc) (Fig. 2.33).

The oasis set for 21 and 23 guage cataract surgery is composed of two I/A handpieces. The instruments have

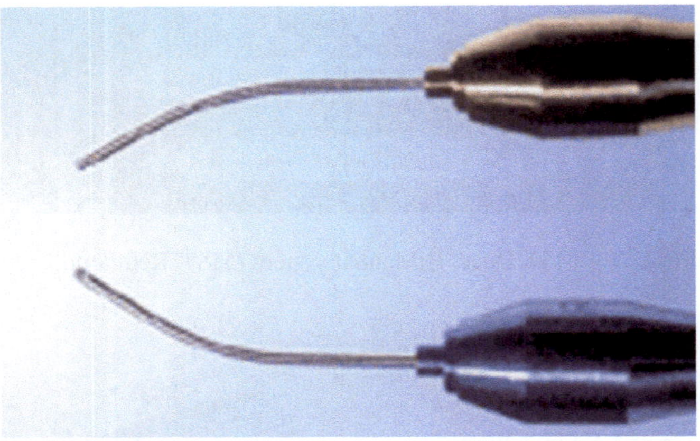

Fig. 2.34 21G Oasis Cataract I/A set (Oasis Medical)

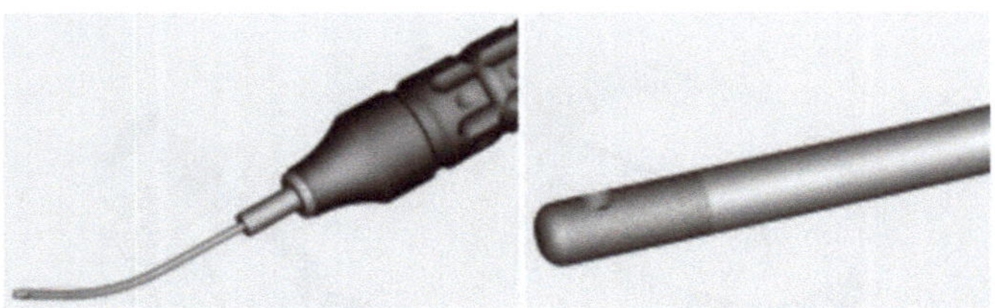

Fig. 2.35 BiManual Max irrigating tip 23G (ASICO LLC)

close-ended curved textured tips. The blue irrigation handpiece has dual oval port with a diameter of 0.5 mm. The gold aspiration handpiece has one round port of 0.3 mm (Fig. 2.34) (Cat. No. 1621, Oasis Medical).

BiManual Max Irrigating Tip is the 23 guage curved bimanual micro irrigating handpiece with dual oval ports of 0.4 mm, with a capsule polisher. Bimanual Micro Aspirating handpiece has an oval 0.3 mm port (Cat. No. AE7-0208 ASICO LLC) (Fig. 2.35).

2.6 MICS Auxiliary Instrument

2.6.1 Scissors

Scissors are useful in complicated cataracts, which may require a cutting within the anterior chamber of the eye. A scissor can, cut delicate membranes, cut adhesions, make iridotomy, and cut fibrosis of the bags. In these cases, Alio's MICS scissors are useful(Cat. No. K4-5351, Katena Inc). This tool has 23 gauge curved shaft with horizontal micro blades (Fig. 2.36).

The 0.6 mm breadth allows for access into the anterior chamber without the need to widen the incision.

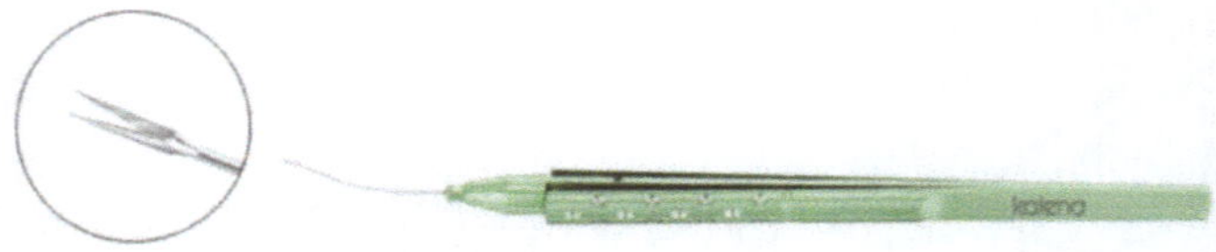

Fig. 2.36 Alio's MICS scissors (Katena Inc)

Its shape allows the comfort of free manipulation in the corner parts of the anterior chamber.

2.6.2 Gas Forced Infusion

In modern cataract surgery, fluidics management becomes a very important element of the surgery. Small diameters of the irrigation and aspiration tools, and the efficacy of the pumps present a huge challenge for maintaining the fluidics. The 20 guage diameter and even the 19 guage inflow diameters can cause problems in delivering the proper amount of the liquid into the eye. However, the problem arises only when the 0.9 or 0.7 mm phaco tip starts to aspire.

The main problems are:

1. Stability of the anterior chamber
2. Stability and control of intraocular pressure (IOP)
3. Stable incision with no leakage
4. High vacuum

To maintain the fluidics, the inflow of the fluid to the anterior chamber should be superior to the outflow. The first step to achieve this balance is to differ the internal diameter of the I/A tools. The aspiration diameter should be smaller than the irrigation one. The efficacy of the Venturi pump is very high and therefore, the danger of the IOP drop and anterior chamber collapse may exist. To solve this problem, gas-forced infusion (VGFI by Alcon) is used. This system controls the IOP and increases the infusion over the gravitation efficiency of the traditional infusion. However, the problem of anterior chamber collapse can still exist. During the tip occlusion, the vacuum rises to a maximum value. After the occlusion brake, the flow is very high without compensation of inflow. This moment is dangerous for anterior chamber stability. There are some post-occlusion surge prevention strategies. Lifting the bottle is insufficient in MICS surgery and hence we need to force infusion with an additional air pump. Phacoemulsification systems such as Accurus (Alcon) or Millennium (Bausch & Lomb) have built-in forced infusion systems to increase infusion. Programing the pump irrigation and aspiration system can decrease the danger of surge after the mass break. Sovereign (AMO) and Infinity (Alcon) have also made it possibile to monitor the vacuum at crisis moments. Other phaco platforms do not have the possibility to raise additional infusion. In this case, we can use additional air pumps, connected to the irrigation bottle, to augment infusion. This combined system is well proved in practice.

2.6.3 Surge Prevention

To prevent the surge during occlusion breaks at higher vacuum level the flow restrictor can be installed between the phacoemulsification handpiece and the aspiration tubing. Stable Chamber System® and Cruise Control™ are the devices that are specially designed for making cataracts in the bimanual microincisional phacoemulsification mode at the high vacuum settings. They have a disposable flow restrictor and a mesh filter against blocking. The lens masses stay on the filter. Restrictor limit the flow. At a vacuum level of 500 mmHg, the anterior chamber does not become shallow, especially if you are working with pressured infusion (Figs. 2.37 and 2.38).

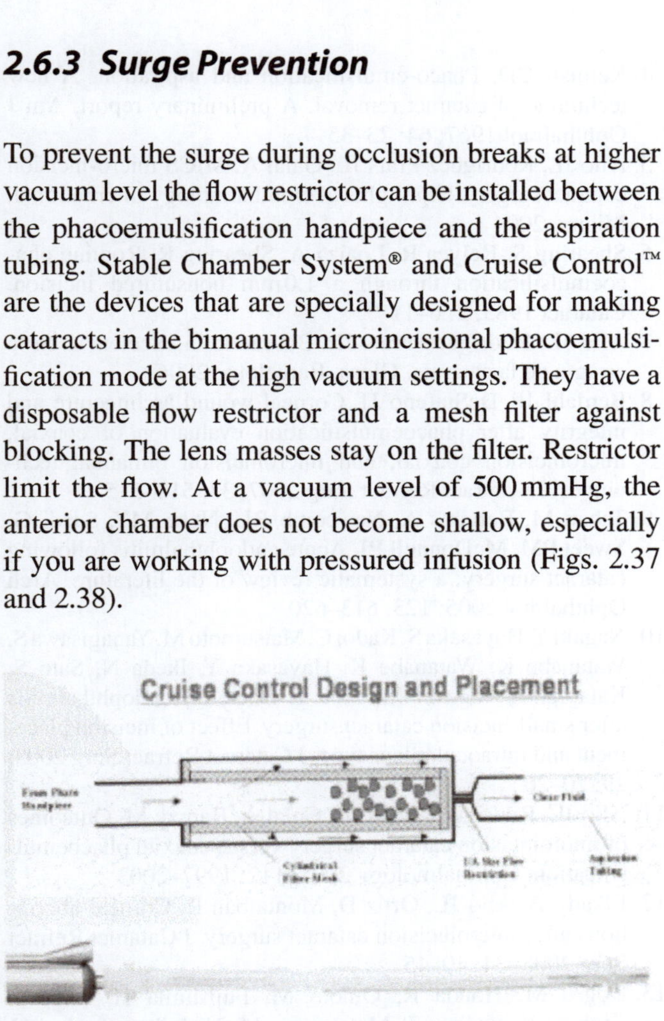

Fig. 2.37 Cruise Control™ system (STAAR Surgical Company Monrovia, CA)

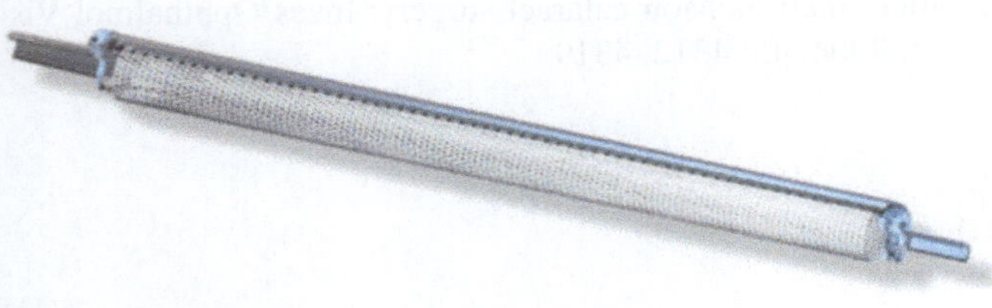

Fig. 2.38 Stable chamber system® (Bausch & Lomb)

2.7 New MICS Instruments

2.7.1 Flat Instruments

The new concept is the idea of plane instruments. Incision with a diameter of 1.5 mm is very susceptible to stretching. The plane instrument idea is to fit the instrument into a natural-shaped wound. The flattened oval profile is better adapted to a linear incision (Fig. 2.39). This type of instrument does not affect the wound border and improves the self-sealing propriety of the incision. Wound integrity is one of the most important factors as it may influence the outcome of the surgery. The tools are adapted to the wound, but the wound is not stressed by the tools. The tissue of the wound is practically untouched. Self-sealing capability of the corneal incision is mainly dependent on wound construction: the angle, the width- to -depth ratio, and multiple-plane construction of incision. Any disturbance in these conditions can affect postoperative healing. The flat instruments do not affect the edges of the tissues of the incision and therefore, the natural process of healing is not disturbed.

Assurance of the proper amount of fluidics in MICS requires a large dimension of the tools. This is the reason for the corneal tissue stress during the operation. Mechanical tissue stress can evoke leakage, astigmatism, and problems with stability of the anterior chamber [13, 14]. Improved tools are required to solve these problems. New Alio's MICS Flat Instruments are made by Katena. The irrigation and aspiration tools have a rectangular cross-section. The change of shape does not influence the fluidics parameters. The fluidic flow of these tools is proper for MICS. The leakage around the tool is absent. Manipulation of the tools is easy and cause only minimal corneal tissue stress. Vertical manipulation does not stretch the wound and the horizontal movements do not press the angle of the wound

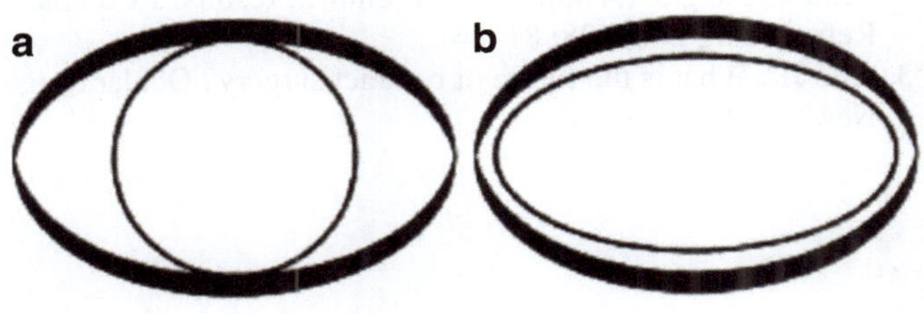

Fig. 2.39 Incision adaptation to the round (**a**) and flat (**b**) instruments

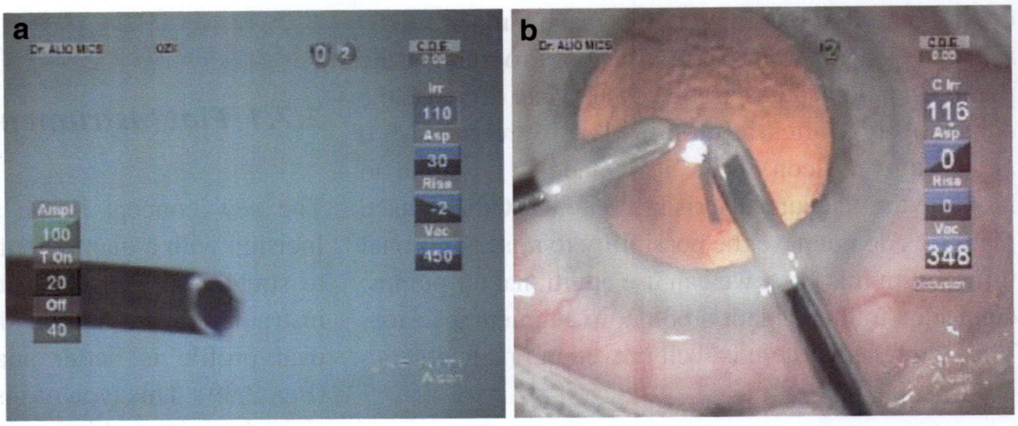

Fig. 2.40 MICS plane instruments: phaco tip (**a**), Alio's Stinger and aspiration cannula (**b**)

because of the trapezoidal shape. This concept of irrigation-aspiration flat tool is a new way of conserving the wound (Fig. 2.40).

Take Home Pearls

- The right choice of instruments will help the surgeon in the transition.
- Watertight incisions, especially during phacoemulsification and proper I/A instruments should be used.
- Fluidics should be improved by increasing the inflow and reducing outflow by use of other specific devices such as cruise control, which now is useful to improve MICS surgery at a high vacuum level.

References

1. Alio JL, Rodriguez-Prats JL, Vianello A, Galal A. Visual outcome of microincision cataract surgery with implantation of Acri.Smart lens. J Cataract Refract Surg 2005; 31: 1549–1556
2. Tsuneoka H, Shiba T, Takahashi Y. Ultrasonic phacoemulsification using a 1.4 mm incision: clinical results. J Cataract Refract Surg 2002; 28: 81–86
3. Alió JL. What is the future of cataract surgery? Ocular Surg News 2006; 17: 3–4
4. Kelman CD. Phaco-emulsification and aspiration. A new technique of cataract removal. A preliminary report. Am J Ophthalmol 1967; 64: 23–35
5. Alio JL, Rodriguez Prats JL, Galal A. MICS micro-incision cataract surgery. Highlights of Ophthalmology International, Miami, 2004
6. Shearing S, Relyea R, Loaiza A, Shearing R. Routine phacoemulsification through a 1.0 mm nonsutured incision. Cataract 1985; 2: 6–11
7. Alió JL, Rodriguez-Prats JL. Buscando la excelencia en la cirugía de la catarata. Glosa, Barcelona, 2006
8. Berdahl JP, DeStafeno JJ. Corneal wound architecture and integrity after phacoemulsification evaluation of coaxial, microincision coaxial, and microincision bimanual techniques. J Cataract Refract Surg 2007; 33: 510–515
9. Taban M, Behrens A, Newcomb RL, Nobe MY, Saedi G, Sweet PM, McDonnell PJ. Acute endophthalmitis following cataract surgery: a systematic review of the literature. Arch Ophthalmol 2005; 123: 613–620
10. Nagaki Y, Hayasaka S, Kadoi C, Matsumoto M, Yanagisawa S, Watanabe K, Watanabe K, Hayasaka Y, Ikeda N, Sato S, Kataoka Y, Togashi M, Abe T. Bacterial endophthalmitis after small-incision cataract surgery. Effect of incision placement and intraocular lens type. J Cataract Refract Surg 2003; 29: 20–26
11. Alio JL, Rodriguez-Prats JL, Galal A, Ramzy M. Outcomes of microincision cataract surgery versus coaxial phacoemulsification. Ophthalmology 2005; 112: 1997–2003
12. Elkady B, Alió JL, Ortiz D, Montalbán R. Corneal aberrations after microincision cataract surgery. J Cataract Refract Surg 2008; 34: 40–45
13. Dogru M, Honda R, Omoto M, Fujishima H, Yagi Y, Tsubota K, Kojima T, Matsuyama M, Nishijima S, Yagi Y. Early visual results with the rollable ThinOptX intraocular lens. J Cataract Refract Surg 2004; 30: 558–565
14. Guirao A, Tejedor J, Artal P. Corneal aberrations before and after small-incision cataract surgery. Inves Ophthalmol Vis Sci 2004; 45: 4312–4319

3 Evolution of Ultrasound Pumps and Fluidics and Ultrasound Power: From Standard Coaxial Towards the Minimal Incision Possible in Cataract Surgery

William J. Fishkind

Core Messages

- Increased capability of the phaco machine permits a considerable individualization of the phaco parameters.
- Through consideration of machine settings, the quality of cataract surgery and its outcomes can be appreciably improved.

3.1 Introduction

Although phacoemulsification machines have undergone continuous improvement, ever-increasing in both, their complexity and safety, one principle remains unchanged: All phaco machines consist of a computer to generate ultrasonic energy, and a transducer to turn these electronic signals into mechanical, acoustical, and cavitational energy. The energy thus produced, is transferred through a hollow needle and will overcome the inertia of the lens to emulsify it. The second of the refined elements of the machine are the "fluidic control systems." These consist of a vacuum generating pump and computer algorithms to control it, phaco needles of varying diameters and configurations, and infusion sources.

3.2 Power Generation

Power is created by an interaction between frequency and stroke length.

W. J. Fishkind
Director Fishkind, Bakewell, Maltzman
Eye Care and Surgery Center
Tucson, Arizona, USA

Frequency is defined as the speed of the needle movement. The manufacturer of the machine determines it. Presently, most machines operate at a frequency between 27,000 cycles per second (Hz) to 50,000 cycles per second. This frequency range is efficient for nuclear emulsification. Lower frequencies become less efficient and higher frequencies create excess heat.

Stroke length is defined as the length of the needle movement. This length is generally 2–6 mils (thousandths of an inch). Most machines operate in the 2–4 mil range. One mil is 25 μm. Therefore, most phaco needles travel a distance of 50–100 μm. Longer stroke lengths and higher frequencies are prone to generate extra heat. The longer the stroke length, the greater is the physical impact on the nucleus, and so, the generation of cavitation energy is greater. When the frequency is higher, the impacts per unit time is more and the physical impact is greater.

3.3.1 Tuning

The central processing unit (CPU) of modern phaco machines recognizes the phaco needle when it passes into different intraocular media. It does this by turning the driver piezo crystals, momentarily, into receiving crystals. The system is most efficient when it is operating

J. L. Alió, I. H. Fine (eds.), *Minimizing Incisions and Maximizing Outcomes in Cataract Surgery*,
DOI: 10.1007/978-3-642-02862-5_3, © Springer-Verlag Berlin Heidelberg 2010

at its resonant frequency. For example, the resistance of the aqueous is less than the resistance of the cortex, which in turn, is less than the resistance of the nucleus. As the resistance to the phaco tip varies, to maintain maximum efficiency, depending on the machine, small alterations in frequency or stroke length are created by the tuning circuitry in the CPU. This is important to minimize the excessive generation of ultrasonic energy, which is harmful to the intraocular contents. The surgeon will subjectively determine good tuning circuitry by a sense of smoothness and power.

3.2.2 Phaco Energy

The actual tangible forces that emulsify the nucleus are thought to be a blend of the "Jackhammer" energy and cavitational energy. The "jackhammer" energy is the physical striking of the needle against the nucleus. Cavitational energy generation is more convoluted. Recent studies indicate that there are two kinds of cavitational energy: low frequency energy and high frequency energy.

3.2.2.1 Low Frequency Energy

Low frequency energy is the frequency of energy that is selected by the manufacturer for the individual machine. As noted above, it is generally 27–50 Hz. It is omni directional and will reflect from surfaces such as the cornea or sclera. It travels over great distances and has no cavitational impact. It is, however, the engine that generates cavitational bubbles. These are the fuel for high frequency energy.

3.2.2.2 High Frequency Energy

Low frequency energy is the dynamic force to generate high frequency energy. When the needle, moving at the lower frequency, excites implosion of cavitational bubbles, high frequency energy is created. In its powerful configuration, transient cavitation will generate a 1-mm cone of energy extending up to 10 mm. from the phaco tip. In its inactive form, sustained cavitation does nothing more than vibrating the cavitational bubbles.

3.2.3 Transient Cavitation

The phaco needle, moving through a liquid medium at ultrasonic speeds, gives rise to intense zones of high and low pressure. Low pressure, created with the backward movement of the tip, pulls dissolved gases out of the solution, thus producing micro bubbles. Forward tip movement then creates an equally intense zone of high pressure. This initiates compression of the micro bubbles until they implode. At the moment of implosion, the bubbles create a temperature of 7,204°C and a shock wave of 5,171,100 mbar. Of the micro bubbles created, 75% implode, amassing to create a powerful shock wave, radiating from the phaco tip perpendicular to the bevel of the phaco tip with annular spread.

However, 25% of the bubbles are too large to implode. These micro bubbles are swept up in the shock wave and radiated with it. Transient cavitation is a violent event. The energy created by transient cavitation exists for not more than 4 ms and extends from the phaco tip in a cone shape distribution, in the immediate vicinity of the phaco tip, and within its lumen. It is this form of cavitation that is thought to generate the energy responsible for emulsification of cataractous material (Fig. 3.1). Additionally transient cavitation is instrumental in clearing nuclear fragments within the phaco needle preventing repetitive needle clogging.

The transient cavitational energy can be directed in any desired direction. The angle of the bevel of the

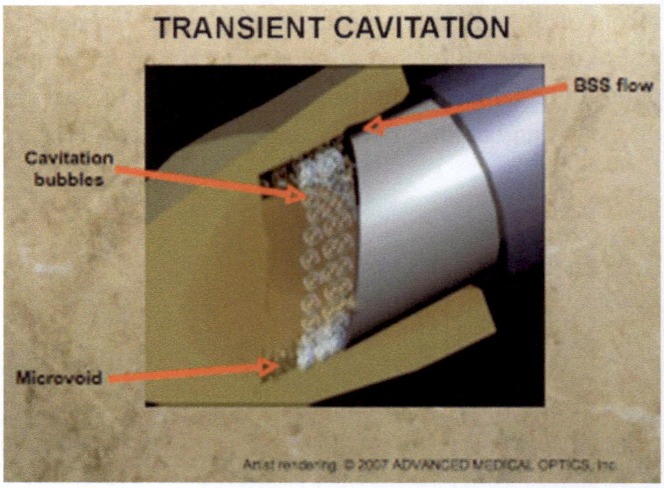

Fig. 3.1 The micro bubbles are visible at the phaco tip. The micro void around the phaco tip is replenished with fresh BSS providing fuel for transient cavitation

phaco needle governs the direction of the generation of shock wave and micro bubbles.

3.2.4 Sustained Cavitation

If phaco is energized beyond 4 ms, transient cavitation, with generation of micro bubbles and shock waves, ends. The bubbles then begin to vibrate, without implosion.

No shock wave is generated. Therefore, other than mechanical energy, no cavitation energy is produced. Sustained cavitation is ineffective for emulsification (Fig. 3.2a).

Water bath, hydrophonic studies indicate that transient cavitation is significantly more powerful than sustained cavitation (Fig. 3.2b). With this information in mind, it would appear that continuous phaco is best used to emulsify the intact nucleus, held in place by the capsular bag, during the sculpting phase of divide and conquer or stop and chop. In this setting, jackhammer energy is most important for emulsification.

Transient cavitation is maximized during micro pulse phaco. This is best used during phaco of the nuclear fragments in the later phase of the above two procedures, or during phaco chop procedures [1].

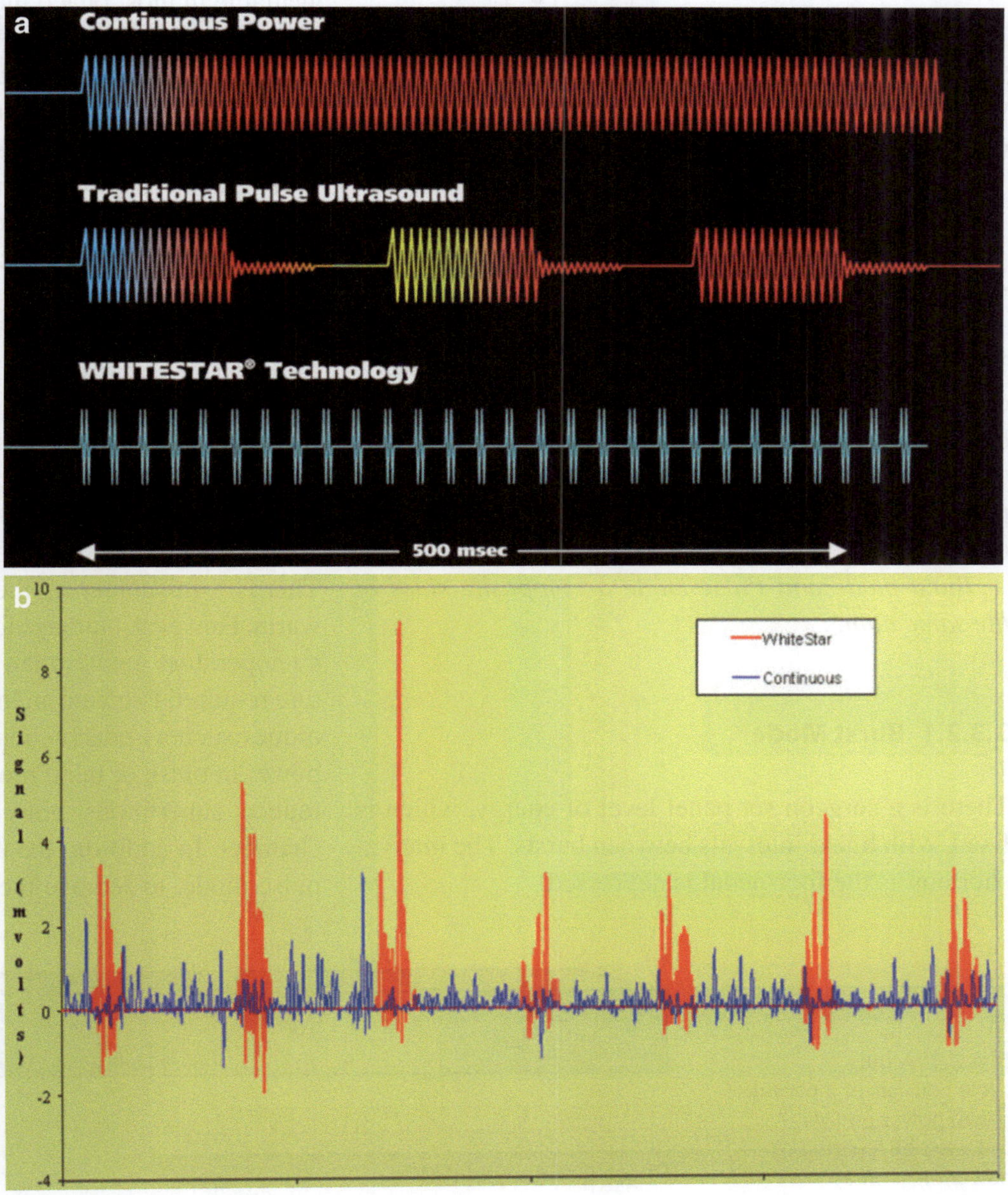

Fig. 3.2 (a) Transient cavitation energy is shown in blue, stabilized cavitational energy shown in *red*. Continuous power: Only the initial energy is transient. The remaining is stabilized energy. In a 50-ms pulse, only the initial 4 ms are transient. In micro pulse phaco, the entire pulse is transient energy. (b) The *x*-axis represents time and the *y*-axis millivolts. The *blue* tracing shows the low power (mv) created during continuous phaco. This is stabilized cavitation. The *red* tracing represents shorts bursts of high power (mv) generated during whitestar phaco. This is transient cavitation

3.3 Modification of Phaco Power

Application of the minimal amount of phaco power/energy necessary for adequate emulsification of the nucleus is desirable. Unnecessary power/energy is a cause of heat with subsequent wound trauma, endothelial cell trauma, trabecular meshwork trauma, and iris trauma with an alteration of the blood-aqueous barrier. Phaco power/energy can be modified by the alteration

1. In stroke length
2. Of duration
3. Of emission

3.3.1 Alteration of Stroke Length

Stroke length is determined by foot pedal adjustment. When set for linear phaco, depression of the foot pedal will increase stroke length and therefore power.

3.3.2 Alteration of Duration

The duration of the application of phaco power has a dramatic effect on overall power delivered. Usage of burst or pulse mode phaco will considerably decrease the overall power delivery. New machines allow for a period of power alternating with a period of aspiration only.

Burst mode and Pulse mode are opposite sides of the same coin.

3.3.2.1 Burst Mode

There is a surgeon set panel level of energy, which is fixed, with linear intervals between bursts. The interval shortens as the foot-pedal is depressed.

3.3.2.2 Pulse Mode

There is a fixed interval between pulses, but linear power, so that as the foot-pedal is depressed, the number (singular) of bursts remain the same but the power is increased.

Micro Pulse (Hyper-Pulse)

Through the development of highly responsive and low mass piezo crystals, combined with software modifications, the manufacturers of phaco machines have shortened the cycle of on and off time. This process, patented by AMO (Advanced Medical Optics) is called "micro pulse" or "Whitestar®." This technology is now available in most phaco machines.

A duty cycle is defined as the length of the time of power on combined with power off. (Fig. 3.3) Within the duty cycle, the duration of on and off time is variable depending on the phase of the procedure.

The short bursts of phaco energy followed by a short period without phaco energy allows two important events to occur. First, the period without phaco energy permits the nuclear material to be drawn toward the phaco tip to increase efficiency. Second, the absence of power allows inflow of the irrigating fluid into the micro cavity between the phaco tip and the nuclear fragment. This renewal of fluid is important to provide new fuel for transient cavitation as well as for the cooling of the phaco tip (Fig. 3.1).

The cool phaco tip has been termed "cold phaco." This is a misnomer as the phaco tip is not cold, but warm. However, studies indicate that it will not develop a temperature greater than 55°C which is the temperature required to create an incision burn [2, 3]. Phaco techniques such as phaco chop utilize minimal periods of power in pulse or burst mode, or micro pulse mode, to reduce superfluous power delivery to the anterior chamber. In addition, the use of pulse mode, or micro pulse mode, to remove the epinucleus provides for an

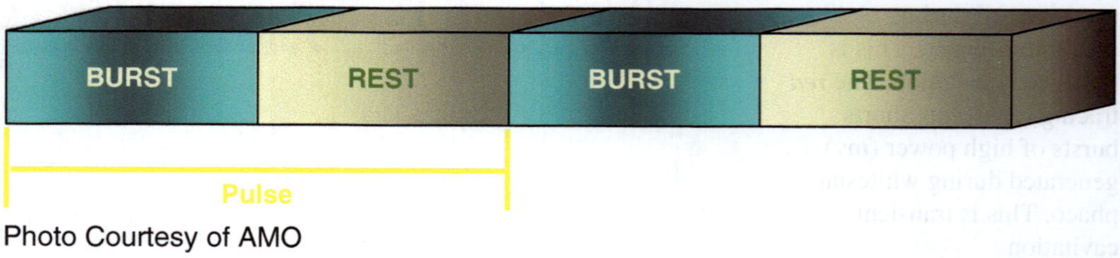

Fig. 3.3 A duty cycle consists of a period of phaco power on (*blue*) followed by a period of power off (*white*)

added margin of safety. When the epinucleus is emulsified, the posterior capsule is exposed to the phaco tip and may move toward it due to surge. Activation of pulse phaco, or micro pulse phaco, will create a deeper anterior chamber to work within. This occurs because, as noted previously, each period of phaco energy is followed by an interval of no energy. During the interval of the absence of energy, the epinucleus is drawn toward the phaco tip, producing partial occlusion, and interrupting outflow. This allows inflow to deepen the anterior chamber immediately prior to the onset of another pulse of phaco energy. The surgeon will recognize the outcome as operating in a deeper, more stable anterior chamber.

Pulse Shaping

This is a modification of varying power duration. By changing the morphology of the power burst in hyperpulse phaco, the power can be delivered with greater effectiveness. Different manufactures have developed different burst morphology.

AMO (Whitestar/Signature) use ICE (increased control and efficiency). A 1-ms punch of power with amplitude of 7% of the preset power maximum is delivered at the beginning of each burst (Fig. 3.4). This "kicker" has two consequences. First, it drives the nucleus away from the phaco tip sufficiently to augment partial occlusion phaco. Second, it allows the phaco tip to accelerate to the preset velocity almost instantly. The result is more effective phaco of the fragments.

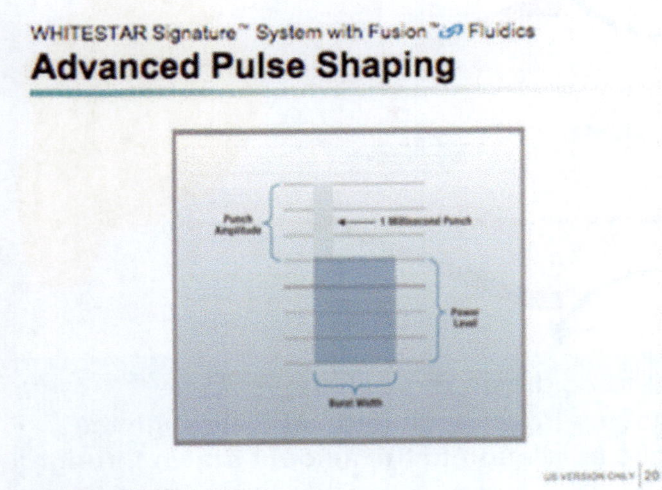

Fig. 3.4 AMO ICE. A 1-µs burst of power at the beginning of the power portion of the duty cycle

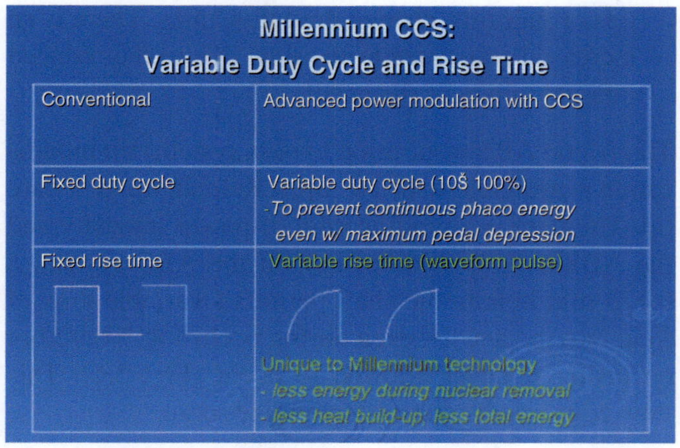

Fig. 3.5 B&L Millennium Pulse Shaping brings power up to preset slowly to decrease the repulsive effect of ultrasonic energy

B&L (Milennium/Stellaris) has taken a different approach. They bring the power up to maximum more slowly (Fig. 3.5). They believe that the slow increase in power enhances partial occlusion by not pushing the fragment away from the phaco tip.

3.3.3 Alteration of Emission

The emission of phaco energy is modified by tip selection. Phaco tips can be modified to accentuate: (1) power, (2) flow, or (3) a combination of both.

1. Power is modified by altering bevel tip angle. The bevel of the phaco tip will focus power in the direction of the bevel. The Kelman tip will produce broad powerful cavitation directed away from the bend in the shaft. This tip is excellent for the hardest of nuclei. New flare and cobra tips direct cavitation into the opening of the bevel of the tip. Additionally, at the point where the wider end of the tip narrows additional cavitational energy is created, thus further emulsifying the lens material as it passes into the shaft of the needle.
2. Power and flow are modified by utilizing a 0° tip. This tip will focus power directly ahead of the tip and enhance occlusion due to the smaller surface area of its orifice. Additionally it is easier to occlude the tip due to the ease of applanation of the tip to the lens material. Small diameter tips, such as 21 gauge

tips or flair tips, change fluid flow rates. There is an increased resistance to the flow due to the reduced internal lumen of the needle.

The Alcon ABS (aspiration bypass system) tip modification is available with a 0° tip, a Kelman tip, or a flare tip. The flare is a modification of power intensity and the ABS a flow modification. In the ABS system, a 0.175-mm hole in the shaft permits a variable flow of fluid into the needle, even during occlusion. Therefore occlusion is never allowed to occur (Fig. 3.6). This flow adjustment serves to minimize surge.

3. Flow can be modified by utilizing smaller diameter tips. These tips have a thin flexible outer sleeve to seal the phaco incision. Coaxial-micro incisional phaco makes use of these tips to accomplish a tight seal and permit a low-flow phaco without the danger of wound stretching and wound burns.

Phaco power energy emulsifies the lens nucleus. The phaco tip must operate in a cool environment and with adequate space to isolate its actions from delicate intraocular structures. This portion of action of the machine is dependent on its fluidics.

3.4 Fluidics

The fluidics of all machines depend upon a balance of fluid inflow and fluid outflow.

Inflow is determined by the bottle height above the eye of the patient, and irrigation tubing diameter. Potentially new improvements will certainly include pressurized infusion systems with anterior chamber pressure sensors in the form of a computer generated virtual anterior chamber to regulate the inflow volume contingent on the outflow volume. One type of pressurized infusion consists of an irrigation bag with two compartments. One compartment contains BSS. The other is pressurized by a pressure pump in the machine to compress the BSS and therefore increases inflow.

Outflow has two components.

1. Unregulated Fluid Outflow: This is determined by the sleeve-incision relationship, as well as the paracentesis size. The incision length selected should create a snug fit with the phaco tip selected. This will result in minimal uncontrolled incisional outflow with resultant increased anterior chamber

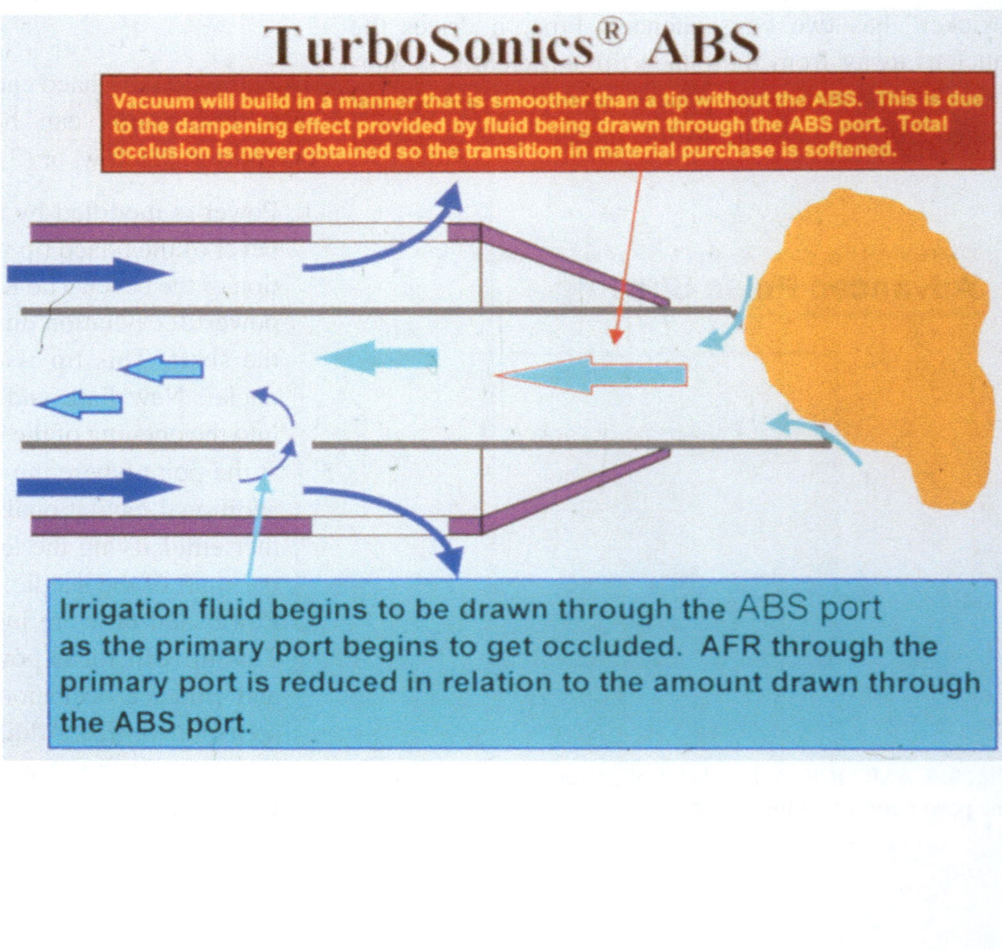

Fig. 3.6 A 0.175-mm hole drilled in the shaft of the ABS tip provides an alternate path for fluid to flow into the needle when there is an occlusion at the phaco tip

stability. The paracentesis should not be unnecessarily large, thereby leading to unnecessary fluid outflow.

2. Regulated Fluid Outflow: This is defined as the fluid, which passes through the phaco needle. The volume of the fluid exiting through the needle is restricted by the needle diameter, length, and configuration. If the diameter of the needle is smaller, less fluid can egress per unit time. Similarly, the tubing diameter and compliance act in an analogous manner. Tubing modifications such as "cruise control" (manufactured by Staar Surgical) can have a potent effect on fluid egress and preserve anterior chamber depth in the face of major potential episodes of surge.

Aspiration rate, (or flow), is defined as the flow of the fluid, measured in cc/min, through the tubing. With a peristaltic pump, it is determined by the speed of the pump. Flow determines how well particulate mater is attracted to the phaco tip. Aspiration level (or vacuum) is defined as the magnitude of negative pressure created in the tubing. It is measured in mmHg. Vacuum is the determinant of how well, once occluded on the phaco tip, particulate material will be held to the tip.

3.5 Vacuum Sources

There are three categories of vacuum sources or pumps. These are flow pumps, vacuum pumps, and hybrid pumps.

1. The primary example of the flow pump type is the peristaltic pump. These pumps allow for independent control of both aspiration rate (flow) and aspiration level (vacuum) (Fig. 3.7).
2. The primary example of the vacuum pump is the venturi pump. This pump type allows direct control of only vacuum level. Flow is dependent upon vacuum level setting. Examples of additional types are the rotary vane and the diaphragmatic pumps (Fig. 3.8).
3. The primary example of the hybrid pump is the AMO Signature peristaltic pump or the Bausch & Lomb Stellaris Peristaltic Pump. These pumps are interesting as they are able to act either like a vacuum or like a flow pump depending on programming.

They are generally controlled by digital inputs creating incredible flexibility and responsiveness.

The challenge to the surgeon is to balance the effect of phaco power intensity, which tends to push nuclear fragments away from the phaco tip, with the effect of

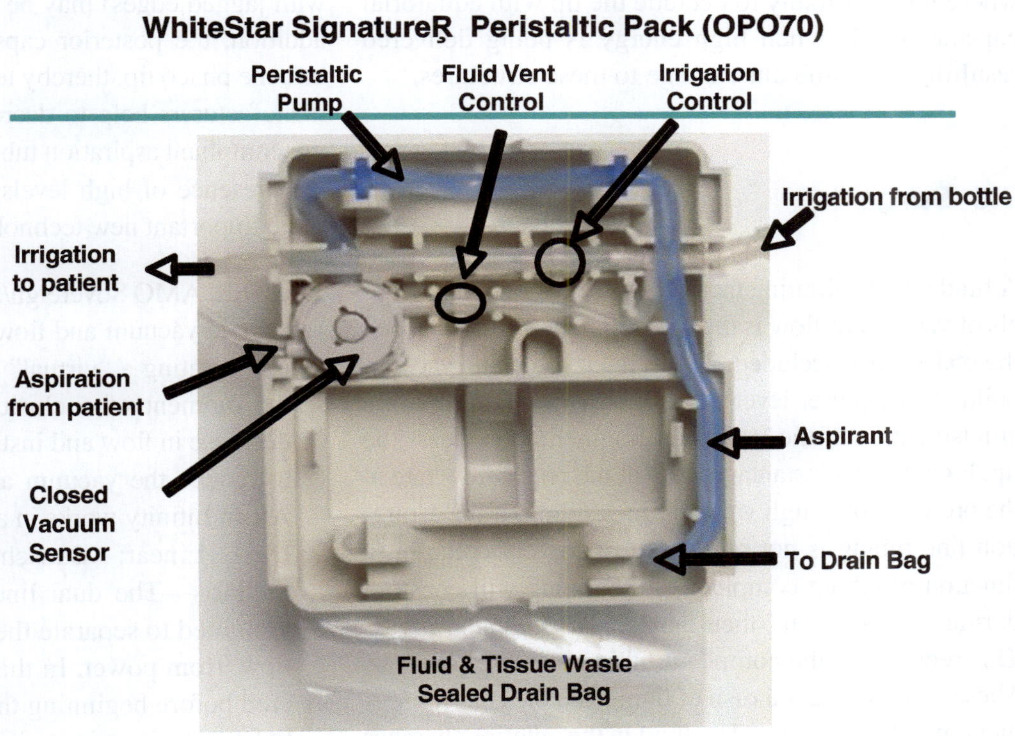

Fig. 3.7 Hybrid Pump. The AMO digital pump. A peristaltic pump with digital controls allows forward, backward, or to and fro movement to precisely control flow. This pump is capable of performing like a venturi or peristaltic pump

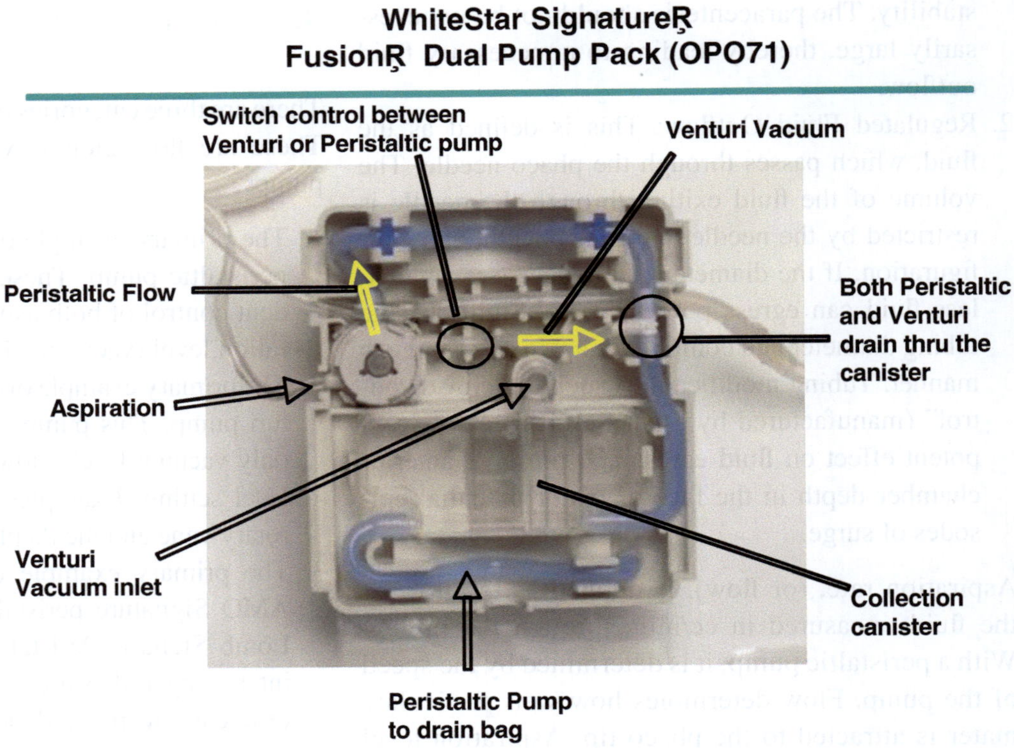

Fig. 3.8 Venturi pump AMO signature venturi pump showing flow based mechanics

flow, which attracts fragments toward the phaco tip, and vacuum, which holds the fragments on the phaco tip. Generally low flow slows down intraocular events, and high vacuum speeds them up. Low or zero vacuum is helpful during sculpting of hard or large nucleus, where it is less likely to occlude the tip with equatorial capsule or iris when high energy is being delivered resulting in significant damage to these structures.

3.6 Surge

A fundamental limiting factor in the selection of high levels of vacuum or flow is the development of surge. When the phaco tip is occluded, flow is interrupted and vacuum builds to its preset level (Fig. 3.9). Vacuum and partial emulsification of the occluding fragment then clears the tip. Flow begins instantaneously at the preset flow rate in the presence of a high vacuum. In addition, if the aspiration line tubing is not reinforced to prevent collapse (a function of tubing compliance) the tubing will constrict during occlusion and then expand on occlusion break. This rebound of the compliant tubing increases outflow. These factors trigger a rush of fluid from the anterior segment into the phaco tip. The fluid in the anterior chamber may not be replaced rapidly enough by infusion, to prevent shallowing of the anterior chamber. Therefore sudden volume reduction in the anterior segment is succeeded by the rapid anterior movement of the posterior capsule. This abrupt forceful stretching of the bag around the nuclear fragments (especially if the fragment is hard with jagged edges) may be a cause of capsular tears. In addition, the posterior capsule can be literally sucked into the phaco tip, thereby tearing it. The phaco machine manufacturers help to decrease the surge by providing noncompliant aspiration tubing. This will not constrict in the presence of high levels of vacuum. The following, more important new technologies are noteworthy:

1. CASE: AMO Sovereign/Signature—Microprocessors sample vacuum and flow parameters 50 times a second creating a "virtual" anterior chamber model. At the moment of occlusion the computer senses the decrease in flow and instantaneously slows the pump to reduce the vacuum and suppress the surge. The Alcon Infinity works in a similar manner (Fig. 3.10).
2. Dual Linear: Bausch & Lomb Millennium/Stellaris—The dual linear foot pedal can be programmed to separate the vacuum, and therefore the flow, from power. In this way, vacuum can be lowered before beginning the mobilization and the partial emulsification of an occluding fragment. Therefore the surge is minimized.

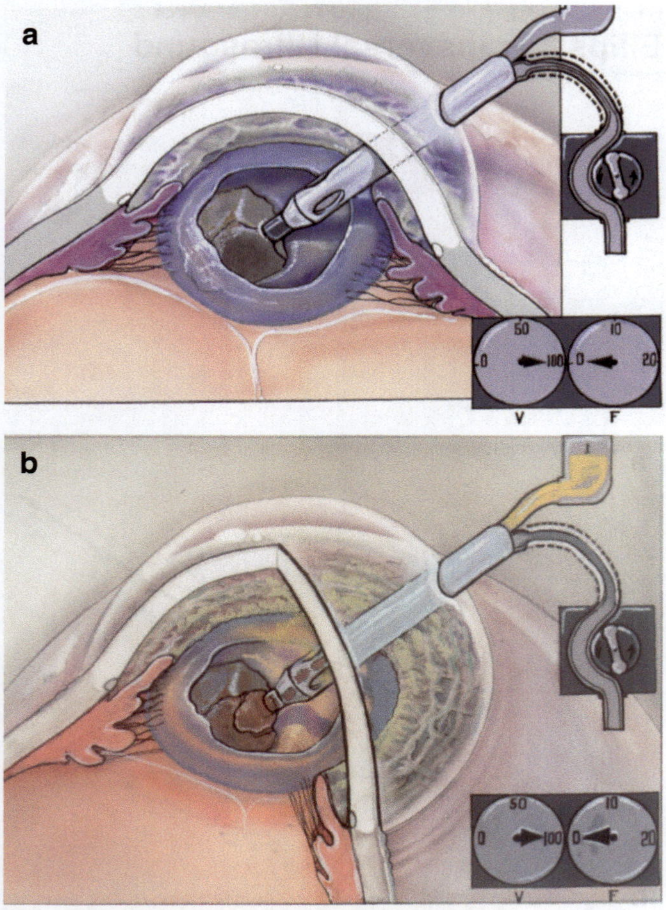

Fig. 3.9 (**a**) Occlusion: vacuum increases to pre set maximum, flow decreases toward zero, tubing collapses. (**b**) Occlusion break: vacuum drops to zero. Flow rapidly increases to preset. Tubing expands. Outflow exceeds inflow. Anterior chamber begins to shallow. Photo courtesy of Thieme Publishers, New York City

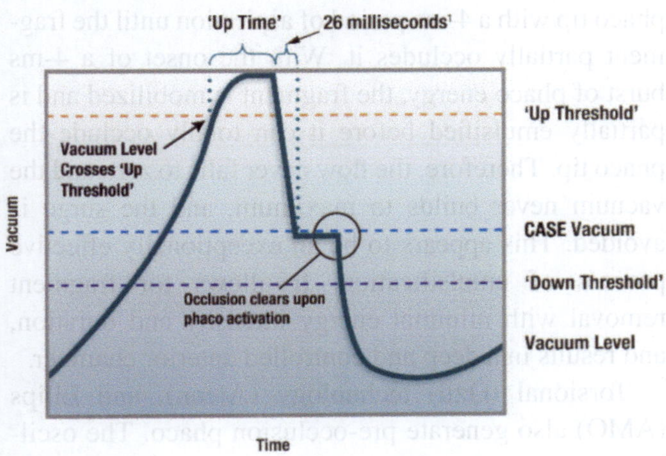

Fig. 3.10 If occlusion should occur CASE changes the pump speed and changes the commanded vacuum at a preset "up" level, "down" level or time

3. Aspiration Bypass System (ABS) Alcon Infiniti/Legacy—The Aspiration Bypass System (ABS) tips have 0.175 mm holes drilled in the shaft of the needle. During occlusion, the hole provides for a constant alternate fluid flow. This will cause dampening of the surge on occlusion break.

3.6.1 Non-Longitudinal Phaco: Modification of Fluid Control by Power Modulations

Three significant trend setting technologies have revolutionized the way the power is modulated. When employing these power modulations, the duration of the power application and the motion of needle movement affect the fluid flow and occlusion. These modulations have an effect on the fluidic balance during phaco which is as important to chamber maintenance and the ease of nuclear fragments removal, as that of the preset vacuum and flow.

1. Micro-Pulse Phaco

As discussed previously, the rapid 4-ms power on cycles maximizes the development of transient cavitational energy. All cavitational energy in the 4-ms burst is capable of emulsifying the tissue. The ensuing 4-ms period of aspiration replenishes the fluid at the phaco tip and cools it. The use of micro-pulse phaco is necessary to create the shift in phaco technique from post-occlusion phaco to partial occlusion phaco.

2. Torsional Phaco (Alcon Infiniti Ozil Handpiece)

Classic phaco has utilized a phaco tip that moves forward and backward, or longitudinally. Torsional phaco is defined as the 32-kHz oscillatory movement of an angled (Kelman) phaco tip which shears nuclear material at the phaco tip. This can be alternated with longitudinal movement of the needle at 44 kHz. The torsional component is linear and the longitudinal component can be micro pulse. The potential flexibility of this system is enormous (Fig. 3.11).

3. Elliptical Phaco (AMO Signature)

In this system the longitudinal movement of the phaco tip at 38 kHz is combined with a transversal motion at 26 kHz. The resultant movement of the needle can be

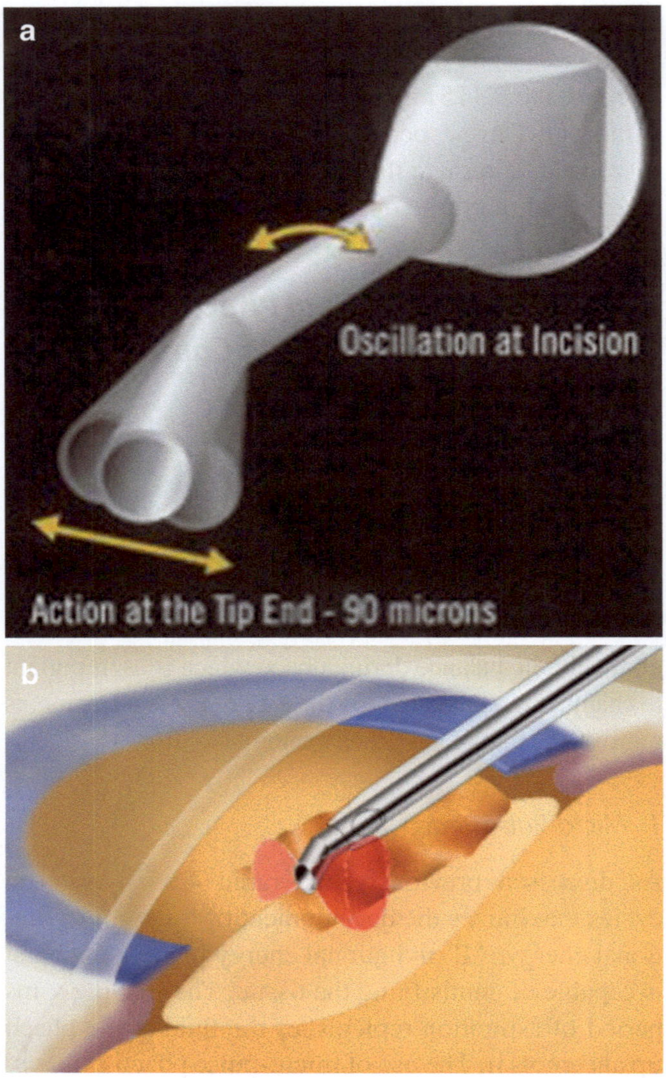

Fig. 3.11 (**a**) Alcon Infinity. Ozil Torsional Handpiece 32 kHz. Oscillatory Movement 44 kHz. Linear Movement. Torsional and longitudinal combined in different ratios. (**b**) Torsional energy spreads laterally like a bow tie shaving the nucleus. Photo courtesy of William J. Fishkind, MD

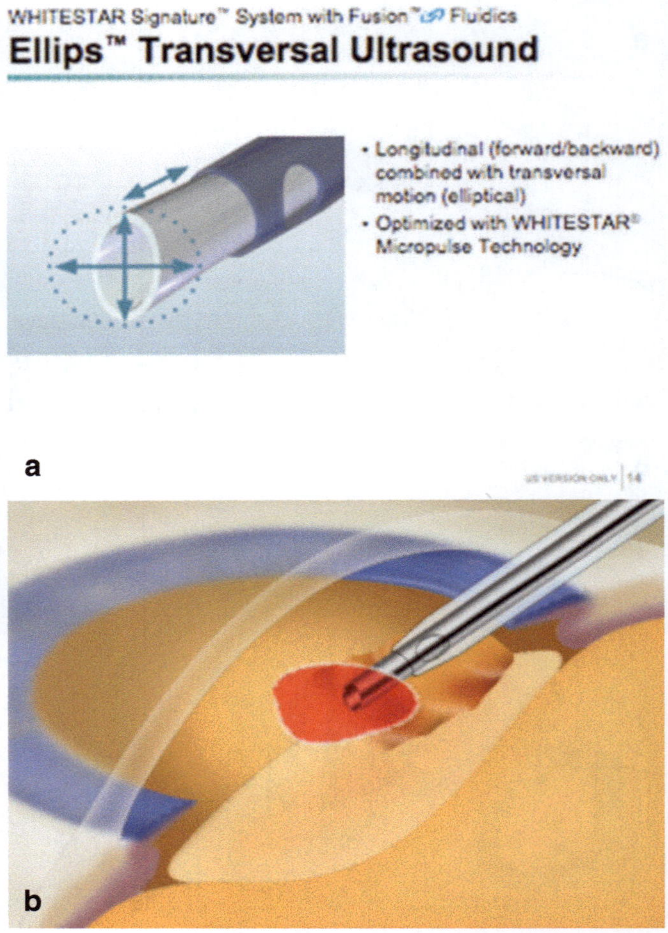

Fig. 3.12 (**a**) AMO elliptical. Phaco tip moves longitudinally, and in a prolate spheroidal manner to shave the nucleus. (**b**) AMO elliptical creates energy in the shape of a prolate spheroid shaving the nuclear material. Photo courtesy of William J. Fishkind, MD

described as prolate-spheroid. (Shaped much like an egg cut in half) (Fig. 3.12).

While the longitudinal phaco cores the nuclear material, the non-longitudinal phaco shaves the nuclear material (Figs. 3.11 and 3.12) This mode of needle movement is a noteworthy variation from other technology, since by its very movement, it generates partial occlusion phaco and therefore lessens the risk of surge.

3.6.2 Partial-Occlusion Phacoemulsification

The way to avoid surge is to prevent total occlusion entirely. By definition, a surge requires total occlusion. In partial-occlusion phaco, micro pulse phaco is the catalyst. The nuclear fragment is brought close to the phaco tip with a 4-ms period of aspiration until the fragment partially occludes it. With the onset of a 4-ms burst of phaco energy, the fragment is mobilized and is partially emulsified before it can totally occlude the phaco tip. Therefore, the flow never falls to zero and the vacuum never builds to maximum, and the surge is avoided. This appears to be an exceptionally effective process of emulsification. It allows for fragment removal with minimal energy intensity and duration, and results in a deep and controlled anterior chamber.

Torsional (Ozil) technology (Alcon), and Ellips (AMO) also generate pre-occlusion phaco. The oscillatory movements of the phaco tip automatically knock the fragments off the phaco tip. Unlike longitudinal phaco where the removal of the tissue is described as coring, the removal with non-longitudinal phaco is described as shaving. Since the oscillatory movement holds the lens material close to the phaco tip without total occlusion, the partial occlusion environment of this system generates remarkable follow-ability and deep, stable, anterior chambers.

3.7 Phacoemulsification Technique and Machine Technology

The patient will have the best visual result when the total phaco energy which is delivered to the anterior segment is minimized [4]. Additionally, phaco energy should be focused onto the nucleus. This will prevent damage to iris blood vessels, trabecular meshwork, and endothelium. Finally, proficient emulsification will lead to shorter overall surgical time. Therefore a lesser amount of irrigation fluid will pass through the anterior segment. The general principles of power management are, to focus phaco energy into the nucleus, vary fluid parameters for efficient sculpting and fragment removal, and minimize surge.

Generally all phaco procedures have two phases. The first is the creation of fragments. This requires sculpting or chopping. The second phase is the removal of the fragments in a controlled approach. Occlusion is mandatory to move the fragments to the iris plane. Fragment removal is assisted by partial occlusion phaco.

All phaco techniques are preceded by capsulorhexis, cortical cleaving hydrodissection, and the removal of the superior cortex and the epinucleus to expose the endonucleus.

3.7.1 Micro-incisional Phaco

The development of micro-pulse and non-longitudinal phaco ("cold phaco") has led to the performance of phaco through increasingly small incisions with tighter irrigation sleeves or no irrigation sleeves.

3.7.2 Bimanual Micro-Incisional Phaco

Two incisions are created 90° apart. Their size is dependant on the instrumentation. Instruments require 1.4–1.1 mm incisions. There is no irrigating sleeve on the phaco tip. The instrumentation for this procedure is important and the relationship between the instrument and incision size is essential. If the wound is too tight, it is difficult to manipulate the instruments. If the wound is too large, excessive outflow leads to chamber shallowing with an unstable anterior segment. In bimanual MICS the instruments can be moved only forward and backward through the incisions without creating corneal distortion. If the instruments are angled in the incision, sufficient corneal distortion occurs and the procedure becomes appreciably more difficult. The problem can be prevented by the construction of trapezoidal incisions where the needle has room to move at the external incision. The irrigating chopper should be parallel to the iris and above it. The inflow current thus created, tends to wash the fragments toward the unsleeved phaco tip. The small incisions cause less disruption of the blood aqueous barrier, and are more stable and secure.Then a new incision is created for IOL implantation. In the future, with the insertion of an intraocular lens (IOL) through the 1.4 mm incision, there should be less disruption of ocular integrity, immediate return to full activities, and less risk of postoperative wound complications (Fig. 3.13).

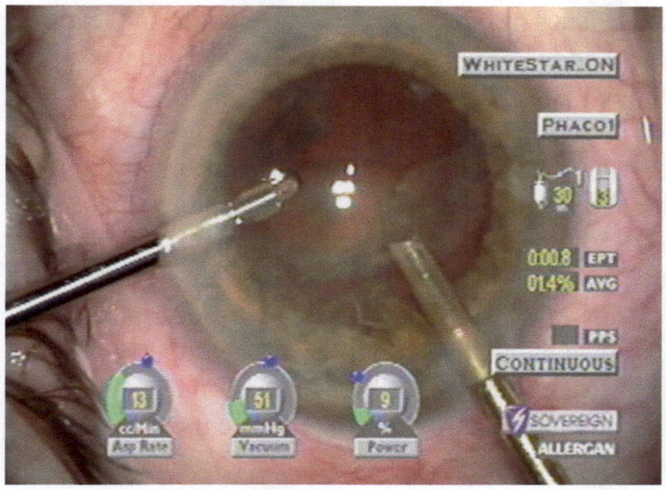

Fig. 3.13 Bimanual Phaco. Irrigating chopper on right. Unsleeved phaco tip on left

3.7.3 Micro-Incisional Coaxial Phaco

A thin walled flared, 21-gauge phaco tip and thinner irrigation sleeve is available for both the Infiniti (Alcon) and Stellaris (Bosch and Lomb) machines, which permits phaco though a 2.2-mm incision with Infiniti and 1.8 mm. with Stellaris. Despite the smaller incision, inflow is adequate to maintain a deep anterior chamber. The procedure has no significant learning curve and therefore is no more difficult than when performed through a 2.8-mm incision.

Both the companies also manufacture a one-piece acrylic IOL and injector, which is capable of implanting the IOL through the 2.2 mm unenlarged incision.

B&L now has a new Akrios hydrophilic acrylic IOL that can be implanted through a 1.8-mm incision.

Sub 2 mm incision phaco is a reality, but not an accepted alternative, at present. When IOLs are available to be introduced through these micro-incisions, the surgical community will embrace the procedure.

3.7.3.1 Irrigation and Aspiration

Similar to phaco, the anterior chamber stability during irrigation and aspiration (I/A) is due to an equilibrium of inflow and outflow. Wound outflow can be minimized by employing a soft sleeve around the I/A tip. Combined with a small incision (2.8–3 mm), a deep and stable anterior chamber will result. Generally, a 0.3-mm I/A tip is used. With this orifice, a vacuum of 500 mmHg and a flow of 20 mL/min is excellent to tease out the cortex from the capsular fornices.

Linear vacuum allows the cortex to be grasped under the anterior capsule with low vacuum and be drawn into the center of the pupil at the iris plane. There, in the safety of a deep anterior chamber, vacuum can be increased and the cortex aspirated.

Bimanual I&A is also a viable procedure. A 21-gauge irrigating cannula provides inflow through one paracentesis while an unsleeved 21-gauge aspiration cannula is used through the opposite paracentesis. The instruments can be easily switched making the removal of the stubborn cortex considerably easier.

3.8 Conclusion

The phaco process is a balance of technology and technique. Awareness of the principles that influence phaco machine settings is a prerequisite for the performance of a proficient and safe operation. Additionally, often during the procedure, there is a demand for modification of the initial parameters. A thorough understanding of the fundamental principles will enhance the capability of the surgeon for an appropriate response to this requirement. It is through this crucial attitude of relentless evaluation of the interaction of the machine and the phaco procedure, that a skillful surgeon will find innovative methods to enhance the technique.

Take Home Pearls

- The capability of the current phaco machines to take advantage of hyper-pulse phaco and non-longitudinal phaco energy, and the enhanced fluid management of pumps and software, has revolutionized the way, phacoemulsification is performed.
- In the past, phaco demanded the occlusion of the tip with inevitable post-occlusion surge.
- Presently the method is partial occlusion, and hence related to this change, the fluid equilibrium in the anterior chamber is significantly different than in the past. With partial occlusion phaco the anterior chamber is notably more stable with negligible surge.
- Software management of energy application and fluidics has superbly augmented the surgeons' command of the stability of the anterior chamber.
- There is, therefore, less risk of torn posterior capsules during surgery and less risk of vitrectomy. This leads to improved outcomes as determined by the rapidity of the return of vision, as well as decreased corneal edema and endothelial cell loss.
- Creative technology in phaco machine design is an enormous enhancement over previous technologies.

Reference

1. Packer M, Fishkind W, Fine IH, Seibel B, Hoffman R (2005) The physics of phaco: a review. J Cataract Refract Surg 31:424–431
2. Donnenfeld ED, Olson RJ, Solomon R, Finger PT, Biser SA, Perry HD, Doshi S (2003) Efficacy and wound-temperature gradient of WhiteStar phacoemulsification through a 1.2 mm incision. J Cataract Refract Surg 29(6):1097–1100

3. Soscia W, Howard JG, Olson RJ (2002) Microphacoemulsification with WhiteStar: a wound-temperature study. J Cataract Refract Surg 28(6):1044–1046
4. Fine IH, Packer M, Hoffman RS Power modulations in new phacoemulsification technology: improved outcomes (2004) J Cataract Refract Surg 30(5):1014–1019

Further Reading

1. Buratto L, Osher RH, Masket S, eds. Cataract Surgery in Complicated Cases. Thorofare, NJ: SLACK Incorporated; 2001.
2. Fishkind WJ, ed. Complications in Phacoemulsification: Recognition, Avoidance, and Management. New York: Thieme Publishers; 2001.
3. Fishkind WJ. Pop Goes the Microbubbles. ESCRS Film Festival Grand Prize Winner, 1998.
4. Fishkind WJ, Neuhann TF, Steinert RF. The Phaco Machine in Cataract Surgery Technique: Complications & Management. 2nd Ed. Philadelphia: W.B. Saunders and Co; 2004.
5. Seibel BS. Phacodynamics: Mastering the Tools and Techniques of Phacoemulsification Surgery. 4th edition Thorofare, NJ: SLACK Incorporated; 2005.
6. "From phaco-cutting to true phacoemulsification." Miyoshi, T. Video competition grand prize winner ASCRS, ESCRS 2007.

4 Coaxial Microincision Cataract Surgery Utilizing Non-Linear Ultrasonic Power: An Alternative to Bimanual Microincision Cataract Surgery

Stephen S. Lane

Core Messages

- Torsional phacoemulsification is a more efficient use of ultrasound than longitudinal phacoemulsification
- Followability of nuclear material is improved with torsional ultrasound
- Torsional phacoemulsification combined with less compliant tubing allows surgeons to use more conservative fluidic settings, lessening the potential for complications
- Torsional phacoemulsification allows for microincisonal surgery (2.3–2.4 mm) through which currently available IOLs can be placed
- Microincisions of 2.2 mm produce negligible surgically induced astigmatism

4.1 Introduction

Charles Kelman's revelation in the dentist chair, leading to the invention of ultrasonic phacoemulsification in 1967, began the relentless march toward ever-smaller incision sizes to be utilized in cataract surgery. The original procedure by Dr. Kelman used a four-pound ultrasound hand piece in a surgical procedure that took 4 h (including 41 min of ultrasound time) and resulted in endophthalmitis and eventual phthisis. It is a testament to the perseverance and ingenuity of many phacoemulsification pioneers that the procedure has evolved to its current state where a cataract can be removed in minutes, and it is one of the safest and most successful surgical methods ever developed.

Each development in phacoemulsification surgery has set the stage for the next. *Kaizen*, a Japanese word meaning gradual, orderly, continuous improvement, exemplifies the persistent ongoing development of both phacoemulsification technology and techniques. In the early days of phacoemulsification, the smaller incision size drove intraocular lens (IOL) technology to develop foldable lenses that would fit through these smaller incisions (usually about 3 mm). As IOL technology evolved, lenses and injector systems were introduced that allowed lens implantation to be performed through smaller incisions, driving phacoemulsification instrumentation technology to allow cataract removal through even smaller incisions. With these current advances, we have come full circle. The advent of a new generation of IOLs and injectors, in combination with increasing patient expectations for excellent uncorrected acuity, the desire to better control the unpredictability of surgically induced astigmatism and the minimization of incision size to prevent incision wound incompetence, allows us now to perform phacoemulsification through incisions that are smaller than most modern IOLs can go through. The challenge, once again, has been to find an IOL that can be placed thru an ultra-small opening (sub-2.0 mm), but importantly not to compromise on the attributes of current IOLs or on the phacoemulsification procedure itself, which is so successfully performed worldwide.

Biaxial microincisional cataract surgery (MICS) performed through two sub-2 mm incisions, using the

S. S. Lane
University of Minnesota, 2950 Curve Crest Boulevard, Stillwater, MN 55082, USA;
e-mail: sslane@associatedeyecare.com

J. L. Alió, I. H. Fine (eds.), *Minimizing Incisions and Maximizing Outcomes in Cataract Surgery*,
DOI: 10.1007/978-3-642-02862-5_4, © Springer-Verlag Berlin Heidelberg 2010

irrigation instrument through one site and an unsleeved phaco tip through the other, became possible several years ago when advances in phacoemulsification power modulation technology helped solve most of the problems associated with heat generation at the incision. While biaxial MICS has many proponents who expound upon its multiple advantages, the procedure has not been widely embraced as other surgeons perceive various drawbacks. These include: a difference in fluidics, a new learning curve, wound damage/distortion, and the logic of performing cataract surgery through a sub-2 mm incision without the availability of a microincision IOL, which would be able to provide high-quality and stable vision with a low risk of posterior capsule opacification (PCO).

Microcoaxial phacoemulsification (2.2 mm incision or smaller) presents the unique characteristics of preserving many of the advantages of coaxial small incision surgery and biaxial MICS, while offering significant advantages over both.

4.2 The Fluidics of Coaxial Microincisional Phacoemulsification

Traditional longitudinal ultrasound requires surgeons to use relatively high aspiration flow and vacuum settings to overcome the repulsive effect of the phaco tip's forward strokes. With coaxial microincisional phaco, fluidic settings need to be decreased to compensate for the reduced irrigation inflow. This decrease in irrigation flow has to be compensated by a similar decrease of aspiration flow and vacuum limit or by raising irrigation bottle height. Therefore, with coaxial microsurgery, there is roughly a 30% decrease of irrigation flow if surgeons switch from a 2.6–2.8 mm incision to a 2.2–2.4 mm incision if the bottle height is not adjusted. If longitudinal ultrasound is utilized with lower settings, efficiency and safety of the procedure might be compromised. High bottle heights can lead to increased fluidic turbulence that can prove problematic during the procedure and jeopardize optimal postoperative results.

A significant decrease of aspiration flow results in a significant decrease of the process of nuclear pieces being attracted to the phacoemulsification tip since the speed of the fluid stream (aspiration flow) determines how fast the nuclear fragment is transported to the phaco

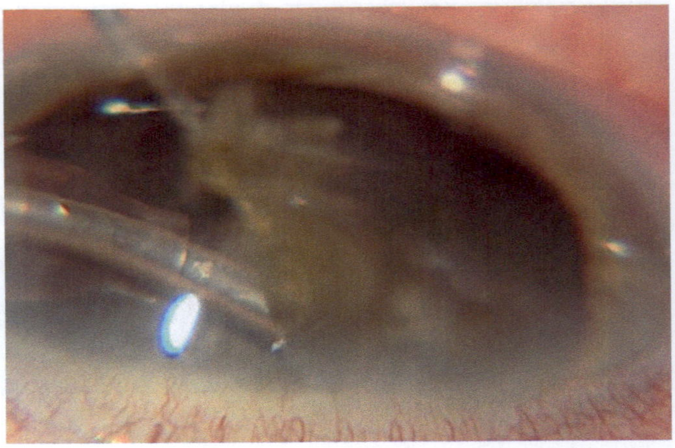

Fig. 4.1 Intraoperative photograph of longitudianl phacoemulsification illustrating repulsion of a nuclear fragment seen just above the phaco tip

tip opening [1]. This is particularly important when one realizes that traditional longitudinal ultrasound does not only emulsify the nuclear material by the forward stroke of the phaco tip, but also repels the nucleus at the same time. This paradox is, in fact, the greatest drawback of longitudinal ultrasound. Longitudinal ultrasound depends on high attractive forces-high aspiration flow and high vacuum to compensate for its intrinsic repulsive forces (Fig. 4.1).

Operating under conditions of high vacuum settings has the potential of increasing the possibility of surgical complications. When occlusion of the phaco tip is broken with a high vacuum by the emulsification of lens material on or in the phaco tip, the immediate return of the peristaltic pump tubing to its original dimension after being contracted by a high vacuum results in a sudden outflow of fluid from the fluid paths and, potentially, the anterior chamber. This could lead to a sudden shallowing of the anterior chamber, contact of the phaco needle with the capsule or other anterior segment structures, and potentially rupture the posterior capsule. This phenomenon is called surge and its severity is determined by the height of the vacuum and the compliance of the tubing. The more compliant (softer, more pliable) the tubing, the more contraction occurs and the worse the surge flow is. The new Intrepid FMS system (Alcon, Fort Worth, TX) increases the rigidity of the aspiration tubing, which reduces the occlusion break surge response significantly. This reduction in tubing contracture improves anterior chamber stability, decreasing the need to adjust flow and vacuum settings or raising bottle heights to very high levels.

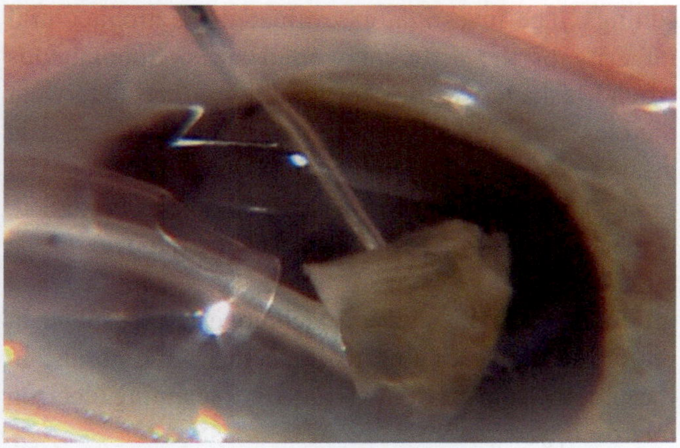

Fig. 4.2 Intraopertive photograph of microincision torsional phacoemulsification illustrating attraction of a nuclear fragment to the tip during the emulsification process

The introduction of torsional ultrasound with its side-to-side ultrasonic sheering motion of the phaco tip has led to a paradigm shift in fluidics management during micro-coaxial surgery. High vacuum is no longer necessary to obtain efficient and effective emulsification as there is no repulsion that the system needs to overcome (Fig. 4.2). This allows surgeons a broader range in vacuum limits and bottle heights than is offered with modulated, longitudinal ultrasound.

Another advantage to lower fluidic settings is that, dispersive viscoelastic is not aspirated and may further protect the delicate intraocular structures during complicated cases. Compared to biaxial MICS, a microcoaxial approach avoids problems with intraoperative fluid leakage and does not require special instrumentation or modifications to the surgical technique that create a learning curve for biaxial MICS. In surgical challenges such as weak zonules, a posterior capsular rupture, or floppy iris syndrome, torsional ultrasound allows us to adjust the fluidics parameters to maintain low pressure fluctuations and reduced turbulence.

Dr. Kerry Solomon [2] developed a model to help determine how the phacoemulsification tip mechanics and intraocular fluidics flow contribute to the improved attractability and followability of nuclear material when using torsional phacoemulsification. The method he developed was based on analysis of the intraoperative dynamics of microcarrier beads suspended in the balanced salt solution (BSS) irrigating fluid. The beads were constructed of a cross-linked polystyrene material that have a collagen surface coating and are very small. They range in diameter from 125 to 212μm and have a surface area of 390 cm^2/g, and a specific gravity of 1.02, which allows them to remain suspended in BSS. In their study, 30 fresh porcine eyes and 16 fresh human globes from bilateral donors (that were not suitable for transplantation) were utilized.

They took the same amount of beads by weight (50 mg) and the same amount of BSS (1.5 mL) and injected them into each eye via the irrigation tubing. The same person performed injections at a steady rate in a standardized way for each eye. After this, phacoemulsification was carried out on each eye using a standardized procedure. A 2.6 mm incision, a vacuum rate with a limit of 350 mg Hg, a bottle height of 90 cm, and the same aspiration flow rate (AFR) of 35 mL/min was used for each case. Ultrasound power was varied so that they could study fluidics through the entire range of power modulation: 100, 50, and 25% to evaluate clearance time of the collagen beads through the anterior chamber. High speed photography was used to evaluate the difference in fluid patterns by computer tracing of ten random beads within the solution. The flow pattern was tracked within the anterior chamber between torsional and pulse traditional ultrasound. Each evaluation was videotaped in real time from the surgeon's view and from a side view and also with a high-speed camera that captures 300 frames/s. The high-speed camera was used to demonstrate different fluidic patterns of bead flow in the periphery and at the central needle tip with and without lens material.

The investigators looked at how long the beads took to clear the system, first using ultrasonic phaco and then using torsional phaco at 25% power, 50% power, and then 100% power. They found that there was a 50% quicker removal of the beads with the torsional vs. conventional ultrasound across the entire range of power modulations.

The high-speed camera footage and bead tracking showed that, with traditional longitudinal phaco, beads were attracted to the tip and then repelled by the pulsing of traditional ultrasound. The beads would then continue to be repelled and travel away from the tip before finally being attracted and cleared from the anterior chamber.

Evaluation of high-speed footage of the torsional fluidics showed little to no repulsion of the beads. Once the beads got in the path of the phaco tip, the beads that were tracked were aspirated into the tip. Analyzing the movement of the beads with nuclear material demonstrated that, once occlusion was broken, the fluidics helped drive the beads in the chamber to the tip as the lens material was absorbed.

Although this cadaver eye model is a preliminary study looking at fluidics, the investigators clearly demonstrated improved fluidics and followability with torsional ultrasound compared to conventional longitudinal ultrasound.

4.3 Incision Size

As ophthalmic surgeons, we know that smaller corneal incisions induce less astigmatism and can self-seal more easily than their larger counterparts. Therefore, in theory, we would be reducing the risk of wound leakage and endophthalmitis [3].

But if the incision size is too small, the surgeon's ability to manipulate instruments can be hindered and the potential benefits are offset. Additionally, the smallest of incisions (1.1–1.2 mm) can limit the movement of instruments and necessitate the use of unsleeved instruments, thereby increasing mechanical and thermal trauma to the wound.

To address the weaknesses of biaxial micro incisions used in bimanual phacoemulsification, some surgeons are suturing their micro incisions while others are making a third incision for IOL insertion. Both of these options offset any advantages of biaxial micro incision surgery. A more ideal system allows surgeons to perform phacoemulsification through micro incisions that will capitalize on the benefits of smaller incision sizes without increasing the downside.

Typical phacoemulsification, as previously described, operates with a longitudinal jackhammer-type motion in conventional ultrasound mode. With torsional ultrasound, the handpiece amplifies the side-to-side oscillatory motion to the phaco tip, which helps minimize the stress to the incision. As a result, the side-to-side shearing motion allows for more efficient emulsification of lens material, greatly reduces repulsion and increases followability. Laboratory and clinical studies have validated these theories.

In one ex vivo study [4], 15 human cadaver eyes were divided into three groups: group one received 2.8 mm coaxial incisions, group two received 2.2 mm coaxial incisions, and group three received 1.2 mm biaxial incisions. All eyes underwent simulated phacoemulsification using longitudinal ultrasound with standard settings. The investigators evaluated the architectural integrity of the different wound sizes. Spontaneous wound leakage was present in all eyes that underwent the biaxial technique, in one eye in the 2.8 mm coaxial group and in none of the eyes in the 2.2 mm coaxial group. Histopathologic examination of the eyes studied, revealed India Ink penetration in all of the eyes in the bimanual group and no eyes in the 2.2 mm coaxial group. The biaxial incision technique also resulted in more qualitative trauma to Descemet's membrane in the endothelium, as demonstrated by scanning electron microscopy.

In addition to improved wound integrity, Sam Masket showed that coaxial micro phacoemulsification performed through a 2.2 mm incision resulted in significantly less induced astigmatism than conventional coaxial phacoemulsification through a 3.0 mm incision.

In the study, all surgeries were performed through a temporally oriented, grooved, clear corneal tunnel incision, using a phaco chop technique and a 1.1 mm flared tip (Alcon Laboratories). This prospective investigation was designed as an intra-patient comparison and included 16 subjects. Astigmatism was measured preoperatively and after 6 weeks with autokeratometry in a masked fashion by a technician. The mean induced astigmatism was 0.10 diopters for the 2.2 mm incision group, which was significantly less then the 0.32 diopters of change in the 3 mm incision group [5].

While the 2.2 mm incision size is smaller than the traditional 3.0–3.2 incision size, there is essentially no learning curve for the surgeon transitioning to this unique instrumentation. Because of the coaxial nature of the procedure, this instrumentation affords stable anterior chambers intraoperatively and excellent postoperative results. A phacoemulsification surgeon can easily transition to this new technique because it is performed with almost identical surgical parameters as for standard coaxial surgery and is amiable to any approach to lens removal, be it chop, divide and conquer, or combinations thereof. 2.2–2.4 mm steel and diamond blades are readily available and enlargement of these wounds is unnecessary with the introduction of new cartridges to inject the thinner aspheric profile IOLs that are commonly used today. The incision size is readily amiable to either a standard capsulorrhexis forceps or a needle and requires no specific instrumentation.

An important advantage of the micro-coaxial technique is that, it affords the thermal protection benefit of having a sleeve over the phaco tip. This feature is especially relevant when operating on more dense cataracts where thermal injury can be a significant concern. While results of multiple studies demonstrate that the presence of a sleeve over the phaco tip helps to protect against thermal injury, use of torsional ultrasound provides an added benefit. A study presented by Richard Mackool showed that the use of torsional ultrasound was associated with a decrease in temperature rise of about 60% compared with longitudinal ultrasound [6].

In summary. the use of 2.2–2.4 mm microincisions creates a stable, hermetically sealed environment, that reduces the likelihood of microbial contamination, thereby reducing the chance of a postoperative infection. This is in keeping with the teachings of Paul Ernest et al. [3], who proved more than a decade ago that square surface incision architecture is more resistant to deformation than other types of incisions. Additionally, incisions limited to this size are astigmatically neutral, which is a critical feature as we try to optimize our postoperative refractive results.

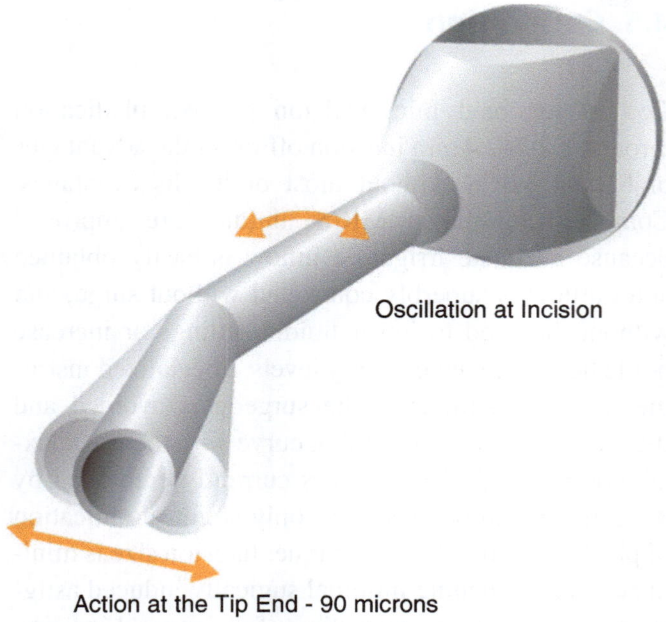

Fig. 4.3 Ultrasonic oscillations within the wound are translated to a side-to-side cutting action at the torsional tip. This minimizes thermal energy at the proximal portion of the phaco needle (at the incision site) while maintaining an efficient cutting action at the tip (Courtesy of Alcon Labs)

4.4 Torsional Ultrasound

For years, surgeons have looked for various methods to reduce the ultrasonic energy used during phacoemulsification. We have learned that ultrasonic energy correlates with corneal endothelial cell density loss, so using less energy would therefore be safer. Previously, this has been achieved using power modulation with pulse and burst ultrasound.

Torsional phacoemulsification using angled phacoemulsification needles is the latest technological advance, combining stable fluidics with a limited irrigation inflow while maintaining a secure wound construction that allows IOL insertion through a 2.2 mm incision. Oscillatory torsional amplitude creates a lateral tip movement that shears lens material and has proven cutting efficiency while at the same time reducing the amount and amplitude of the thermal energy needed (Fig. 4.3). The interesting characteristic about torsional ultrasound is what is taking place at the actual phaco tip. The oscillation at the hub, occur with the frequency of 32,000 cycles per second. With a standard Kelman style tip (approximately 20°) this translates into an actually horizontal excursion as opposed to a longitudinal excursion. The maximum horizontal excursion is 3.5 mills or 90 μm, which is almost exactly the maximum excursion with longitudinal phaco.

Compared to traditional phacoemulsification, torsional ultrasound cuts more efficiently. In torsional phaco there is a shearing effect as the tip moves to the right and to the left. In other words, 100% of the cycle is devoted to the emulsification process. In contrast, traditional ultrasonic phacoemulsification delivers less than 50% effective longitudinal energy as half the energy is lost on the back stroke. In addition, there is less heat and, hence, less thermal damage to the wound. In essence, there is less energy delivered into the eye which allows surgeons to effectively use smaller incisions, whose architecture remains unchanged throughout the procedure giving pristine incisions. This, in turn, means almost no surgically induced astigmatism and rapid healing.

Finally, angulation of the tip greatly aids in visualizing the dynamics occuring between the tip and the lens material at the distal end of the needle. The reason for this is that, unlike longitudinal phaco where movement is forward/backward, in torsional phaco the movement is from side to side, hence resulting in better visualization. This is of particular importance in difficult cases with small pupils or floppy irides.

4.5 Conclusion

Coaxial torsional microincision phacoemulsification through a 2.2–2.4 mm incision offers all the advantages of biaxial MICS without most of its disadvantages. Compared to biaxial MICS, fluidics are improved because adequate irrigation inflow is easily obtained and outflow is superbly controlled without surge, and without the need to lower fluidic settings or increase bottle heights to unnecessary levels. Specialized instrumentation unfamiliar to the surgeon is avoided and there is essentially no learning curve with the use coaxial MICS. Surgical techniques currently employed by the surgeon can be used with only slight modification of phacoemulsification technique. Incision size is minimized accomplishing minimal sugically induced astigmatism, maximizing protection of the corneal incision site and attaining a watertight, hermetically sealed wound to guard against endophthalmitis. Additionally current IOLs can be placed with an injector through the unenlarged 2.2 mm incision. Finally, torsional ultrasound improves cutting efficiency, minimizes the amount of energy delivered to the eye, thereby greatly reducing the chance of incisional wound burn. The synergism of torsional ultrasound when combined with the advanced fluidic system described represents a new chapter in the long history of cataract removal that is likely to endure well into the future.

Take Home Pearls

- Use low-compliance tubing to decrease surge and improve overall fluidics
- Use a Kelman or angled phacoemulsification needle to improve torsional efficiency
- Hundred percent torsional amplitude is a very efficient cutting instrument and can emulsify even the most dense nuclei
- A 2.2 mm unenlarged temporal incision creates no surgically induced astigmatism
- The smaller (0.9 mm) Kelman phaco needles, when used in combination with torsional ultrasound, provide more room in small pupil cases and improve the efficiency of nuclear assembly and removal

References

1. Seibel B. Phacodynamics: Mastering the Tools and Techniques of Phacoemulsification Surgery. Slack Thorofare, NJ, 2004
2. Solomon K. Unique model illustrates fluidic flow during torsional phaco. Ophthalmology Times 2006; 31:56–58
3. Ernest PH, Fenzyl R, Lavery KT, Sensoli A. Relative stability of clear corneal incisions in a cadaver eye model. J Cataract Refract Surg 1995; 21:1:39–42
4. Berdahl JP, DeStafeno JJ, Kim T. Corneal wound architecture- and integrity after phacoemulsification evaluation of coaxial, microincisional coaxial, and microincision bimanual techniques. J Cataract Refract Surg 2007; 33:510–515
5. Masket S. Coaxial 2.2mm microphaco technique reduces surgically induced astigmatism. Ophthalmology Times 2006; 31:1–2
6. Mackool RJ. Lens removal/torsional phacoemulsification: advantages of nuclear ultrasound. In: Annual ASCRS Symposium on Cararact, IOL, and Refractive Surgery, San Francisco, CA, 17–22 March 2006

5 Technology Available

Rupert Menapace and Silvio Di Nardo

5.1 How to Better Use Fluidics with MICS

Rupert Menapace and Silvio Di Nardo

Core Messages

- Decreasing the downsizing the incision size for coaxial phacoemulsification does not necessarily mean that the efficiency and quality of the fluidics and the emulsification properties decrease.
- In this chapter, we will show how a tip/sleeve design, which is optimized according to the physical laws, allows for excellent fluidics and emulsification.
- Down-sizing clear corneal incisions to less than 2 mm significantly enhances corneal topographical neutrality and wound deformation stability.
- A funnel-shaped wound configuration reduces tissue stress by oar locking during phaco and facilitates instrument insertion. This is especially true for the CO-MICS 2-style phaco tip with its narrow shaft and its sleeve running flush with the protruding head.

5.1.1 *Physical Considerations*

Historically, cataract operations have been performed using many different techniques and instruments. Till date, there is no standardized method: Incision architecture and size, choice of phaco tip and irrigation sleeve, and method of removing the nucleus and cortex are three examples where the surgeon can choose between various options. It depends on the surgeon's skills and preferences, but also on non-medical arguments such as tradition and teaching.

A good understanding of the physical properties may help each surgeon to choose his/her own appropriate technique and to develop the most efficient way for cataract surgery. Understanding the fluidics is a prerequisite for the efficient use of the evolving microphacoemulsification instrumentation. In the following sections, the physical dependencies of aspiration efficiency, chamber stability, and holdability are detailed.

R. Menapace (✉)
Department of Ophthalmology
Medical University Vienna, Vienna General Hospital
Waehringer Guertel 18-20, A 1090 Vienna, Austria
e-mail: rupert.menapace@meduniwien.ac.at

5.1.1.1 Aspiration Efficiency

There are two different pumps in use for cataract surgery: *vacuum*-controlled pumps (e.g. Venturi) and

J. L. Alió, I. H. Fine (eds.), *Minimizing Incisions and Maximizing Outcomes in Cataract Surgery*,
DOI: 10.1007/978-3-642-02862-5_5, © Springer-Verlag Berlin Heidelberg 2010

flow-controlled pumps (e.g. peristaltic). The Venturi pump induces a vacuum in a rigid vacuum container, while with the peristaltic pump the vacuum is produced by a wheel containing ball bearings that milks fluid out of the tubing. The vacuum "propagates" through the tube and induces a flow if the needle is not occluded. The total flow depends on the applied vacuum p_{asp}, the anterior pressure $p_{a.c.}$, and the flow resistance R. Mathematically the flow Φ can then be expressed by the following formula:

$$\frac{p_{a.c} - p_{asp}}{R} = \Phi.$$

The flow resistance R depends on the design of the particular instrument and the tubing. *For smaller diameter tips, for example, the resistance increases. Therefore, a higher vacuum is needed in order to obtain the same flow.* On a Venturi pump the vacuum can be set to a higher value, and on a peristaltic-pump it may be necessary to increase the vacuum limit to obtain the same flow rate. In Fig. 5.1, the relation between the vacuum (Y-axis) and the induced flow (X-Axis) is plotted for two different needles. The data of the red curve have been taken with a traditional 19-gauge needle, and the blue curve has been recorded with a CO-MICS microincision needle from Oertli Instruments. The slope of the two curves corresponds to the resistance R, and the data confirm the higher resistance value for the smaller needle. If, with a peristaltic pump, the vacuum limit is not adequately raised, the pump sensor will prematurely stop the pump, as a result of which the preset flow rate will not be reached.

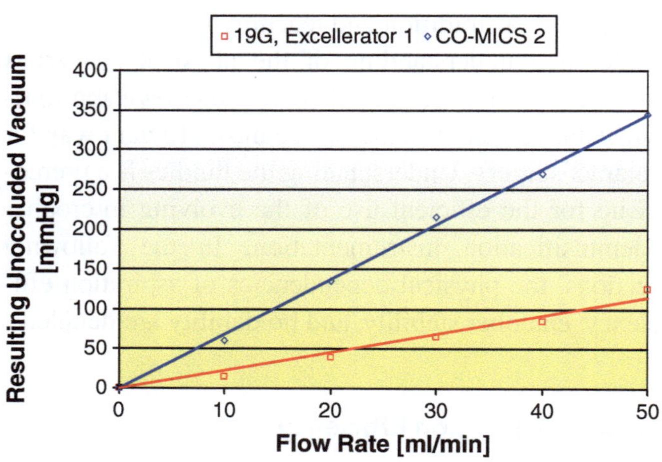

Fig. 5.1 The relation between the flow in the non-occluded case and the necessary vacuum is plotted

In order to achieve the same efficiency of aspiration, the vacuum has to be raised by 100–150 mmHg during quadrant removal.

5.1.1.2 Chamber Stability

The stability of the chamber is one of the most important issues in cataract surgery, since chamber instability or collapse may result in endothelial and capsular damage. To avoid this, it is important that the pressure inside the eye never falls below atmospheric pressure. In such a case, the anterior chamber will collapse and, as a result, the corneal endothelial will be damaged. The natural anterior overpressure of up to 20 mmHg ensures a certain reserve for chamber stability. Ideally, this limit is never underrun, not even during an operation. The course of overpressure over time graphically corresponds to the area beneath the actual pressure and the critical pressure and may be termed "stability band" for better clearness.

The critical point for chamber stability is the moment where the occlusion breaks. This situation may be simulated on an artificial "eye". (A rigid plastic chamber with an integrated sensor to measure the intraocular pressure is used.) For the experiment, a vacuum of 600 mmHg is built up during the simulated occlusion, using a peristaltic pump. Then, the occlusion is broken at the time t_{brk} and the pressure is measured inside the "eye" as a function of time. The maximum vacuum inside the eye p_{stb} is a measure of chamber stability. In Fig. 5.2, the data are shown for a traditional 19-gauge tip and the CO-MICS microincision tip from Oertli Instruments, both used in a coaxial instrument.

The measurement shows that the maximum drop of the pressure is higher for the traditional 19-gauge tip (approximately 135 mmHg below atmospheric pressure) as compared to the CO-MICS tip (55 mmHg). This measurement demonstrates that the smaller tip has a better chamber stability than the larger one when using the same vacuum settings. This result is explained by the fact that not only the irrigation line but also the aspiration line does have a considerably larger flow resistance. A high vacuum does not induce poor chamber stability when using a small aspiration tip, because the aspiration flow is kept small by the large flow resistance.

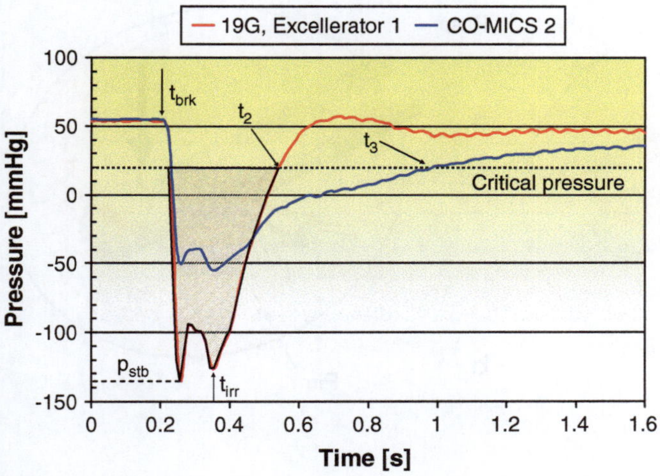

Fig. 5.2 The dynamics of the pressure in an artificial "eye" is plotted. The atmospheric pressure has been subtracted and corresponds to 0 mmHg in this figure. The critical pressure of 20 mmHg approximately matches the natural pressure inside the human eye

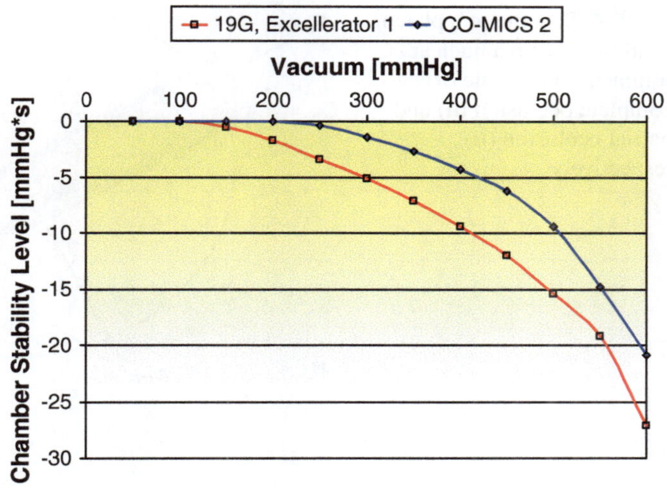

Fig. 5.3 The time-integrated vacuum (chamber stability level) is plotted on the *Y*-axis for various vacuum settings of the pump (*X*-axis). The blue line corresponds to the CO-MICS tip, and the red line is a traditional 19-gauge tip

The curve further shows that the dynamics of the traditional 19-gauge needle is much faster than the one of the CO-MICS. The irrigation line in the traditional 19-gauge system provides sufficient BSS-flow to restore the anterior chamber pressure within the shortest time (steeply rising slope between t_{irr} and t_2). In the case of CO-MICS, it takes longer to re-establish this pressure. This is explained by the cross section of the space between the tip and the sleeve, which is greater with a 19-gauge as compared to a CO-MICS system.

Apart from determining the highest vacuum value p_{stb}, there is another measure for chamber (in-)stability. It corresponds to the time-integrated vacuum inside the eye. For a given stability-limit, the (negative) pressure is "summed up in time" whenever it is lower than the critical limit. In this measurement, the critical limit has been set to 20 mmHg, close to the natural eye pressure. The integrated vacuum corresponds to the area between the curve and the critical limit, which is the shaded area in Fig. 5.2 for the traditional 19-gauge tip. The value of this area is measured for various vacuum settings of the pump. The results are shown in Fig. 5.3.

For all vacuum settings of the pump, the chamber stability level, (defined in the way described above), is clearly better for the CO-MICS tip than for the traditional 19-gauge tip. For the CO-MICS tip, the vacuum can be increased by approximately 100 mmHg to obtain the same amount of stability.

> As a conclusion one can state that the chamber stability of the small diameter needle is better when working with the same vacuum limit. In order to achieve a certain flow rate, the vacuum has to be raised by approximately 100–150 mmHg. Then the chamber stability is comparable to the traditional 19-gauge instrumentation.

5.1.1.3 Holdability

The holdability describes a property of the system during an occlusion. The holdability is defined as the force with which the nuclear fragment is firmly attached to the tip. It must be distinguished from the followability, which describes the streaming characteristics towards the tip.

The holding force *F* depends on the vacuum in the aspiration line, on the size and geometry of the phaco tip, and on the degree of occlusion (Fig. 5.4).

The following calculations apply for a fully occluded phaco tip. Partial occlusion will reduce the holdability considerably. In case of perfect occlusion, the pump does not induce a flow but a constant vacuum p_{asp} that equals the vacuum generated at the location of the pump. The general formula for calculating the force *F* that results from a pressure *p* acting on a surface with area *A*, is as follows:

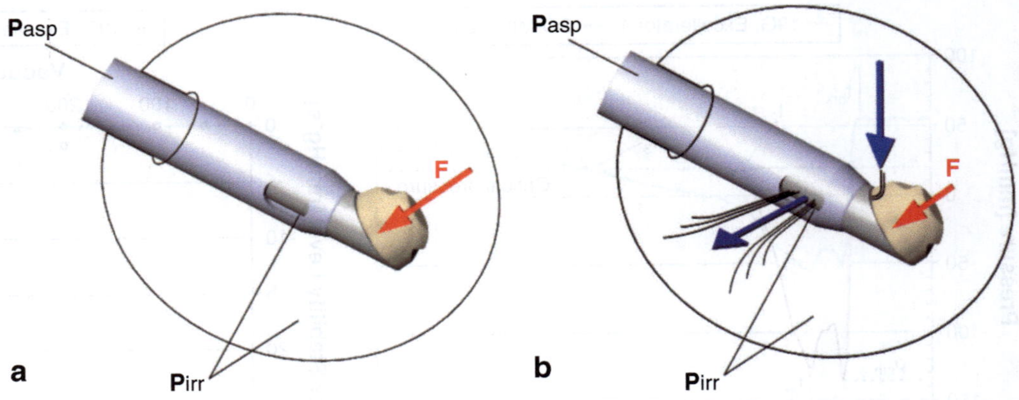

Fig. 5.4 Scheme of a phaco hand piece with a nuclear fragment in the state of complete occlusion (**a**) and partial occlusion (**b**), respectively

$$F = p \cdot A.$$

In the specific setting of the phacotip within the eye, the term p can be identified with the pressure difference between the two sides of the nuclear particle (the phaco tip on the one hand and the pressure in the anterior chamber on the other). In this case, the pressure in the anterior chamber equals the pressure induced by the irrigation bottle. It therefore depends on the height of the irrigation bottle measured with respect to the patient's eye.

A is the surface of the needle opening. Therefore, the holding force can be expressed as a function of the pump vacuum p_{asp} and the anterior chamber pressure $p_{a.c.}$ which is given by the height of the irrigation bottle,

$$F = (p_{a.c} - p_{asp}) \cdot A.$$

Writing the irrigation pressure as a function of bottle height h finally leads to the expression

$$F = (\rho \cdot g \cdot h - p_{asp}) \cdot A,$$

where ρ is the density of BSS and g, the acceleration of gravity. The formula shows that there are three different ways to increase the holdability:

- Increasing the bottle height h
- Increasing the vacuum settings of the pump (both peristaltic and Venturi)
- Increasing the tip area A

When increasing the bottle height, both the holdability and the chamber stability can be optimized. However, the increase of the bottle height is limited by medical aspects (high intraocular pressure and leaking of the incisions).

An increased vacuum in the aspiration line raises the holdability too. However, the vacuum cannot be set too high due to its negative influence on the chamber stability. Here, a compromise has to be found between the two effects, but priority has to be given to the chamber stability.

The third option for an increased holdability is the use of a bigger needle opening. Here, either the tip diameter or the bevel angle can be increased. The diameter of the needle is limited by the incision size. The relation between the diameter and the area (flat cut) is given by the formula for a circle

$$A_0 = \frac{d^2}{4} \cdot \pi.$$

The dependence on the bevel angle α is given by the following formula

$$A_a = \frac{1}{\cos(a)} \cdot A_0.$$

This is shown in Fig. 5.5.

Oertli Instruments has chosen a new solution for the latest generation of micro incision tips. In Fig. 5.6, two designs are illustrated: on the lower picture (b), a traditional phaco tip is shown. It has an inner diameter of 0.57 mm and a bevel angle of 30°. On the upper picture (a), the latest generation of the

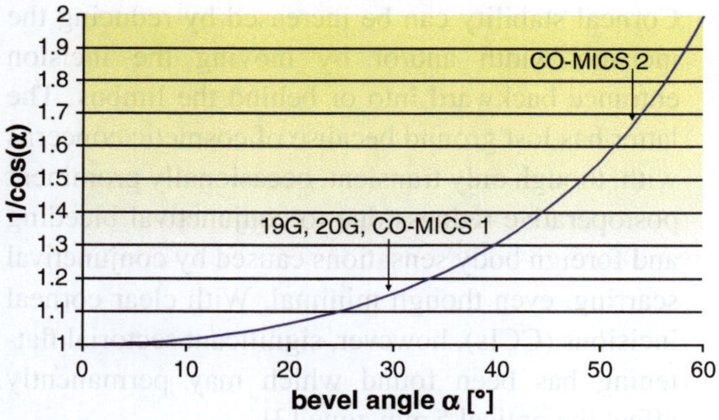

Fig. 5.5 Increase of the surface area of a phaco needle as a function of the cut angle

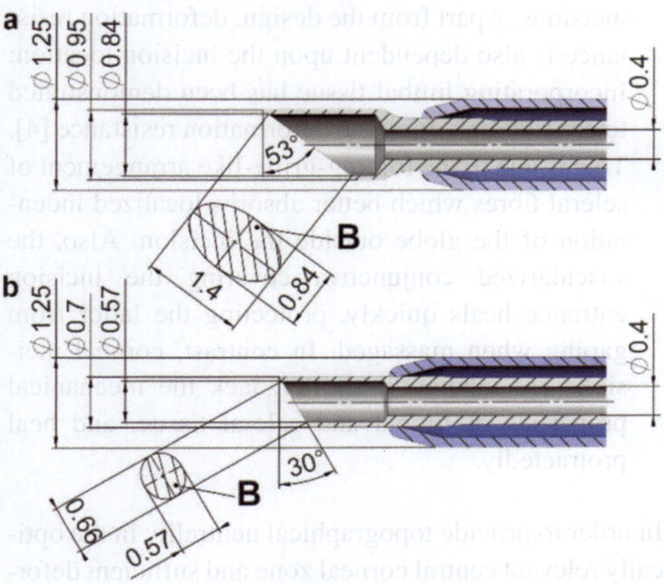

Fig. 5.6 Difference between **(a)** a CO-MICS 2-tip from Oertli Instruments and **(b)** a traditional tip design (CO-MICS 1). Both the diameter and the bevel angle α are maximized to obtain an optimum holdability in the CO-MICS 2 design

Oertli CO-MICS tip is drawn. A staged outer tube diameter allows for an increased opening area. It maximizes the inner diameter of the tip opening (0.84 mm) while keeping the outer diameter (at the location of the elastic sleeve) at a minimum. In addition, the bevel angle of 53° leads to the same holdability as a 19-gauge tip with an angle of 30°.

This design has two advantages:

- The thin wall of the metal tubing at the head and the angled cut both maximize the area of the frontal tip opening and thus the holdability.
- The reduction of the external metal tube diameter along the shaft allows adding a sleeve such that the total size of the tip–sleeve combination is the same as for a traditional CO-MICS tip.

The holding force can now be written as a function of the four parameters: bottle height, aspiration vacuum, diameter of the needle, and bevel angle (h, p_{asp}, d and α)

$$F = (\rho \cdot g \cdot h - p_{asp}) \cdot \frac{d^2}{4} \cdot \pi \cdot \frac{1}{\cos(\alpha)}.$$

As an example, the holdability should be calculated for the following, realistic parameters: bottle height $h = 70$ cm, aspiration vacuum $p_{asp} = -400$ mmHg (−53328.8 Pa). The density of water is $\rho = 1{,}000\,\mathrm{kg/m^3}$ and the gravitational constant equals $g = 9.81\,\mathrm{m/s^2}$. The values for the holdability are given in Newton.

D(mm)	Holdability as a function of internal tip diameter and bevel angle		
	0°	30°	53°
1 (19G)	0.047	0.055	0.079
0.75 (20G)	0.027	0.031	0.044
0.84 (CO-MICS2)	0.033	0.039	0.055

As a conclusion, one can say that the holdability is increased by lifting the irrigation bottle, by applying a high vacuum, and by choosing a needle with a large internal diameter and a large bevel angle. When replacing a 19-gauge or 20-gauge tip by a smaller one, the vacuum should be enhanced in order to obtain the same flow rate. This increase in vacuum further increases the holdability. An angled cut, for example, the CO-MICS 2-tip again raises the holdability.

What is "*vacuum*"? What is "pressure"?

In ophthalmic surgery all pressure values are measured relative to the atmospheric pressure. For example, an intraocular pressure of 15 mmHg means that the pressure inside the eye is 15 mmHg higher than the atmospheric pressure. Or on the other hand, the aspiration pump displays a vacuum of 300 mmHg if the pressure inside the tubing is 300 mmHg lower than the ambient pressure. Therefore, we could either consider this value as a vacuum or as a negative pressure of 300 mmHg. The two points of view are equally correct. As a conclusion: A vacuum is a negative pressure. Therefore, the pressure difference $p_{a.c.}-p_{asp}$ can also be written as $p_{a.c.}+vac_{asp}$, where vac_{asp} is the aspiration vacuum.

5.1.2 Surgical Considerations

What can be done by the surgeon to fully exploit the emulsification potential of phaco tips specifically designed for microincisional cataract surgery (MICS), while preserving maximum incisional and corneal stability, avoiding tissue trauma or incisional leak, and provide optimal chamber stability for the protection of the endothelium and the posterior capsule?

With biaxial phaco tips, exact dimensioning of the incision size is crucial, since tissue trauma will ensue when incision size is too small, and collateral leak will result when it is too wide. The advantage of the coaxial phaco approach is the protection of the peri-incisional tissue from mechanical distension and thermal shrinkage [1, 2], and the lack of fluid loss through the space between the rigid metal tip and the incisional slit. With a stab incision, any tilting of the phaco instrument will jeopardize the safety of the procedure: With a biaxial instrument, the metal tip will either compromise the integrity of a tightly fitting incision or result in significant and variable collateral infusion leak. Such leak will not only jeopardize the chamber stability, but also endothelial integrity: The turbulences quickly wash away the protective viscoelastic layer from the endothelium, exposing the latter to the bombardment by emulsified nuclear particles carried along with the fluid stream. On the other hand, tilting a coaxial instrument may cause chamber collapse by pinching off the sleeve.

To avoid this, special attention must be paid to the details of incision construction:

5.1.2.1 Incision Configuration

Generally, incisions have to be designed in such a way as to provide for maximum topographical stability of the cornea and deformation resistance of the incision when digitally massaged.

- Corneal stability can be increased by reducing the incision width and/or by moving the incision entrance backward into or behind the limbus. The latter has lost ground because of cosmetic concerns with, though only transient, occasionally prominent postoperative redness due to conjunctival bleeding and foreign body sensations caused by conjunctival scarring, even though minimal. With clear corneal incisions (CCIs), however, significant sectorial flattening has been found which may permanently affect the optical 5 mm zone [3].
- Incision stability is dependent upon the width and length of the incision. It increases as the incision narrows and the tunnel lengthens. Inherently, CCIs cannot be made as long as limbo- or sclerocorneal incisions. Apart from the design, deformation resistance is also dependent upon the incision location: Incorporating limbal tissue has been demonstrated to considerably increase deformation resistance [4]. This is due to the folding-grille-like arrangement of scleral fibres which better absorbs localized indentation of the globe outside the incision. Also, the vascularized conjunctiva covering the incision entrance heals quickly, protecting the latter from gaping when massaged. In contrast, corneal incisions are inherently shorter, lack the mechanical properties of limbal and scleral tissue, and heal protractedly.

In order to provide topographical neutrality in the optically relevant central corneal zone and sufficient deformation stability, defined as the patient's inability to reopen the incision tunnel even with intense digital massaging in the temporal palpebral fissure, CCIs must be downsized as much as possible.

Detailed attention must be paid to the design of small CCIs in order to not only optimize the postoperative deformation stability, but also to allow for easy and atraumatic insertion of instrumentation (phaco and injector tip), to avoid damage of the tissue and specifically of the corneal lip when a non-sleeved phaco tip is used, and to provide unimpeded infusion inflow when a sleeved phaco tip is moved to the sides or downwards.

In a parallel-walled tunnel, any deviation of a coaxial phaco tip from the tunnel axis will inevitably compress the sleeve, jeopardizing chamber stability, especially after occlusion break. With a non-sleeved biaxial phaco tip, any off-axis manipulation of the tip will result in mechanical deformation and potential damage of the incision by oarlocking or, with a wider incision, in varying fluid leakage depending on the angle of offset between instrument and incision axis. To avoid this, CCIs must be designed funnel-shaped. The narrow end of the funnel will then act as the pivot point providing for a tight fit of the sleeve while offering freedom of tip movement without deforming the incision or sleeve, respectively. Since it is the diameter of the smallest section of the tunnel rather than a small diameter of the whole tunnel that is critical, the deformation stability of a funnel-shaped incision is not reduced compared to a parallel-walled tunnel.

In principle, the funnel may open up internally or externally. Though both may be applied, there are well-defined advantages and disadvantages of both options to be considered:

- *Internally* widening funnel: It is created by fully entering the chamber with the blade. After partially retracting it, the inner aspect of the tunnel is extended towards both sides in a funnel-shaped manner by again advancing the blade and pushing the cutting edge to the left and right while sparing the tunnel entrance. This incision design has the advantage of avoiding pinching of the sleeve of a coaxial phaco tip and maximally protecting the inner corneal lip from overextension and mechanical damage when a non-sleeved instrument is used. As the main downside, however, such an incision configuration impedes the insertion of instruments, particularly that of injector cartridge tips for lens injection, that are not adequately conical and bevelled.
- *Externally* widening funnel: It is created by not fully advancing a blade with a total width that is larger than that of the inner incision. There are blades available with a cross-mark of a defined length. The blade is advanced until the visible penetration line in Descemet´s membrane coincides with the mark on the front side of the blade below. This incisional architecture has the advantage of facilitating docking or insertion of instruments, especially during lens injection. The downside is that – though the Descemet´s membrane is very robust and elastic – it may be overextended or torn, compromising the sealing properties of the internal corneal valve. Also, endothelial damage may result from direct stripping or indirectly by creating radiating stress folds.

The current popularity of externally widening funnels is mainly nourished by the lack of instrumentation with appropriate tip designs making it cumbersome to snugly thread them into the incisional canal. The gradual introduction of strongly bevelled micro-incisional phaco tips and injector cartridges with an oval cross section will eventually allow to take full advantage of the benefit from the Descemet's membrane- and endothelium-preserving properties of internally widening funnels.

Conventional coaxial phaco tips require a larger incision due to the addition of a soft infusion sleeve. The overall diameter has been reduced by downsizing the metal tip. This, however, reduces phacoemulsification efficiency as explained above. When using modified designs with a trumpet-shaped and strongly bevelled head and a narrow shaft accommodating a sleeve with a diameter hardly larger than that of the metal tip head itself (e.g. CO-MICS 2 tip), phacoemulsification efficiency comparable to a standard 20-gauge tip can be achieved while only requiring a 1.4 mm funnel-shaped incision for unimpeded infusion flow. The increased flow resistance of the narrow shaft inherently acts as surge break which allows working with extremely high vacuum settings. Biaxial phaco instrumentation cannot profit from such a design since the incision size required depends on the segment with the largest diameter, which is the tip head. Reducing the size of the shaft without adding a sleeve would cause considerable leakage and, thus, chamber turbulences and instability. Therefore, a separate surge protector must be interpolated into the infusion line (e.g. "StableChamber®", Bausch & Lomb).

With the large front opening of strongly bevelled tips and the particular fluidics coming with narrow-shaft designs, the surgical technique must also be adjusted for maximum efficiency.

5.1.2.2 Phaco Technique

Generally, highly efficient phacoemulsification requires permanent full tip occlusion. With a peristaltic pump, a high flow rate provides for quick attraction and apposition of nuclear chunks to the phaco tip and for quick subsequent vacuum rise. However, full circumferential sealing of the tip opening by the nuclear chunk is required if the maximum vacuum level has to be reached within the shortest time possible and maintained during phacoemulsification. In order to achieve such docking, low phaco power should be used to allow for full circumferential coupling. With suboptimal sealing between the chunk and the tip, the chunk may be pushed away from the tip when using higher phaco power, which has been termed "chatter".

For the physical reasons detailed above, a strong bevel compensates for the reduced holdability of the smaller diameter of MICS phaco tips. This has been implemented in the Oertli CO-MICS 2 tip. However, increasing lumen and bevel inherently counteracts ease of occlusion ("occludability"). Therefore, Such a tip design requires surgical adaptation of the surgical technique:

Nuclear disintegration ("divide"): For the popular chop technique, tips with a larger diameter and a weaker bevel are most adequate. The former guarantees for a strong grasp of the nucleus required during the chopping manoeuvre. The latter avoids tilting or slipping of the nucleus chunk. By simply reducing the diameter of a conventional tip for micro-incisional phacoemulsification, holdability is inherently reduced, since the latter is proportional to the area of the tip opening. This can be compensated by increasing the bevel angle of the tip. However, the latter is counterproductive regarding the chopping procedure, since the chunk may easily slip off the bevel when an oblique vector force is exerted by the chopper. Therefore, the chopping technique is less appropriate for such a tip.

With a *medium to hard nucleus*, a modified dividing technique is recommended that may be termed "direct crack" in analogy to the "direct chop" technique: With the pump set at a low vacuum level and the bevel directed to the side and away from the phaco spatula, the tip is directed downward right towards the centre of the nucleus. No more energy is used than necessary to allow the tip to penetrate the nucleus without pushing on it. A second or third pass may be done when the tip gets stuck in a hard nucleus. After having reached the bottom of the nucleus, the phaco spatula is deeply inserted in between the phaco tip and the trough wall, and both instruments are then moved sideward which usually results in a nasal crack, which is then extended temporally (with surgeon sitting on temporal side) and usually ends up in the complete division of the nucleus into two halves (Fig. 5.7a). During this combined manoeuvre, the sideward tilted tip acts like a sharp blade that easily cuts through the nucleus, and as a blunt spatula when dividing the nucleus. Then, the well-hydrodissected lens contents are rotated by 90° increments, and two halves are split into quadrants in a similar way.

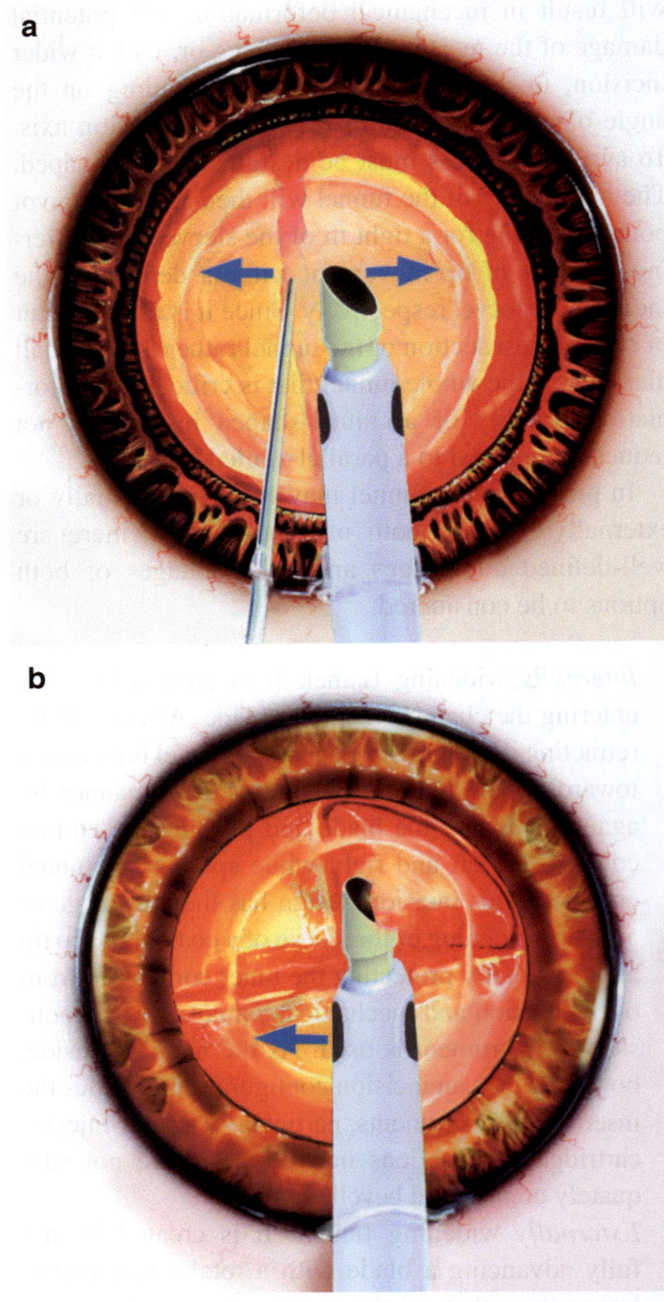

Fig. 5.7 (**a**) "Direct crack": With the bevel directed to the side and away from the phaco spatula, the tip is directed downward right toward the centre of the nucleus. After having reached the bottom of the nucleus, the phaco spatula is deeply inserted in between the phaco tip and the trough wall, and both instruments are then moved sideward which usually results in a distal crack that is then extended proximally. (**b**) The sideward turned tip opening is approached to the flank of the quadrant and docked to it by aspirating it with high flow and vacuum, slightly activating the phaco power to make the tip edge dig into the lens material. When full occlusion is obtained, the phaco power is linearly modulated to emulsify the quadrant, using not more power than necessary for aspiration

Quadrant aspiration ("conquer"): When all four quadrants are separated, phacoaspiration is initiated. Other than with conventional tips the bevel of the CO-MICS *2*–style tip is turned sideward. Instead of engaging a nasal quadrant at its apex, it is approached to its flank and docked to it by aspirating it with high flow and vacuum, slightly activating the phaco power to make the tip edge dig into the material. When full occlusion is finally obtained, the phaco power is linearly modulated to emulsify the quadrant, using not more power than necessary for aspiration (Fig. 5.7b).

With a *soft lens* mass, a trough is created step by step with the bevel oriented upward, as with the conventional technique, which allows good visual control of the depth reached. If the mass is too soft and cohesive to allow subsequent nucleus division, the bevel may be turned sideward and docked to each half which is then aspirated with flow and vacuum set at a high level, usually resulting in a collapse of the lens contents. Alternatively, the tip may be docked to the lens equator with the bevel pointing centrally, and the whole lens mass aspirated with low phaco power while it rotates in a spiral fashion.

It is important that, when working with the bevel turned sideward, the fluid outlets of the sleeve must be aligned with the bevel so as to direct the outflow horizontally in order to preserve the adherent viscoelastic layer, and thus protect the endothelium.

5.1.2.3 Infusion-Assisted High-Flow High-Vacuum Phacoaspiration (Hybrid Phaco)

As stated, emulsification efficiency is highly dependent on the coupling force between the phaco tip and the nuclear chunk. If not appropriate, emulsification efficiency is suboptimal and nuclear chatter may ensue. Setting the vacuum at a very high level carries the risk of chamber flattening due to the surge following occlusion break. This is mitigated by the surge-reducing effect of a narrow segment placed within the tubing. This can be inserted behind the phaco handpiece as realized in the Bausch & Lomb Stellaris® phaco equipment ("StableChamber®"), or integrated in the phaco tip as in the Oertli® CO-MICS 2 tip. Surge may also be counteracted by elevating the infusion bottle. However, excessive infusion pressure exerts considerable stress on ocular structures and blood flow [5]. Therefore, an additional infusion line may be used that complements the coaxial inflow. An anterior chamber maintainer has been used to accomplish this. However, an additional paracentesis is required, and the tubing interferes with free globe mobility. Alternatively, an infusion handpiece of a biaxial phaco or I&A set may be used as an "infusion spatula" inserted through the pre-existing paracentesis instead of a conventional phaco spatula. Since this approach combines micro-coaxial and biaxial features, it may be termed "Hybrid phaco". The additional influx provided by the infusion spatula supplements the flow provided by the sleeve to a considerable extent. The abundant surplus of infusion allows for vacuum levels as high as 600 mmHg and flow rates of up to 40 mmHg even with a moderately elevated bottle, while the chamber stays rock-solid when occlusion breaks. The tip of the infusion handle is inserted only when nuclear division is completed. It serves as a blunt spatula to manipulate the nuclear pieces towards the tip opening, and is positioned between the posterior capsule and the tip when occlusion break is imminent in order to mechanically protect the posterior capsule should chamber flattening occur (Fig. 5.8a). The additional use of an appropriate high-flow infusion spatula (Fig. 5.8b) has proven to significantly enhance phacoemulsification efficiency during the phase of quadrant conquering: Energy consumption as expressed by the integrated phaco time displayed by the machine was reduced by more than one half (by 53.3%). Fluid consumption from the bottle was increased by one fourth (25.8%) which reflects the enhanced followability provided by the high flow. (Preliminary data from prospective randomized intraindividual comparison study with 30 patients [6, 7]. Fluidic settings: 20 ml/min and 400 mmHg without, and 35 ml/min and 600 mmHg with infusion spatula, respectively). Turbulences during aspiration are confined to a smaller space around the phaco tip, and nuclear chunks or emulsified lens material are immediately re-grasped or aspirated by the tip, which should minimize the risk of endothelial trauma.

In conclusion: With MICS, special attention has to be paid to the details of incision construction. The reduced holdability of a smaller-diameter tip can be compensated by increasing the bevel angle. The trumpet-shaped head of the CO-MICS 2 coaxial tip additionally boosts phaco energy transfer by increasing the projection area of the frontal plane without requiring a larger incision for the sleeve, since the reduced shaft diameter allows the sleeve to run flush with the head

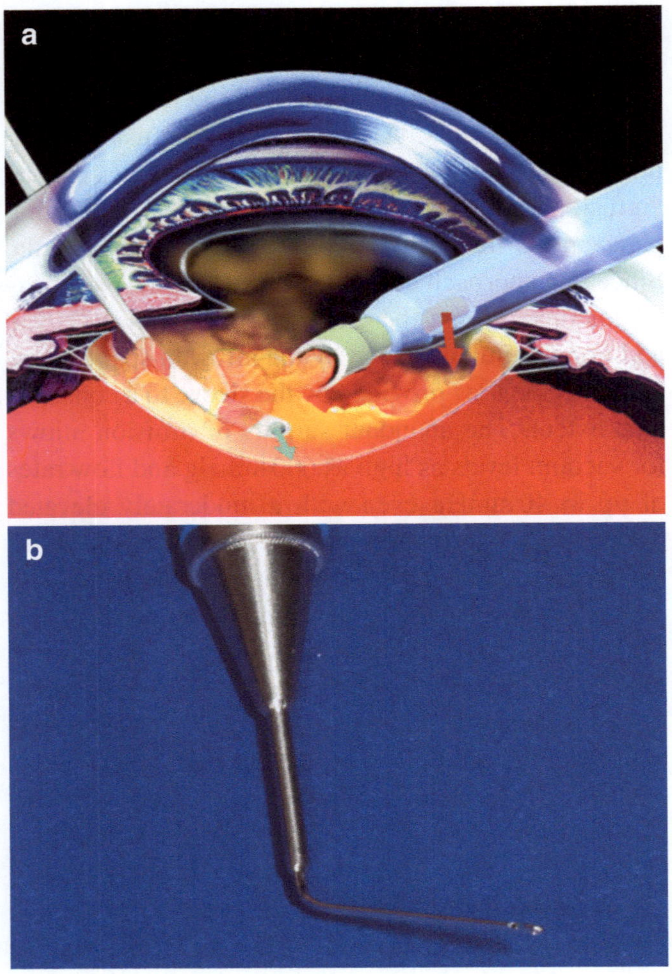

Fig. 5.8 (**a**) "Infusion spatula": When nuclear division is completed, the tip of a high-flow infusion handle is inserted to boost irrigation. It also serves as a blunt spatula to manipulate the nuclear pieces towards the tip opening, and is positioned between the posterior capsule and tip when occlusion break is imminent in order to mechanically protect the posterior capsule should chamber flattening occur. (**b**) Prototype of infusion spatula with oval cross-section and low-resistance shaft for maximum through-put of infusion fluid (Geuder, Germany)

along. The internal step from tip head to shaft significantly enhances the efficiency of the phaco tip and avoids tip obstruction ("clogging") by nuclear pieces. To be efficient, this requires adaptations in the phaco technique. With strongly bevelled tips, direct nuclear cracking has turned out to be the most appropriate technique. For both the divide and conquer manoeuvres, the bevel is turned sideward. An additional infusion handle inserted through the side-port allows for very high vacuum and flow settings and *saves* phaco time and energy. This provides for both maximum efficiency and safety of phacoemulsification procedure.

5.1.2.4 The OS3 and CataRhex SwissTech Platforms

The Oertli OS3 and Oertli CataRhex SwissTech platforms (Fig. 5.9) support both coaxial and bimanual MICS. While (sleeveless) bimanual MICS requires adjustments of fluidics and "cool phaco" power settings, which are readily available on these platforms by simply pressing the CMP cool micro pulse button, coaxial MICS with the Oertli CO-MICS tip needs an increase of the vacuum only.

However, in our experience the coaxial approach to MICS has two major advantages: (1) The sleeve seals the wound, thereby preventing fluid outflow. With sleeveless phaco tips, fluid loss is not only inevitable but also variable depending upon the relative orientation of the tip with regard to the wound. This leads to pressure fluctuations within the chamber which may be difficult to counterbalance and carry the risk of a chamber collapse in case of occlusion break. (2) The sleeve protects the surrounding wound tissue from mechanical and thermal damage [1, 2]. With sleeveless phaco tips, the wound slit must be kept as narrow as possible to provide a tight fit and thus avoid excessive fluid outflow. This may lead to tissue damage especially when instrument manipulation in a tight incision causes oar locking of the wound. Other advantages of coaxial MICS are improved fluidics as dealt with in Sect. 3.2 in Chap. 3 "How to better use fluidics in MICS". Use of OS3 and CataRhex SwissTech platforms is therefore described for coaxial MICS only.

Equipment

No specific software or special tubing-system or other modification is required to do coaxial MICS with the OS3 and CataRhex SwissTech platforms. The CO-MICS 2 (Oertli) phaco tip and sleeve are mounted to the Oertli Hexadisq phaco hand piece. The front side of the sleeve must be positioned as illustrated in Fig. 5.10.

When appropriately adjusted, the front of the sleeve seals with the backside of the tip head, avoiding anteriorly directed inflow. With traditional tips, this coaxial inflow tends to push fragments away from the tip. With the CO-MICS 2 tip, the irrigation fluid inflow is essentially confined to the side openings.

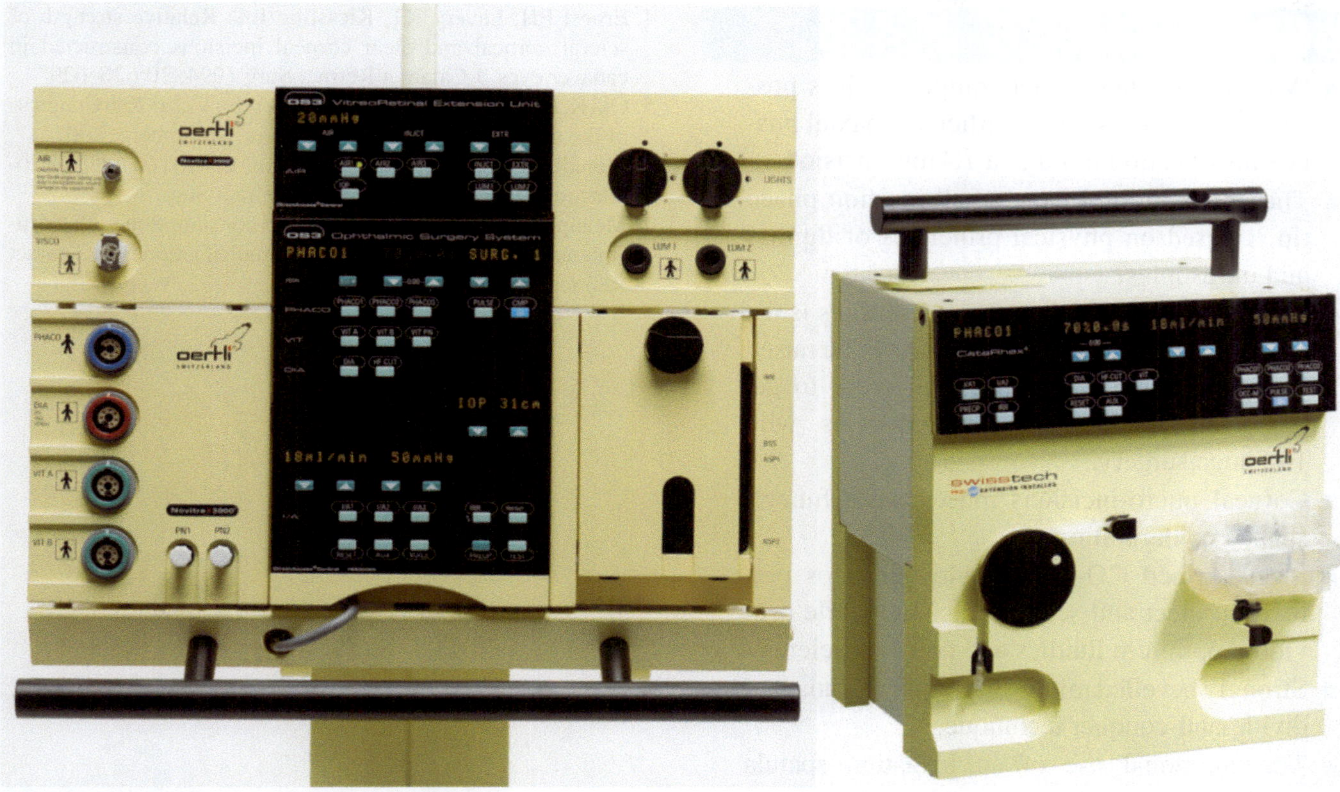

Fig. 5.9 The Oertli OS3 surgery unit, here with the vitreoretinal extension (left); and the Oertli CataRhex SwissTech platform

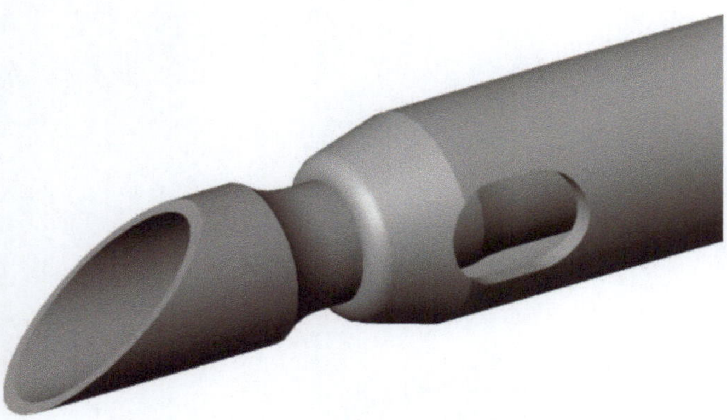

Fig. 5.10 Positioning of the sleeve in the Oertli CO-MICS 2 instrumentation

Machine Settings

CO-MICS 2 works equally well with the venturi or the peristaltic pump of the OS3 platform. A venturi surgeon can stay with the venturi pump, a peristaltic surgeon with the peristaltic pump. In both cases the vacuum limit alone needs to be changed. Here are the rules of thumb:

- Do not change your flow settings (ml/min peristaltic) or venturi rise time (% venturi)
- For grooving: increase the vacuum level by 50 mmHg (peristaltic and venturi)
- For fragment removal: increase the vacuum level by 150 mmHg (peristaltic and venturi)
- Phaco power and modulation needs no adjustment, keep your preferred values and modulation mode.
- After the first CO-MICS surgery, take into consideration, the possibility of further increasing the vacuum levels and flow rate.

Do not be afraid of working with high vacuum levels. CO-MICS 2 provides for excellent chamber stability and suppresses surges. The behaviour is very different from standard 2.8 mm incision tips, and is much smoother and more "forgiving".

The CO-MICS 2 tip provides for astonishing phacoemulsification efficiency and chamber stability, inherent reduction of surge upon occlusion break and optimally preserves the integrity and self-sealing properties of the wound.

Take Home Pearls

- With up-to-date cataract equipment, it is possible to perform safe and efficient coaxial phacoemulsification through a 1.4 mm incision.
- The optimization of the small-incision phaco tip is based on physical principles of fluidics and ultrasonics.
- The only change in the machine settings is the vacuum limit: the vacuum limit has to be raised by approximately 150 mmHg in order to get the same quality and efficiency as with 19-gauge surgery.
- Corneal micro-incisions must have a funnel-shaped configuration.
- Sleeve-armed CO-MICS-style microtips perfectly protect and seal the incision while providing optimum fluidics and power efficiency.
- Strongly bevelled micro-tips require an adapted divide-and-conquer technique.
- The additional use of an irrigation spatula ("hybrid phaco") allows to safely perform high-flow high-vacuum phaco and thus dramatically reduces phaco power consumption.

Acknowledgement The measurements in graphs Figs. 5.1–5.3 were conducted at Oertli Instruments, Inc. in Berneck, Switzerland. The drawings in Figs. 5.7–5.9 have been provided by "Highlights of Ophthalmology", Panama.

Financial disclosure: The principal author has no financial interest in any of the materials or equipments mentioned. Dr Di Nardo is the R&D manager at Oertli Instruments Inc. in Berneck, Switzerland.

References

1. Berdahl JP, DeStefano JJ, Kim T. Corneal wound architecture and integrity after phacoemulsification: evaluation of coaxial, microincisional coaxial and microincisional bimanual techniques. J Cataract Refract Surg 2007; 33:510–515
2. Johar SRK, Vasavada AR, Praveen MR, et al. Histomorphological and immunofluorescence evaluation of bimanual and coaxial phacoemulsification incisions in rabbit. J Cataract Refract Surg 2008; 34:670–676
3. Vass C, Menapace R. Computerized statistical analysis of corneal topography for the evaluation of changes in corneal shape after surgery. Am J Ophthalmol 1994; 118:177–184
4. Ernest PH, Lavery KT, Kiessling LA. Relative strength of scleral corneal and clear corneal incisions constructed in cadaver eyes. J Cataract Refract Surg 1994; 20:626–629
5. Oki K. Normal tension cataract surgery. In: Video 20th Congress of the German Ophthalmic Surgeons, Nuremberg, 2007
6. Menapace R. Technique of "infusion-assisted coaxial microphacoemulsifaction". J Cataract Refract Surg
7. Menapace R. Time, energy and fluid consumption with "infusion-assisted coaxial microphacoemulsifaction". J Cataract Refract Surg

5.2 How to Use Power Modulation in MICS

Randall J. Olson

Core Messages

- Safety and efficiency in phacoemulsification can conflict.
- Comparisons, such as percent power, are meaningless if not standardized.
- The incidence of wound burn can vary from 0.2 to 0.03% depending on approach and ultrasound power modulation.
- Machine-indicated parameters may not be very accurate.
- The control of anterior chamber depth associated with post-occlusion surge can vary dramatically depending on the parameters chosen, between machines and between patients, even when using the same machine and parameters.

5.2.1 Introduction

Phacoemulsification of the cataract is all about two core elements: (1) efficiency, and (2) safety. Unfortunately, improved efficiency can result in decreased safety; therefore, maximizing both is an important process, which will increase the speed of cataract removal without sacrificing safety. A full understanding of how energy modulation works to enhance both safety and efficiency is the subject of this chapter and has been an ongoing research effort for the last several years on behalf of my research group at the John A. Moran Eye Center, at the University of Utah, in Salt Lake City, UT.

R. J. Olson
Department of Ophthalmology and Visual Sciences, Moran Eye Center, University of Utah School of Medicine, 65 N Medical Drive, Salt Lake City, UT 84132, USA
e-mail: randall.olson@hsc.utah.edu

5.2.2 What Do Phacoemulsification Machines Really Do?

Our original interest in this was generated due to the statements made about comparisons of machines that were not physically possible. It was unlikely that physics had been thrown out of the window and, therefore, some core assumptions could not be correct. Our early work looked at measuring actual power output and determining actual vs. machine-indicated parameters. What we learned is that flow can be different from what is indicated on the machine [1–3], in particular if flow restrictors are in place, such as Cruise control (STAAR Surgical, Monrovia, CA). We also found that vacuum can be off by as much as 23% and that features such as a bypass port in the phaco needle (ABS, Alcon Surgical, Fort Worth, TX) decreases the actual vacuum at the tip by an average of 7.5% [4]. While some of this may not seem clinically important, it certainly is important in any comparative studies between different machines. Our clinically most important early finding is that percent power had no correlation between any of the machines, including the two Alcon machines, Infiniti and Legacy. Furthermore, the power output with and without a load varied even more dramatically among different machines: with Millennium and Stellaris (Bausch & Lamb, Beverly Hills, CA) and Sovereign and Signature (Advanced Medical Optics, Santa Ana, CA), all power-based, as the foot pedal increases, the power increases; and with Legacy, being stroke length-based, the power is varied to maintain the stroke length, such that the power, even without changing the foot pedal under a load, can change dramatically.

Infiniti, interestingly, is not the same as Legacy and is somewhere between the two different extremes (Table 5.1) [1, 3].

So using percent power for any type of comparison between machines is impossible because it is different for every machine we have tested so far. For instance, a common comparison would be testing the machines in water, and based upon our work, Legacy at 100% power would be the same as Infiniti at 67%, Sovereign at 43%, and Millennium at 36%.

5.2.3 The Concept of Unoccluded Flow Vacuum

We also noted that there was quite a difference in the vacuum necessary to maintain flow, particularly as

Table 5.1 Temperature Increase (*C*) at 1 min per 20% increment of power increase (40% divided by 2, 60% by 3) for four phacoemulsification machines with 20 ml/min of free flow (*n* ❑ 25 for each category)

Machines	Unweighted	Weighted	Ratio of weighted/ unweighted
Millennium	5.67 ❑ 0.51	6.80 ❑ 0.80	1.202
Sovereign	4.59 ❑ 0.70	5.65 ❑ 0.72	1.232
Infiniti	2.79 ❑ 0.62	3.96 ❑ 0.311	1.423
Legacy	1.99 ❑ 0.49	4.27 ❑ 0.761	2.153

p ❑ 0.0001 for all unweighted vs. weighted comparisons and for all vertical comparisons except: $_1p$ ❑ 0.06, $_2p$ ❑ 0.34, and $_3p$ ❑ .0016. The weight used was 200 g. Sovereign and Legacy data from [5]

Table 5.2 A Comparison of actual vacuum created at the actual flow for the range of 26 through 36 ml/min of flow in 2-ml/min steps (0.9-mm tip used), for the Alcon Infiniti (INF) and Legacy (LEG), Bausch and Lomb Millennium Peristaltic (MILL-P) and Venturi (MILL-V), and AMO Sovereign (SOV), also with Staar Cruise control (SOV-CC) [6]

Machine	Comparison value
SOV	1.0 ± 0.07
LEG	1.16 ± 0.08
INF	1.16 ± 0.06
MILL-P	1.52 ± 0.03
MILL-V	1.81 ± 0.05
SOV-CC	2.44 ± 0.07

For all comparisons, $p < 0.0001$ except LEG to INF ($p = 0.75$). Sovereign is used as the reference with the mean set at 1.0 for each 2-ml/min step. Millennium is only compared through 34 ml/min limit of actual range tested and Sovereign with Cruise Control through 32 ml/min of flow (also limit of actual range tested). Sovereign and Legacy values from reference number 1. *INF* Alcon Infiniti phacoemulsification machine; *LEG* Alcon Legacy phacoemulsification machine; *MILL-P* Bausch & Lomb Millennium phacoemulsification machine with peristaltic vacuum; *MILL-V* Bausch & Lomb Millennium phacoemulsifi-cation machine with venturi vacuum; *SOV* AMO Sovereign phacoemulsification machine; *SOV-CC* AMO Sovereign phacoemulsification machine with the Staar Cruise Control attached to the aspiration line

flow increased above 30 ml/min of actual flow. It has generally been assumed in peristaltic vacuum systems that vacuum is zero until there is occlusion of the tip, at which point vacuum will build up. What we found is that once flow went above 20 ml/min,

active vacuum was needed to maintain that level of flow, in particular with 20-gauge tips. With a flow restrictor such as Cruise Control, the unoccluded vacuum measured at the tip was greater than what we have measured with Venturi flow systems with similar flow [3]. This unoccluded flow vacuum may be a safety concern at higher flow. At the very least, at high flow we need to be aware that there is likely to be significant active vacuum at the tip without occlusion, so one must be careful when working near the capsule or iris (Table 5.2).

5.2.4 The Intricacies of Ultrasound Power Modulation

An additional area of our research deals with power modulation. Pulsing ultrasound with a variable on-time and off-time has been around for a long time; however, there was evidence accruing that very short pulses, first pioneered by Sovereign White Star, with on-times in the 4–6 ms range, seemed to provide additional efficiency and were potentially protective of wound burn as we showed in early eye bank eye studies [7, 8]. Other papers using percent power to compare machines suggested that very short pulses like signature White Star were not better temperature-wise than long pulses in Legacy; however, we can easily explain those results based on the fact that percent power has no meaningful correlation between these two machines [1, 3]. That still left unanswered the issue of any safety or efficiency advantages with these very short on-times.

One comparative study looked at Sovereign with and without the use of White Star. This multicentered study, in which we participated, did show that these very short on-times did clinically and statistically significantly decrease the amount of energy necessary to complete a case. Furthermore, we did show significantly less corneal endothelial cell loss with White Star [9].

With regard to wound burns, we found that the overall amount of heat produced, whether with long or short ultrasound pulse, made no difference; the only issue of importance was the percent of on-time (i.e., if ultrasound is on half the time you produce half the heat) [1]. This is no surprise, as it fits the law of thermodynamics, and cannot explain any wound burn safety protection from these very short ultrasound pulses (Fig. 5.11).

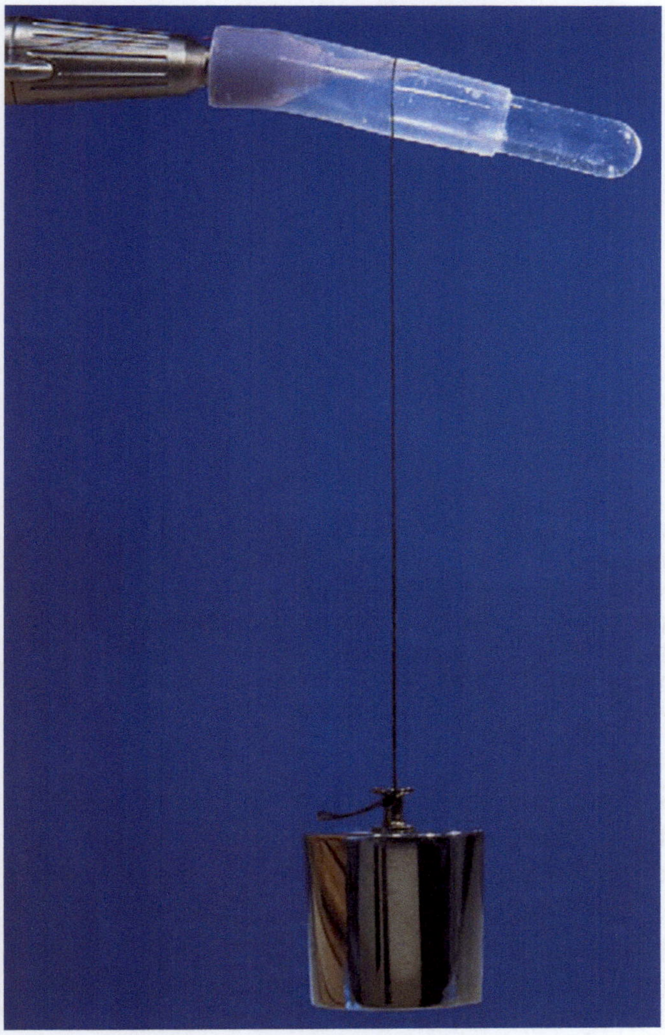

Fig. 5.11 A weight is hung with 5-0 Prolene suture around the artificial test chamber at the same point throughout, producing consistent friction of the sleeve against the phaco tip [10]

5.2.5 The Variable Incidence of Wound Burn Rates

Because no large study had ever been done with regard to wound burn, and we had no idea how common a problem this might be, we decided that the best thing to do was to survey the problem. Wound burn occurs when the collagen is heated by the phaco tip to 60°C, or higher, at which time a burn will occur in a matter of seconds. Many people call wound edema, which can result from localized endothelial destruction, wound burns; therefore, we defined this as increased astigmatism, and actual traction lines around the wound showing collagen were permanently shortened by the increase in temperature. By conducting a survey in the northwestern United States we were able to show that the incidence of wound burn was about 1:1,000 and indeed did vary between machines with Sovereign and Millennium statistically less than Legacy ($p = 0.014$) with regard to overall wound burn. When looking at the technique, we also found that chopping, in particular vertical chopping, was safer than either a carousel or divide-and-conquer approach ($p = 0.003$). The most important finding, however, was that the very short power modulations (i.e., White Star, hyper pulse, or ultra pulse) decreased wound burn in comparison to continuous ultrasound by eightfold ($p = 0.0001$), and in a multivariate analysis showed the strongest relationship to wound burn protection (Table 5.3) [12]. So, if indeed the duty-cycle (the amount of time on) is the only thing that is important in regard to heat generation, then why would this be protective?

Table 5.3 Survey response rates and phacoemulsification wound burn rates as reported by surgical approach, phacoemulsification unit, and usual settings [11]

Surgeries		Wound burns	Wound burn rate (per 1,000)
Surgical approach			
Divide and conquer1	41,125	53	1.29
Carousel2	10,057	12	1.19
Horizontal chop	11,359	7	0.62
Vertical chop3	11,554	3	0.26
Other	2,487	0	0
1 vs.3 ($p = 0.003$)			
2 vs.3 ($p = 0.009$)			
Phaco unit			
Legacy1	46,416	54	1.16
Millennium	5,140	2	0.39
Sovereign2	20,885	11	0.56
Other	4,141	8	1.93
1 vs.2 ($p = 0.014$)			
Unit setting			
Continuous1	23,899	42	1.76
Pulse2	8,685	12	1.38
Burst3	18,588	16	0.86
WhiteStar4	19,260	5	0.26
1 vs.3 ($p = 0.013$)			
1 vs.4 ($p < 0.0001$)			
2 vs.4 ($p = 0.0004$)			
3 vs.4 ($p = 0.013$)			

Cavitational energy peaks after a few seconds of ultrasound and rapidly drops to a low steady state. So very short pulses of ultrasound create more cavitational energy than continuous ultrasound at the same power setting. Furthermore, one of the great inefficiencies of ultrasound utilization is chatter where the longitudinal stroke repels the lens particle and no emulsification occurs. These very short on-times do not allow for much chatter because during the off-phase, flow and vacuum can recapture the particle at the tip ready for the next ultrasound pulse. So these two means of using energy more efficiently, which we have documented, result in less ultrasound time necessary to remove a cataract [9]. There would also be a commensurate protection from thermal injury.

Another possible way in which thermal injury is prevented is thermal inertia. This represents the lag time before heat is transferred to the tissue. If your on-time is brief and the off-time allows cooling, then this is another possible thermal protective mechanism for these very short pulses. By looking at the differences in heat creation in vitro, vs. 100μm from the tip in eye bank eyes, we showed that there was about 11% thermal inertia in an eye bank model for protection of wound burn [13]. At a wound burn temperature of 60°C, an energy saving of 11% would equate to 6.6°C for short vs. long ultrasound pulses. Thermography work of the wound has shown that dangerous temperatures are easily reached, so a 10% temperature saving could often spell the difference between a safe case and a wound burn.

A newer power modulation is torsional ultrasound, where the phaco tip sweeps laterally, rather than longitudinally. This virtually eliminates chatter and, as a result, improves efficiency. Furthermore, with the needle rotating in the wound rather than moving longitudinally, there is less friction generated at any power setting. A concern is that rather than using 10–15% energy, many use torsional ultrasound at the 90–100% energy setting, at which point thermal advantages may not be apparent. We do not have any study looking at wound burns with torsional ultrasound, so all of this is conjecture. One clinical finding is that torsional ultrasound does increase clogging of the phaco needle, so many surgeons add short bursts of longitudinal ultrasound, especially with harder cataracts, to minimize this clogging.

5.2.6 Measuring the Amplitude of Post-Occlusion Surge

An underlying reason in determining the accuracy of phacoemulsification instrumentation has been the measurement of post-occlusion surge (POS). POS is the result of the inherent elasticity of the system, such that when the occlusion is broken, the release of this elasticity will result in a sudden inflow of fluid into the phaco tip and at its most severe presentation, will completely evacuate the anterior chamber. The parameters I safely use today on the machine I first used over 30 years ago would evacuate the entire anterior chamber after each occlusion break! Obviously things have changed dramatically over the years and an example of some of the breakthroughs to control POS are small-bore, thick-walled, low-compliance tubing to minimize this elastic rebound, and constant monitoring of the vacuum level through computerized pumps, which not only stop when the required vacuum level is reached, but can also change direction at the start of POS.

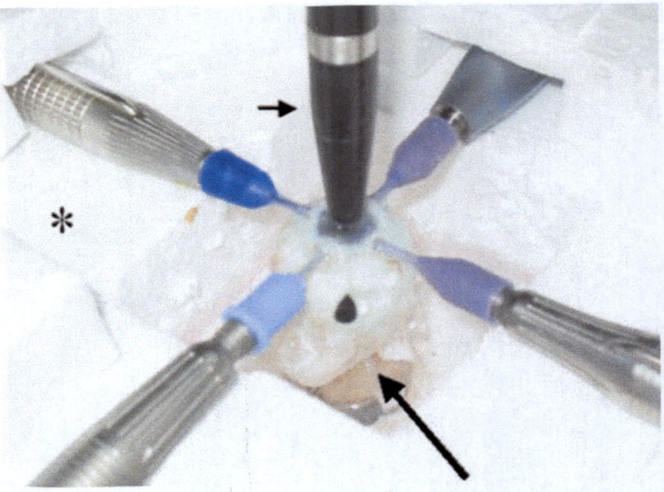

Fig. 5.12 Experimental setup for postocclusion surge studies: human eye-bank eye is sitting in a 35 ml syringe (*big arrow*), which is fixated in the center of a styrofoam box (*asterisk*). The phaco tips are inserted in the eye through scleral tunnel incisions placed 90° apart and the wounds are sealed with cyanoacrylate glue. The A-scan probe, which is fixated on a burette arm holder, is sitting 1 mm above the cornea (*small arrow*) [14]

We decided that the clinically most relevant way to look at POS was to measure the anterior chamber collapse in eye bank eyes (Fig. 5.12). This is the most noticeable problem, and movement of the capsule toward the phaco tip is the most dangerous scenario we encounter. By placing multiple instruments into the same eye we could have a very fair comparison of each of the instruments. Furthermore, with our work on machine accuracy, we could adjust each of the machines; so we are comparing actual parameters and not machine-indicated parameters, which could bias the results.

Our first comparison was between Infiniti, Legacy, Millennium and Sovereign. We did find that all four machines were statistically significantly different from each other, with Millennium being the best of the lot followed closely by Sovereign, then Infiniti, and the clear outlier being Legacy, which had twice as much POS as Infiniti. We then looked at different parameters and found, not surprisingly, that if you elevate the bottle, you decrease POS, and also if you elevate flow, you increase POS. In fact, we found that Legacy with the appropriate parameters was as good as any of the other machines. We were very surprised to find that changing from a 20-gauge to a 19-gauge phacoemulsification needle for Sovereign and Infiniti almost tripled the level of POS; so this is another way to tame POS by moving to a 20-gauge needle. We found that the ABS port used with Infiniti and Legacy did improve POS dramatically for Legacy, but did not have a statistically significant effect on Infiniti, showing that the machines clearly behaved differently in how they respond to POS [15].

We were interested in POS suppression with Cruise Control and found that it did not seem to have much of an effect where POS was minimal such as with Millennium; however, in machines such as Legacy, we did have a significant effect. When we went to Millennium with a Venturi pump, however, the impact was dramatic, with POS decreased by at least fivefold and probably closer to tenfold [16].

With Stellaris (Bausch & Lomb) and Signature (Advance Medical Optics) new to the market, we then compared these machines. We looked at very aggressive parameters, which would be a low bottle height of 60 cm, a 19-gauge needle, and the maximum vacuum that we can obtain at our altitude of about 550 mmHg and the maximum flow attainable by all of the machines. Because the machines were new, we did look at flow and found that when trying to get 60 ml/min, Stellaris had the least flow; when it said 60 ml/min, it was at 53.5 + 0.0 ml, followed by Infiniti at 55.8 ± 0.4 ml/min, and the closest to actual was Signature at 58.5 ± 0.0 ml/min. All of them were very close with regard to vacuum, with Stellaris overestimating vacuum (526 ± 3.3 mmHg actual vs. 550 mmHg machine-indicated vacuum), Infiniti closest to the actual (551.6 ± 3.5 mmHg actual vs. 550 mmHg machine-indicated vacuum), and Signature actually underestimating the vacuum (569.4 ± 6.0 mmHg actual vs. 550 mmHg machine-indicated vacuum).

So in POS comparisons of these machines in two eye bank eyes, we found that Stellaris and Signature were quite similar to each other and both had half or less POS than Infiniti (Fig. 5.13). Signature had a small edge over Stellaris, which was statistically significantly different in one of the eye bank eyes. With regard to the amount of vacuum required to produce flow, the clear outlier was Signature, which required approximately half the vacuum to provide the same amount of high flow as Infiniti or Stellaris (Fig. 5.14).

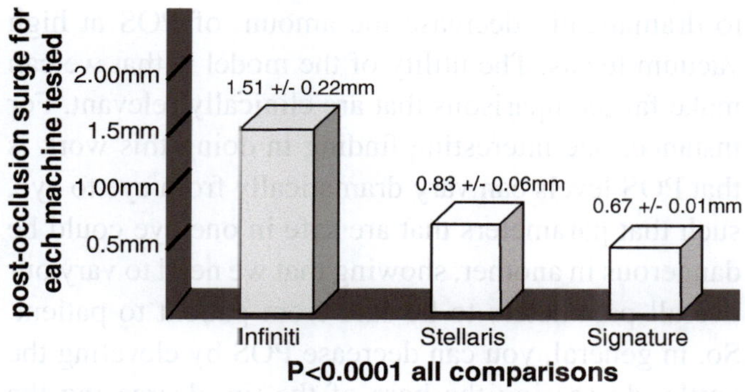

Fig. 5.13 Bar graph demonstrating postocclusion surge comparisons (in millimeters) in a 81-year-old human cadaver eye using three phacoemulsification machines. Vacuum was at 400 mmHg (actual), flow was at 40 ml/min (actual), bottle height was at 70 cm, and 19-gauge tips were used (n = 20 for each machine) [17]

Additional work is ongoing for the refinement of our model. Because minor variations with regard to the size of the phacoemulsification needles can have a big impact with regard to our measurements, we are now using a stopcock to run all the machines through the same hand piece and the same phaco needle. This will be used to compare the new cassettes that have come out with Infiniti to improve their overall POS, and also for comparisons of the new vacuum-based pumps in both Stellaris and Signature, which are said

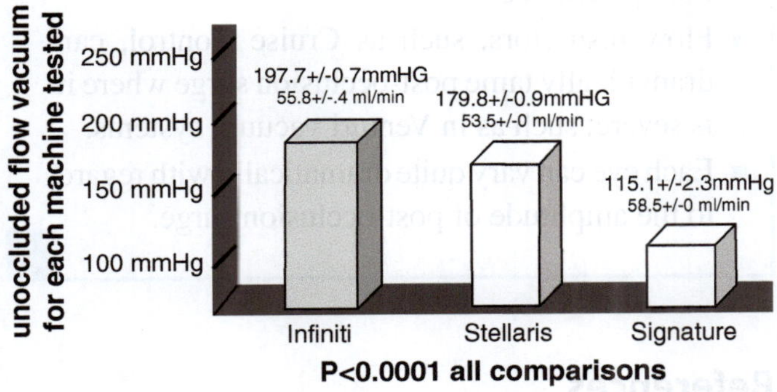

Fig. 5.14 Bar graph demonstrating, with the machines set at 550 mmHg vacuum (actual), 60 ml/min machine indicated flow, 60 cm bottle height, and with 19-gauge tips to measure actual flow, the mean vacuum (actual) necessary to maintain that flow for three phacoemulsification machines (n = 10 for each machine)s [18]

to dramatically decrease the amount of POS at high vacuum levels. The utility of the model is that we can make fair comparisons that are clinically relevant. For instance, one interesting finding in doing this work is that POS levels can vary dramatically from eye to eye, such that parameters that are safe in one eye could be dangerous in another, showing that we need to vary our overall parameters to be safe from patient to patient. So, in general, you can decrease POS by elevating the bottle, decreasing the bore of the tip, decreasing the flow of the instrument and/or decreasing vacuum. It also turns out that the POS protectors such as the ABS tip for the Alcon systems and Cruise Control may, but not always, help in controlling POS.

In conclusion, it is important to understand the machine as well as the parameters used to optimize both efficiency and safety. From the work, as outlined, it is clear as to what can be done to optimize safety. Furthermore, very short ultrasound pulses at 4–6 ms with variable on–off times do improve efficiency with additional safety documented with regard to wound burn and corneal protection. Torsional ultrasound also improves efficiency with the virtual elimination of chatter and may protect against wound burn.

Take Home Pearls

- Do not rely on the machine-indicated values as they may be inaccurate.
- Very short bursts of ultrasound and a vertical chopping approach are very protective of wound burn.
- Post-occlusion surge can be minimized by raising the irrigation bottle, decreasing flow and maximum vacuum, and moving to a smaller-bore phaco needle.
- Flow restrictors, such as Cruise Control, can dramatically tame post-occlusion surge where it is severe, such as in Venturi vacuum systems.
- Each eye can vary quite dramatically with regard to the amplitude of post-occlusion surge.

References

1. Adams W, Brinton J, Floyd M, et al (2006) Phacodynamics: an aspiration flow vs vacuum comparison. Am J Ophthalmol 142:320–322
2. Bradley, Olson RJ (2006) A survey about phacoemulsification incision thermal contraction incidence and causal relationships. Am J Ophthalmol 141:222–224
3. Britton JP, Adams W, Kumar R, et al (2006) Comparison of thermal features associated with 2 phacoemulsification machines. J Cataract Refract Surg 32:288–293
4. Fishkind W, Bakewell B, Donnenfeld ED, et al (2006) Comparative clinical trial of ultrasound phacoemulsification with and without the WhiteStar system. J Cataract Refract Surg 32:45–49
5. Floyd MS, Valentine JR, Olson RJ (2006) Fluidics and Heat Generation of Alcon Infiniti and Legacy, Bausch & Lomb Millennium, and Advanced Medical Optics Sovereign Phacoemulsification Systems. AJO 142:387–392 ([3] Table 1)
6. Floyd MS, Valentine JR, Olson RJ (2006) Fluidics and Heat Generation of Alcon Infiniti and Legacy, Bausch & Lomb Millennium, and Advanced Medical Optics Sovereign Phacoemulsification Systems. AM J Ophthalmology 142: 387–392 ([3] Table 4)
7. Floyd MS, Valentine JR, Olson RJ (2006) Fluidics and heat generation of Alcon Infiniti and Legacy, Bausch & Lomb Millennium and Advanced Medical Optics Sovereign phacoemulsification systems. Am J Ophthalmology 142: 387–392
8. Georgescu D, Payne M, Olson RJ (2007) Objective measurement of postocclusion surge during phacoemulsification in human eye bank eyes. Am J Ophthalmology 143:437–440.
9. Olson MD, Miller KM (2005) In-air thermal imaging comparison of Legacy AdvanTec, Millenium, and Sovereign WhiteStar phacoemulsification systems. J Cataract Refract Surg 31:1640–1647
10. Brinton JP, Adams W, Kumar R, Olson RJ. (2006) A comparison of Legacy and Sovereign phacoemulsification machine thermal ratios using different ultrasound power settings. JCRS 32: 288–293 [1] Figure 2
11. Bradley MJ, Olson RJ. (2006) Results from a wound burn survey. AJO 141: 222–224 [10] The Table
12. Olson RJ, Jin Y, Kefalopoulos G, et al (2004) Legacy AdvanTec and Sovereign WhiteStar: a wound temperature study. J Cataract Refract Surg 30:1109–1113
13. Payne M, Waite A, Olson RJ (2006) Thermal inertia associated with ultrapulse technology in phacoemulsification. J Cataract Refract Surg 32:1032–1034
14. Georgescu D, Payne M, Olson RJ. (2007) A typical comparative set-up for four phacoemulsificiation machines in the same eye-bank-eye. AJO 143:437–440 [12] The Figure
15. Soscia W, Howard JG, Olson RJ (2002) Microphacoemulsification with WhiteStar. A wound-temperature study. J Cataract Refract Surg 28:1044–1046
16. Wade M, Isom R, Georgescu D, et al (2007) Efficacy of Cruise Control in controlling postocclusion surge with Legacy and Millenium venturi phacoemulsification machines. J Cataract Refract Surg 33:1071–1075
17. Georgescu D, Kuo AF, Kinard KI, Olson RJ. (2008) A Fluidics Comparison of Alcon Infiniti, Bausch & Lomb Stellaris, and Advanced Medical Optics Signature Phacoemulsification Machines. AJO 145:1014–1017 [14] Figure 3
18. Georgescu D, Kuo AF, Kinard KI, Olson RJ. (2008) A Fluidics Comparison of Alcon Infiniti, Bausch & Lomb Stellaris, and Advanced Medical Optics Signature

Phacoemulsification Machines. AJO 145:1014–1017 [14] Figure 1

19. Wade M, Isom R, Georgescu D, Olson RJ. (2007) The impact of Cruise Control on Millennium with the venturi pump is clearly evident. 33: 1071–1075 [13] Figure 3
20. Georgescu D, Kuo AF, Kinard KI, et al (2008) A fluidics comparison of Alcon Infiniti, Bausch & Lomb Stellaris, and Advanced Medical Optics Signature phacoemulsification machines. Am J Ophthalmology 145:1014–1017
21. Mackool RJ, Sirota MA (2005) Thermal comparison of the AdvanTec Legacy, Sovereign WhiteStar, and Millenium phacoemulsification systems. J Cataract Refract Surg 31:812–817

5.3 MICS with Different Platforms

5.3.1 MICS with the Accurus Surgical System

Arturo Pèrez-Arteaga

Core Messages

- While performing MICS with the Accurus machine, the fluidics are improved, because of the advantages of fluidics control for posterior segment surgery in addition to those for anterior segment surgery.
- The use of internal forced infusion incorporated in the Accurus machine is a very efficient tool, especially when using incision sizes of less than 1 mm.
- The internal forced infusion has the advantage of maintaining a constant positive intraocular pressure, thereby avoiding the surge
- The key to using forced infusion is to obtain a fluid rate of 45 ml/min as a minimum, with the irrigating chopper or cannula that the surgeon is accustomed to use. There is no single parameter for all devices. Settings must be individualized.
- The force of infusion can be preprogrammed and so the surgeon is able to switch between two different forces with only the foot-pedal, avoiding the need for touching the panel or the remote control.

5.3.1.1 Introduction and Historic Background

The Accurus surgical system has proved to be a magnificent tool to perform microincisional cataract surgery (MICS) because of their specific features. It was conceived by Alcon engineers as an hybrid system, containing distinctive attributes described to work

A. Pèrez-Arteaga
Centro Oftalmològico Tlalnepantla, Vallarta 42, Tlalnepantla, Mèxico, 54000, Mèxico
e-mail: drarturo@prodigy.net.mx

mainly for posterior segment surgery (vitreo-retinal procedures), but also the necessary characteristics to perform anterior segment procedures (cataract surgery and anterior vitrectomy). So when it was released in the surgical market for the first time, it was mainly used for the posterior segment surgery, and the features for cataract surgery were secondary, utilized as an accessory or auxiliary device.

When MICS was conceived for the first time by authors like Professor Jorge Aliò and Prof. Amar Agarwal, one trouble to solve was the amount of fluid incoming the eye during the phacoemulsification procedure, because the irrigating chopper has less irrigation rate than the irrigation sleeve (it has small diameter) [1–6]. So for the first time, some systems were adopted, like elevation of the bottle, use of a wider irrigation line, or even a double-bottle system, with the objective to increase the fluid incoming inside the eye and avoid surge. At that time Sunita Agarwal, from India [7], described the use of an external air pump to "push" the air inside the eye in an active way, avoiding in this way, the use of passive methods (that utilize the gravity force) to increase the incoming fluid; this method was called *external forced infusion* [8]. Nevertheless, to incorporate an external air pump was not an easy approach, because it must be calibrated in an "empirical" way, according to the diameter of the instrumentation and the amount of vacuum utilized, until the exact amount of fluid to avoid surge was obtained; furthermore, most of the air pumps utilized to create external forced infusion were not created initially for ophthalmic purposes, creating this way less confidence among the ophthalmic surgeons. At that time, we realized that the Accurus machine contained an air pump inside (conceived for posterior segment surgery, but with the possibility to be incorporated to the anterior segment procedures); so we started to work with the objective to obtain the ideal pressure according to the instrumentation utilized to perform MICS. It worked, and it worked really nice. The use of an air pump that is inside the phaco machine to actively push the fluid inside the eye and avoid in this way the surge in MICS procedures was called *internal forced infusion* (Fig. 5.15) [8–12].

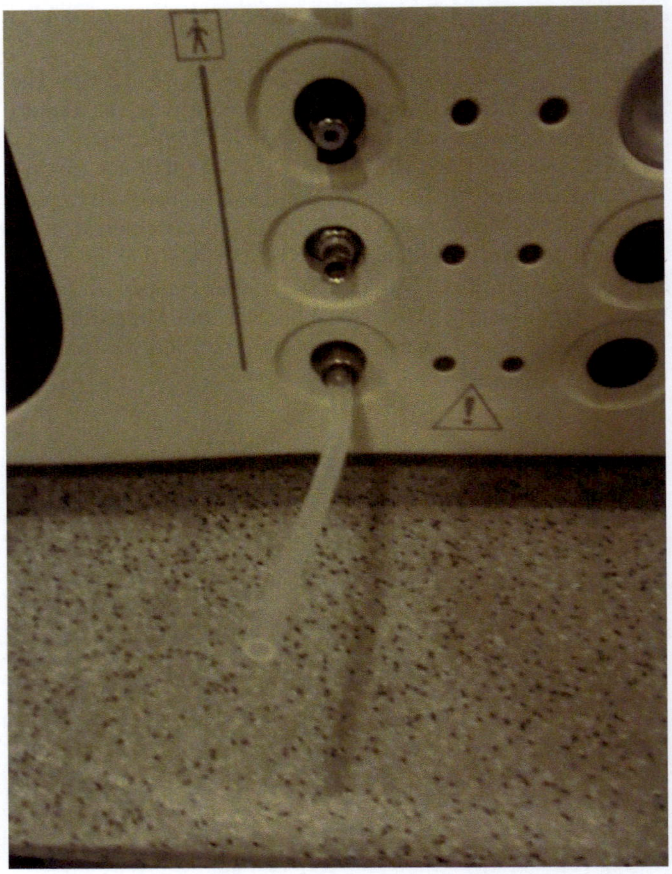

Fig. 5.15 Air Pump in the Accurus Surgical System. It is used in MICS to create Internal Forced Infusion

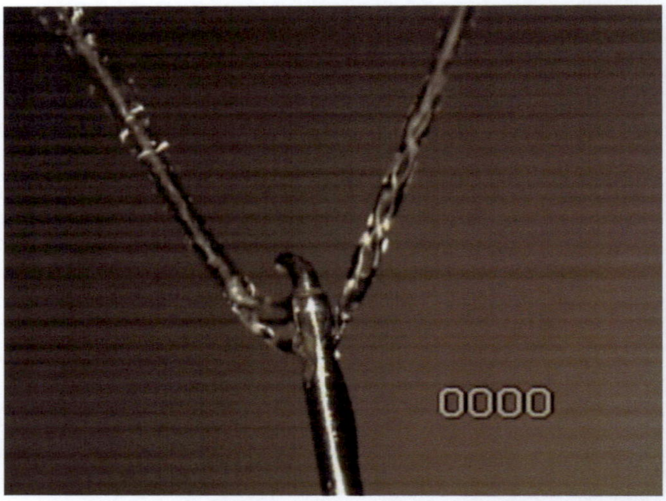

Fig. 5.16 Internal Forced Infusion active through an Alio's Irrigating Chopper

The main advantages of internal forced infusion are as follows:

1. It actively pushes fluid inside the air by creating an active air cushion inside the bottle (Fig. 5.16).
2. It can be digitally controlled at the same panel that contains the phacoemulsification settings (Fig. 5.24).
3. The parameters can be modified during the procedure according to the particular needs of the case (Figs. 5.21, 5.23 and 5.24).

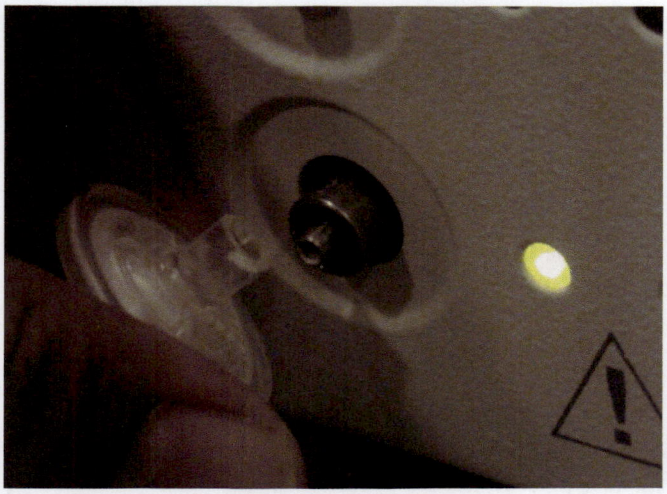

Fig. 5.17 Exit of Air in the front panel of the Accurus Surgical System with its Air Filter

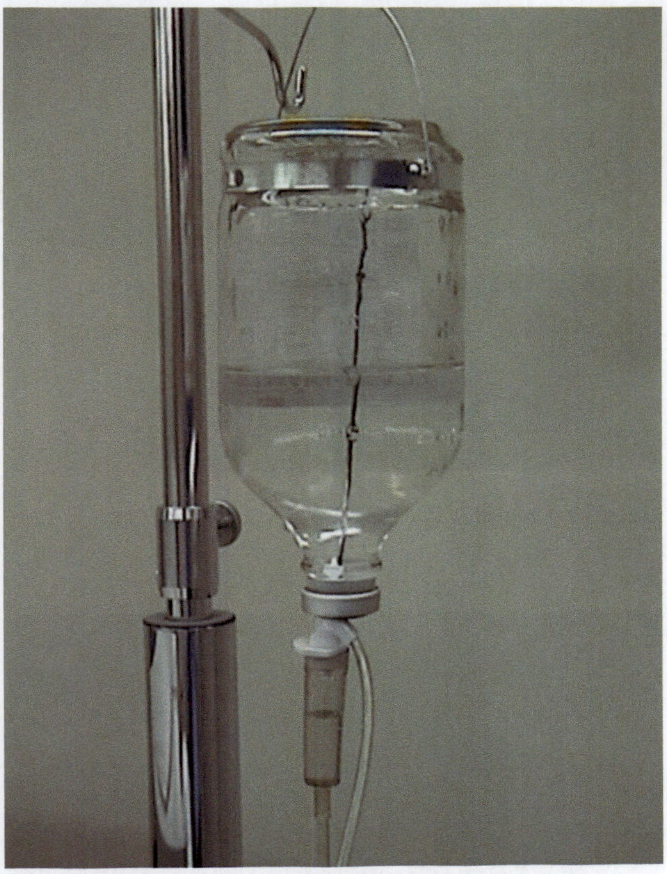

Fig. 5.18 Metal needle contained in the AVGFI System to avoid bubbles formation inside the bottle

4. The air pump is inside the same phaco machine; so there is no need to obtain it as an additional device (Fig. 5.17).

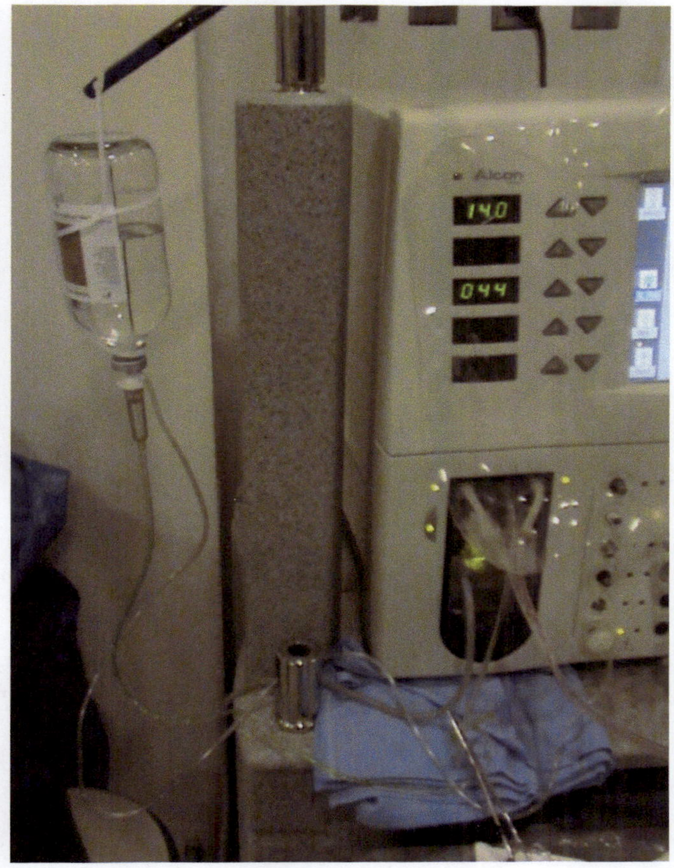

Fig. 5.19 Exit of Air in the front panel of the Accurus Surgical System with its Air Filter and the system armed

Internal forced infusion can be created with some other phaco machines that contain an air pump inside, like the Millenium Surgical System (Bausch & Lomb) [10] or the Oertly Phaco-Vitrectomy machine. Most of them are also hybrid systems, working for anterior and posterior segment surgery. Currently, new systems like Stellaris (Bausch & Lomb) are incorporating active air pump systems to improve fluidics performance.

5.3.1.2 Surgical Features of the Accurus Surgical System Useful for MICS Procedures

1. Internal air pump

The air pump is located inside the Accurus machine and the exit of air is located in the front panel in the lower portion of the machine (Fig. 5.17). An air filter must be placed to connect the air line to the bottle, with the objective to avoid contamination of the intraocular

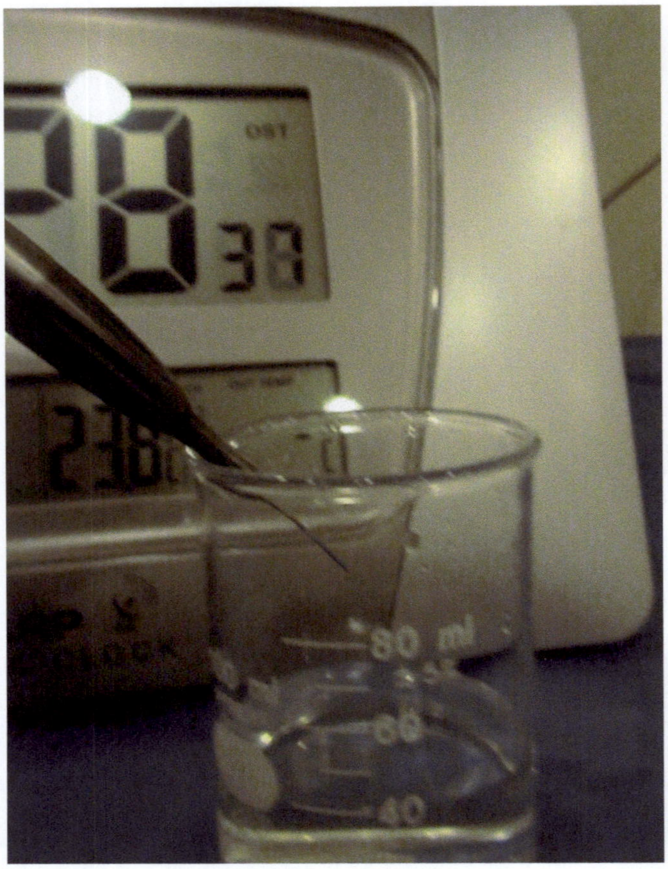

Fig. 5.20 Measure of the Rate of Infusion

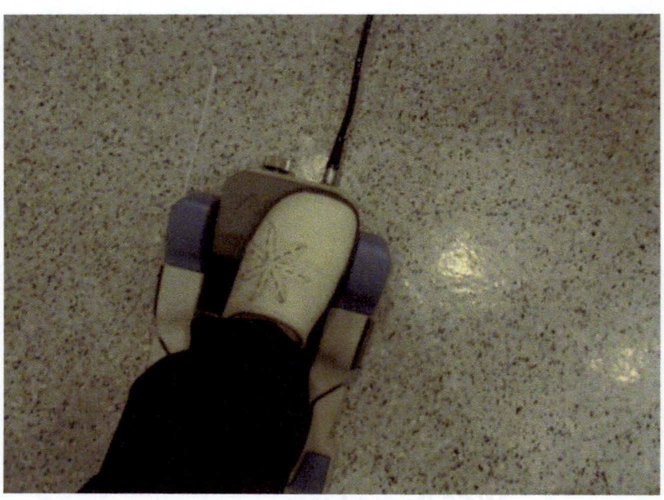

Fig. 5.21 Change of two pre-settings of Forced Infusion with the foot-pedal during surgery

solution (Fig. 5.19). This air filter is provided by Alcon within the disposable system named anterior vented gas forced infusion system (AVGFI) [11]. This AVGFI system contains an air filter, a plastic-tubing air line, a

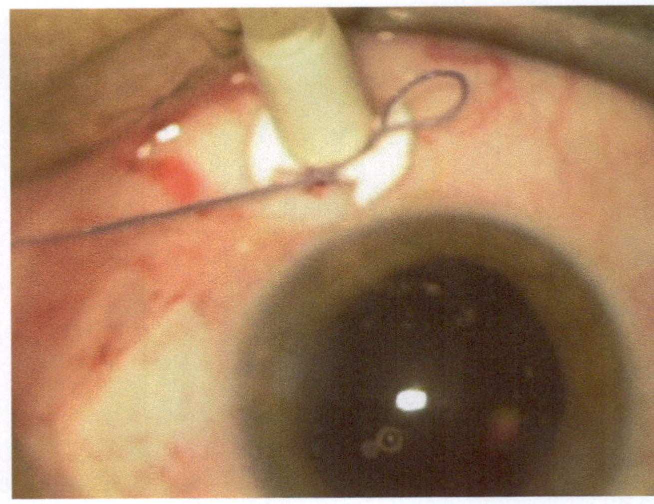

Fig. 5.22 Combined procedure, MICS & Posterior Vitrectomy. Note the corneal incisions and the absence of the lens

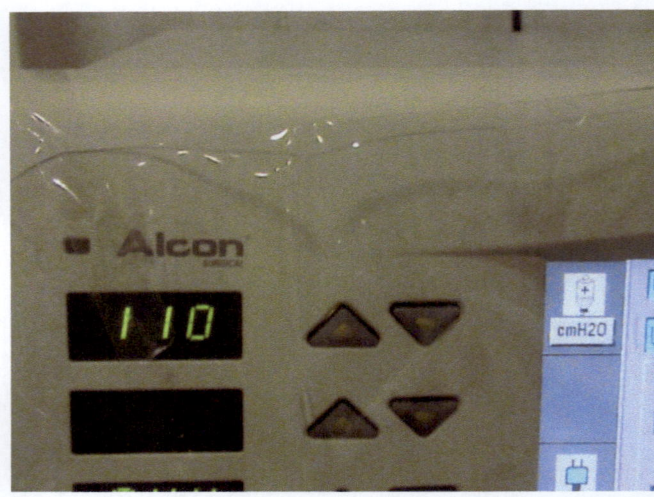

Fig. 5.23 Control of Air Pressure. Set at 110 cmH_2O

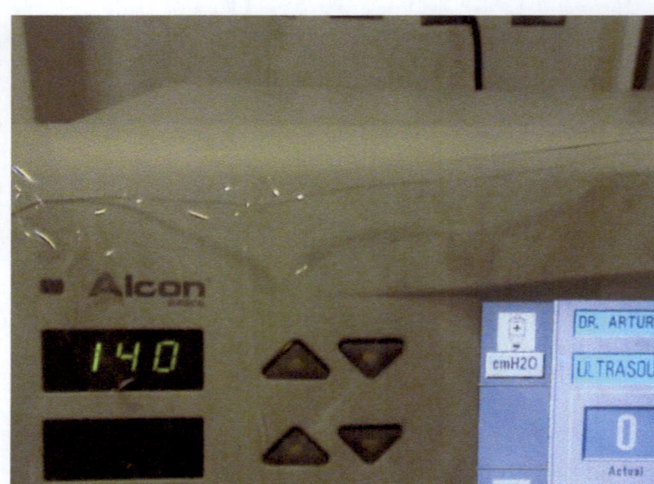

Fig. 5.24 Control of Air Pressure. Set at 140 cmH_2O

metal needle that goes inside the bottle to avoid the formation of bubbles (Fig. 5.18), a drip chamber, and the plastic-tubing line for the infusion of intraocular solution.

The control of the amount of air expulsed by the air pump to create forced infusion is at the upper portion of the panel (Fig. 5.23); it can be digitally preset manually at the panel or at the remote control of the phaco machine. Two different settings can be programmed (Figs. 5.24 and 5.22) when starting; the Accurus machine has the advantage of allowing the surgeon to switch between both established forces of infusion during the surgery through the foot-pedal, with just a movement of the foot (Fig. 5.21), without the need to loose precious time changing the parameters at the panel or at the remote control [11].

With this system, the air exits from the air pump through the air filter, goes through the air tubing, enters to the bottle through the metal needle, forms a cushion inside the bottle according to the established force, and pushes the fluid through the drip chamber and the plastic line until the fluid reaches the irrigating device (chopper or cannula) located at the end of the line (Fig. 5.25). All of the mentioned parts of the system and their work conform to the system of internal forced infusion; it works with active hydrostatic force.

The rate of infusion will experience variations according to the force of air and the diameter of the irrigation device. The rate is measured by the amount of fluid that exits the irrigation device per unit of time (rate = ml × min). An ideal rate to perform a safe MICS procedure is around 45 ml/min (Fig. 5.20). The surgeon must keep in mind that when performing surgery, two more parameters must be taken into account (conforming both the outgoing fluid): the force of vacuum and the leakage through the incisions. So the surgeon must know the machine, the parameters, the instrumentation, and the construction of incisions, in order to maintain the surgery within the limits of safety [7, 8, 12, 13].

The air pressure is measured in the Accurus machine in centimeters of water (cmH_2O), but can also be converted to millimeters of mercury (mmHg) according the preferences of the surgeon (Figs. 5.23 and 5.24). Also the surgeon must notice that for the creation of forced infusion, it is better to have the intraocular solution in a glass bottle (Fig. 5.18), so that the resistance of the material allows a true pressure; otherwise, the plastic bags have too much compliance in comparison to the glass bottle and important differences in the hydrostatic pressure can be found, leading the possibility of surge during the surgery.

2. Phaco settings

The Accurus surgical system contains different phaco modalities, all of them corresponding to longitudinal energy. No torsional ultrasound has been incorporated to this machine by Alcon engineers until the time of writing this chapter; maybe this will happen in the near future. Nevertheless, the ultrasonic modalities are the same as that of other phaco machines; linear, continuous, pulsed, burst, or microburst, all depending on the software integrated in each machine.

The phaco tip can be used as the surgeon is accustomed to; nevertheless, we must remember that the ABS tips are not useful, because they may have leakage outside the eye, leading to important surge. An angled Kelman tip can be very useful; even if the Accurus machine does not have torsional ultrasound, the angle of the tip can facilitate the fragmentation of nuclear pieces [8].

New hand pieces, new tips, and new ultrasonic modalities are released time to time by the companies in order to increase the safety and efficacy of ultrasonic power; this parameter should always be updated.

3. Venturi-based aspiration system (so named because of Giovanni Battista Venturi)

Many surgeons worldwide are afraid to use venturi systems to create aspiration because they feel less controllable in comparison to peristaltic pumps. Many phaco machines have only peristaltic systems, but with time, the venturi system has been adopted by some other machines, and some of them are hybrid, containing both. The Accurus surgical system contains a venturi system to produce aspiration, and is very well digitally controlled; it has the advantage of being a direct system not depending on the compliance of the tubes and the movement of a peristaltic pump; when you want to stop, it really stops, and does not keep vacuum inside the tubes. Also the reflux does not depend upon the movement to the opposite side of the peristaltic pump, because it only pushes fluid in a reverse mode through the same aspirating tube; so it is a really controlled reflux, just exactly like the vitreoretinal surgeons are accustomed to use. Once the surgeon starts to work with venturi systems, he/she will

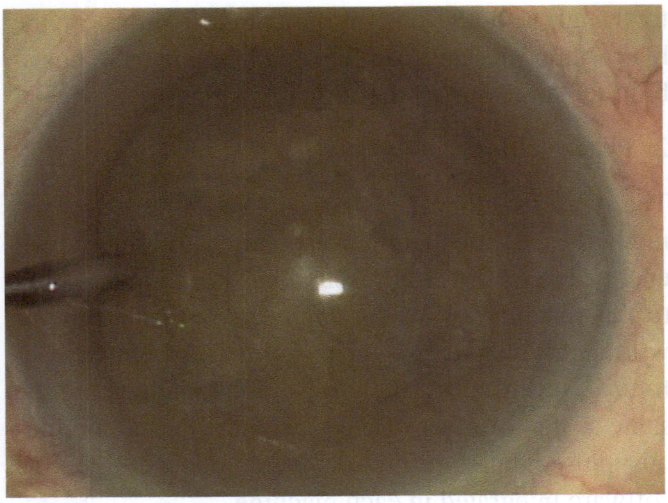

Fig. 5.25 Irrigating cannula with Forced Infusion active inside the anterior chamber. The bottle height is less important

feel confident and will see the advantages of direct vacuum technology over the peristaltic pumps. MICS works well with high vacuum levels, in particular, if you have the "no-surge insurance" that allows the forced infusion.

4. Amphibian possibilities (anterior segment only, posterior segment only, or combined procedures)

This is another important advantage of the Accurus system; it allows you to perform combined procedures (phacoemulsification and posterior vitrectomy) at the same surgical time (Fig. 5.22), with the same machine, decreasing this way, the risk of a second procedure for some patients (e.g., diabetic group), but also allowing economical benefits. It has a powerful vitrectomy system, which means a tremendous advantage in case of vitreous loss and the need of anterior vitrectomy; it can be done in a biaxial approach and with high cut parameters without the need to change machines (Fig. 5.26). This is not possible in other systems used for phacoemulsification only. So this system increases the possibilities of the vitreous management (planned or unplanned), allowing this way to an important increase in the safety of the procedure and for the patient.

5. Economical features

There are many points of view to approach the economical reasons for performing MICS with an Accurus, far away from the medical reasons:

- A combined procedure for anterior and posterior segment at the same surgical time decreases the surgical cost.
- The anterior and posterior segment surgeons can also work in different days, making the machine useful and working every day.
- If desired, the cassette system of this machine can be easily disassembled, allowing the surgeon to resterilize it for each and every case in a safe way, thereby decreasing the cost of a cassette per procedure mandatory in other phaco systems.

5.3.1.3 Surgical Parameters for MICS with Accurus

1. Irrigation

Because the surgeon is working with forced infusion, it has to be remembered that the bottle height is now not important. The bottle should be placed at the level of the machine, at the site described by the manufacturer (Fig. 5.25); the bottle height will not change while the forced infusion is at work. Nevertheless, some surgeons like to work MICS with the Accurus surgical system without the use of forced infusion utilizing only passive infusion (gravity force) to irrigate inside the eye; but we believe that this particular feature of this system must be in use in every case of MICS since it increases the control.

The initial parameter will depend upon the diameter of the irrigation device; the same amount of forced infusion (e.g., 110 cmH_2O) will lead to more infusion rate (ml/min) in a wider irrigation device (e.g., 19 G irrigating chopper) when compared with a

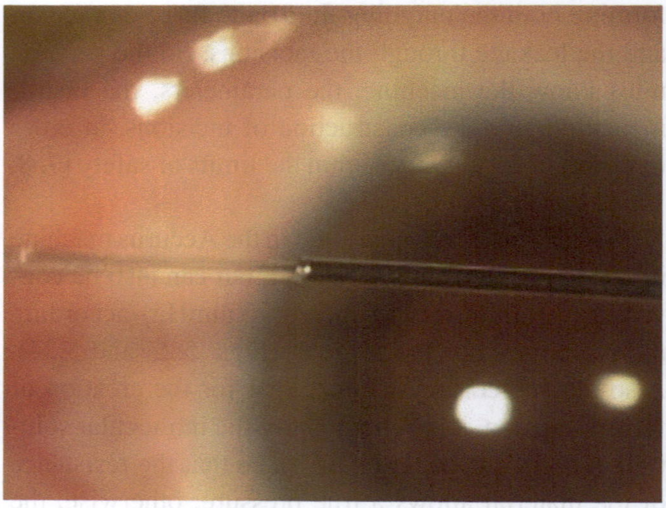

Fig. 5.26 Change of parameters and instrumentation with the same machine for many purposes

small diameter irrigation device (e.g., 22 G irrigating chopper) (Fig. 5.16). So we strongly recommend *to determine the forced infusion needed to obtain a desired infusion rate with the diameter of instrumentation available for the surgeon.* An ideal parameter of reference is 45 ml/min (Fig. 5.24); so before starting to operate, connect your AVGFI, preset the forced infusion at the determined measure (e.g., 100 cmH_2O), collocate your irrigating chopper at the end of the line, and switch-on the irrigation, measuring in a graduated glass the amount of fluid outgoing within 1 min (or 30 s multiplied by two). If you obtain less than 45 ml in a minute, increase the pressure (e.g., 110 cmH_2O) and measure again; if you obtain more than 45 ml, decrease the pressure (e.g., 90 cmH_2O) and measure again. Establish and register this parameter for each irrigating device (chopper or cannula) that you have, even if they are of the same measure, because sometimes the lumen size can vary according to different models and manufacturers. Once you have the amount of pressures needed for each of your irrigating devices, you are ready to start.

Even so, we can recommend some initial parameters according to the size of the irrigation devices: 90–100 cmH_2O for 19 G, 100–110 cmH_2O for 20 G, 110–120 cmH_2O for 21 G, and 120–140 cmH_2O for 22 G. Remember that when you experience surge you can increase the amount of forced infusion during surgery, and so you can preset two parameters at the panel of the machine and then switch between them with the foot-pedal (Fig. 5.21).

When you enter the anterior chamber and the incisions have been properly made and even the irrigation is switched-on, an equilibrium of pressures will be established between the air cushion inside the bottle, and the intraocular pressure (IOP); so you will not obtain any irrigation or any leakage (Fig. 5.27); it means that you have the right pressure and you can start with your sleeveless phacoemulsification; the fluid incoming will compensate just the fluid outgoing, and during the periods of no-aspiration, there will be no fluid incoming the eye (just like how the fluids work in a posterior vitrectomy procedure). An advantage of MICS, in particular with diameters less than 1 mm, is that the amount of total fluid utilized is by far less in comparison to the co-axial procedures.

2. Aspiration

Because it works with venturi system, it has no parameters regarding a peristaltic pump (aspiration rate); so the only one parameter to control vacuum is the amount of suction expressed in mmHg. If you do not feel confident enough to work with high vacuum levels, a good value for starting can be something between 150 and 200 mmHg. As you start to feel confident, you can increase the parameters to higher values like 250 and 300 mmHg.

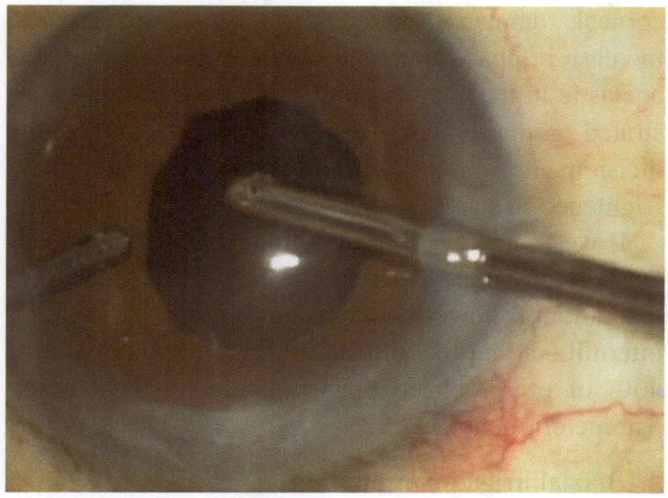

Fig. 5.27 Biaxial Anterior Vitrectomy. Balance of pressures between the irrigating force and the anterior chamber

The advantage of working with high vacuum levels is the decrease in the ultrasonic time and power, because the vacuum force acts as the main force to aspirate the nuclear pieces; this concept increases in value, in particular, when using Kelman tips that helps to produce a mechanical disruption of the pieces and of course if prechop techniques are applied before starting ultrasonic force.

3. Phacoemulsification

If a Stop & Chop technique is going to be performed and so sculpting the nucleus is under the surgical program, 25–35% of lineal phaco power is a good way to start in a continuous mode, followed by intermittent phaco (pulse or burst), just like the surgeon is accustomed to operate with any other phaco machine. If prechop techniques are in the field, no continuous phaco will be needed, and only the intermittent modes will be in use.

Even though many detractors of this technique have mentioned about the increase in the incidence of corneal thermal burns (because of the sleeveless phaco needle), it has been demonstrated in many publications of editors and contributors to this book that it is not true; the sleeveless surgery is not the cause of the corneal damage; deficient incision architecture, increase in phaco time and power, persistence of viscoelastic in the chamber and surge have been demonstrated as the main causes of corneal damage at the incision site; so the learning surgeon must not be frightened to start.

If we follow the current definition of phacoemulsification for cataract surgery (mechanical nuclear fragmentation followed by phacoaspiration assisted by intermittent and low ultrasonic force), a maximum of 40% of preset phaco power should be the starting parameter of choice.

4. Biaxial irrigation/aspiration

You can have preprogrammed parameters for the time to switch to I/A mode. Because the aspirating cannula has a smaller internal diameter than the phaco tip, less amount of irrigation and more amount of aspiration are needed; *remember to test the rate as an initial point of departure*. For biaxial I/A sets going from 19 to 22G, ideal starting parameters are 80–100 cmH_2O of forced infusion and 350–400 mmHg of vacuum; this can allow you to have a positive IOP again, no surge, enough aspirating force and fluid incoming just compensating the fluid outgoing. If the technique (in particular, suitable incisions construction) is properly done, the entire I/A can be done with no more than 20–25 ml of saline intraocular solution.

5. Biaxial anterior vitrectomy

You can also preprogram your parameters for an eventual vitreous loss. You should always keep in mind that you are operating under a biaxial approach and have a high performance machine for posterior segment surgery (unfortunately not possible when operating with an exclusive anterior segment machine); so do not try to perform the anterior vitrectomy in a coaxial approach because you will loose the entire sense of the surgery; do it in a biaxial mode (Figs. 5.25 and 5.27).

Insert the instruments (irrigation-vitrector) as you like: cornea–cornea, sclera–cornea, cornea–sclera, or sclera–sclera, but take advantage of the biaxial approach. You are working in a closed environment, the forced infusion pushes the vitreous behind the iris plane, you can have access to 360° and the positive IOP is always present. Good parameters to start may be 60–80 cmH_2O of forced infusion (remember always to decrease the infusion when your posterior capsule is broken), 150–200 mmHg of vacuum and 800 cuts per minute; with some particular posterior vitrectors, in combination with the software inside the phaco machine, you can perform more than 1,500 cuts per minute. The high speed biaxial vitrectomy is an advantage that you can only obtain with a hybrid machine; so do not let it go when needed.

5.3.1.4 Final Considerations

As you have noticed after reading this chapter, the Accurus surgical system has some specific features that can increase the safety of your MICS procedure, and can also allow the converting surgeons to transit through a smooth learning curve:

1. Digitally controlled air pump for infusion system.
2. Possibility to preprogram two different infusion pressures for different steps of the surgery, controlled in the foot-pedal by the surgeon (only one machine with this feature in the market).
3. No need to depend upon the force of gravity to create infusion, in particular, in ultra-small incision surgery.
4. Safe mode for resterilization of the cassette because of an easy disassembly.
5. Phacoemulsification features as in many other phacoemulsification machines worldwide.
6. High vacuum system.
7. Digitally controlled direct venturi system to create vacuum.
8. Direct and instantaneous reflux created with the same system, not depending upon a peristaltic pump.
9. Digitally controlled, high speed, biaxial anterior vitrectomy for cases of vitreous loss.
10. Possibility to perform combined procedures (cataract surgery plus posterior virectomy).
11. Posterior vitrectomy complete system if needed in the same surgical time (e.g., nucleus or IOL drop into the vitreous cavity).

Take Home Pearls

- The use of fluidics control utilized for posterior vitrectomy to the cataract surgery is an important advancement in modern-day cataract surgery, particularly in MICS.
- Only the machines that have posterior segment surgery and that can perform phacoemulsification (hybrid systems), are able to make full use of the advantages of the internal forced infusion.
- MICS becomes easier and safer for the surgeon when the fluid inflow into the eye is larger than the fluid outflow, even when using high vacuum, in the Accurus machine.
- Remember to be sure to preprogram your settings according the diameter of your irrigating devices, phaco needles and aspirating cannulas, before starting to operate, in order to avoid unwanted surgical surprises. You must individualize the parameters according the instrumentation that you use in MICS.

References

1. Agarwal A, Agarwal A, et al Phakonit phacoemulsification trough a 0.9 mm corneal incision. J Cataract Refract Surg 2001; 27:1548–1552
2. Agarwal A, Agarwal A, et al Phakonit: lens removal trough a 0.9 mm incision. J Cataract Refract Surg 2001; 27: 1531–1532
3. Agarwal A, Agarwal S, Agarwal A. Phakonit and laser phakonit: lens removal trough a 0.9-mm incision. Phacoemulsification, laser cataract surgery and foldable IOL's. Jaypee, New Delhi, India, 2000; 204–216
4. Tsuneoka H, Shiba T. Feasibility of ultrasound cataract surgery trough a 1.4 mm incision. J Cataract Refract Surg 2001; 27:934–940
5. Agarwal A. Bimanual 0.9 mm approach to phaco promises astigmatic neutral cataract surgery and faster rehabilitation. Eurotimes, 2003
6. Alió J. MICS ready to go. Ocular Surgery News, 2003
7. Prakash DP. Cutting phaco sleeve permits ultra-small incision surgery. Ocular Surgery News, 2003
8. Pèrez-Arteaga A. Step by step to biaxial lens surgery. Jaypee, India, 2008
9. Pérez-Arteaga A. Accurus forced infusión good for MICS. Ocular Surgery News, 2003
10. Pérez-Arteaga A. Bottle infusión tool of the millennium surgical system for phakonit. Ocular Surgery News, 2003
11. Pérez-Arteaga A. Anterior vented gas forced infusion of the accurus surgical system for phakonit. J Cataract Refract Surg 2004; 30:933–935
12. Chang D. High vacuum bimanual phaco attainable with STAAR cruise control. Ocular Surgery News, 2003
13. Vejarano LF, Tello A, Vejarano A. Phakonit incisions and use of a pressurized inflow system. J Cataract Refract Surg 2004; 30(5):939
14. Agarwal A, et al Bimanual phaco. Mastering the phakonit/MICS technique. SLACK, New Jersey, 2004
15. Agarwal A. Microphakonit surgery performed with 0.7-mm tip. Ocular Surgery News (Europe/Asia Pacific edition), 2005
16. Alió J. What is the future of cataract surgery? Ocular Surgery News (Europe/Asia-Pacific Edition), 2006
17. Alió JL, Harold Freydell, Virgilio Centurión, Norberto Amado. En Discusión: La importancia de la fluídica en la facoemulsificación. Ocular Surgery News (Latin America Edition), 2006
18. Gonzalez JM. MICS instrumentation growing in versatility, variety. Ocular Surgery News (U.S. Edition), 2004
19. Piechocki M. Surgeons await IOLs, tools for microincision surgery. Ocular Surgery News (Europe/Asia-Pacific Edition), 2003
20. Robert J. Weinstock. Advanced sleeveless microphaco: 700 micron M.I.C.S. ASCRS 2007, San Diego, CA
21. Alió J, Rodríguez-Pratz JL, Galal A, Ramzy M. Outcomes of microincision cataract surgery versus coaxial phacoemulsification. Ophthalmology 2005; 112:1997–2003

5.3.2 Using the Alcon Infiniti and AMO Signature for MICS

Richard Packard

Core Messages

- Both the Infiniti and the Signature will allow the surgeon to perform CMICS and BMICS.
- Understand the ultrasound delivery technology and choose a phaco needle suitable for your needs. The Infiniti has Ozil and the Signature has Ellips.
- Fluidics requirements will depend on the phaco tip in use and so adjust them accordingly to achieve best results. Smaller needles need higher settings.
- Remember about leakage from incisions which is critical in both CMICS and BMICS. Excessive leakage will cause the surgeon to alter fluidics settings unnecessarily.
- Once the cataract has been removed, wound-assisted lens insertion is necessary to enable incision size to be kept at a minimum.

5.3.2.1 Introduction

With the improvements in modulated ultrasound delivery and fluidics, smaller and smaller incisions for cataract surgery have become a reality for most surgeons. This chapter describes the way this author uses two of the machines (Alcon Infiniti and AMO Signature) that have been leading the move to MICS, whether it is biaxial or coaxial. The technology for ultrasound and fluidics as well as phaco tips available on these two machines will be discussed in different clinical situations using these smaller incisions.

5.3.2.2 Technology on the Alcon Infiniti

The Infiniti was introduced in 2003 with micropulsing and microburst capability, which means that ultrasound energy could be delivered in pulses of a few milliseconds. These could be used either as a continuous stream of these very short pulses of variable length and interval or at an increasing frequency up to a predetermined level. Both micropulse and microburst can be used in a linear manner to preset maximum power. The longitudinal tip movement which is traditional had torsional movement added to it in 2005. This appears to be a more efficient way of removing tissue, as there is almost no repulsion and better followability with lower aspiration flow settings. In addition, Alcon have now added the ability to set a lower as well as a higher threshold for power. This torsional phaco called Ozil is delivered in a linear manner but is measured differently from traditional phaco power; therefore, the power used is recorded as CDE (cumulative delivered energy). Ozil can be used as a continuous stream or in micropulse or burst mode. The author has reported that least energy is used in Ozil microburst mode at the expense of slightly increased foot pedal time in foot position three when compared with continuous Ozil. Micropulse Ozil seems to be the least efficient of the three modes. Although some recommend the use of a burst of longitudinal power in front of the torsional for denser nuclei, this author has not found it necessary. In order for Ozil to work effectively, some form of curved phaco needle is required to allow for the rotatory movement of the tip.

5.3.2.3 Setting Up the Infiniti for MICS

The parameters used depend on a number of different factors; the most import are, however, the phaco tip and the preferred irrigating chopper in case BMICS is used. Of course the height of the irrigation bottle will also influence the amount of fluid available to keep the anterior chamber stable. This author usually keeps the setting at 110 mm but the actual height, to be fully accurate, must be related to the position of the patient's eye.

5.3.2.4 Importance of Tip Size on Machine Fluidics Settings with the Infiniti

Alcon are offering a number of tip options for the Infiniti to be used for MICS and Ozil. However, the company is aiming at 2.2 mm incisions using CMICS as its flagship approach. Accordingly, there are both tips and sleeves

R. Packard
Prince Charles Eye Unit, Windsor, England
e-mail: mpacker@finemd.com

matched for this. The Ultra sleeve comes in two versions, a green one for the 1.1 mm Flared Kelman tip and a pink one for the 0.9 mm Tapered Kelman, Mini-flared Kelman, Mini-flared 12° with up and down bevel tips. These are all ABS (aspiration bypass system) tips with a small hole drilled on the side that is supposed to assist in occlusion break control. These are not suitable for BMICS, however, because of the ABS port which may suck up the iris. All of the above tips have some sort of restriction in their diameter along the shaft to increase resistance to lessen the impact of occlusion break on the anterior chamber stability. The need for these sorts of changes is driven by the lower amounts of irrigation fluid entering the eye due to smaller incision sizes. The selection of CMICS tip becomes even more complicated as the 0.9 mm tips are available in both a 30 and 45° bevel. One of the disadvantages of restricted tips is clogging, particularly when harder cataracts are emulsified. In order to overcome this, a 45° tip which is a more efficient cutter works best. This author prefers to use a 30° Kelman non ABS non restricted tip for CMICS using the green Ultra sleeve (Fig. 5.28). The reasons for this are:

1. No clogging
2. Better tissue hold with less vacuum due to no leakage by the tip
3. Easier occlusion of 30° tip for chopping
4. Excellent cutting with Ozil

In order to improve fluid flow into the eye through the smaller incision, the author has designed a new tip for CMICS which can also be used for BMICS; it works

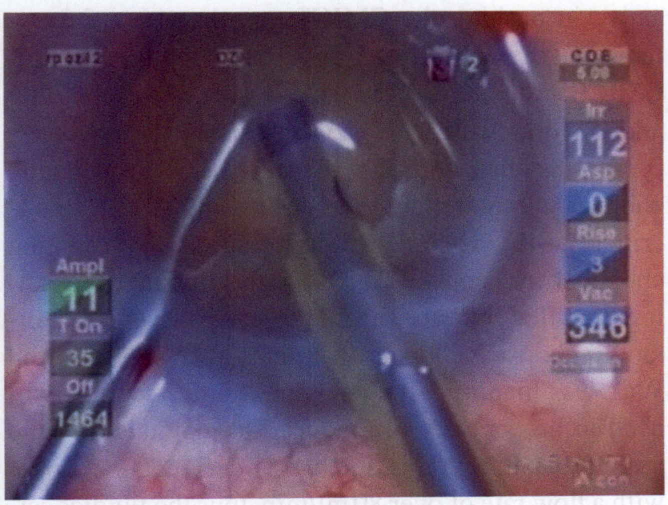

Fig. 5.28 0.9 mm Kelman tip in 2.2mm incision

with all phaco platforms. The basic shape is the standard 0.9 mm Kelman tip, but the overall diameter is reduced to 700 µm and the wall is very thin with an internal diameter of 570µm.

Owing to different internal diameters and the presence or absence of ABS with these different tips, the fluidics settings will vary to achieve the most efficient tissue removal and at the same time a stable anterior chamber. Table 5.4 summarizes the settings, this author uses for CMICS with these tips. The Infiniti has a function called Dynamic Rise which speeds or slows the pump speed on occlusion, according to the surgeon's preference for a particular case or their skill level. The

Table 5.4 Settings for the Infiniti using a variety of tips available for CMICS and BMICS

Tip	Sleeve	Sculpting setting	Segment removal setting
1.1 mm Flared Kelman ABS	Ultra green	Vacuum 50 mmHg aspiration flow rate (AFR) 20 ml/min	Vacuum 300 mmHg AFR 25 ml/min Dynamic Rise 2
0.9 mm Tapered Kelman Microtip ABS	Ultra pink	Vacuum 60 mmHg AFR 25 ml/min	Vacuum 400 mmHg AFR 28 ml/min Dynamic Rise 3
0.9 mm Mini-flared Kelman ABS 30 and 45°	Ultra pink	Vacuum 60 mmHg AFR 25 ml/min	Vacuum 400 mmHg AFR 35 ml/min Dynamic rise 3
0.9 mm Mini-flared 12° ABS 30 and 45°	Ultra pink	Vacuum 60 mmHg AFR 25 ml/min	Vacuum 400 mmHg AFR 35 ml/min Dynamic rise 3
0.9 mm Kelman Microtip non ABS 30°	Ultra green	Vacuum 50 mmHg AFR 25 ml/min	Vacuum 350 mmHg AFR 28 ml/min Dynamic rise 3
700 µm Kelman non ABS 30°	Ultra pink	Vacuum 70 mmHg AFR 26 ml/min	Vacuum 400 mmHg AFR 30 ml/min Dynamic rise 3

settings that this author uses are included in the table. A Dynamic Rise of 3 will cause the pump speed to go up by 100% on occlusion to speed the time taken to reach maximum preset vacuum.

There is going to be a new sleeve called the Nano sleeve for CMICS at 1.8 mm, which the author has used extensively, and works very well with the same fluidics settings when the Mini-flared and 700µm tips are used (Fig. 5.29).

In order to assist further with minimizing the effects of post occlusion surge, Alcon have introduced new thicker, less compliant tubing as part of a whole package called Intrepid.

As with all MICS, getting the incision size right to minimize fluid leakage is critical which applies as much to CMICS as BMICS. The main source of leakage in CMICS is the side port incision. Accordingly, the author has designed a special, double ended, second instrument with a thickened shaft (Fat Boy Chopper, Duckworth and Kent, England) to fill the side port and lessen leakage (Fig. 5.30).

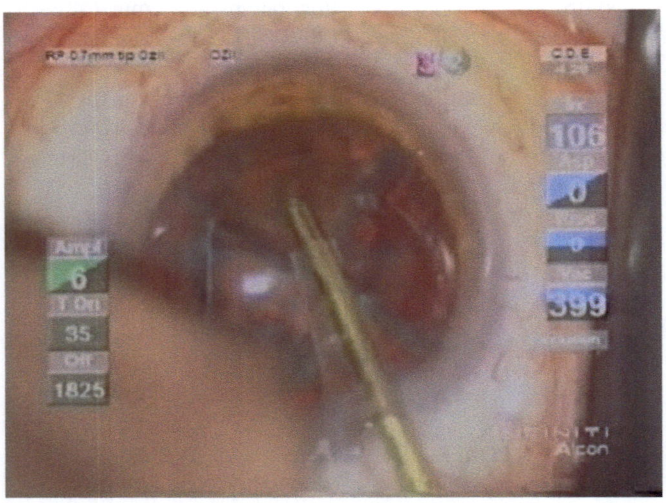

Fig. 5.29 700µm Kelman tip in action with Fat Boy chopper

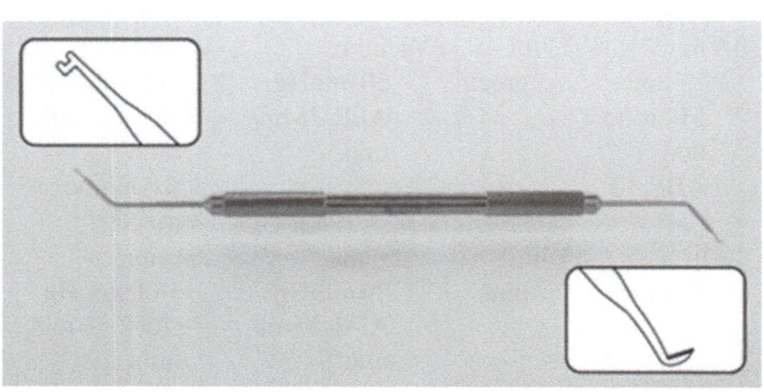

Fig. 5.30 Fat Boy chopper

This instrument is very versatile for cracking and chopping all sorts of hardness of cataract.

5.3.2.5 Setting the Ultrasound Power and Modulation with the Infiniti for MICS

In order to perform both types of MICS safely, it is important to use some form of power modulation to minimize heat rise in the wound. Although this is more important in BMICS, it becomes more of an issue in CMICS than conventional coaxial phaco because of the thinner sleeve and tighter wound. Ozil, even in continuous form, produces much less heat rise in the tip than longitudinal phaco. The author uses it in continuous linear form with a preset maximum of 50% for soft and medium nuclei and 100% for dense ones. This is just to sculpt a small hole in the nucleus to allow the Kelman tip to bury deep in the nucleus for chopping. For the actual chopping and segment removal the settings are changed to microburst Ozil as mentioned above. The on time for the burst is 35 ms and the off time when the foot pedal is fully depressed is 40 ms. The maximum power is set at 100%. This sort of setting will produce CDE readings of the order of 2–3 for soft cataracts, 6–7 for medium and up to 25 for really dense ones. Using continuous Ozil for segment removal will lead to much higher energy usage which is not necessary.

5.3.2.6 The Infiniti and BMICS

Although Alcon as a company have been much more active in pushing the CMICS agenda with a 2.2 mm incision, the Infiniti can be used perfectly well for BMICS. The author first used it in that way in 2004 and it works well with Ozil also using the non ABS 0.9 mm Kelman tip. As with all BMICS, an irrigating chopper is required and the design and size of this is critical to the machine settings (Fig. 5.31). Irrigating choppers vary considerably as to the amount of irrigating fluid that they are capable of releasing. It is important to choose a chopper that gives at least 60 ml/min. With less than this, the machine fluidics settings will need to be considerably reduced to maintain a stable anterior chamber. This author has designed a chopper with a flow rate of over 80 ml/min, thus the fluidics settings as in Table 5.4 do not need altering.

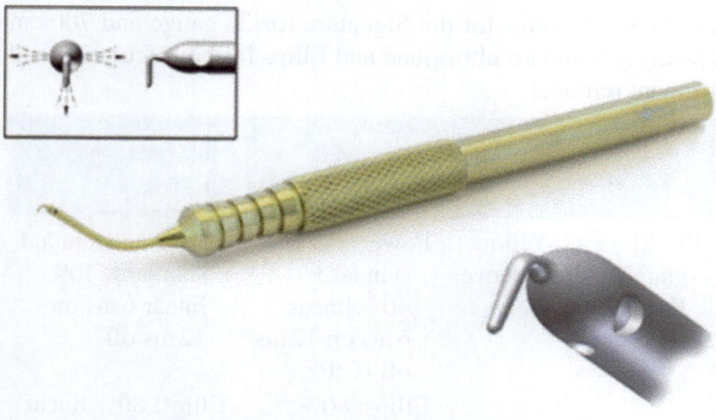

Fig. 5.31 Packard irrigating chopper (Duckworth and Kent, England)

As with all BMICS, part of the balance is about getting the incision sizes right for the instruments going into the eye. The 0.9 mm phaco needle goes through 1.4 mm incision and the chopper through 1.6 mm both of these being the internal diameter of the wound. Ideally a trapezoidal wound should be created to allow instrument movement without damaging the wound and making closure at the end of the operation an issue.

5.3.2.7 Technology for MICS on the AMO Signature

In 2001 on the AMO Sovereign phaco machine, the previous model to the Signature, White Star power modulation using micropulsing was introduced for the first time. This was then further modified 2 years ago with ICE (increased control and efficiency). This was a means of adding a 1 ms punch at the beginning of each pulse of phaco energy at a higher power. The punch could be programmed to stay the same as the energy increases, or be either increased or decreased as the rest of the energy is increased. The object was to allow for enhanced cavitation by pushing a piece of nucleus away and allowing BSS (balanced salt solution) to enter the space created. Since cavitation largely occurs above 70% power settings and certainly this author uses only 40% power settings, it is debatable whether, even if this actually takes place, it is beneficial. It would be difficult to show any difference between the various settings for ICE that would help this debate. As on the Sovereign there is a range of pulse settings. It is useful to be able to use different settings for the tip in both occluded and unoccluded modes. The note of ultrasound delivery changes as the tip occludes and long before the maximum preset vacuum is reached. There is no dedicated sleeve for CMICS available for the Signature; however, the existing yellow sleeve works well with an incision size of 2.2 mm. This is of course not important for BMICS where the sleeve is irrelevant, except to reduce spray from the phaco needle.

Issues around repulsion of nuclear material which had been a driver for other systems have also been addressed on the Signature by the introduction of a lateral movement of the phaco needle; here, it is also accompanied by a longitudinal movement. 50% of the available power goes to longitudinal and 50% to lateral movement. This is called Ellips™ to describe the sort of movement that the tip is making. It does not require a Kelman style needle to work unlike torsional movement on the Infiniti. The division of the power delivered into two components means that the settings need to be altered considerably. Approximately double the settings are recommended, i.e., if the longitudinal setting is for 40% power, raise this to 80% for Ellips. Further, the pulse settings need to be altered to have a much higher duty cycle to be able to sculpt hard nuclei and get good burying of the tip for chopping, to remove hard nuclei. This author's initial experience has indicated good followability compared to longitudinal alone and reduced repulsion. However the ability to cut into dense nuclei and bury the tip even with a Kelman phaco tip does not, with current settings, seem to be as good as conventional longitudinal phaco on the Signature, when pulse settings with White Star are used. As with Ozil on the Infiniti, using the Ellips technology in continuous mode works better for some parts of nuclear removal, such as sculpting and starting to bury the phaco needle for chopping.

The Signature has a development of the fluidics control seen originally on the Sovereign called CASE (chamber stabilization environment). Here in order to help post occlusion surge, the chosen vacuum in segment removal mode can be held for a time limited period of up to 3 s. Various thresholds can be set for different events in the raising and lowering of vacuum. This can be done on the screen of the Signature in an active manner by moving a cursor. It customizes the machine responses to the individual surgeon's technique and needs in a given operative situation (Fig. 5.32).

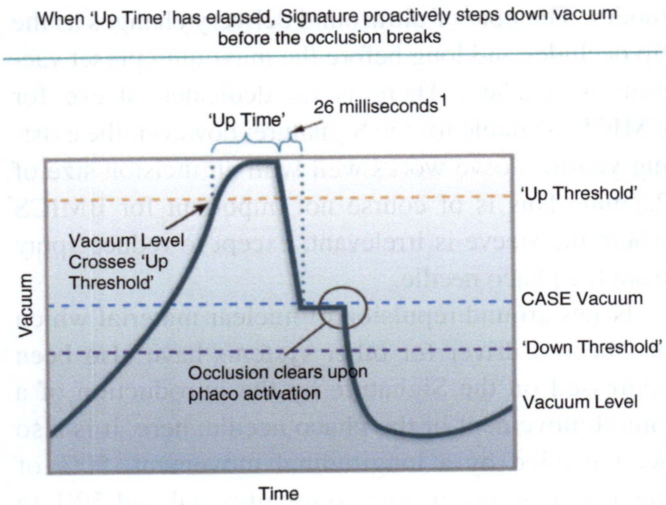

Fig. 5.32 Proactive vacuum adjustment using CASE

5.3.2.8 Applying Signature Technology to CMICS and BMICS

A standard 30° 20 gauge Kelman style needle supplied by AMO was used initially for both C and BMICS. Latterly the 700∝m needle mentioned above has been tried, which works very well. The settings for both C and BMICS are the same but again are tip specific (Table 5.5).

As can be seen from the table, the settings available are varied and many. This table sets out only the basics for each type of ultrasound delivery Standard longitudinal and Ellips transversal. To set up the machine for these settings is relatively straight forward but initially may require some help from a company representative. These settings will work well for all grades of cataract with one exception. For soft/medium nuclei the sculpting setting is used to chop, as this is sufficient vacuum to hold the nucleus without pulling it through the phaco needle. Once the nucleus is chopped, the higher settings are used to remove the nucleus. The author calls this the "soft chop" technique. Both Standard and Ellips ultrasound will work well to get the desired occlusion in this way.

Both the Infiniti and the Signature work well for CMICS and BMICS (Figs. 5.33 and 5.34). This author is currently implanting the Acrysof IQ as his lens of choice for these small incisions using the D cartridge and the Duckworth and Kent single handed injector through a 1.8 mm incision with the Infiniti for B and CMICS, and the Signature for BMICS. CMICS with the Signature is done currently through 2.2 mm incisions due to lack of a suitable sleeve for anything smaller.

Table 5.5 Settings for the Signature for 20 gauge and 700∝m tips using Standard ultrasound and Ellips for both sculpting and segment removal

Tip	Sleeve	Sculpting	Chopping and segment removal
30° 20 gauge Kelman style	Yellow sleeve	Power standard: 40% linear 6 ms on 12 ms off (C:F) Ellips: 80% linear continuous Vacuum: 60 mmHg Aspiration: 25 ml/min	Power unoccluded standard: 40% linear 6 ms on 12 ms off Ellips: 80% linear continuous Occluded Standard: 40% linear four long pulses per second of C:F Ellips: 80% linear six short pulses per second Maximum vacuum: 350 mmHg CASE vacuum 300 mmHg Aspiration: 28 ml/min
30° 700∝m Kelman style	Yellow sleeve	Power settings as above Vacuum: 70 mmHg Aspiration: 30 ml/min	Power settings as above Maximum vacuum: 400 mmHg CASE: 320 mmHg Aspiration: 30 ml/min

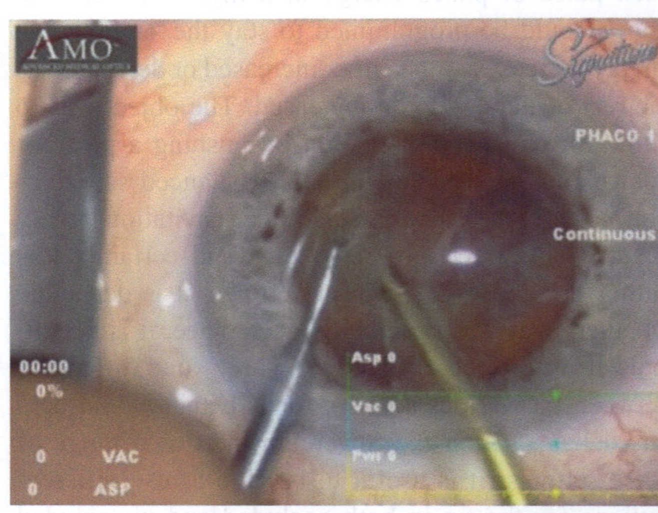

Fig. 5.33 CMICS using 700∝m tip and Signature

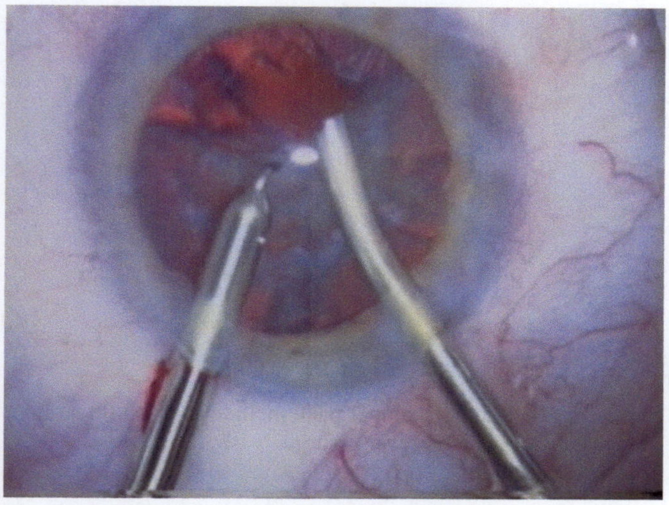

Fig. 5.34 BMICS with Signature

Take Home Pearls

- Appropriate choice of incision size, tip size, ultrasound and fluidics settings is essential for successful MICS with either the Infiniti or Signature phaco machines.
- Wound-assisted lens insertion with minimal enlargement with BMICS and none with CMICS completes the procedure with both these machines.

5.3.3 MICS with Different Platforms: Stellaris Vision Enhancement System

Mark Packer, I. Howard Fine, and Richard S. Hoffman

Core Messages

- Innovative design concepts incorporated into the Stellaris Vision Enhancement System make it a superlative choice for MICS. These concepts include monitoring and maintenance of fluidic parameters, millisecond level surgeon control of ultrasound power and ergonomic comfort and adaptability for any surgical technique.
- The Stellaris Vision Enhancement System is safe and effective for BMICS and CMICS.
- The advantages of BMICS include enhanced surgical flexibility and control made possible by separation of inflow and outflow.
- The CMICS solution enables the incision to be decreased to 1.8 mm without any change in the current coaxial phaco technique.

5.3.3.1 Innovations in Phacoemulsification

The Stellaris Vision Enhancement System (Bausch & Lomb, San Dimas, CA) represents revolutionary progress in phacoemulsification technology (Fig. 5.36). Building on the success of the Millennium, which has offered both Venturi and peristaltic pumps with dual linear foot pedal control, the Stellaris incorporates multiple advances in design. Innovative Stellaris System technology includes the Advanced Flow Module that allows intraoperative toggling between flow and vacuum modes, and also accurately monitors and maintains targeted vacuum levels and intraoperative aspiration rate; the StableChamber Pack, containing small diameter

M. Packer (✉)
Oregon Health & Science University, Drs. Fine, Hoffman and Packer, 1550 Oak Street, Eugene, OR 97401, USA
e-mail: mpacker@finemd.com

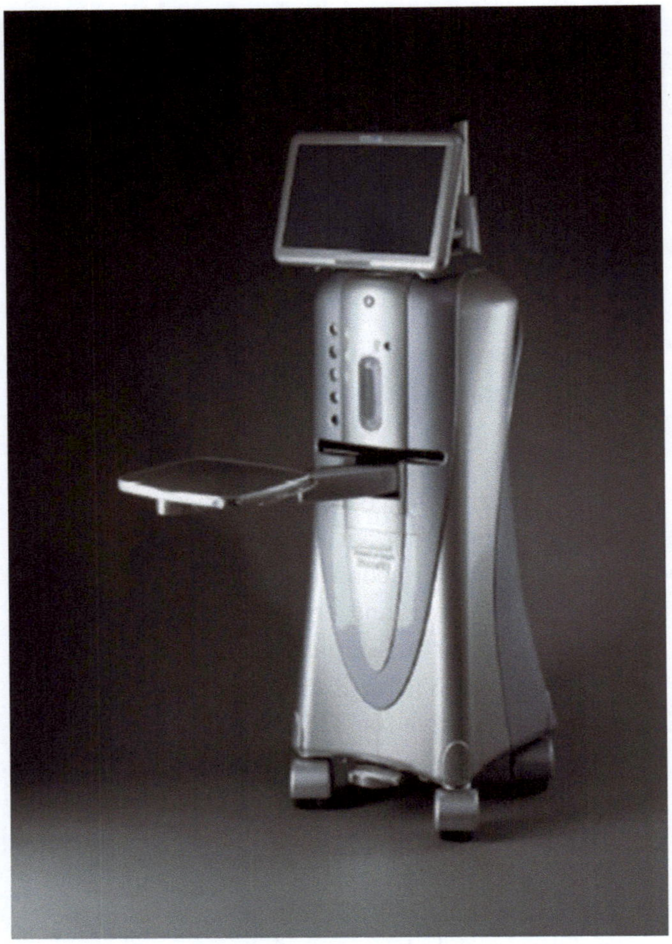

Fig. 5.35 The Stellaris vision enhancement system presents a sleek and flexible design

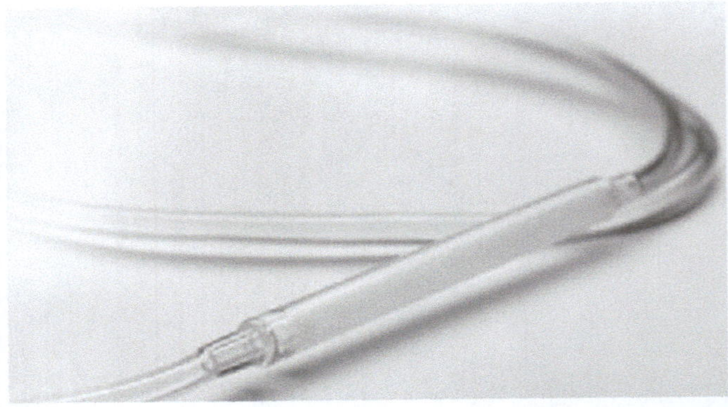

Fig. 5.36 The StableChamber pack includes a mesh filter and a flow restriction which prevents surge

tubing that increases resistance for high vacuum and steady low flow with internal mesh designed to capture material and prevent clogging; CustomControl Software II that permits millisecond range modulation ultrasound control and variable duty cycle application of 28.5 kHz ultrasound for optimized cavitation and rapid emulsification with minimal thermal loading; Bluetooth wireless dual linear foot pedal for instantaneous surgeon control of aspiration and ultrasound; and a light and agile six-crystal configuration handpiece for enhanced ergonomics and balance. These advances in technology provide real advantages for Micro Incision Cataract Surgery, both biaxial and coaxial.

The Stellaris provides solid chamber stability with EQ (equalizing) Fluidics Management Technology in vacuum or flow modes through equalization of aspiration and irrigation. This innovative system allows surgeons to equalize aspiration and irrigation for solid chamber stability in flow and vacuum modes when using advanced MICS techniques. Sensing technology accurately maintains preset vacuum and aspiration flow throughout the procedure for smooth, safe, and efficient material removal. The unique EQ technology monitors vacuum levels in flow mode, and precisely measures and controls vacuum when in vacuum mode for predictable performance. EQ-sensing technology monitors and adjusts flow to pre-emptively reduce the effects of postocclusion surge. Once occlusion breaks, Stellaris regulates the Flow in the aspiration line stabilizing the anterior chamber for increased control and safety.

In addition, the StableChamber pack controls flow for added chamber stability in high vacuum settings preferred for C and BMICS (Fig. 5.36). The pack essentially consists of small diameter tubing integrated into the aspiration line that increases resistance for high vacuum and steady low flow. Internal mesh designed to capture material and prevent clogging minimizes variability in steady state flow. The flow restriction in the StableChamber pack, together with the EQ-sensing technology that monitors and maintains stable pressure for predictable surgery, provides exceptional post occlusion surge responsiveness for rapid return to equalized state for solid chamber stability.

The Stellaris also features unique integration of latest-generation centrifugal pump and valve technology for responsiveness and aspiration efficiency that exceeds the performance of earlier Venturi systems. Advanced sensing technology accurately monitors and maintains targeted vacuum levels and intraoperative aspiration rate. These features safely increase the vacuum limit from 550 to 600 mmHg. Also, the Stellaris eliminates the need for an external gas supply by using an all-electric design. Additional safety features in the fluidics include real-time display of cassette fluid volume via an optical sensor, increased capacity 300 ml cassette and SureLock locking irrigation connectors.

On the power delivery side, the unique six-crystal handpiece is ergonomically designed for excellent balance, and accurately and consistently focuses on efficient cutting dynamics at the nucleus (Fig. 5.37). The CustomControl Software II permits millisecond level control of ultrasound application, with optimized 28.5 kHz frequency cavitation for rapid emulsification. Precise control of power modulation for customized energy wave patterns results in low overall phaco time.

Overall ultrasound energy released in the eye correlates with handpiece operating frequency – the higher the frequency, the higher the energy dose.

The lower 28.5 kHz frequency allows for optimized cavitation and rapid emulsification with minimal thermal loading. Also, an increased stroke length permits more efficient cutting of the nucleus.

Dual linear simultaneous foot pedal control of aspiration and ultrasound enhances surgical safety (Fig. 5.38).

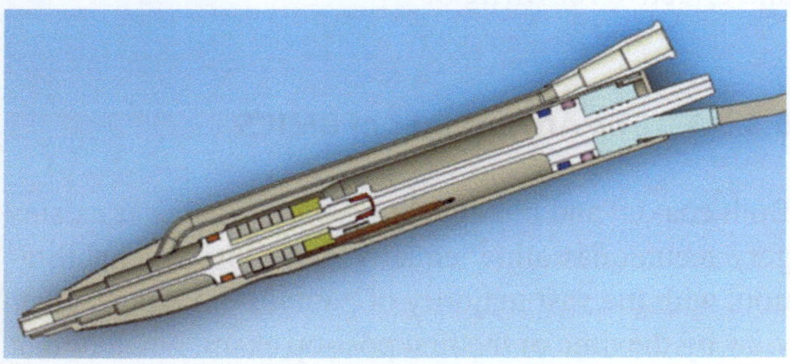

Fig. 5.37 The ergonomic six crystal handpiece is easy to hold and manipulate

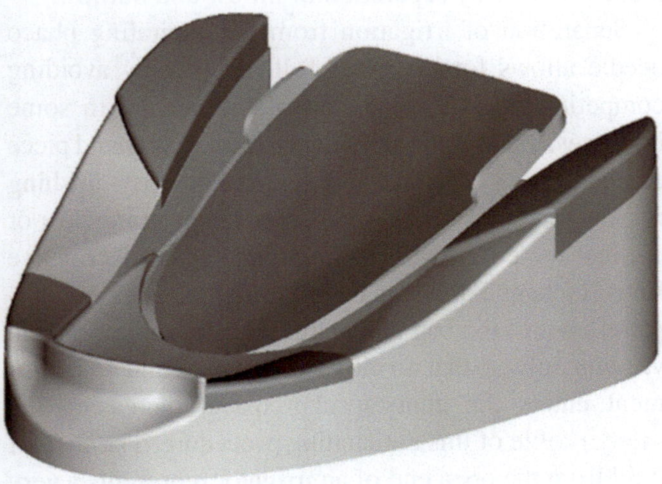

Fig. 5.38 The wireless dual linear foot pedal increases flexibility in the OR and provides increased surgical control

Both the surgeon and OR staff will enjoy the convenience and freedom of the Wireless Dual-Linear foot pedal. There is instantaneous response and control of critical intraoperative surgical parameters with no discernible lag. Of course, preprogrammable foot pedal settings are customizable to surgeon technique.

An intuitive interface and video overlay allows for ease of use by OR staff for set up and priming and fast OR turnaround. The Stellaris features a modular design for easy upgrades, and TruLink Customer Support Network connectivity. These features taken together make the Stellaris a truly twenty-first century phaco machine.

5.3.3.2 Evaluating the Stellaris Vision Enhancement System

In order to assess the facility of use, safety and efficacy of the Stellaris Vision Enhancement System for bimanual micro incision cataract surgery, we undertook a prospective study of 30 unselected eyes of 26 patients presenting for cataract surgery with a single surgeon (MP) using the Advanced Flow System Vacuum Emulation (Table 5.6). Outcome measures included surgical time, Effective Phaco Time and Average Phaco Power, frequency of complications and uncorrected visual acuity at the first postoperative visit (either the same day or the next day).

The patient population was representative of our practice and included 13 women and 13 men with a mean age of 64.2 ± 8.3 years. The mean nucleus grade was 1.4 + NS. Among the group of subjects there were four eyes with a history of LASIK, one eye with pseudoexfoliative glaucoma, eye with pigment dispersion syndrome, one eye with strabismic amblyopia, two eyes with epiretinal membrane.

The surgical technique employed our current standard methods. The evolution of these techniques for bimanual micro incision phaco may be reviewed in a variety of publications [1–4]. Briefly, two single-plane 1.2–1.4 mm trapezoidal incisions are made with a diamond knife about 60° apart in the temporal clear cornea. Aqueous is exchanged for a dispersive viscoelastic and a continuous curvilinear capsulorhexis is constructed with pinch type forceps. Following hydrodissection and hydrodelineation the nucleus is impaled, chopped and mobilized utilizing one of a variety of 20 gauge irrigating choppers and a 30° beveled straight phaco needle.

Table 5.6 Parameters for BMICS with the Stellaris advanced flow system vacuum emulation

Phaco		IA		IA Viscoelastic removal	Vit	
	Chop	Flip	IA	BI/COAX	Hi speed	Regular (pneum)
Power (%)	20 Linear (waveform not enabled)	20 linear			Cut rate: 1,500 cpm	Cut rate: 600 cpm
Mode	30 pps	Fixed burst duration: 10 ms Interval: 30 ms			(Yaw to turn cutter on/off)	
Duty cycle (%)	30	25				
Vac (yaw for max)	125–325	250–325	500 Linear	500 Fixed	150 Linear	150 Linear
Flow	NA	30 Fixed	NA	30	30 Fixed	25 Fixed
Vacuum response	2	2				
Bottle ht	140	140	140	140/80	75	50
In programs	Lin vac ACF	Fixed flow linear vac	Linear fac	Linear flow fixed vac		

Dr. Packer, B & L Stellaris Bi-manual Advance Flow System-vac, October 3 2007
Choose: packer afm vac
Vit – vitrectomy; Pps – pulses per second; Ht – high

Epinucleus management permits simultaneous extraction of cortex in the great majority of cases. The capsule and anterior chamber are filled with a cohesive viscoelastic and limbal relaxing incisions are performed if indicated for the correction of keratometric astigmatism [5]. LRIs are performed prior to intraocular lens (IOL) insertion at 90% depth and the10 mm optical zone, following the Nichamin nomogram. A single plane temporal clear corneal incision is constructed and the posterior chamber IOL is placed in the capsule, usually by means of an insertion device (shooter). The residual viscoelastic is irrigated and aspirated from the eye. The corneal stroma is hydrated at each incision site and a Seidel test is performed to insure a watertight closure.

Of the 30 eyes in our study, 12 (40%) were implanted with presbyopia correcting IOLs (5 ReZoom, 4 crystalens and 2 ReStor). Sixteen eyes (53%) were implanted with cornea customized-aspheric IOLs (9 Tecnis, 4 AcrySof IQ and 3 SofPort AO). Ten eyes (30%) had Limbal Relaxing Incisions. The mean surgery time from start to end was 19.7 ± 5.5 min. The Mean Effective Phaco Time measured 0.77 ± 1.58 s, and the Average Phaco Power was 2.04 ± 2.25%. There were no complications.

At the first postoperative visit, the mean uncorrected visual acuity measured 20/30 (excluding eyes with preexisting pathology and prior surgery). 75% of eyes read 20/40 or better, 63% 20/30 or better, 53% 20/25 or better and 32% 20/20 or better. We concluded that the Stellaris Vision Enhancement System is safe and effective for BMICS.

5.3.3.3 The Advantages of BMICS

Both coaxial and bimanual micro incision cataract surgery techniques allow equally rapid visual rehabilitation, with the vast majority of patients enjoying a clear view by the time of the first post-op exam, whether that exam is conducted on the day of or the day after surgery [6]. We prefer the bimanual technique primarily because of the enhanced surgical flexibility and control made possible by separation of inflow and outflow.

Separation of irrigation from the aspirating phaco needle allows for improved followability by avoiding competing currents at the tip of the needle. In some instances, the irrigation flow from the second hand piece can be used as an adjunctive surgical device – flushing nuclear pieces from the angle or loosening epinuclear or cortical material from the capsular bag. In Refractive Lens Exchange, the lens material may be washed completely out of the bag and extracted with aspiration and vacuum only, so that no ultrasound is used and no instrument enters the endocapsular space, increasing the safety profile of this demanding procedure. The flow of fluid from the open end of an irrigator represents a very gentle instrument which can mobilize material without trauma to delicate intraocular structures.

Another benefit of a separate infusion stream comes to bear in polishing the posterior capsule. Focusing the flow of fluid on the posterior capsule and putting the tissue on stretch facilitates capsule polishing with either a roughened or silicone-covered aspiration tip. The taut posterior capsule shows less inclination to become entrapped in the aspiration port, and the subcapsular plaque material is more easily stripped away.

Perhaps the greatest advantage of the bimanual technique lies in its ability to remove subincisional cortex without difficulty. As originally described by Brauweiler [7], by switching infusion and aspiration hand pieces between two symmetric incisions, 360° of the capsular fornices are easily reached and cortical clean-up can be performed quickly and safely. The ability to switch hands also represents a significant advantage to instructors of phacoemulsification, who may find that they must take over a case from a resident with opposite handedness [8].

Bimanual phaco also provides significant advantages in complication management. If the posterior capsule is compromised during surgery, the first goal of the surgeon is to maintain stability of the anterior chamber to prevent both posterior migration of lens material and anterior prolapse of the vitreous. By maintaining infusion in the anterior chamber, it becomes safer to reach posteriorly with the phaco needle, aspiration tip, or vitrector, to remove residual lens tissue. Irrigation need never be brought down into the capsule where it may dislodge lens tissue, enlarge the capsular tear or engage the vitreous. Hypotony is avoided at all times by keeping the flow of irrigation constant, much in the same way that an anterior chamber maintainer works [9]. Once all lens material has been evacuated from the eye, viscoelastic may be injected prior to removal of the irrigator so that the vitreous face remains under tamponade.

Utilization of bimanual phaco for refractive lens exchange and routine cataract surgery also offers an advantage of maintaining a more stable intraocular environment during lens removal. This may be especially important in high myopes who are at a greater risk for retinal detachment following lens extraction [10]. By maintaining a formed and pressurized anterior chamber throughout the procedure, there should be fewer tendencies for anterior movement of the vitreous body with a theoretically lower incidence of posterior vitreous detachment occurring from intraoperative manipulations. Future studies will need to be performed in order to document a significant reduction in posterior segment morbidity utilizing this method of lens removal.

Some of the major advantages we have seen from bimanual phaco do relate to incision size, for example, there has been an improvement in control of most of the steps involved in endocapsular surgery due to increase chamber stability. Since viscoelastics do not leave the eye as easily through these small incisions, the anterior chamber is more stable during capsulorhexis construction and there is much less likelihood for an errant rhexis to develop. This added margin of safety is particularly noticeable in cases of zonular compromise such as pseudoexfoliation, traumatic zonular dialysis and status post glaucoma filtering surgery, as well as in cases of intumescent cataract and nanophthalmos with a very shallow anterior chamber [11]. The added chamber stability can also make a difference in control of the capsulorhexis in high myopia with an extremely deep anterior chamber and floppy capsule. The adoption of bimanual techniques has also served as a catalyst for instrument manufacturers, who have developed delicate, exquisite forceps for the construction of the capsulorhexis.

References

1. Fine IH, Packer M, Hoffman RS. Transition to bimanual microincision phaco. In: Garg A, Pandey SK, Chang DF, Papadopoulos PA, Maloof AJ (eds). Advances in Ophthalmology Interactive CD-ROM. New Delhi, Jaypee Brothers, 2005
2. Hoffman RS, Fine IH, Packer M. Bimanual micro-phacoemulsification. In: Alio JL, Rodriguez Prats JL, Galal A (eds). MICS: Micro-Incision Cataract Surgery.El Dorado, Panama, Highlights of Ophthalmology International, 2004
3. Packer M, Fine IH, Hoffman RS. Bimanual ultrasound phacoemulsification. In: Fine IH, Packer M, Hoffman RS (eds). Refractive Lens Surgery. Heidelberg, Springer, 2005, pp 193–198
4. Fine IH, Hoffman RS, Packer M. Optimizing refractive lens exchange with bimanual micro-incision phacoemulsification. J Cataract Refract Surg 2004; 30: 550–554
5. Tehrani M, Mamalis N, Hoffman RS, Fine IH, Dick B, Packer M. Surgical correction of astigmatism. In: Gills JP (ed). A Complete Surgical Guide for Correcting Astigmatism: An Ophthalmic Manifesto. Thorofare, NJ, Slack, 2003
6. Packer M, Fine IH, Hoffman RS. Bimanual microincision phacoemulsification. In: Fine IH (ed). Perspectives in Lens & IOL Surgery. EyeWorld 2006; 11(2): 60–63; 72
7. Brauweiler P. Bimanual irrigation/aspiration. J Cataract Refract Surg 1996; 22: 1013–1016
8. Smith JH. Teaching bimanual microincision cataract surgery in a residency program. Symposium on Cataract, IOL and Refractive Surgery, ASCRS, Washington, DC, 19 April 2005

9. Blumenthal M. Use and results using the new ACM. Symposium on Cataract, IOL and Refractive Surgery, ASCRS, Washington, DC, 18 April 2005
10. Colin J, Robinet A, Cochener B. Retinal detachment after clear lens extraction for high myopia: seven-year follow-up. Ophthalmology 1999; 106: 2281–2284
11. Olson R. Viscoelastic to the rescue. In: Obstbaum SA (moderator), Advances in Cataract Surgery: Devices, Applications, Techniques. Ophthalmology Times Supplement 3, 1 April 2004; 29: 12–13

Take Home Pearls

- For the BMICS and CMICS surgeon, the Stellaris Vision Enhancement System offers improved efficiency and safety with superior ergonomic design and flexibility.
- Although smaller incision size has advantages, such as greater chamber stability and reduction of induced astigmatism, we feel that the greatest advantage of BMICS stems from the separation of infusion and aspiration.

Surgical Technique – How to Perform a Smooth Transition

6

Mark Packer, Jennifer H. Smith, I. Howard Fine, and Richard S. Hoffman

Core Messages

- The advantages of micro incision phaco outweigh any increased difficulty or complications that occur during a surgeon's early experience with the technique.
- The many advantages of biaxial micro incision phaco are easily accessible to the skilled cataract surgeon.

The advantages of micro incision phaco outweigh any increased difficulty or complications that occur during a surgeon's early experience with the technique. These advantages include enhanced chamber stability thanks to a near-perfectly closed system, better followability due to the separation of infusion and aspiration, access to 360° of the anterior segment with either infusion or aspiration by switching instruments from one hand to the other, ability to use the flow of irrigation fluid as a tool to move material within the capsular bag or the anterior chamber (particularly from an open-ended irrigating chopper of the manipulator), and significantly decreased chances of vitreous prolapse in case of a posterior capsular tear, zonular dialysis, or subluxed cataracts because of the maintenance of a pressurized stream of irrigation from above.

The many advantages of biaxial micro incision phaco are easily accessible to the skilled cataract surgeon. Micro incision IOLs, already available outside the United States, will soon create a rush to these enhanced techniques. But regardless of the final incision size required for IOL insertion, micro incision phaco stands on its own as a superior technique.

M. Packer (✉)
Oregon Health & Science University, Drs. Fine, Hoffman and Packer, 1550 Oak Street, Suite 5, Eugene, OR 97401, USA
e-mail: mpacker@finemd.com

Separation of irrigation from the aspirating phaco needle allows for improved followability by avoiding competing currents at the tip of the needle. In some instances, the irrigation flow from the second handpiece can be used as an adjunctive surgical device – flushing nuclear pieces from the angle or loosening epinuclear or cortical material from the capsular bag. In Refractive Lens Exchange, the lens material may be washed completely out of the bag and extracted with aspiration and vacuum only, so that no ultrasound is used and no instrument enters the endocapsular space, thus increasing the safety profile of this demanding procedure. The flow of fluid from the open end of an irrigator represents a very gentle instrument which can mobilize material without trauma to delicate intraocular structures.

Another benefit of a separate infusion stream is in scrubbing troublesome plaques from the posterior capsule (Fig. 6.1). Focusing the flow of fluid on the posterior capsule and putting the tissue on stretch facilitates capsule polishing with either a roughened or silicone-covered aspiration tip. The taut posterior capsule shows less inclination to become entrapped in the aspiration port, and the subcapsular plaque material is more easily stripped away.

Perhaps the greatest advantage of the biaxial technique lies in its ability to remove subincisional cortex without difficulty. As originally described by Brauweiler, by switching infusion and aspiration hand

J. L. Alió, I. H. Fine (eds.), *Minimizing Incisions and Maximizing Outcomes in Cataract Surgery*,
DOI: 10.1007/978-3-642-02862-5_6, © Springer-Verlag Berlin Heidelberg 2010

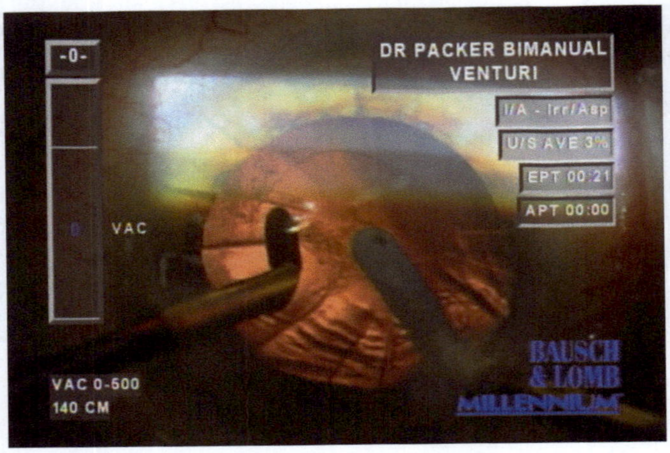

Fig. 6.1 Utilizing xenon slit-beam illumination highlights this posterior subcapsular plaque. The stream of irrigation fluid from the irrigating chopper is directed posteriorly to put the capsule on stretch, while the silicone sleeved aspiration tip is used to scrub away the material

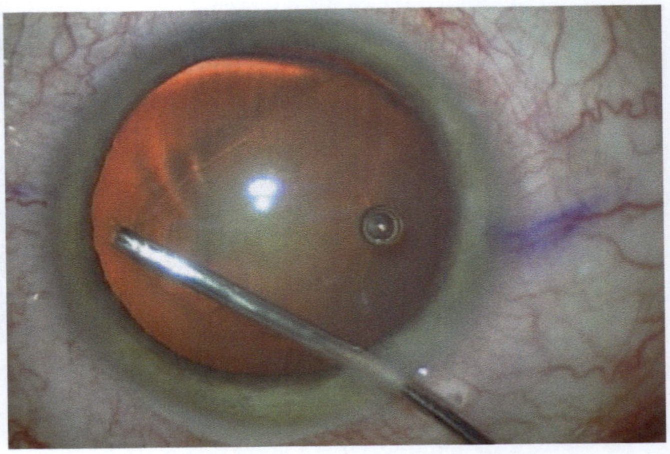

Fig. 6.2 The capsulorhexis is nearly complete in this eye with a history of trauma and 90° of zonular dialysis visible temporally. The wrinkling of the capsule is a clear sign of the absence of tension. Nevertheless, because of the increased control allowed by the micro incisions which do not allow prolapse of the viscoelastic, the capsulorhexis will be centered, round, and smaller in diameter than the IOL

pieces between two micro incisions, 360° of the capsular fornices are easily reached and cortical clean-up can be performed quickly and safely. The ability to switch hands also represents a significant advantage to instructors of phacoemulsification, who may find that they must take over a case from a resident with opposite manual dominance.

Utilization of Biaxial Micro Incision Phacoemulsification for refractive lens exchange and routine cataract surgery, as we have described, offers an enormous advantage of maintaining a more stable intraocular environment during lens removal. This may be especially important in high myopes who are at a greater risk for retinal detachment following lens extraction. By maintaining a formed and pressurized anterior chamber throughout the procedure, there should be fewer tendencies for the anterior movement of the vitreous body, with a theoretically lower incidence of posterior vitreous detachment occurring from intraoperative manipulations. Future studies need to be performed in order to document a significant reduction in posterior segment morbidity utilizing this method of lens removal.

Some of the major advantages we have seen from Biaxial Micro Incision Phaco do relate to incision size, for example, there has been an improvement in the control of most of the steps involved in endocapsular surgery due to increased chamber stability. Since viscoelastics do not leave the eye easily through these small incisions, the anterior chamber is more stable during capsulorhexis construction and there is much

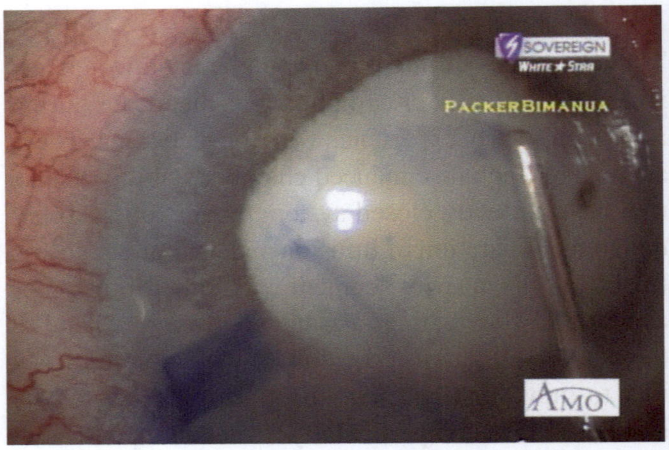

Fig. 6.3 Capsular dye and micro incisions help to control the capsulorhexis in this eye with a hypermature cataract

less likelihood for an errant rhexis to develop. This added margin of safety is particularly noticeable in cases of zonular compromise such as pseudoexfoliation, traumatic zonular dialysis and status post glaucoma filtering surgery, as well as in cases of intumescent cataract and nanophthalmos with a very shallow anterior chamber (Figs. 6.2 and 6.3). The added chamber stability can also make a difference in the control of capsulorhexis in high myopia with an extremely deep anterior chamber and floppy capsule. The adoption of Micro Incision techniques has also served as a catalyst for instrument manufacturers, who have developed delicate, exquisite forceps for the construction of the capsulorhexis. The result has been unparalleled surgical control. Hydrodelineation and hydrodissection can also be performed more efficiently by virtue of a higher level of pressure building in the anterior chamber, prior to the eventual prolapse of viscoelastic through the Micro Incisions.

In order to reap the benefit of these advantages strict attention to detail is required. The first technique to master is the construction of the incision. There is a variability in incision size among surgeons who employ 20, 19 gauge and even 18 gauge instrumentation. We prefer 20 gauge because we feel it offers greater control. Because the outer diameter of the 20 gauge tip is 0.9 mm, the circumference of the tip is 2.8 mm and the incision must measure 1.4 mm. An incision smaller than 1.4 mm stretches and tears, causing loss of self-sealability. These micro incisions are converted from a line to a circle upon introduction of the tip, and we want them to resume the configuration of a line when the tip is withdrawn. Compromise of the corneal collagen by stretching or tearing will reduce the likelihood that the incision will resume its virgin architecture at the end of the case. This can be minimized by using only trapezoidal-shaped incisions. There are now available from a variety of manufacturers, diamond and metal knives specially designed for the construction of 20 or 19 gauge incisions. It behooves the surgeon to purchase and learn to use this instrumentation, whether constructed of steel, diamond or other material.

Capsulorhexis construction represents the initial hurdle in the biaxial learning curve. However, micro incision capsulorhexis forceps permit a greater degree of precision and control, so much so that we advocate their use with any size of incision. The pinch type initiation of the capsulorhexis is particularly valuable in cases of zonular compromise since the forces acting on the capsule remain balanced. Even with a severely wrinkling capsule due to traumatic zonular dialysis, these extraordinarily delicate forceps permit moment-by-moment control of the capsulorhexis. With new technology IOLs, such as the crystalens (Bausch & Lomb, San Dimas, CA), we have found capsulorhexis size to be an important determinant of the final lens position and, therefore, of postoperative refractive status. Using micro incisions enhances the precision of capsulorhexis construction not only because of the improvements in instrumentation, but also because there is no tendency for the chamber to shallow as often occurs with a 2.5 mm incision due to burping of the viscoelastic.

There is an increased risk of losing control of the capsulorhexis in highly myopic eyes with very large, floppy capsules. Due to the extremely long anterior chamber depth in these eyes, the angle of approach to the anterior capsule is much steeper. If one notices that the capsulorhexis is tearing out further peripherally than one would like, a simple technique for capsulorhexis recovery involves laying down the flap and pulling centripetally. This maneuver redirects the capsulorhexis centrally [1]. In extreme cases, it may be necessary to cut the flap with scissors and begin the tear a new.

The goal of cortical cleaving hydrodissection as described by Howard Fine is to lyse the equatorial capsular–cortical connections, which will generally allow aspiration of the cortex, along with the mobilization of the epinucleus [2]. Hydrodelineation is performed to allow free mobility of the endonucleus within the epinuclear shell, allowing endocapsular nuclear disassembly within the safety cushion of the epinucleus. Hydrodissection and hydrodelineation may be performed just as they are with standard small incision surgery; the micro incisions do allow egress of the viscoelastic during this step so that there is not an increased risk of blowing out the posterior capsule due to overpressurization. It is of note that the intraocular pressure during hydrodissection, as measured in the vitreous cavity of a cadaver eye, varies around means of 78–223mmHg, regardless of whether a standard small incision or a micro incision is employed [3]. These were among the highest pressures we recorded during the entire phacoemulsification and IOL implantation procedure. Clearly, if the viscoelastic is prevented from exiting the eye, there is adequate pressure to rupture the capsule. This represents a special concern to users of high zero shear viscosity OVDs, who should insure that a path for egress is prepared with a track of balanced salt solution from the cannula tip to the incision.

A variety of irrigating choppers are now available for micro incision surgery. The method of placing the blade or the paddle of the chopper through the incision is not always immediately apparent. With the canoe paddle shaped Tsuneoka chopper (Du-02317, MicroSurgical Technologies, Redmond, WA), for example, the paddle must be placed parallel to the incision, inserted into the chamber and then rotated to allow full entry. Surgical videos are generally available from industry for instructional purposes. Placing the phaco tip through the incision may also be harder than it first appears. A 30° tip may be inserted into the incision bevel down, and then rocked gently from side to side to permit passage into the chamber.

The surprising fact about horizontal and vertical chopping techniques with biaxial phaco is how little they differ in terms of hand movement from the standard small incision coaxial phaco. Seeing the bulkier irrigating chopper in the eye and getting used to the heavier feel in one's hand represent the major differences; the actual chopping techniques are the same. The stream of irrigation fluid from the chopper or manipulator can function as an efficient tool within the eye and is one of the most significant advantages of biaxial phaco, which is a key reason we do not want to go back to coaxial phaco. In particular, washing subincisional endo- or epinuclear material into the range of the phaco tip permits enhanced safety and control. A great example is Refractive Lens Exchange with an accommodative IOL in high myopia, probably the situation in which we are most concerned about maintaining the integrity of the capsule. Not only would compromising the capsule increase the risk of posterior segment complications, but it may also result in an inability to implant the IOL of choice for the procedure. With biaxial RLE, no instrument other than a cannula and a stream of fluid ever need enter the endolenticular or endocapsular space; we can hydroexpress the soft lens material into the anterior chamber with the stream of the irrigation fluid and carousel it safely from the eye with fluidics alone [4]. Thanks to cortical cleaving hydrodissection, we can achieve a clean capsule without ever placing an aspiration tip below the level of the capsulorhexis. The absence of ultrasound energy allows for the safest, minimally invasive procedure. The margin of safety is further enhanced by this approach.

If there is a breach of the posterior capsule, residual lens material can generally be removed while maintaining irrigation in the anterior chamber and disallowing vitreous prolapse. With biaxial phaco, we have the option of switching from a phaco tip to an aspirator to a vitrector if necessary, without ever compromising chamber stability. The approach, once a tear is recognized, consists of continuous irrigation in the anterior chamber while the lens material is removed from the bag. Once the bag is clean, a dispersive viscoelastic is injected at the level of the posterior capsule while irrigation is still maintained; only when the viscoelastic has fully tamponaded the break and filled the chamber is the irrigator removed. The IOL can then be inserted into the ciliary sulcus and capsule through a standard temporal clear corneal incision between the microincisions. In the case of sulcus placement, the optic is pushed posteriorly through the capsulorhexis prior to final clean up. In compromised posterior capsules, residual viscoelastic is removed from the anterior chamber with a vitrector. Once the viscoelastic is removed, the kenalog technique described by Scott Burke is utilized to insure a completely vitreous-free environment in the anterior segment.

We have found this technique to be simple, efficacious, and safe, since most of the lens extraction is occurring in the plane of the iris, away from the posterior capsule and the corneal endothelium. Whether surgeons employ 18 or 21 gauge incisions, the principle advantages of B-MICS Phaco arise from the separation of infusion and aspiration. No matter how small the incision, these advantages cannot be achieved with coaxial techniques.

B-MICS: Take Home Pearls

- Details are very important with this technique – it is not very forgiving. Carefully follow an experienced B-MICS surgeon's recommendations for settings and phaco tips specific to your phaco machine.
- Balancing inflow and outflow is critical. Most initial difficulties relate to chamber stability and fluid dynamics.
- Conversation with an experienced B-MICS surgeon is extremely helpful – both for preparation before and for troubleshooting after the initial cases.
- Surgical equipment representatives are additional good resources for technical information and optimization of power and fluidic parameters.
- Have a phaco machine surgical representative present in the OR for the first few cases to adjust the machine settings during surgery as needed. This leaves the nurses/techs free to concentrate on the new procedure steps and equipment. A representative with B-MICS experience is best of all.
- Decrease aspiration flow rates for initial B-MICS cases because, due to the smaller caliber of the irrigator, effective aspiration flow rates are higher with B-MICS than in coaxial phaco. This results in faster movement of material within the eye at a given aspiration setting.

- Decrease the vacuum setting for initial B-MICS cases to help prevent chamber fluctuations due to post-occlusion surge. Once the flow parameters are worked out and the chamber is stable, vacuum can be gradually increased.
- The phaco tip is used without a sleeve, but it is useful to place a cut-off sleeve on the phaco handpiece to prevent spraying of BSS during ultrasound. The sleeve must be cut off very close to the hub – if the stump of the sleeve is longer than about 1 mm, it can limit the phaco tip's excursion into the eye.
- Initially, B-MICS makes nuclear disassembly easier in some aspects and more difficult in others. It is made easier by improved chamber stability and followability, and it is made more difficult by the bulkier irrigating choppers and smaller, more restrictive incisions. Once adjusted to the instruments and smaller incisions, however, B-MICS is a superior technique for nuclear disassembly.

References

1. Little BC, Smith JH, Packer M (2006) Little capsulorhexis tear-out rescue. J Cataract Refract Surg 32:1420–1422
2. Fine IH (2000) Cortical cleaving hydrodissection. J Cataract Refract Surg 26(7):943–944
3. Khng C, Packer M (2004) Intraocular pressure during phacoemulsification [poster]. In: XXII Congress of the European Society of Cataract and Refractive Surgery, Paris, 18–22 September 2004
4. Fine IH, Hoffman RS, Packer M (2004) Optimizing refractive lens exchange with bimanual microincision phacoemulsification. J Cataract Refract Surg 30:550–554

6.1 Pupil Dilation and Preoperative Preparation

Mark Packer, I. Howard Fine, and Richard S. Hoffman

Core Messages

- Management of small pupil may be successfully accomplished by means of any one or a combination of the following techniques:
  - Pharmacologic mydriasis
  - Viscomydriasis
  - Pupillary stretching techniques
  - Pupil ring expanders
  - Iris surgery
- Preoperative preparation accomplishes multiple goals, including infection prophylaxis. Preventing infection is a multi-factorial process involving positioning, prepping, and draping of the patient, and the use of antibiotics as well as surgical technique.

6.1.1 *Managing the Small Pupil*

The pupil that dilates poorly or is fibrosed or hyalinized is frequently associated with complications during cataract surgery. With endolenticular techniques, especially with nucleofractis procedures and chop techniques [1–4], pupils do not need to be as large as previously required. This is because, much of the procedure takes place in the endolenticular space, within the center of the capsulorhexis, rather than at the equator of the lens as in anterior chamber phacoemulsification [5] and nuclear tilt pupillary plane phacoemulsification techniques [6]. However, there are still numerous instances in which the pupil is inadequate to allow the surgeon to proceed and some form of manipulation or surgery is required.

M. Packer (✉)
Oregon Health & Science University, Drs. Fine, Hoffman and Packer, 1550 Oak Street, Suite 5, Eugene, OR 97401, USA
e-mail: mpacker@finemd.com

6.1.2 Techniques that Depend on the Manipulation of the Pupil

The surgeon may tailor the initial pharmacological intervention for pupillary mydriasis in cataract surgery to achieve greater dilation. The use of phenylephrine 10% and cyclopentolate 2% will sometimes produce more effective mydriasis than lower concentrations of these or other agents, especially when administered in multiple doses over 1 h. The use of preoperative non-steroidal anti-inflammatory agents, such as flurbiprofen sodium 0.03% (Ocufen, Allergan) or suprofen 1.0% (Profenal, Alcon) mitigates any intraoperative pupillary constriction. Additionally, preservative-free epinephrine 1:10,000 may increase the diameter of the pupil, when injected into the anterior chamber at the start of surgery.

A viscoelastic device, particularly a high molecular weight product, can increase mydriasis by applying direct mechanical pressure on the pupillary margin during instillation. When poor mydriasis is due to the presence of posterior synechiae and there is adequate zonular support, the surgeon may insinuate the viscoelastic cannula between the anterior capsule and the pupillary margin and then inject the viscoelastic in order to disrupt the irido-capsular adhesions. The cannula is angled in a tangential fashion to create a viscoelastic wave, which will dissect the synechiae. Multiple injection sites may be utilized to free the pupil fully. Following dissection of the synechiae, additional dispersive viscoelastic may be injected in the center of the pupil to achieve even greater dilation of the pupillary margin.

Frequently, the pupil can be manipulated with the phacoemulsification handpiece. One can retract the proximal portion of the pupil through the incision with the sleeve on the phacoemulsification handpiece, and effectively enlarge its size. This technique requires a great deal of skill and may result in thermal injury with chafing of the pupil and focal depigmentation of the iris. Additional advantage can be obtained by using the second handpiece, in such a way as to stretch the pupil in front of the phacoemulsification tip, once again enlarging the pupil for adequate visualization of structures, just under the margin of the pupil. In other circumstances, a portion of the lens may be manipulated through the pupil to maintain the pupil in a semi-dilated state. The protruding portion of the nucleus can then be consumed by the phacoemulsification handpiece before repositioning the nucleus within the pupil.

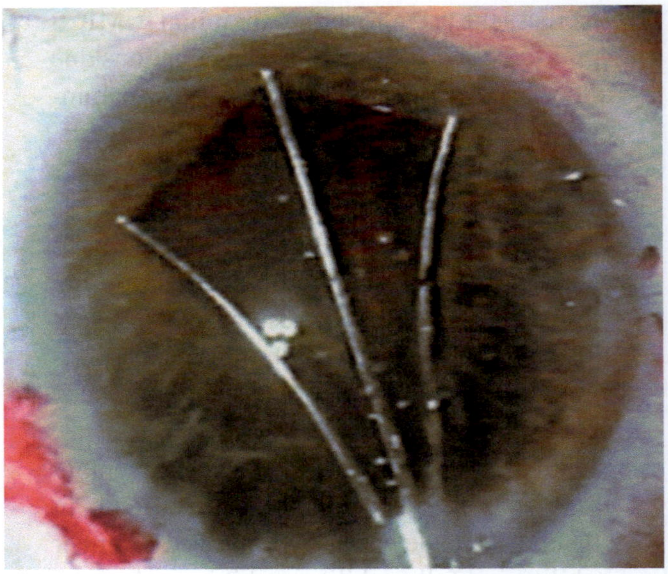

Fig. 6.4 The Beehler pupil dilator effectively stretches the pupil to a diameter of 6–7 mm by creating tiny microsphincterotomies

The surgeon may accomplish mechanical stretching of the pupil with a variety of instruments. Frye [7] has taught a technique that he attributes to Keener of Indianapolis, Indiana. Here, two hooks engage the pupillary margin at opposite points and apply steady, gentle pressure across the full extent of the anterior chamber to produce a pupillary diameter of 5–6 mm. A second stretch placed orthogonal to the first increases the diameter further. Viscoelastic protects the anterior lens capsule during this maneuver.

Alternatively, the Beehler pupil dilator (Moria #19009) is uniformly applicable in front of small pupils. Inserted through a 2.5-mm single plane clear corneal incision, it usually stretches the pupil to 6–7 mm, while creating tiny microsphincterotomies circumferentially around the pupil (Fig. 6.4). The pupil can then be mechanically reduced at the end of the procedure with a Lester hook supplemented with an intraocular miotic agent. Pupils enlarged in this manner maintain a good cosmetic appearance and an ability to react to light, but may require a miotic agent for some time after cataract surgery to prevent the formation of irido-capsular synechiae.

Recently, we have seen a renewed interest in the use of iris hooks as described by McReynolds [8]. Mackool [9] has designed self-retaining titanium hooks that can be placed through paracenteses, so that the pupil can be positioned and held in a widely dilated state in a triangular or square shape, to adequately perform phacoemulsification, regardless of the initial size of the pupil. Although this procedure is somewhat time-consuming and results in considerable fluid loss from the eye, as a result of leakage through the paracenteses during phacoemulsification, it is an effective method of pupillary dilation and visualization of the structures for phacoemulsification. De Juan designed disposable nylon hooks with an adjustable silicone retaining sleeve that can be used through smaller paracenteses. Although more expensive, they may offer some additional advantages as reported by Nichamin [10], particularly the facilitation of hook removal through the paracentesis incisions.

Pupil ring expanders represent another option in the surgical armamentarium for small pupil cases. The Hydroview Iris Protector Ring (Grieshaber) forms a compressed oval in its dehydrated state. It can then be placed in the anterior chamber through a 3-mm incision and inserted into the small pupil. This hydrogel device expands with hydration, and captures the pupillary margin by means of flanges. The ring can be manipulated to expand the pupil as it hydrates. The device then remains in place for the entire surgical procedure, including implantation of the intraocular lens. The Graether silicone pupil expansion ring (Eagle Vision, Inc., Memphis, TN) offers another injectable option for maintaining dilation.

The Morcher Pupildilator Type 5S is a solid polymethylmethacrylate (PMMA) ring that is placed at the pupillary margin and expands the pupil through 300° of even tension, thus reducing the likelihood of iris sphincter tears and postoperative pupillary deformity. The ring may be introduced into the anterior chamber with forceps and then placed within the pupillary margin with a small hook. The central segment of the ring is manipulated into position, first in apposition to the distal pupillary margin, and then the ends of the ring are placed with the aid of eyelets on the ring. Following implantation of the intraocular lens, the ring is removed by first freeing the ends from their point of apposition with the pupil by means of the small hook and again placed in each eyelet. The ring may then be withdrawn from the anterior chamber with forceps. An injection device is also available for the ring from Geuder (Figs. 6.5 and 6.6).

The Malyugin Ring (MicroSurgical Technologies) features an innovative design that resembles a four-cornered paperclip (Fig. 6.7). It is placed in the eye with an injector and can also be removed with the same injector, by freeing the proximal corner of the device with a hook and then grasping it with the retractable arm of the injector.

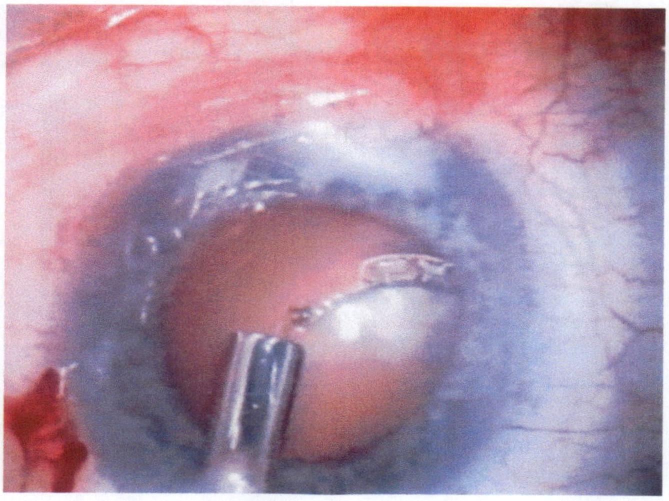

Fig. 6.5 The Morcher Pupildilator may be injected via a device available from Geuder, as seen in this case of floppy iris

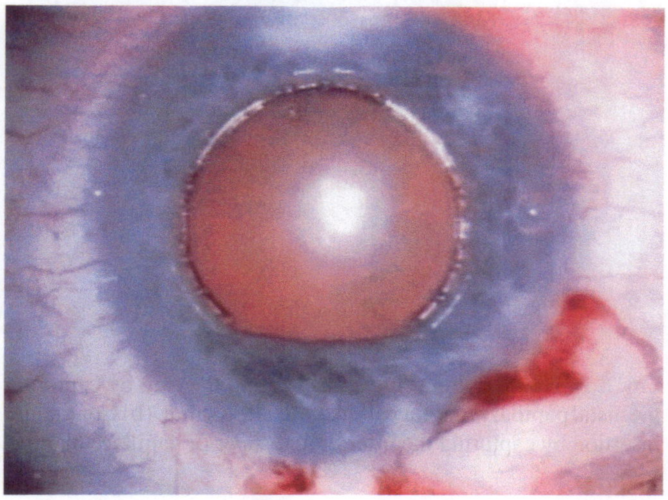

Fig. 6.6 The Morcher pupildilator in place, permitting capsulorhexis and the completion of the surgery

6.1.3 Iris Surgery

A variety of techniques using iris surgery enable the enlargement of the pupil. A proximal sphincterotomy can be performed by grasping the superior sphincter and pulling it out of the incision. A small segment of the sphincter can be excised, after which the iris is repositioned [11]. While this procedure results in a

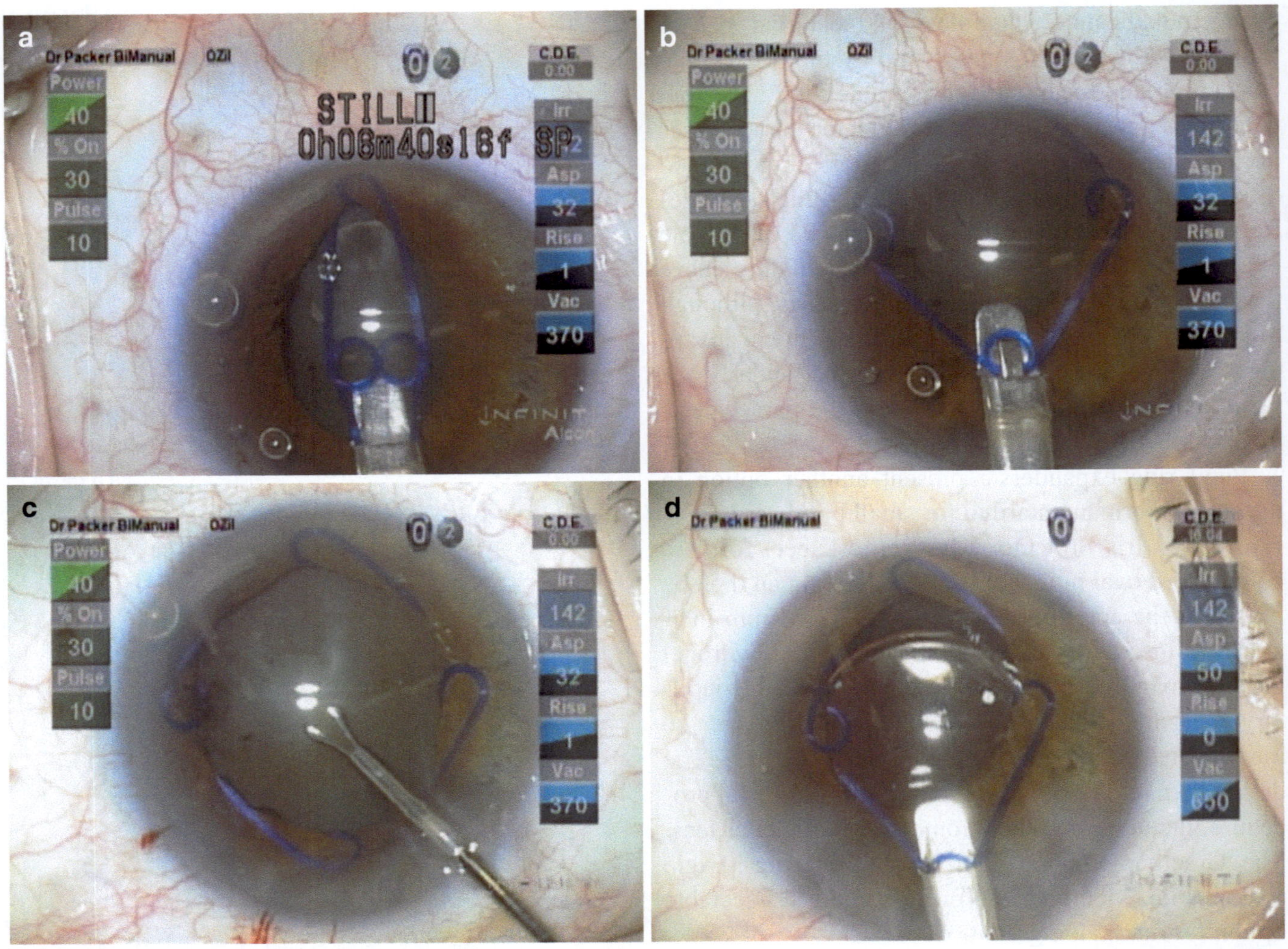

Fig. 6.7 The Malyugin ring: (**a**) Inserting the ring by capturing the distal papillary margin within the leading spiral. (**b**) Continuing insertion by capturing the inferior and superior papillary margins in the ring. (**c**) Capsulorhexis with the ring in place. (**d**) Removing the ring at the conclusion of the case by grasping the proximal spiral with the retractable arm of the injector

permanently enlarged pupil that may be somewhat oval in shape, it does frequently achieve adequate dilation for the completion of the surgery. This has been found especially useful in glaucoma patients undergoing cataract surgery, and may be combined with a small inferior sphincterotomy.

Superior sector iridectomy is frequently performed for pupillary enlargement. However, this technique subjects the patient to glare and other undesirable retinal images postoperatively, because of the permanently enlarged pupil and the potential for edge effects from lenses and haptics, uncovered by the prominently enlarged pupils.

A modification of the superior sector iridectomy, which tends to give adequate dilation for surgery and yet, is less of a problem postoperatively, is the superior midiris iridectomy followed by sphincterotomy. This allows the pillars of the iris to come together more closely following the completion of the surgery, than that done by sector iridectomy.

Many surgeons use a suture to close the sphincterotomy at the completion of the surgery, hoping to avoid potential sources of glare and trying to achieve a more cosmetically acceptable appearance, postoperatively. These sutures may be preplaced through the clear cornea. The posterior loop is drawn out of the peripheral iridectomy with a hook prior to sphincterotomy. Alternatively, the suture may be placed through the clear cornea at the end of the surgical procedure. The ends are drawn out of the cataract incision and tied in the same way as originally described by Worst and reported by Drews [12].

Masket [13] has described a technique for using a preplaced suture in the inferior or distal portion of the iris, drawing a loop of the central segment of the suture out of the incision, and then performing a sphincterotomy inferiorly or distally. After the implantation of the intraocular lens, the ends of the suture are drawn out of an inferior or distal limbal self-sealing paracentesis and tied. This can dramatically increase exposure to the area in which most of the phacoemulsification takes place. Exposure is increased specifically at the distal portion of the capsulorhexis and the capsular bag, just under the distal capsular flap. This suture can restore an acceptable cosmetic appearance to the pupil postoperatively and remove the potential for unwanted glare.

An additional iris surgical procedure for pupillary enlargement is the pupilloplasty technique of Fine [14]. After lysing synechiae, partial-thickness sphincterotomies are made using Rappazzo scissors (Storz Instruments, E-1961-A) either through the paracentesis or through the cataract incision. The sphincterotomies cut full thickness through approximately one half the width of the musculus sphincter pupillae at each of the eight sites. Following sphincterotomies, each of the sites is stretched to the root of the iris. The author believes that this results in fracturing of the hyalinized fibrotic portions of the pupil and,stretching only the residual circular muscle in the pupil that was not transected. This technique usually achieves 6–7-mm pupil diameters, regardless of the initial size of the pupil. At the completion of the phacoemulsification and implantation procedure, a Lester type hook is used to mechanically return the pupil to as small a configuration as possible. The patient should use miotic drops and ointments postoperatively, to keep the pupil small and to avoid synechiae from the sphincterotomy sites to the anterior edge of the capsulorhexis. This technique tends to achieve an excellent cosmetic appearance postoperatively and also allows for more normal physiologic behavior of the pupil.

Osher has described pupillary membrane dissection [15] as a technique to allow the dilation of the pupil to an adequate diameter. This procedure involves meticulous dissection with a bent needle or microforceps to free and remove a fibrotic pupillary membrane. This technique is time-consuming and may produce some bleeding, but has proved to be a valuable aid in the management of some cases of small pupil.

In conclusion, phacoemulsification in the presence of a small pupil, continues to pose a challenge to the surgeon. However, the diverse techniques for the management of these pupils, present us with options for reducing complications in these cases, to the standard low complication rate.

6.1.4 Preoperative Preparation and Infection Prophylaxis

The state of the art of infection prophylaxis in cataract and refractive surgery continues to evolve, and therefore the standard of care remains a moving target. A plethora of reports have appeared in the scientific literature, which surgeons must weigh and consider. As a starting point, it is critical to realize that any data analysis should take into account, the multifactorial pathogenesis of postoperative infection. Studies which retrospectively review a case series, may easily fall prey to narrative fallacy and confounding errors. As David Chang recently pointed out, "... we must be cautious about making practice recommendations based solely on retrospective population studies with multiple covariables" [16].

6.1.5 Evaluating Risk

In the wake of the European Society of Cataract and Refractive Surgeons' multicenter study of endophthalmitis, the Cataract Clinical Committee of the American Society of Cataract and Refractive Surgeons performed an on-line survey to characterize current practices among the members [17]. Of the 1,312 respondents, 90% reported an infection rate of less than one in one thousand. In general, the published incidence of endophthalmitis after cataract surgery in the peer-reviewed literature, ranges from a low of less than one in five thousand, [18] to a high of about three in one thousand [19]. The risk of severe visual loss from endophthalmitis following cataract surgery has been put at one in six thousand [20]. For LASIK, the risk of infectious keratitis has been reported to be about one in three thousand [21].

For cataract surgery, factors which increase the risk of postoperative infection have been identified. Oliver Schein has pointed out that "consistent findings have been, excess risk associated with corneal incisions, age (especially over 80 years), and loss of posterior capsular integrity..." [22]. He notes that the "modest" increased risk associated with corneal incisions "can be mitigated by expertise (i.e., close attention to wound construction and integrity)." This statement echoes closely whathas been said in the past [23].

In terms of prophylaxis, several approaches have demonstrated a reduced risk of infection. The use of povidone-iodine antisepsis has probably received the most universal support [24]. Chemoprophylaxis has demonstrated efficacy by various routes, and is widely employed. In the ASCRS survey, 88% of the surgeons used preoperative topical antibiotics and 98% used postoperative topical antibiotics. Intracameral antibiotic administration also received support: 30% of surgeons reported using this route either via irrigation or by direct injection. Subconjunctival administration can also be effective, although it is perhaps less appealing to surgeons performing clear corneal surgery with topical anesthesia, due to the stinging and pain it may engender [25]. Whatever the method is, killing bacteria on the ocular surface and inside the eye has value in the prevention of infection.

6.1.6 Assessing Your Approach

In the year 2004, David Allen and his colleagues presented a series of seven cases of endophthalmitis that occurred in a single surgeon's practice during a 27 week period [26]. This surgeon's incidence of infection rose precipitously to 1.6%. The surgeon stopped operating at this point. Statistical analysis suggested that these cases represented a true outbreak. After examining a variety of potential causative factors, including the timing of cases, nursing staff, equipment, patient risk factors and microbiology, they determined that the "only common contributory factor in each case was the surgeon." A review of the surgeon's technique determined that two weeks prior to the occurrence of the first case, the earlier practice of administering a subconjunctival antibiotic injection at the conclusion of surgery, had been discontinued. Following this analysis, the surgeon resumed his use of subconjunctival antibiotic injections and enjoyed a zero incidence of endophthalmitis in the subsequent 1,350 cataract operations he performed.

This cautionary tale demonstrates how a systematic investigation into an outbreak of infection, led to the correct causative factor. When infection strikes, surgeons should first determine if the event represents a random and statistically expected event. If it does not, investigation is warranted to determine the cause. Casting a wide net by reviewing all the potentially relevant factors in an outbreak of infection increases the likelihood of finding the culprit. This approach is analogous to the one that is undertaken in looking for the source of outbreaks of noninfectious postoperative inflammation, such as TASS [27] and DLK [28].

Assigning the correct significance to the results of the published studies, as they apply to local conditions represents a second important lesson from this paper. At the time, subconjunctival injections were deemed "possibly relevant but not definitely related to clinical outcome" in Ciulla's evidence-based update [8]. However, an earlier report had suggested a possible link [29]. Nevertheless, the key to understanding the outbreak lies in the fact that the subconjunctival injection represented the *only* antibiotic prophylaxis employed by this surgeon. Discontinuing the injection meant dispensing with all chemoprophylaxis. In a different setting, for example, the one where the surgeon uses topical antibiotics both pre and postoperatively, the discontinuation of subconjunctival antibiotics might not be significant.

Recently, Ng et al. performed a retrospective study of endophthalmitis in Western Australia from 1980 to 2000 by examining 205 cases of postoperative infection, and four time-matched randomly selected controls for each case. The authors found a significant impact from antiseptic preparation and subconjunctival antibiotic injection. Interestingly, antisepsis was nearly universal in both cases and controls, while subconjunctival injection was about 50/50 in controls and 30/70 in cases. Postoperative topical antibiotics were also nearly universal in both groups, while intracameral antibiotics were rare in both groups. Ironically, therefore, the power of the study to detect a significant difference for subconjunctival injections was higher than its power to detect a difference for antisepsis or topical antibiotics. The fact that, it did still find a difference for antisepsis confirms again the importance of povidone-iodine, and the fact that it did not find a difference for topical antibiotics does not mean that they are worthless.

Turning to wound location, Ng et al. did not find a significant difference between cases and controls based on scleral, limbal or clear corneal incisions. In a recent thorough review of the literature, Lundstrom concluded

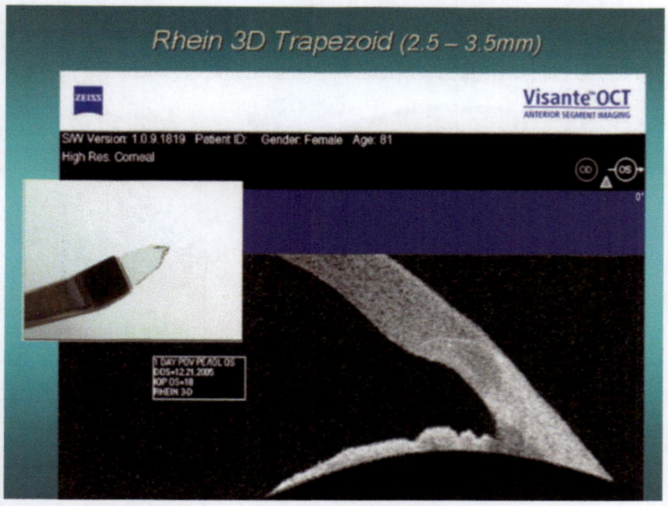

Fig. 6.8 Optical coherence tomography of the anterior segment (Visante, Carl Zeiss Meditec, Dublin, CA) demonstrates the profile of a temporal clear corneal incision constructed with the 3D Trapezoidal diamond (Rhein Medical, Tampa, FL). The incision is constructed by placing the tip of the blade just anterior to the corneal vascular arcade and directing the knife toward the corneal apex in a single planar motion. The differentially beveled blade is designed to create a tunnel that is 2 mm in chord length

that, “There is no conclusive evidence of the relationship between clear corneal incision and endophthalmitis” [30]. Nevertheless, a clear corneal incision design and construction appear to be less forgiving than scleral tunnel incisions [31]. When reviewing the potential causes for infection, a leaky wound with hypotony represents a clear avenue for the introduction of bacteria into the eye. The use of correct architecture and the attainment of a Seidel negative closure are critical for the prevention of infection (Fig. 6.8) [32]. A single suture should be placed if necessary. Incision construction represents an important area for examination, when faced with an increased incidence of infection or if self-sealing cannot be routinely obtained.

6.1.7 Preventing Infection, Step by Step

Infectious disease subspecialists generally consider pathogenesis in terms of both, the resistance of the host and the virulence of the etiologic agent. Most cases of postsurgical endophthalmitis are related to normal flora of the eyelids and the ocular surface, for example, *Staphylococcus epidermidis*. Gram negative organisms, such as *Pseudomonas aeruginosa*, though capable of more rapid destruction of tissue, occur less frequently. While the etiology remains fairly consistent, host factors may vary widely. The patient’s age remains as the most significant factor s. However, thorough examination of the ocular adnexa, with special attention to signs of blepharitis, eyelid malposition and lacrimal insufficiency or obstruction, forms an important step in assessing infection risk. Initial treatment with eyelid hygiene for blepharitis or definitive surgical treatment of ectropion or nasolacrimal duct obstruction makes sense, prior to cataract or refractive lens surgery. Less obviously, treatment of dry eye syndrome (e.g., with topical cyclosporine) prior to surgery may improve the quality of the tear film and strengthen its defensive mechanisms. The presence of poor or partial blinking due to a facial palsy may indicate a need for increased lubrication with artificial tears in the perioperative period. Consideration of host factors such as these may lead to special precautions in the setting of reduced resistance to infection.

Preoperative antibiotic prophylaxis to sterilize the ocular surface remains a mainstay of infection prophylaxis. Many surgeons begin topical antibiotics, especially a fourth generation fluoroquinolones, moxifloxacin or gatifloxacin, up to three days prior to surgery. Additional topical antibiotic is often administered in the immediate preoperative period along with mydriatic agents and nonsteroidal anti-inflammatory drops. Topical antibiotic administration is frequently continued following the surgery for a period of one to two weeks. Some surgeons have adopted perioperative oral antibiotic prophylaxis, as fluoroquinolones exhibit excellent penetration into the vitreous body.

Sterile preparation of the eye for the surgery forms the most critical aspect of infection prophylaxis, as has been shown by the nearly universal adoption of povidone-iodine. Important considerations for draping include, optimal ergonomic access to the eye, complete sequestration of the lids and lashes, and maintenance of fluid drainage away from the surgical field. Critical aspects of intraoperative technique include incision construction and avoidance of complications. In particular, compromise of the capsular bag is recognized as posing increased risk of infection. Surgeons should consider the use of intracameral antibiotic agents, either in the irrigation solution or as an injection into the anterior chamber. At the conclusion of surgery, the incision, whether clear corneal, limbal or scleral, must be checked for watertight closure, following the adjustment of the

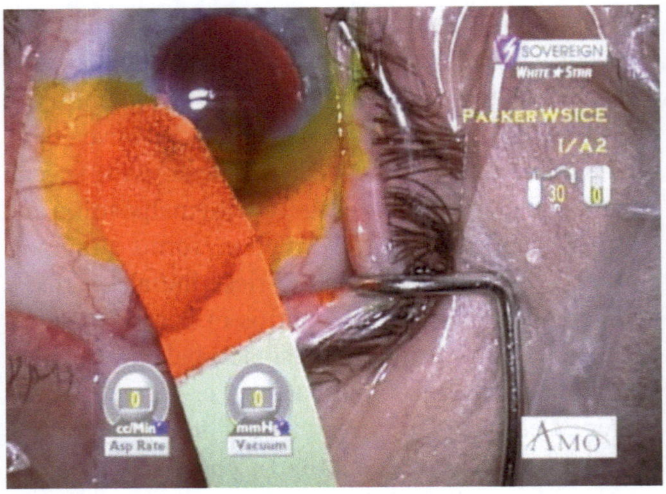

Fig. 6.9 Seidel test is performed at the conclusion of the surgery after the intraocular pressure has been adjusted to a physiologic level. If persistent leakage occurs, stromal hydration is performed. Massage of the corneal surface with the side of a cannula sometimes facilitates the apposition of the roof and the floor of the incision, leading to sealing. Occasionally, a 10-0 nylon suture is required to effect closure

intraocular pressure to physiologic levels (Fig. 6.9). A leaky incision requires stromal hydration, massage or suture closure. Removal of the lid speculum and drapes should be accomplished without putting pressure on the eye. The postoperative exam is performed 2–24 h after surgery, and the patient is instructed to call the doctor immediately if there is increased pain and decreased vision.

6.1.8 Sample Protocol Outline

1. Topical fourth generation fluoroquinolone antibiotic (e.g., gatifloxacin or moxifloxacin), four times a day beginning three days prior to surgery, and continuing for two weeks after surgery.
2. Preoperative pledget solution (placed on the eye in surgical holding area)

Proparacaine 0.5%/phenylephrine 10%/tropicamide 1%/ flurbiprofen 0.3%/cyclopentolate 2%/gatifloxacin 0.3%

3. Sterile preparation
   - Site prepped: quarter face
   - Solution used on skin: 5% betadine
   - Solution used in eye: 5% ophthalmic betadine with BSS rinse

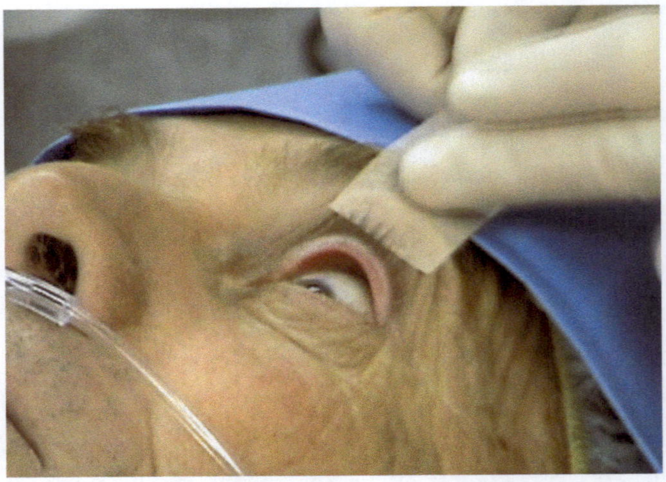

Fig. 6.10 Following sterile preparation of the skin, the upper eyelid is retracted with a 1 × 5 in. suture strip (Derma Sciences TP-1105). The strip is placed as close to the eyelid margin as possible

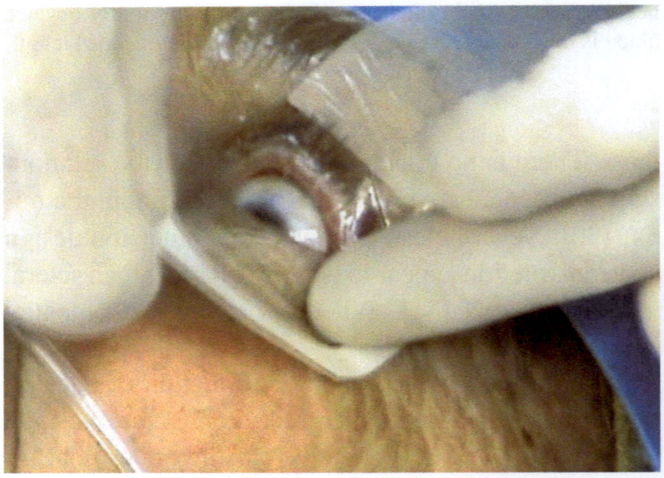

Fig. 6.11 The upper and lower eyelashes are covered with one Tegaderm, cut in half (3M NDC 8333-1624-05)

4. Irrigation solution

500 mL BSS with 0.5 mg epinephrine 1:1,000, 4 mg gentamicin, 10 mg vancomycin

5. Draping protocol (Figs. 6.10–6.12)
   - The eye should be dried around with a 4 × 4
   - Disposable drape towel should be placed across the forehead
   - The upper eyelid should be retracted with 1 × 5 in. suture strip and the strip should be placed as close to lid margin as possible (Derma Sciences TP-1105)

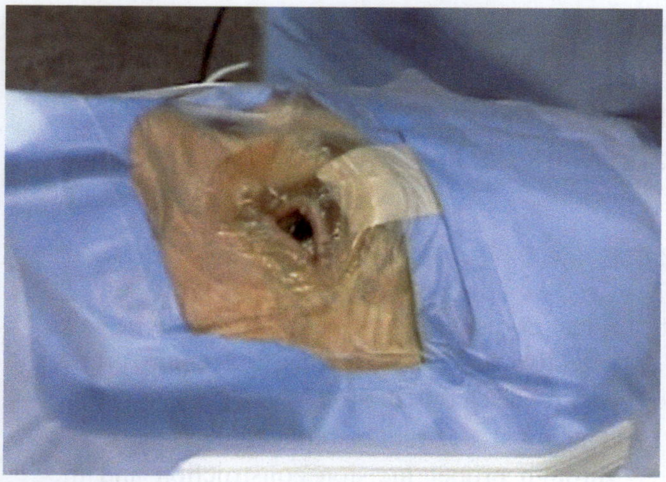

Fig. 6.12 The operative eye is covered with an ophthalmic drape. This drape is fenestrated and has an attached fluid collection pouch (Allegiance #7445 48″ × 68″)

- The upper and the lower eyelashes should be covered with Tegaderm. One Tegaderm, cut it in half, should be used. (3M NDC 8333-1624-05)
- The operative eye should be draped with the ophthalmic drape which is fenestrated and has an attached fluid collection pouch (Allegiance #7445 48 × 68 in.)

6. Immediate postoperative drops

Gatifloxacin 0.3%, pilocarpine 2%, diclofenac, prednisolone acetate 1%, genteal gel

6.1.9 A Careful, Critical Eye

A surgeon's primary challenge in preventing endophthalmitis consists of keeping a critical perspective on infection prophylaxis. Many reports are heard and multiple studies are seen, some of which contain relevant information and provide thoughtful insights. We should always evaluate the conclusions and opinions of others in the light of our own experience. The best way to build knowledge is to document outcomes; as human beings we are generally too much concerned with the results of our most recent or most unusual experiences. Documenting outcomes and tracking one's own data allows an objective measure of risk as well as the potential to improve results by following up on alterations in protocol and technique, after they are made.

Take Home Pearls

- Expanding the small pupil facilitates phacoemulsification; the techniques described here should be used in a stepladder approach, tailored to the severity of the condition.
- Preventing infection requires a multifactorial analysis of the present practices and an aggressive adoption of the best methods.

References

1. Gimbel HV (1991) Divide and conquer nucleofractis phacoemulsification: development and variations. J Cataract Refract Surg 17:281–291
2. Shepherd JF (1990) In situ fracture. J Cataract Refract Surg 16:436–440
3. Fine IH, Maloney WF, Dillman DM (1993) Crack and flip phacoemulsification technique. J Cataract Refract Surg 19: 797–802
4. Fine IH (1998) The choo-choo chop and flip phacoemulsification technique. Oper Tech Cataract Refract Surg 1(2):61–65
5. Kelman CD (1979) Phacoemulsification in the anterior chamber. Ophthalmology 86:1980–1982
6. Kratz RP, Colvard DM (1979) Kelman phacoemulsification in the posterior chamber. Ophthalmology 86:1983–1984
7. Frye LL (1992) Pupil stretch maneuver. Course No. 454 (Modern Phaco/ECCE Implant Surgery: XII). American Academy of Ophthalmology, Dallas, TX
8. McReynolds WU (1976) Pupil dilator for phacoemulsification. In: Emery JM, Paton D (eds) Current concepts in cataract surgery, selected proceedings of the first biennial cataract surgery congress. CV Mosby, St. Louis
9. Mackool RJ (1992) Small pupil enlargement during cataract extraction: a new method. J Cataract Refract Surg 18(5): 523–526
10. Nichamin LD (1993) Enlarging the pupil for cataract extractions using flexible nylon iris retractors. J Cataract Refract Surg 19:795–796
11. Fishkind WA, Koch PS (1991) Managing the small pupil. In: Koch PS, Davison JA (eds) Textbook of advanced phacoemulsification techniques. Slack, Thorofare, NJ, pp 79–90
12. Drews RC (1984) Straight needle technique. In: Emery JM, Jacobson AC (eds) Current concepts in cataract surgery, selected proceedings of the eight biennial cataract surgical congress. Appleton-Century-Crofts, Norwalk, CT
13. Masket S (1992) Preplaced inferior iris suture method for small pupil phacoemulsification. J Cataract Refract Surg 18(5):518–522
14. Fine IH (1994) Pupilloplasty for small pupil phacoemulsification. J Cataract Refract Surg 20:192–196
15. Osher RH (1991) Pupillary membranectomy [Videotape]. Audiovisual J Cataract Implant Surg 7(3)

16. Chang DF (2007) Reducing the risk of endophthalmitis after cataract surgery. J Cataract Refract Surg 33(12):2008–2009; author reply 2009
17. Chang DF, Braga-Mele R, Mamalis N, Masket S, Miller KM, Nichamin LD, Packard RB, Packer M (2007) ASCRS Cataract Clinical Committee. Prophylaxis of postoperative endophthalmitis after cataract surgery: results of the 2007 ASCRS member survey. J Cataract Refract Surg 33(10): 1801–1805
18. Buzard K, Liapis S (2004) Prevention of endophthalmitis. J Cataract Refract Surg 30(9):1953–1959
19. Nichamin LD, Chang DF, Johnson SH, Mamalis N, Masket S, Packard RB, Rosenthal KJ (2006) American Society of Cataract and Refractive Surgery Cataract Clinical Committee. ASCRS white paper: what is the association between clear corneal cataract incisions and postoperative endophthalmitis? J Cataract Refract Surg 32(9):1556–1559
20. Lundström M, Wejde G, Stenevi U, Thorburn W, Montan P (2007) Endophthalmitis after cataract surgery: a nationwide prospective study evaluating incidence in relation to incision type and location. Ophthalmology 114(5):866–870
21. Solomon R, Donnenfeld ED, Azar DT, Holland EJ, Palmon FR, Pflugfelder SC, Rubenstein JB (2003) Infectious keratitis after laser in situ keratomileusis: results of an ASCRS survey. J Cataract Refract Surg 29(10): 2001–2006
22. Schein OD (2007) Prevention of endophthalmitis after cataract surgery: making the most of the evidence. Ophthalmology 114(5):831–832
23. Fine IH (2003) Clear corneal cataract incisions require attention to detail. In: Packer M, Hoffman RS (eds) Cataract corner. Ophthalmology Times (15 January 2003) 28(2):12–13
24. Ciulla TA, Starr MB, Masket S (2002) Bacterial endophthalmitis prophylaxis for cataract surgery: an evidence-based update. Ophthalmology 109(1):13–24
25. Ng JQ, Morlet N, Bulsara MK, Semmens JB (2007) Reducing the risk for endophthalmitis after cataract surgery: population-based nested case-control study: endophthalmitis population study of Western Australia sixth report. J Cataract Refract Surg 33(2):269–280
26. Mandal K, Hildreth A, Farrow M, Allen D (2004) Investigation into postoperative endophthalmitis and lessons learned. J Cataract Refract Surg 30(9):1960–1965
27. Mamalis N, Edelhauser HF, Dawson DG, Chew J, LeBoyer RM, Werner L (2006) Toxic anterior segment syndrome. J Cataract Refract Surg 32(2):324–333
28. Hoffman RS, Fine IH, Packer M, Reynolds TP, Bebber CV (2005) Surgical glove-associated diffuse lamellar keratitis. Cornea 24(6):699–704
29. Lehmann OJ, Roberts CJ, Ikram K, Campbell MJ, McGill JI (1997) Association between nonadministration of subconjunctival cefuroxime and postoperative endophthalmitis. J Cataract Refract Surg 23(6):889–893
30. Lundström M (2006) Endophthalmitis and incision construction. Curr Opin Ophthalmol 17(1):68–71
31. Masket S (2005) Is there a relationship between clear corneal cataract incisions and endophthalmitis? J Cataract Refract Surg 31:643–645
32. Fine IH, Hoffman RS, Packer M (2007) Profile of clear corneal cataract incisions demonstrated by ocular coherence tomography. J Cataract Refract Surg 33(1):94–97

6.2 Incisions[1]

I. Howard Fine, Richard S. Hoffman, and Mark Packer

Core Messages

- Clear corneal incisions have proven to be safe, effective, and advantageous, and require proper and precise construction.
- The most desirable architecture is achieved through proper incision construction and the use of trapezoidal knives;
- Postoperative endophthalmitis prophylaxis requires not only proper incision construction and architecture, but also the use of antibiotics, precise surgical technique, and the testing of incisions at the end of the procedure.

The role of unsutured clear corneal incisions for cataract surgery in the apparent increased incidence of postoperative endophthalmitis is under intense scrutiny and the literature is not conclusive [2–9].

Clear corneal incisions, which involve an incision in the plane of the cornea with a length equal to 2.0 mm, were first described in 1992 [10] and continue to be constructed in essentially the same manner in practice today. In 1992, the incisions were wide as 4.0 mm, but more recently the maximum width is 3.5–3.8 mm, if not sutured. Figure 6.13 shows an artist's view of what the profile of clear corneal incisions was thought to look like. Part A shows the single plane incision and its apparent inherent lack of stability as one surface can easily slide over another. Charles Williamson, from Baton Rouge, innovated an alteration of the incision,

[1]Portions of this chapter were originally published as Fine et al. [1].

I. H. Fine (✉)
Oregon Health & Science University, Drs. Fine, Hoffman and Packer, 1550 Oak Street, Suite 5, Eugene, OR 97401, USA
e-mail:hfine@finemd.com

which involves a shallow, perpendicular groove prior to incising the cornea into the anterior chamber (Part B). David Langerman, deepened the perpendicular groove with the belief that it would lead to greater stability (Part C). These grooved incisions have been abandoned by the authors in favor of a paracentesis-style incision due to gaping of the groove and the difficulties associated with persistent foreign body sensation and the pooling of mucus and debris in the gaping groove. More importantly, the grooved incisions represent a disruption in the fluid barrier created by the intact epithelium, which allows for a vacuum seal as a result of endothelial pumping.

The artist's view of these incisions has perpetuated till today, as seen in Fig. 6.14 [11], and has a similar architecture to the drawing in Fig. 6.13, with the explanation of how these incisions open as a result of hypotony. In fact, since the pressure within a fluid acts perpendicular to all surfaces, there would be a greater amount of pressure lifting the roof of the incision off the floor of the incision under conditions of eye pressure, than the smaller area against which intraocular pressure would be pushing to help close the incision. However, as will be seen, this view of the incision architecture is erroneous, with respect to clear corneal incisions.

The initial incision construction technique began with a blade applanated to the surface of the globe, with the point at the edge of the clear cornea and the blade advanced for 2.0 mm in the plane of the cornea before incising Descemet's membrane (Fig. 6.15). These early incisions were made with knives with straight sides; however, these were subsequently replaced by trapezoidal-shaped knives in order to be able to enlarge the incision without violating the architecture by cutting sideways. From the onset of the use of clear corneal incisions, stromal hydration of the incisions, which thickens the cornea, forcing the roof of the incision onto the floor of the incision, and facilitating endothelial pumping to the upper reaches of the cornea, was strongly advocated. Testing the seal of the incision with a Seidel test using fluorescein was also strongly advocated [12]. These practices have not changed since 1992, except for the elimination of the depression of the posterior lip of the incision.

We examined the profile of clear corneal incisions using the Zeiss Visante Optical Coherence Tomography (OCT) anterior segment imaging system. This technology allowed the first view of the clear corneal incision in the living eye in the early postoperative period. All previous views were in autopsy eyes sectioned through the incision, which introduces artifacts. Figure 6.16 shows an example of the corneal periphery in a control eye which includes the anterior chamber angle. The regularity of the corneal epithelium blending in the conjunctiva and the clear corneal stroma blending into sclera can be clearly seen.

All clear corneal incisions were made by one surgeon (IHF). The OCT images of each operative eye were taken on the first postoperative day, within 24 h of cataract surgery, and are representative of multiple images from multiple patients. Incision width is defined as the measurement parallel to the limbus. Incision length is the distance, in a straight line, between the external incision and the entrance through Descemet's membrane. Several types of knives were used to create the clear corneal incisions during cataract surgery.

Figures 6.17 through 6.25, which were taken on the first postoperative day , show that clear corneal incisions constructed in the way as described are actually curvilinear, not a straight line as seen in the artists' depictions. It is an accurate incision with an arc length, which is considerably longer than the chord length originally estimated for the length of the incision. It is very important to note that the architecture of the incision allows for a fit, not unlike tongue and groove paneling, which adds a measure of stability to these incisions and makes sliding of one surface over the other considerably less likely.

All clear corneal incisions demonstrated a similar, arcuate architecture, even though they were constructed using a variety of blades. Figures 6.17 and 6.18 show clear corneal incisions made with the Rhein 3D Trapezoidal blade (#05-5088, Rhein Medical, Tampa Fl). The BD Kojo Slit (BD Medical-Ophthalmic Systems, Franklin Lakes, NJ, #372032) is a metal blade that is curved in the direction of the width of the incision. This creates an arcuate incision paralleling the curvature of the peripheral cornea with a chord length, whose width is considerably smaller than the arcuate incision in the dimension, tangential to the limbus itself, which may add a greater degree of stability. Once again, the very advantageous architecture of the incision, as constructed by the BD blade, is observed in Fig. 6.23. It is interesting to note once again, that the arc length is considerably longer than the chord length and is probably a hyper-square incision in that it is only 2.0 mm wide. Advantageous architecture can be achieved with any of the blades provided the construction of the incision is properly performed.

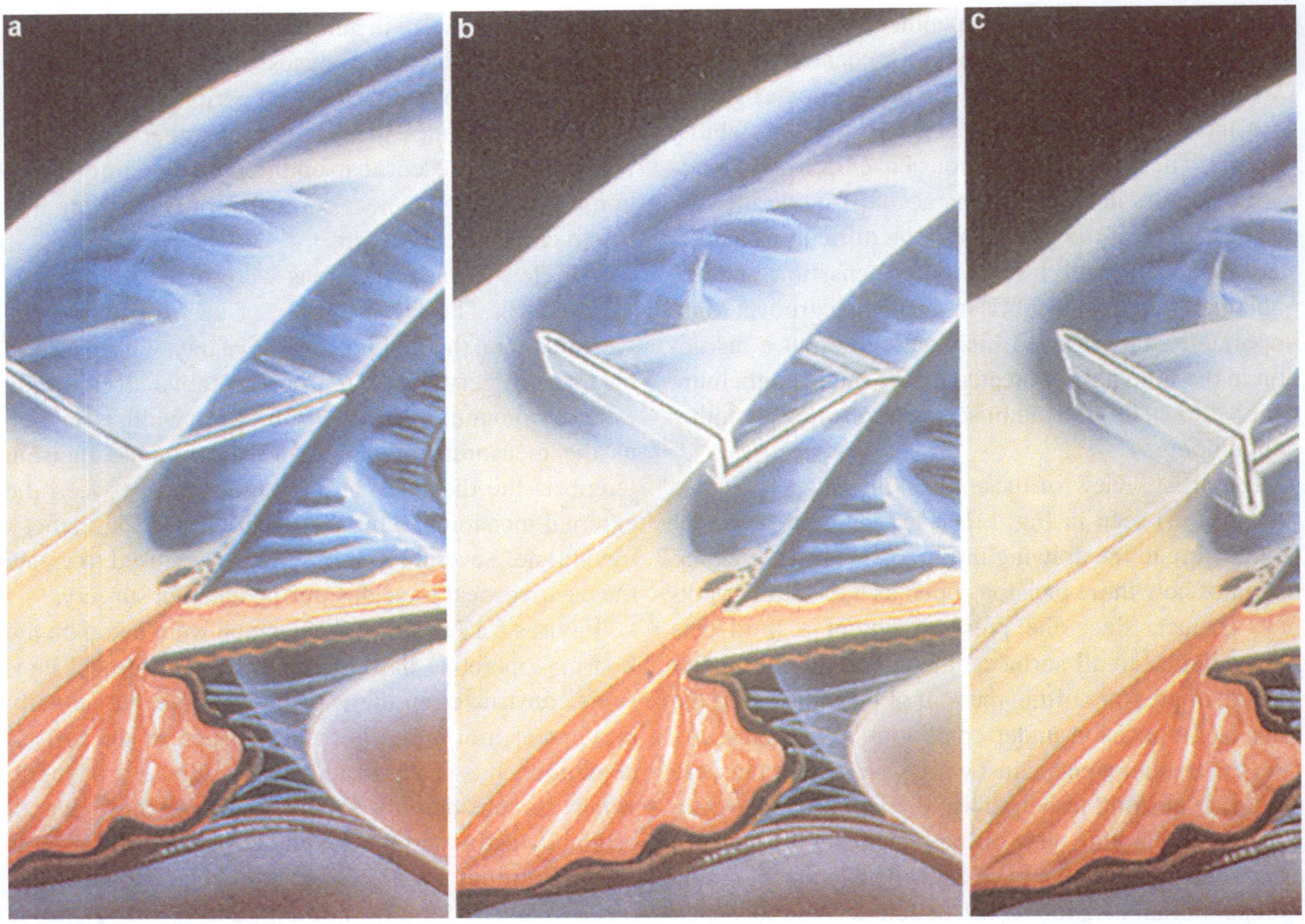

Fig. 6.13 Artist's interpretation of cross sectional view of clear corneal incisions circa 1992

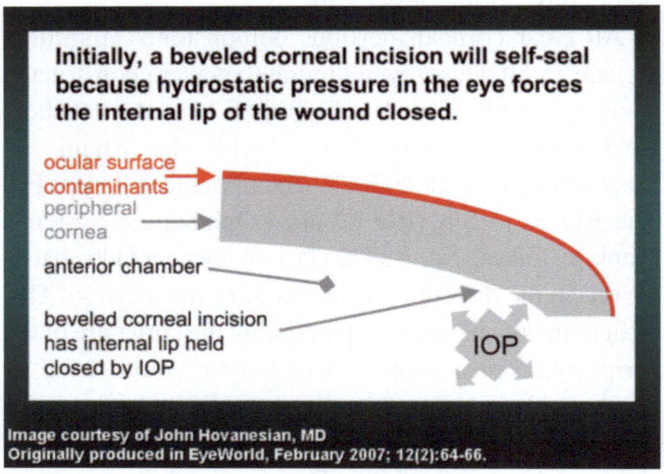

Fig. 6.14 Another artistic interpretation of cross sectional view of clear corneal incisions from the February 2007 issue of EyeWorld

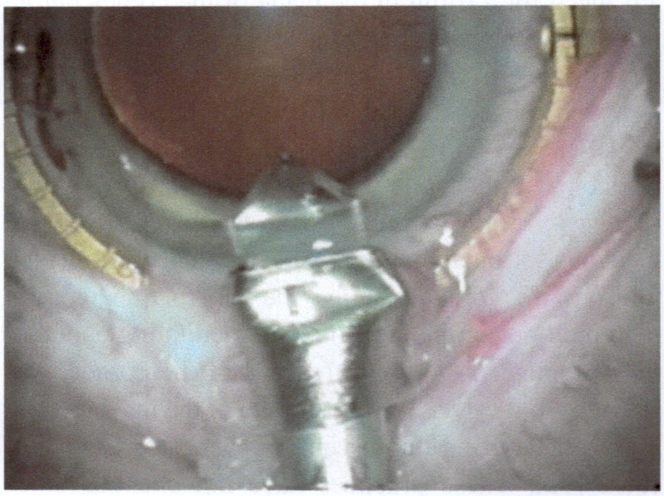

Fig. 6.15 Clear corneal incision construction, circa 1992, with the blade completely inserted

Figure 6.18 shows an incision that was made with a 300 μm groove at the external edge of the incision prior to incision construction. The incision itself has a curved or arcuate configuration, but the gaping of the external groove, which is noted on the first postoperative day, is accompanied by a similar offset of the internal lips of the incision, which appears to be somewhat less stable than a paracentesis-style incision.

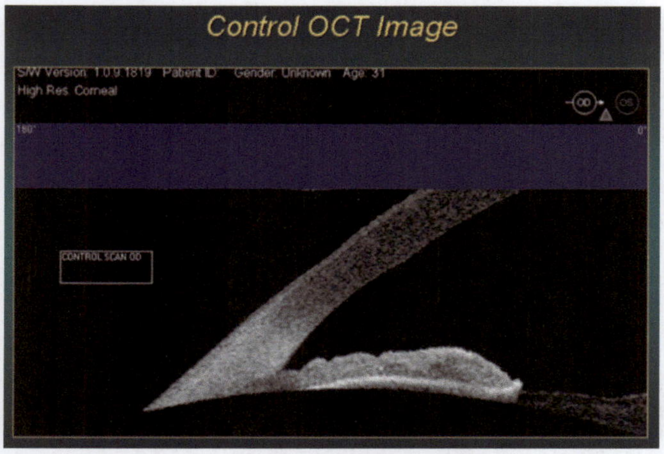

Fig. 6.16 OCT image of a control eye showing the corneal periphery including the anterior chamber angle

These images demonstrate the persistence of stromal swelling from stromal hydration on the first postoperative day, which, according to many critics of clear corneal incisions, disappeared within an hour or two. To confirm that the swelling is due to stromal hydration rather than surgical trauma, OCT images were taken of cases in which there was no stromal hydration of the incision. As demonstrated in Fig. 6.26, which is representative of an incision which did not undergo stromal hydration, there is less thickening around the incision and some gaping of the internal lip of the incision.

Finally, each figure also has the intraocular pressure recorded at the time of the postoperative visit. Many of these are hypotonous and yet are perfectly well sealed, which contradicts the current thinking regarding incision architecture and hypotony [11].

A surprising finding was that proper incision construction resulted in a longer incision than the chord length that was measured and in greater stability (like tongue in groove paneling) of the incision. Another surprising finding was that stromal swelling does

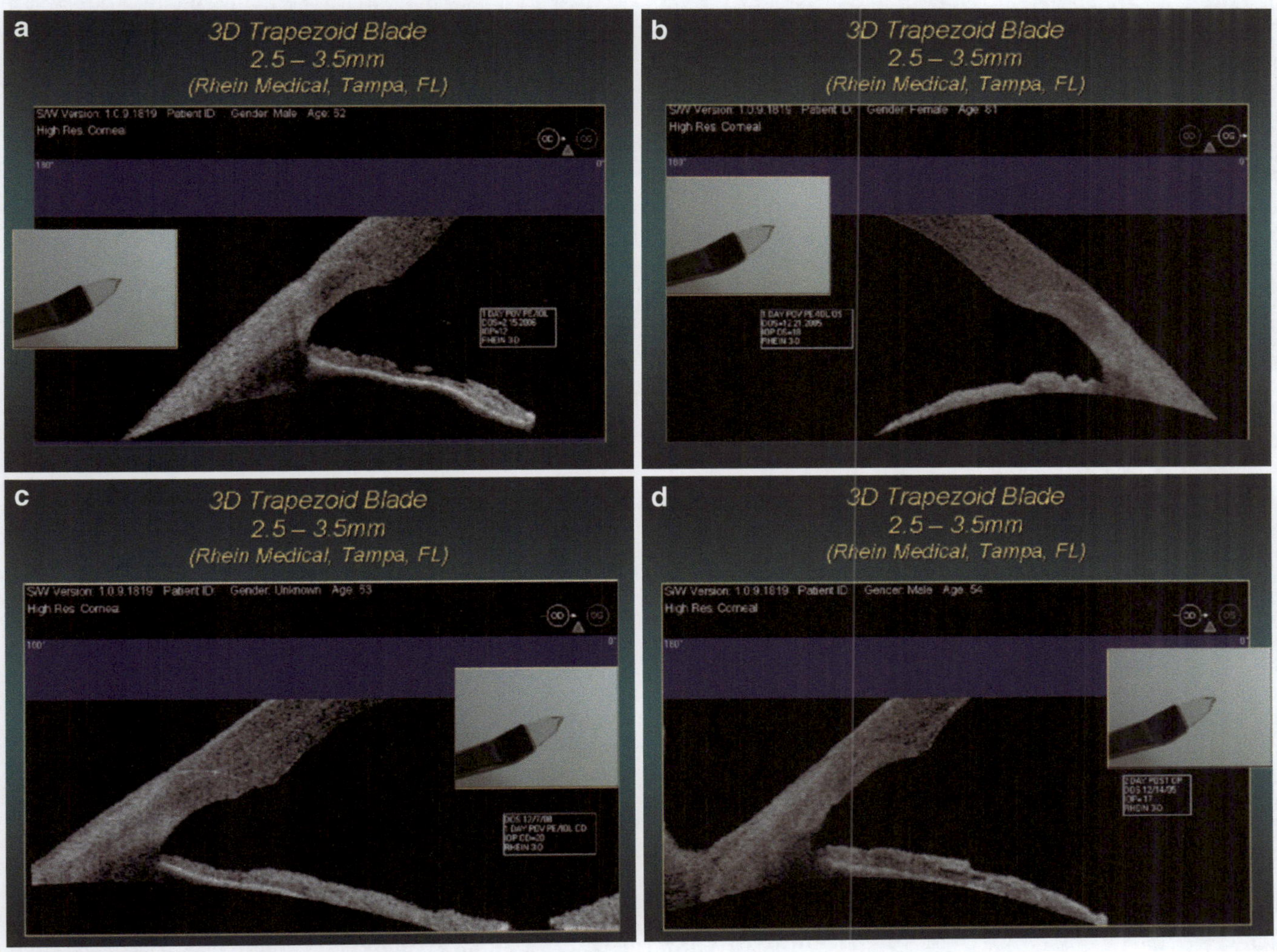

Fig. 6.17 (**a–d**) OCT images of clear corneal incisions made with the Rhein 3D Trapezoidal 2.5–3.5 mm Blade. Image of the blade is inset

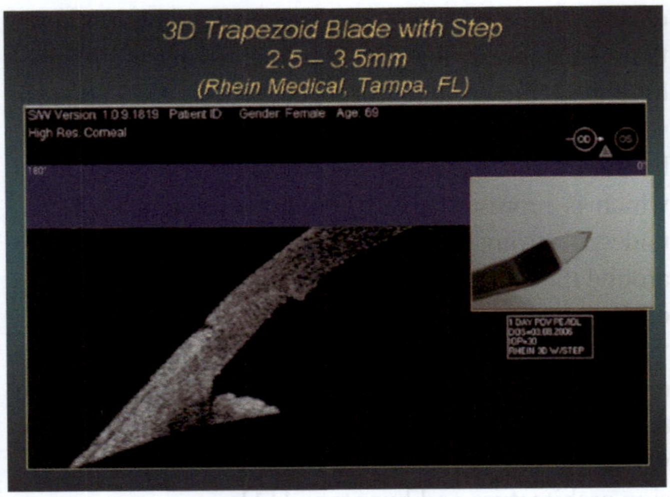

Fig. 6.18 OCT image of a clear corneal incision with a 300 µm groove at the external edge of the incision. Image of the Rhein 3D blade is inset

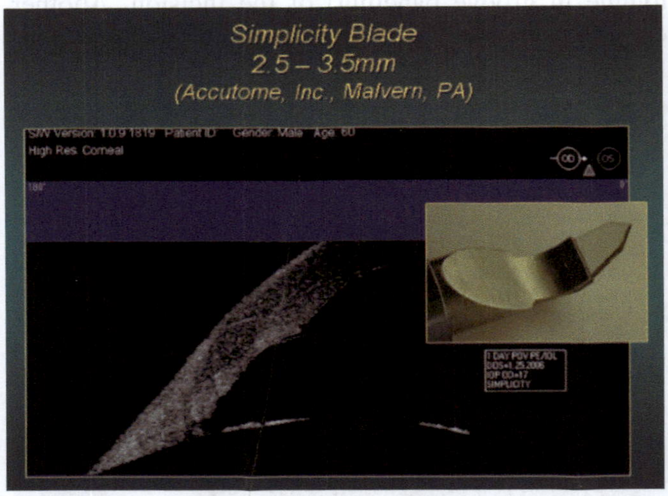

Fig. 6.19 OCT image of clear corneal incision with the Accutome Simplicity 2.5–3.5 mm blade. Image of the blade is inset

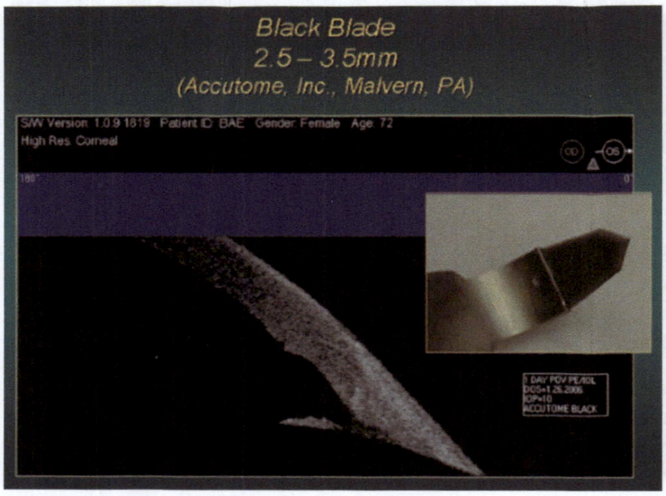

Fig. 6.20 OCT image of clear corneal incision with the Accutome Black 2.5–3.5 mm Blade. Image of the blade is inset

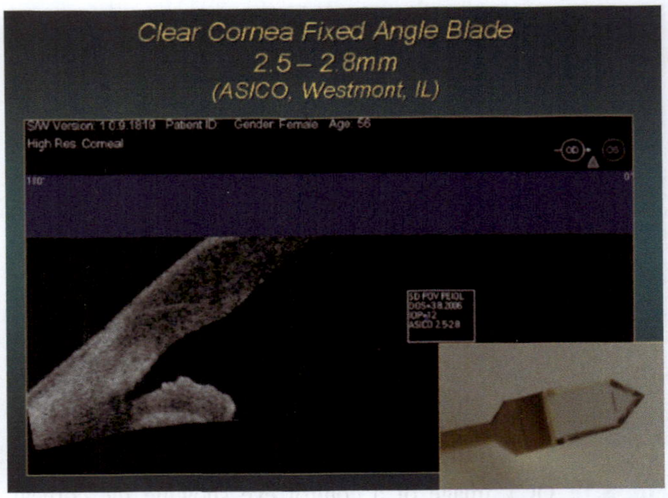

Fig. 6.21 OCT image of clear corneal incision with the ASICO Clear Cornea Fixed Angle 2.5–2.8 mm blade. Image of the blade is inset

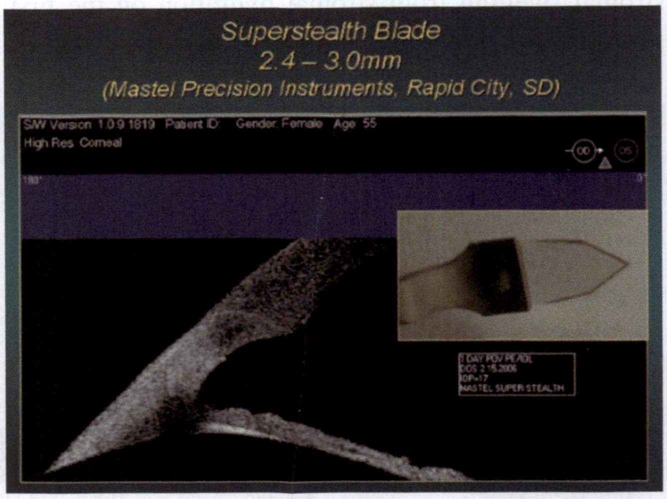

Fig. 6.22 OCT image of clear corneal incision with the Mastel Superstealth 2.4–3.0 mm blade. Image of the blade is inset

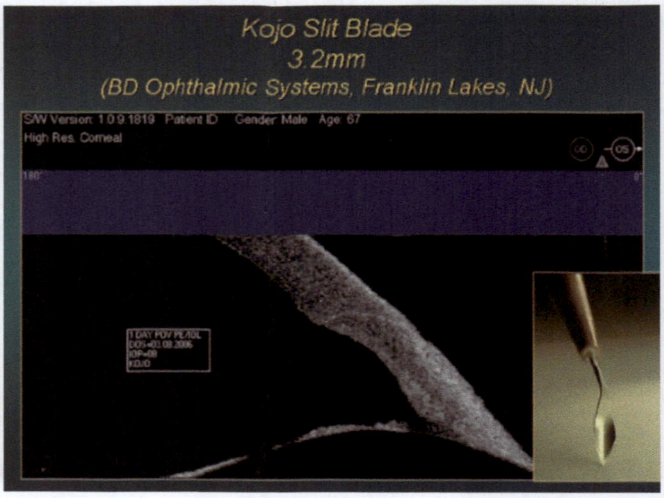

Fig. 6.23 OCT image of a clear corneal incision made with the BD Kojo 3.2 mm slit blade. Image of blade is inset

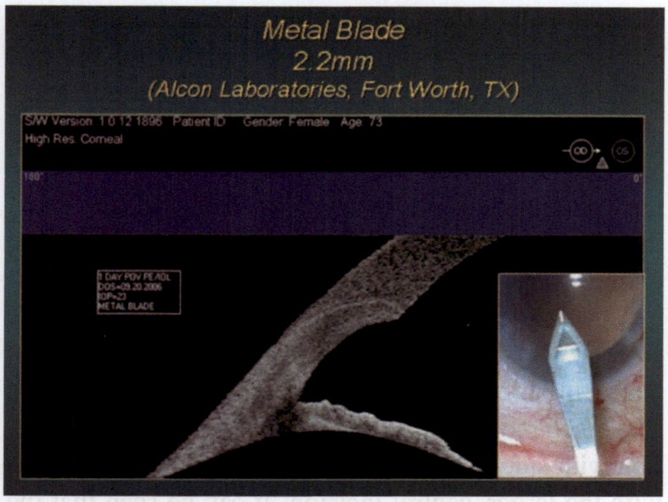

Fig. 6.24 OCT image of a clear corneal incision made with an Alcon 2.2 mm metal blade. Image of blade is inset

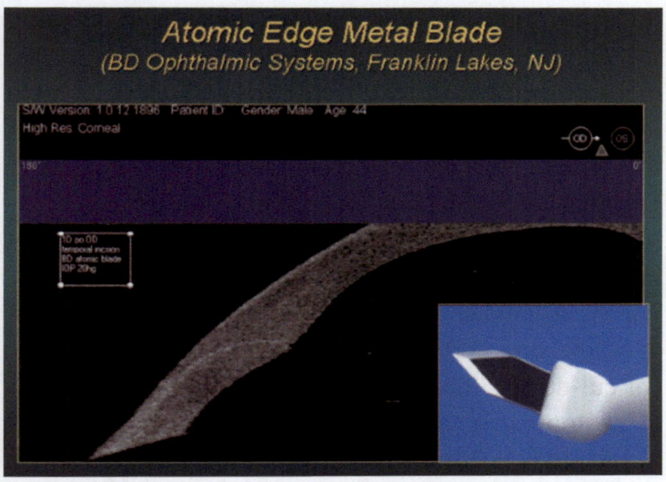

Fig. 6.25 OCT image of a clear corneal incision made with a BD Atomic Edge metal blade. Image of blade is inset

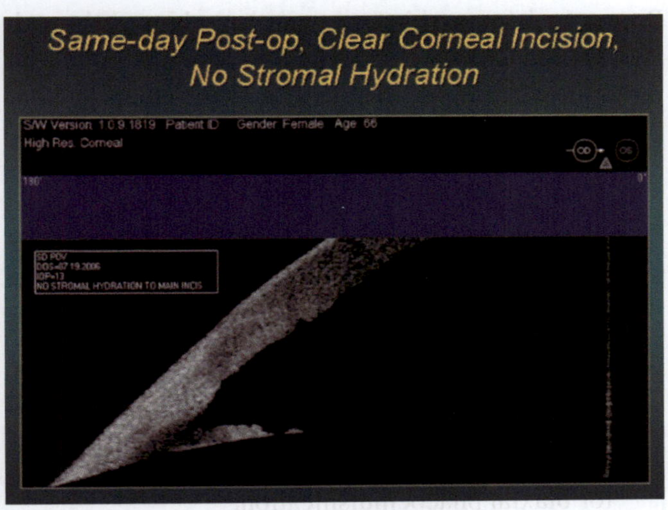

Fig. 6.26 OCT image of a clear corneal incision that did not receive stromal hydration

indeed last for at least 24 h. These findings demonstrate some of the characteristics that the authors believe to have contributed to an added measure of safety in clear corneal incisions that, in conjunction with other prophylactic measures, can result in the absence of endophthalmitis.

Endophthalmitis prophylaxis involves a large number of factors including proper preoperative antibiotic regime; preparation of the surgical field including Betadine and draping over the lashes and meibomian orifices; incision construction; surgical technique including atraumatic surgery; power modulations to avoid heating the incision; avoiding grasping the roof of the incision with a toothed forceps which would abrade the epithelium and disrupt the fluid barrier for endothelial pumping; incision closer; testing for leakage; and postoperative antibiotics. The authors have gone for longer than 15 years and over 13,000 cases without a *single* case of infectious endophthalmitis.

Attention to all of the details for endophthalmitis prophylaxis is essential. However, incision construction leading to proper architecture is of primary importance among all of the variables that are part of endophthalmitis prophylaxis. This is the same conclusion that was made in a recent white paper by the American Society of Cataract and Refractive Surgery (ASCRS) [13]. It is important to recognize that all clear corneal incisions are clearly not the same.

An incision in the plane of the cornea with a chord length of at least 2 mm appears to give uniquely advantageous architecture for adequate self-sealability.

6.2.1 Side-Port Incisions

Bimanual microincision phacoemulsification is being performed for over seven years and it has been found that the side-port incisions, through which irrigating choppers are used in one hand and an unsleeved phacoemulsification needle in the other, are a little more difficult to seal, compared to coaxial side-port incision. Attention has recently been directed towards possible damage to side-port incisions as a result of the use of an unsleeved phaco tip [14–17]. It is important to note that these investigators have not completed a learning curve in bimanual microincision phacoemulsification and so some of what is demonstrated may be the result of their novice status with respect to this technique. However, as a result of our study of clear corneal cataract incisions, we decided to look at our side-port incisions and we were quite surprised to find that many of them did not contain the architecture that we preferred, but were closer to the architecture demonstrated in the artist's depictions of clear corneal incisions (Fig. 6.27a, b).

As a result of our studies of these incisions, we began to take the same amount of time, effort, and precision in side-port incision construction as we do in our larger incisions. In this way, by making more careful and longer incisions, it was possible to achieve exactly the same architecture in side-port incisions (Fig. 6.28a–f). Each of these figures contain an incision location as depicted in the circle in the right-hand upper corner, where the bottom of the circle represents the temporal periphery and the meridian of the incision is located by the arrow as seen from the surgeon's perspective, sitting temporally. Within the box in the lower left-hand corner, the hand for which paracentesis was made is indicated. In each instance, all right hand incisions were the ones through which the unsleeved phaco needle was placed, and all left-hand incisions were the ones through which the irrigating chopper was placed.

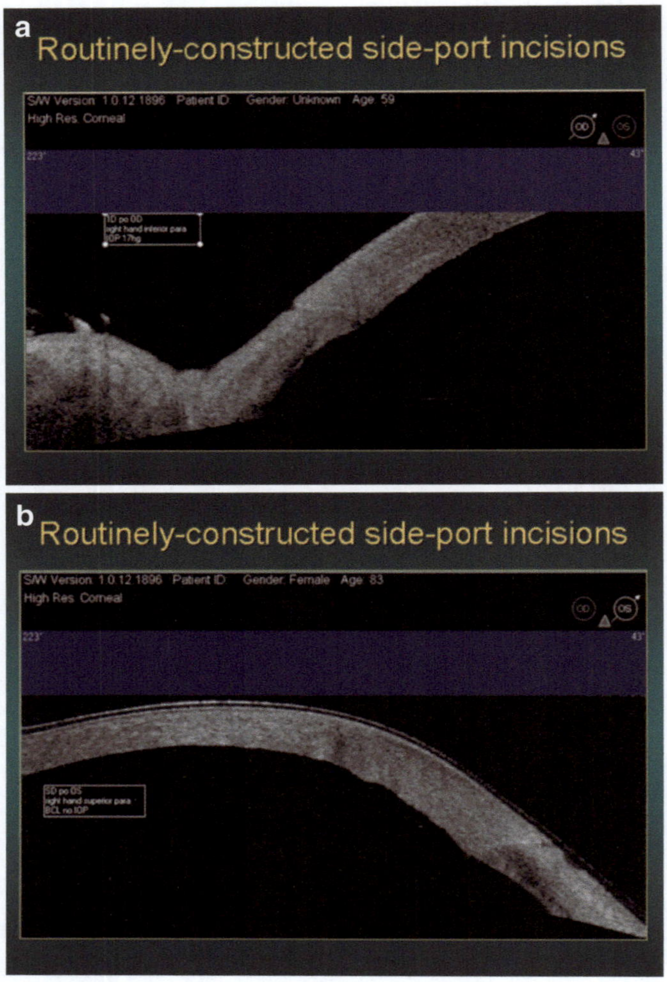

Fig. 6.27 (**a**, **b**) OCT images of routinely-constructed side-port incisions. For (**b**), the bandage contact lens, which was applied due to an epithelial abrasion at the incision cite, is clearly visible

The last three figures (Fig. 6.29a–c) show a single case in which refractive lens exchange was done. The beautiful architecture of the side-port incisions, which seal much more easily, can be seen, as incision construction with side-ports have been done in the same way as with the larger, central incision. It can be seen that the implantation incision, through which a Synchrony IOL was injected, was a self-sealing 3.8 mm incision.

The examination of side-port incisions with OCT forces us to recognize that proper incision architecture for side-port incisions requires the same, appropriate incision construction as for temporal clear corneal incisions. The blade must be advanced in the plane of the cornea for an adequate length (approximately 1.5 mm) before incising Descemet's membrane.

For most surgeons, the transition to clear corneal incisions also involved transition to temporal surgery. For right-handed, coaxial surgeons operating on left eyes, the side-port incision is in the inferior conjunctival cul-de-sac. The role of inferior side-port incisions in postoperative endophthalmitis has been raised. A recent study documented that there was indeed, a much greater incidence of postoperative endophthalmitis in clear corneal cataract surgery in left eyes compared to right eyes [18].

Cataract surgery begins with incision construction. Proper incision architecture can be achieved through appropriate incision construction which requires an unfailing attention to details, for both temporal clear corneal and side-port incisions.

Take Home Pearls

Clear corneal incisions

- Are safe, effective, advantageous, and cosmetically desirable
- Require accurate construction and architecture
- Need to be very precise even for microincisions for biaxial phacoemulsification.

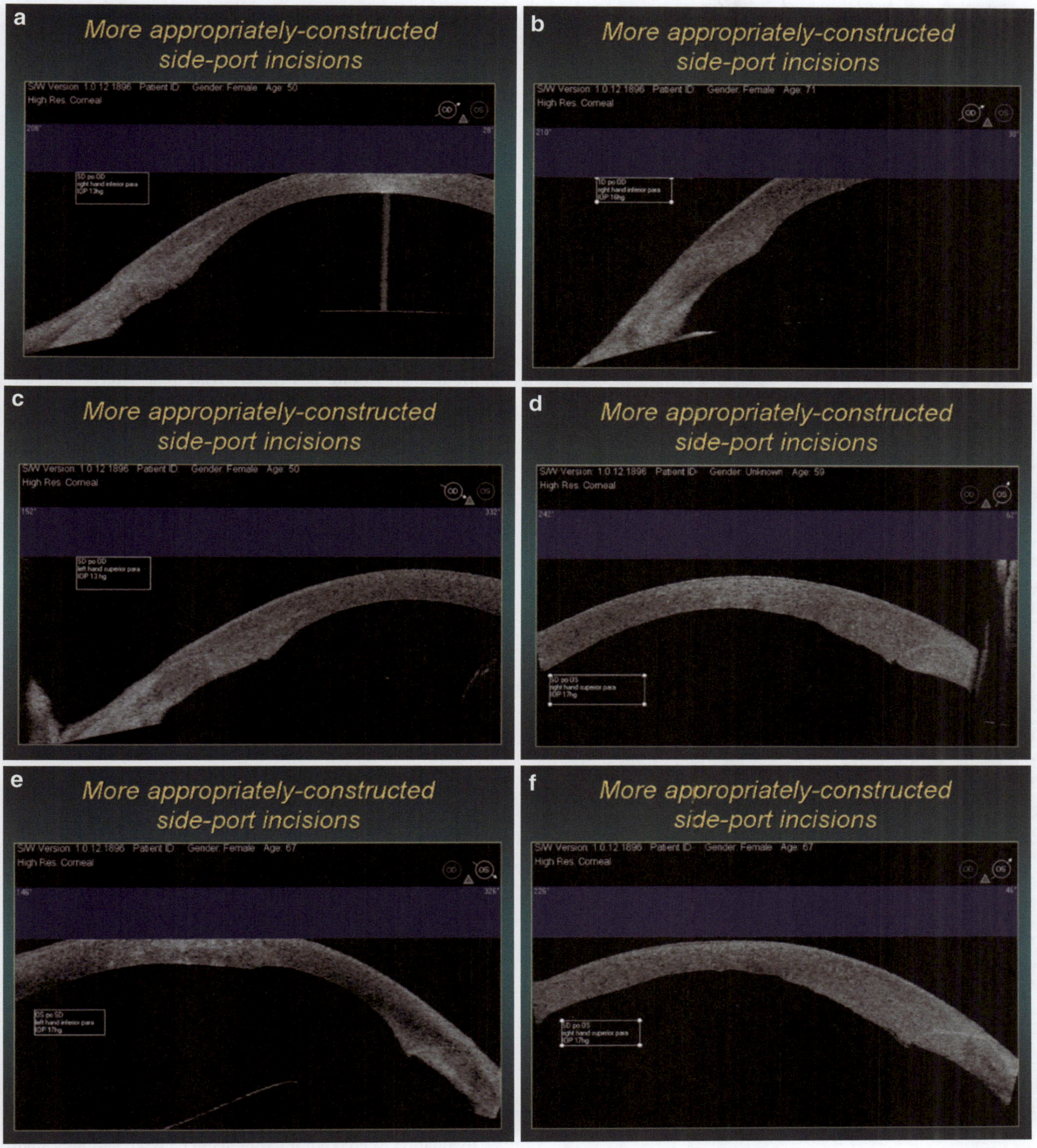

Fig. 6.28 (**a–f**) OCT images of more appropriately-constructed side-port incisions

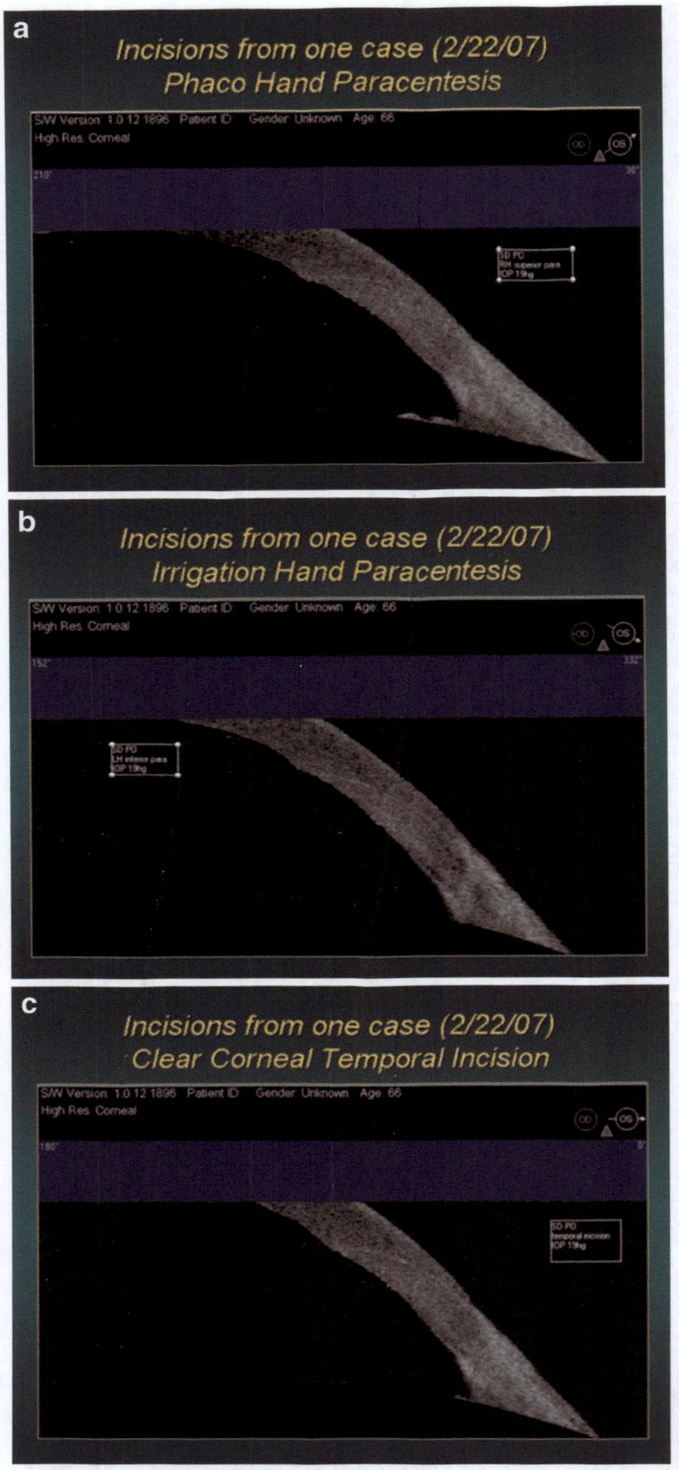

Fig. 6.29 OCT images of incisions from one case: (**a**) Phaco side-port incision; (**b**) Irrigating side-port incision; (**c**) Clear corneal temporal IOL implantation incision

References

1. Fine IH, Hoffman RS, Packer M (2007) Architecture of clear corneal incisions demonstrated by optical coherence tomography. Highlights Ophthalmol 35(4):2–4; 6–9 (Reprinted with permission from Highlights of Ophthalmology)
2. Cooper BA, Holekamp NM, Bohigian G, Thompson PA (2003) Case-control study of endophthalmitis after cataract surgery comparing scleral tunnel and clear corneal wounds. Am J Ophthalmol 136:300–305
3. Nakagi Y, Hayasaka S, Kadoi C et al (2003) Bacterial endophthalmitis after small-incision cataract surgery; effect of incision placement and intraocular lens type. J Cataract Refract Surg 29:20–26
4. Eifrig CW, Flynn HW, Scott IU, Newton J (2002) Acute-onset postoperative endophthalmitis: review of incidence and visual outcomes (1995–2001). Ophthalmic Surg Lasers 33:373–378
5. Miller JJ, Scott IU, Flynn HW Jr, Smiddy WE, Newton J, Miller D (2005) Acute-onset endophthalmitis after cataract surgery (2000–2004): Incidence, clinical settings and visual acuity outcomes after treatment. Am J Ophthalmol 139(6):983–987
6. Monica ML, Long DA (2005) Nine-year safety with self-sealing corneal tunnel incision in clear cornea cataract surgery. Ophthalmology 112(6):985–986
7. Masket S (2005) Is there a relationship between clear corneal cataract incisions and endophthalmitis? J Cataract Refract Surg 31(4):735–741
8. Mollan SP, Gao A, Lockwood A, Durrani OM, Butler L (2007) Postcataract endophthalmitis: incidence and microbial isolates in a United Kingdom region from 1996 through 2004. J Cataract Refract Surg 33(2):265–268
9. Ng JQ, Morlet N, Bulsara MK, Semmens JB (2007) Reducing the risk for endophthalmitis after cataract surgery: population-based nested case-control study. Endophthalmitis population study of western Australia sixth report. J Cataract Refract Surg 33(2):269–280
10. Fine IH (1992) Self-sealing corneal tunnel incision for small-incision cataract surgery. Ocular Surgery News 10(9): 38–39
11. Realini T (2007) Wound construction key to avoiding endophthalmitis. EyeWorld 12(2):64–66
12. Fine IH (1994) Clear corneal incisions. Int Ophthalmol Clin Spring 34(2):59–72
13. White Paper ASCRS Cataract Clinical Committee (2007) Special Report: Association between CCI and endophthalmitis. EyeWorld (suppl). Available at: www.eyeworld.org/ewweeksupplementarticle.php?id=187&strict=&morphologic=&query=association%20between%20CCI%20and%20endophthalmitis. Accessed 16 May 2007
14. Vasavada AR (2005) Phaco tips and corneal tissue. Cataract Refract Surg Today 5(Suppl):9–10
15. Weikert M, Koch D (2005) Phaco wounds study. Cataract Refract Surg Today (Suppl):11–13
16. Berdahl JP, DeStafano JJ, Kim T (2007) Corneal wound architecture and integrity after phacoemulsification: Evaluation of coaxial, microincision coaxial, and microincision bimanual techniques. J Cataract Refract Surg 33: 510–515
17. Osher RH, Injev VP (2007) Microcoaxial phacoemulsification: Part 1: laboratory studies. J Cataract Refract Surg 33(3): 401–407
18. Colin S Tam MD (2008) Ophthalmology Times (15 August 2008) 33(16)

6.3 Thermodynamics[1]

Alessandro Franchini, Iacopo Franchini, and Daniele Tognetto[2]

Core Messages

- Prevention of thermal injury to corneal incisions requires:
- Proper machine settings
- Proper incision construction
- Management of viscoelastic substances
- Proper irrigation flow
- Optimal manipulation of the phaco tip within the incision
- Tip design
- Proper surgical technique

6.3.1 Introduction

Since its introduction in the 1960s by Charles Kelman, ultrasonic phacoemulsification has achieved high standards, both in safety and efficiency. However, the dream of the ophthalmologist

working in the anterior segment is to perform phacoemulsification through an incision small enough to be truly, astigmatically neutral. Decreasing the incision size has been limited by the need for a sleeve around the phaco tip and a fluid flow through the incision in order to avoid increased temperatures at the incision site that could result in corneal or scleral burns [1–3]. In the 1990s, a number of pioneers suggested alternative sources of energy with the hope of reducing the temperature of the tip. Lasers have been a focus of this investigation [1].

[1]Rewritten by I. Howard Fine

[2]The Authors have no proprietary or financial interest in any product or device discussed in this paper and have not received any payment as a reviewer or evaluator.

A. Franchini (✉)
Eye Institute, University of Florence, Viale Morgagni 85-50134 Florence, Italy
e-mail: oculist@unifi.it

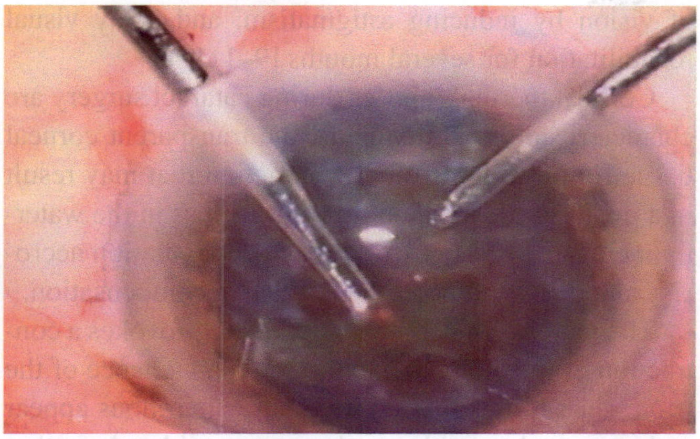

Fig. 6.30 Erbium:YAG laser microincision cataract extraction

In 1993, we began working with the erbium:YAG laser for cataract extraction [4]. Temperature increases with laser phacoemulsification were very slight, allowing us to move to a biaxial technique in which the irrigation was separated from the laser/aspiration handpiece , which makes it possible to carry out cataract surgery through two 1.0 mm incisions (Fig. 6.30).

Unfortunately, laser phacoemulsification is not as efficient as ultrasound phacoemulsification, particularly with nuclei of a density greater than 2+. In dense nuclei, the procedure can take three times longer with the erbium:YAG laser, when compared to that of ultrasound phacoemulsification.

Since our early work with the erbium: YAG laser, there has been an evolution in ultrasound phacoemulsification. The introduction of power modulations, especially ultrapulse technology, has represented one of the most important innovations in cataract surgery. In fact, the so-called cold ultrasound has made it possible to achieve the dream of microincision, uniting the safety of laser and the efficiency of ultrasound, in the same machine. This new technology produces very rapid microbursts of energy followed by microrests that allow the phaco tip to cool. This significantly reduces the amount of energy expended in the eye [5]. It has been shown in both clinical [6] and cadaver eye [7] studies, that the temperature at the wound site with cold ultrasound does not achieve the necessary levels to produce a wound burn under clinically applicable conditions.

6.3.2 Corneal Thermal Damage

Today, incision wound burns occur in less than one patient out of 1,000 [8], but they can degrade the quality of vision by inducing astigmatism, and delay visual rehabilitation for several months [9–11].

Corneal thermal injuries during cataract surgery are characterized by whitening of the transparent corneal tissue followed by stromal contraction that may result in a misfit of the incision lips, with a loss in the watertight closure [12]. In extreme cases, coagulation necrosis can occur with potential corneal decompensation.

The increase in corneal temperature provokes a contraction of the alpha helix with the maintenance of the triple helix tertiaris structure. These alterations appear to be corneal wrinkles and are reversible. A further increase in temperature creates a destruction of the collagen matrix tertiaris structure. These alterations create a loss of the corneal clarity and determine nonreversible damage [13].

The surgeon often becomes aware of this when the damage is already irreversible.

The denaturization of the collagen fibers occurs after 18 s at a temperature of 63°C (145°F), after 1 s at 100°C (212°F), and 0.001 s at a temperature of 200°C (392°F) [13].

The first thermal changes in the cornea do not occur below a temperature of 40°C [please provide reference].

6.3.3 Heat Generation

The standard ultrasonic handpiece produces a longitudinal movement of the tip. The power generated by the tip is the product of the frequency and the stroke length.

The frequency is the number of tip movements within unit time and is measured in Kilohertz (KHz; 1,000 cycles per second).

All of the phacoemulsifiers today operate at a frequency between 35 and 45 KHz; the higher the frequency, the higher is the risk of thermal damage [14]. The frequencies used today represent the best compromise to achieve emulsification efficiency and thermal safety.

The frequency can vary during phacoemulsification due to the changing load at the tip (i.e., the size, the shape and the density of lens material occluding the tip). All of the modern machines have a software that regulates either the resident frequency or the stroke length.

The stroke length is the length of the tip movements and is measured in thousandths of an inch (mil). Today all the machines operate in a range between 2 and 4 mil which again, represent the best compromise between emulsification efficiency and thermal safety.

The longitudinal movements emulsify the lens material by the application of mechanical, cavitational, thermal, and acoustical energy. The mechanical energy (jackhammer) is due to the hit of the needle against the lens material. The cavitational energy results from the gas bubbles which are formed by the backstroke of the tip, creating a relative vacuum. With vaporization of some of the fluid, the gas bubbles are the fuel that generates cavitational energy. The next forward movement of the tip compresses the bubbles resulting in their implosion.

There are two types of cavitation energy. First is the transient cavitation, which is characterized by high-energy implosion of the cavitation bubbles. Second is the stable cavitation,which occurs when the bubbles begin to vibrate with fewer collapses and dramatically reduced release of energy.

6.3.4 Factors that Contribute to Thermal Incision Damage

The following factors can contribute to an increase in the temperature of the tip and to the genesis of the incision burns:

(a) Energy emission – amount and pattern of how the energy is delivered
(b) Incision – incision construction and possible constriction of the sleeve
(c) Viscoelastic devices and possible occlusion of the aspiration line
(d) Irrigation flow
(e) Position of the tip inside the incision
(f) Tip design
(g) Surgical technique

6.3.4.1 Energy Emission: Amount and Pattern of How the Energy Is Delivered

Over the past 10 years, the evolution of technology with power modulations and pulse shaping (Fig. 6.31) has allowed us to work utilizing less energy.

Continuous phaco mode produces the highest energy, pulse and burst modes reduce the energy, and finally, the ultrapulse mode reduces the energy significantly.

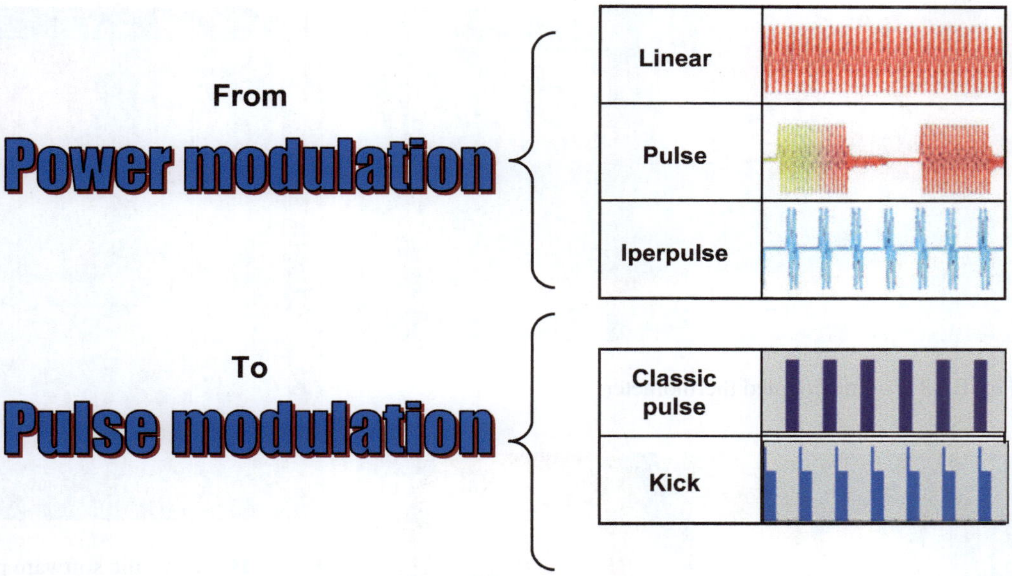

Fig. 6.31 Energy emission

Micropulse settings (6 µs on, and 12 µs off) produces less frictional heat at the incision site than the pulse setting (50 ms on, and 50 ms off), which maintain the same emulsification efficiency [15].

This is true in vivo even when in micropulse mode, the phaco time off is equal to phaco time on. In vitro, there isn't a significant difference in temperature between ultrapulse (6 µs on, 6 µs off) and pulsed energy (50 µs on, 50 µs off), when the ratio of phaco on/phaco off, is 1 [16].

The concept of thermal inertia means that the shorter pulse has a slower propagation in biological tissues [17]. This effect reduces the penetration of heat by only 10% and so does not explain the limited increase in temperature generated by ultrapulse mode. Therefore, other factors have also been involved, specifically the features of how ultrasound energy works.

It has been hypothesized that shorter phaco on time produces a decrease in repulsion of the nuclear fragments from the tip at each pulse. This allows an increase in followability and holdability, with an enhancement of the jackhammer effect due to the near continuous contact of the fragments with the tip.

Another hypothesis is that micropulse generates only transient cavitation, which is the most energetic, and therefore an efficient component of cavitational energy. In fact, when the pulse lasts for more than a few microseconds, the transient cavitation gives way to stable cavitation. Stable cavitation is less efficient than transient cavitation and a bigger part of energy is dissipated as heat [18].

During recent years, we have moved from the concept of pulse modulation to the concept of shape modulation. In this case, the ultrasound emission is characterized by the so called "kick," which is an impulse that lasts for 1 mm sec and which is 12% more powerful than the maximum power of the rest of the pulse. Therefore, the "kick" can be defined as an increase in power in the first microsecond of the duty cycle. The power of the "kick" can be the same in all duty cycles, or can be programmed to produce an increase or a decrease throughout the "on" time.

The "kick" physically separates the nuclear material from the phaco tip allowing the creation of a microvoid between the occluded tip and the nuclear material. The microvoid allows fresh balanced salt solution (BSS) to get between the phaco tip and the nuclear material, and results in the generation of transient cavitation and an increased release of energy without an increase in temperature. Therefore, the efficiency of the emulsification is increased.

In the year 2006, a new concept of ultrasonic movements was introduced to decrease the heat generation while maintaining or increasing the phaco efficiency by torsional movements of the tip at a frequency of 32 KHz.

Many years ago, a similar idea of lateral movements was introduced, but the low frequency of the sonic movements (100–400 Hz) was insufficient to guarantee efficiency.

The reduction of the frequency by 20% and of the stroke length by 50%, make it possible for the torsional movements to use less energy and generate a lower increase in temperature [19] which is estimated to be 60% of the temperature rise with standard longitudinal movements of the tip [20].

The lens is efficiently emulsified by a mechanical effect that is different from the jackhammer effect,

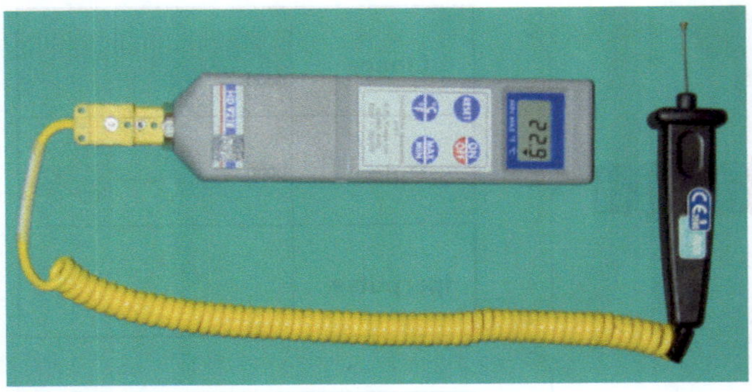

Fig. 6.32 Thermocoupled thermometer

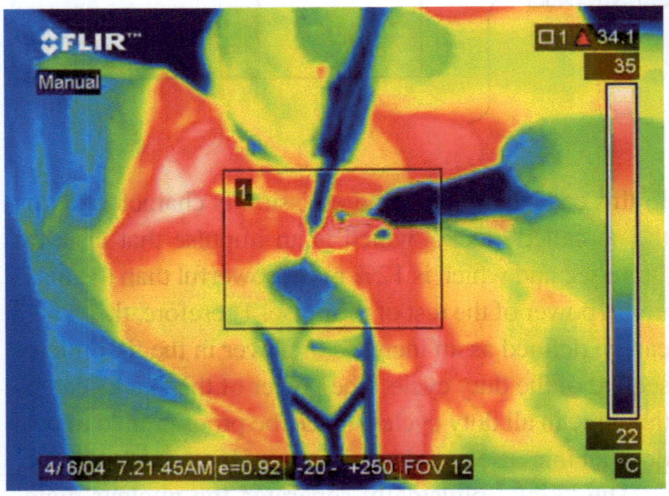

Fig. 6.33 Infrared thermal image

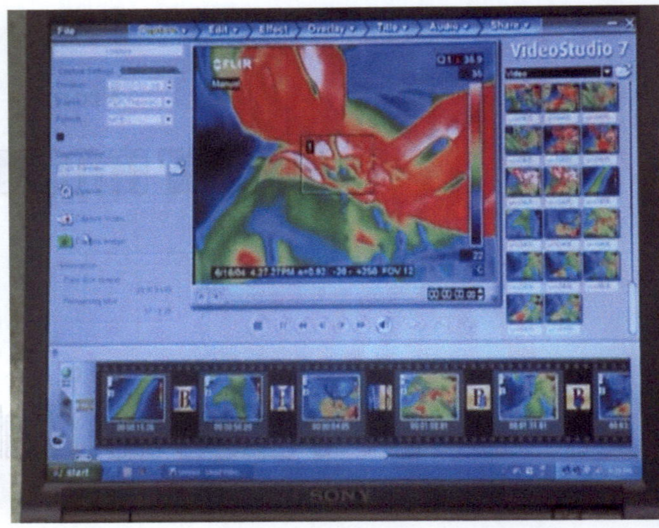

Fig. 6.34 A specific software processes the image in real time

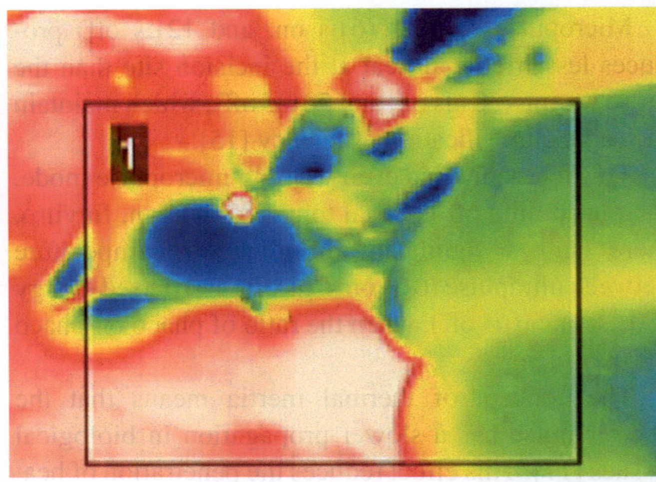

Fig. 6.35 Tip temperature over 45°C

since the tip continuously shears the lens without repelling it. However, the role of cavitation in torsional emulsification requires further investigation [21].

Recently, a software has been introduced that combines the lateral tip movement with the longitudinal movement resulting in an elliptical cutting surface. This maintains the continuous advantage of cavitational energy.

The temperature at the tip and at the incision site have been studied in vivo, initially using a thermocoupled thermometer and then thermal imaging. The thermocoupled thermometer (Fig. 6.32) is characterized by a digital thermometer connected to a sensor which can be placed on the incision or directly connected to the tip. Despite being accurate, these thermometers do not allow the full range of movement during surgery. Therefore, in recent years, infrared cameras and specific software (Fig. 6.33) have been used, creating thermographic, color images of the ocular surface, where it is possible to detect minimal temperature changes and precise temperature measurements in real time (Figs. 6.34 and 6.35).

Using these instruments, many authors have tried to compare different machines at different settings and different surgical conditions. This is impossible because parameter settings on different machines do not correlate with each other [14, 22, 23] (See Sect. 5.2 in Chap. 5). Other factors such as incision outflow are impossible to standardize.

6.3.4.2 Incision: Incision Construction and Possible Constriction of the Sleeve

Generally, incisions need to be of the appropriate width to minimize incision outflow (with microincision cataract surgery) without compressing the sleeve, and appropriate length (usually 2.0 mm) to allow self-sealability. Trapezoidal-shaped incisions allow more maneuverability of the tip without stressing or tearing the incision.

6.3.4.3 Viscoelastic Devices and Possible Occlusion of the Aspiration Line

There are no indications that the use of different ophthalmic viscodevices (cohesive, dispersive, etc.) is more often linked to higher incision temperatures. The aspiration line may become clogged by an ophthalmic viscodevice, which would then block irrigation flow. When this occurs with the phaco power on, the heat is no longer dissipated (Fig. 6.36a, b). Increased heat may also result from cavitation bubbles being trapped in viscoelastic divice and blocking out flow, as well as, perhaps, the liberation of free radicals during phacoemulsification, which may have a minimal, theoretical impact [24].

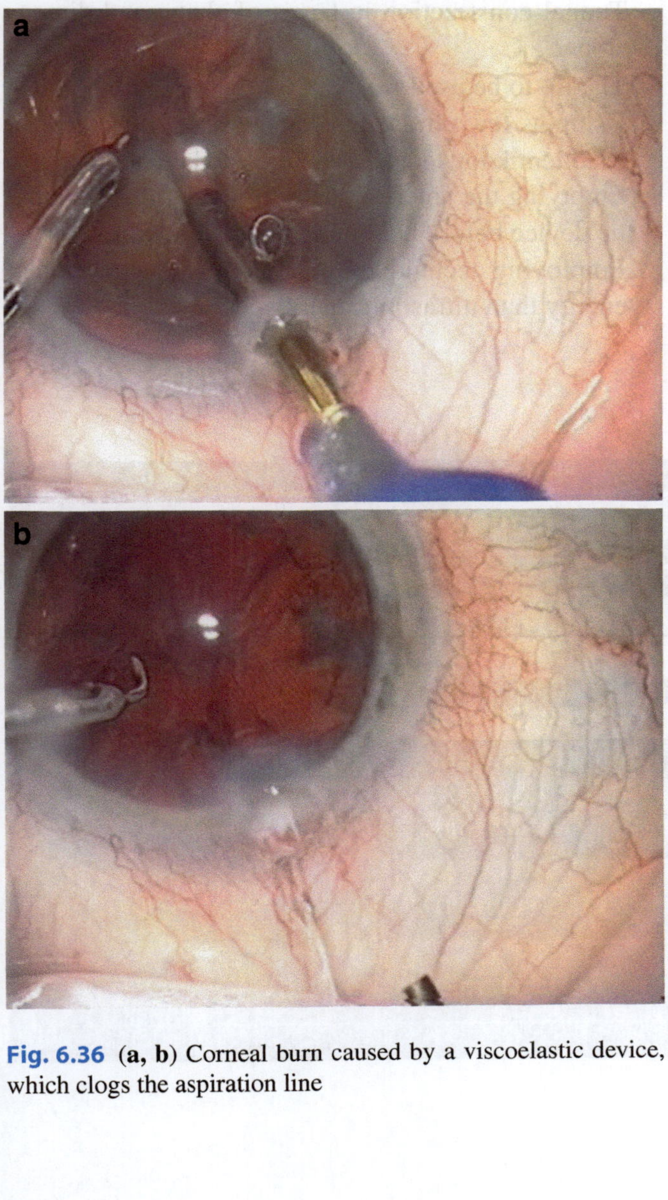

Fig. 6.36 (a, b) Corneal burn caused by a viscoelastic device, which clogs the aspiration line

Prior to entering foot position 3, surgeons should aspirate some viscoelastic divice from the front and the top.

6.3.4.4 Irrigation Flow

Cooling of the irrigating fluid should have some effect on reducing the temperature at the tip; however, this practice has been discontinued in the US with the advent of power modulations. Increasing the bottle height may result in some increased incisional out flow at the cost of increasing intraocular pressure, which may, under some conditions, exceed intraluminal profusion pressure in the ophthalmic artery [25].

6.3.4.5 Position of the Tip Inside the Incision

Movement of the phacoemulsification handpiece during the surgical procedure can result in compression of the tip against the sleeve, with a resultant transmission of heat to the incision itself. Therefore, movements have to be appropriate and ergonomic with a consideration of the possibility of transmitting heat to the incision (Fig. 6.37–6.38).

6.3.4.6 Tip Design

Increasing the lumen of the sleeve, compared to the size of the phaco tip, may result in greater amounts of

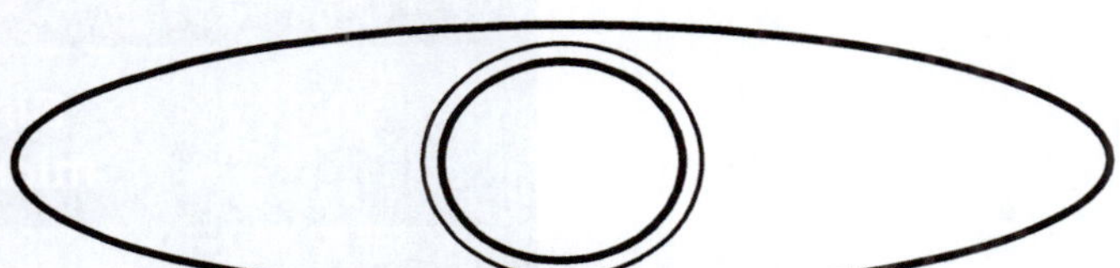

Fig. 6.37 A well centered tip inside the incision (the space between the tip and the sleeve and the space between the sleeve and the incision-wall are maintained)

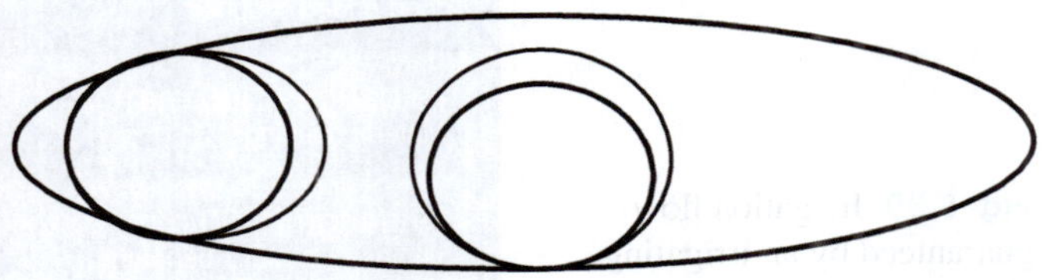

Fig. 6.38 When the tip is pushed toward the incision wall, the tip is in contact with the sleeve and the sleeve, with the incision-wall

irrigation and greater cooling, and less potential for the compression of the tip to block irrigation flow. An aspiration bypass tip can avoid excessive increase in temperature at the incision site because of the lack of complete occlusion of the tip and the absence of flow during occlusion. The use of an angled phaco tip, such as the Kelman tip, gives accessibility to the endolenticular material with less tilting of the tip and therefore, greater protection against thermal injury [26] (Fig. 6.38).

6.3.4.7 Surgical Technique

Chopping techniques utilize less ultrasound energy in general, because they use mechanical forces in the form of chopping to disassemble the nucleus compared to ultrasound energy grooving, in preparation for cracking. There are some studies that indicate that biaxial microincision cataract surgery results in increased thermal damage [27, 28]; however, other studies [6, 7, 29–33] have not found a significant difference in the temperature at the incision using a sleeveless technique compared to a sleeved one. Although early irrigating choppers had less flow than conventional coaxial systems, the more modern irrigating choppers and larger lumens have flows that are comparable to coaxial microincision cataract surgery [34] (Fig. 6.39).

6.3.5 Conclusion

In the past, corneal burns during phacoemulsification have represented an important problem, which has partially delayed the complete diffusion of this surgical procedure. To a greater extent, the fault can be placed on the machines which delivered too much energy for too long.

With the improvement of scientific knowledge in ultrasonic emission, it has been possible to have even more efficient machines that are able to use lesser energy[35–40].

For this reason, during recent years, the occurrences of corneal burns has been much more occasional and can no longer be put down to any machine malfunction, but to a series of surgeon's distractions.

The surgeon who prepares to perform an ultrasonic phacoemulsification must know that, apart from a valid and well-set machine, it is also necessary to pay attention to a number of other factors:

- Tunnel construction in terms of shape and dimension
- The tip to be used
- Using as few ultrasounds as possible by having an excellent knowledge of the foot pedal adopted
- Emptying the anterior chamber from the viscoelastic device before beginning phacoemulsification
- Employing techniques that use more mechanical energy than ultrasonic energy

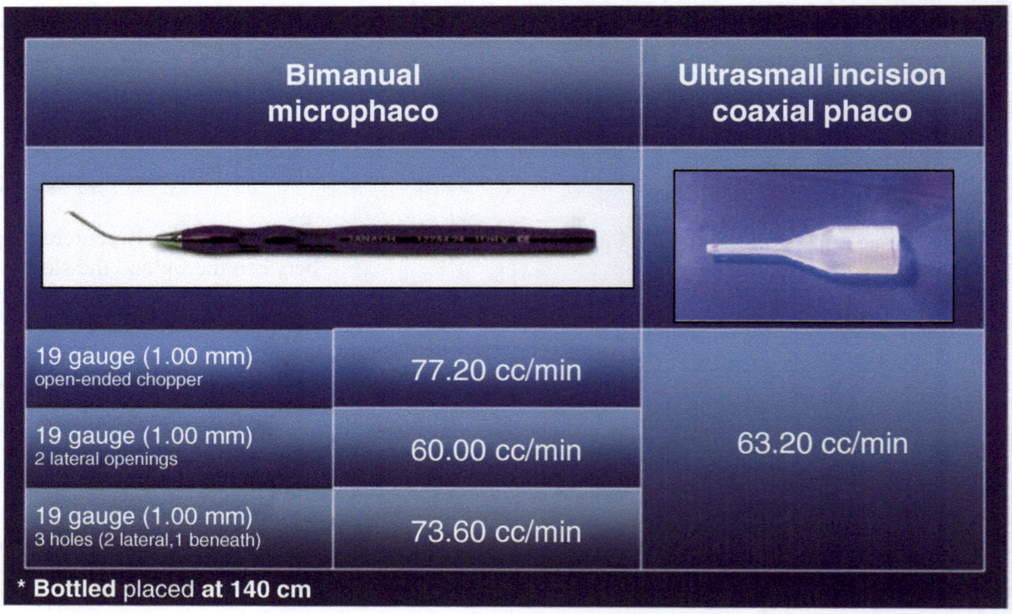

Fig. 6.39 Irrigation flow guaranteed by an irrigating chopper and an ultrasmall sleeve

By observing the points listed above, corneal burns in phacoemulsification can become a thing of the past.

Take Home Pearls

- In order to Avoid Thermal Damage due to Corneal Incisions, the following factors should be paid attention.
- Accurate incision construction and architecture
- Tip design appropriate for the particular procedure being done
- Use of power modulations with decreased energy delivered
- Careful control of the foot pedal to avoid prolonged time in foot position 3
- Need to aspirate OVD prior to commencing in foot position 3
- Using surgical techniques that depend more on mechanical forces for disassembly of the nucleus rather than grooving and cracking.

References

1. Benolken RM, Emery JM, Landis DJ (1974) Temperature profiles in the anterior chamber during phaco-emulsification. Invest Ophthalmol 13:71–74
2. Hwang DG, Smith RE (1981) Corneal complications of cataract surgery. Refract Corneal Surg 7:77–80
3. Wirt H, Heisler J-M, Domarus DV (1995) Phacoburns: experimental study for evaluation of risk factors. Eur J Implant Refract Surg 7:275–278
4. Franchini A, Zamma Gallarati B, Vaccari E (2001) 5 anni di esperienza nella erbio facolaseremulsificazione ed altre applicazioni cliniche. Atti della Fondazione G.Ronchi 2:211–237
5. Fishkind WJ (2002) Multisite comparative study of the current Sovereign power control system with the WhiteStar control system. In: Symposium on Cataract, IOL and Refractive Surgery, Philadelphia, PA
6. Donnenfeld ED, Olson RJ, Solomon R et al (2003) Efficacy and wound-temperature gradient of Whitestar phacoemulsification through a 1.2 mm incision. J Cataract Refract Surg 29:1097–1100
7. Soscia W, Howard JG, Olson RJ (2002) Microphacoemulsification with WhiteStar: a wound temperature study. J Cataract Refract Surg 28:1044–1046
8. Bradley MJ, Olson RJ (2006) A survey about phacoemulsification incision thermal contraction incidence and causal relationship. Am J Ophthalmology 141: 222–224
9. Khodabakhsh AJ, Zaidman G, Tabin G (2004) Corneal surgery for severe phacoemulsification burns. Ophthalmology 111:332–334
10. Majid MA, Sharma MK, Harding SP (1998) Corneal scleral burn during phacoemulsification surgery. J Cataract Refract Surg 24:1413–1415
11. Sugar A, Schertzer RM (1999) Clinical course of phacoemulsification wound burns. J Cataract Refract Surg 25:688–692
12. Osher RH (2005) Shark fin: a new sign of thermal injury. J Cataract Refract Surg 31:640–642
13. Enest P, Rhem M, Mc Dermott M et al (2001) Phacoemulsification conditions resulting in thermal wound injury. J Cataract Refract Surg 27:1829–1839
14. Fishkind WJ (2000) Phacoemulsification technology: improved power and fluidica. Chapter 9. In: Wallace RB (ed) Refractive cataract surgery and multifocal IOLs. Slack; Thorofare, NJ, p 87
15. Olson MD, Miller KM (2005) In-air thermal imaging comparison of Legacy AdvanTec, Millenium, and Sovereign WhiteStar phacoemulsification systems. J Cataract Refract Surg 31:1641–1647
16. Brinton JP, Adams W, Kumar R et al (2006) Comparison of thermal features associated with 2 phacoemulsification machine. J Cataract Refract Surg 32:288–293
17. Payne M, Waite A, Olson RJ (2006) Thermal inertia associated with ultrapulse technology in phacoemulsification. J Cataract Refract Surg 32:1032–1034
18. Schaeffer ME (2004) Demonstration of cavitation effects in phacoemulsification devices. In: ASCRS Symposium, San Diego, CA
19. Liu Y, Zeng M, Liu X et al (2007) Torsional mode versus conventional ultrasound mode phacoemulsification. Randomized comparative study. J Cataract Refract Surg 33:287–292
20. Mackool RJ (2007) Phaco arena: to sleeve or not to sleeve; this is the question. In: Course presented at the Congress of the American Society of Cataract and Refractive Surgery, San Diego, CA
21. Boukhny M (2003) Phaoemulsification tips and sleeves. In: Buratto L, Werner L, Zanini M, Apple D (eds) Phacoemulsification principles and techniques, 2nd edn. Slack, Thorofare NJ, pp 247–254
22. Braga-Mele R (2006) Thermal effect of microburst and hyperpulse settings during sleeveless bimanual phacoemulsification with advanced power modulations. J Cataract Refract Surg 32:639–642
23. Olson RJ, Jin Y, Kefalopoulos G et al (2004) Legaci AdvanTec and Sovereign WhiteStar: A wound temperature study. J Cataract Refract Surg 30:1109–1113
24. Takahashi H (2005) Free radical development in phacoemulsification cataract surgery. Nippon Med Sch 72:4–12
25. Franchini A (2007) Signature: discovering new frontiers in creating a stable environment during cataract surgery. In: Paper presented at the XXV Congress of the ESCRS, Stockholm
26. Vasavada AR, Mamidipudi PR, Minj M (2004) Relationship of immediate intraocular pressare rise to phaco-tip ergonomics and energy dissipation. J Cataract Refract Surg 30:137–143
27. Berdahl J, DeStefano J, Kim T (2007) Corneal wound architecture and integrity after phacoemulsification. Evaluation

of coaxial, microincision coaxial and microincision bimanual techniques. J Cataract Refract Surg 33:510–515
28. Vasavada AR (2005) Phaco tip and corneal tissue; histomorphology and immunochemistry reveal the effects of sleeveless and sleeved tip. Cataract Refract Surg Today (Suppl):9–10
29. Alió J, Rodríguez-Prats JL, Galal A et al (2005) Outcomes of microincision cataract surgery versus coaxial phacoemulsification. Ophthalmology 112:1997–2003
30. Assaf A, El-Moatassem Kotb AM (2005) Feasibility of bimanual microincision phacoemulsification in hard cataracts. Eye 21:807–811
31. Soscia W, Howard JG, Olson RJ (2002) Bimanual phacoemulsification through 2 stab incisions; a wound-temperature study. J Cataract Refract Surg 28: 1039–1043
32. Tsuneoka H, Shiba T, Takahashi Y (2001) Feasibility of ultrasound cataract surgery with a 1.4 mm incision. J Cataract Refract Surg 27:934–940
33. Tsuneoka HT, Shiba Takahashi Y (2001) Wound temperature during ultrasmall incision phacoemulsification. Nippon Ganka Gakkai Zasshi 105:237–243
34. Franchini A (2006) Bimanual microphacoemulsification vs. ultra-small incision coaxial phacoemulsification. In: Paper presented at the Congress of ASCRS, San Francisco, CA
35. Alzner E, Grabner G (1999) Dodick laser phacolysis: thermal effects. J Cataract Refract Surg 25:800–803
36. Floyd M, Valentie J., Coombs J et al (2006) Effect of incisional friction and ophthalmic viscosurgery devices on the heat generation of ultrasound during cataract surgery. J Cataract Refract Surg 32:1222–1226
37. Mackool R, Sirota MA (2005) Thermal comparison of the AdvanTec Legaci, Sovereign WhiteStar, and Millenium phacoemulsification systems. J Cataract Refract Surg 31:812–817
38. Miyajima HB, Shimmura S, Tsubota K (1999) Thermal effect on corneal incisions with different phacoemulsification ultrasonic tips. J Cataract Refract Surg 25:60–64
39. Osher RH, Injev VP (2006) Thermal study of bare tip with various system parameters and incision size. J Cataract Refract Surg 32:867–872
40. Tsuneoka H, Shiba T, Takahashi Y (2002) Ultrasonic phacoemulsification using a 1.4 mm incision: clinical results 22. J Cataract Refract Surg. 28:81–86

6.4 Using Ophthalmic Viscosurgical Devices with Smaller Incisions

Steve A. Arshinoff[1]

Core Messages

- Understanding the rheology of cataract surgery steps greatly facilitates micro incision surgery, whether coaxial or biaxial.
- Before using an ophthalmic viscosurgical device (OVD) in any situation, a clear idea of the method of removing it at the end of the case, is necessary.
- OVD techniques need only minor modification to accommodate microincision surgery. Awareness of the actual purpose of each OVD in a given situation is a critical factor.
- Generally speaking, smaller incisions seal better, making all OVD techniques more stable and easier to perform.
- While a single OVD may be excellent in uncomplicated routine cataract surgery, variations of soft shell and ultimate soft shell techniques make difficult cases much easier.
- It is never too early or too late in the cataract procedure to alter or correct an OVD strategy.

6.4.1 Introduction

Routine cataract surgery, by phacoemulsification and intraocular lens implantation, is regarded as a quick, mature and relatively simple procedure. However, when the sequential steps of the procedure are

[1]Declaration: SAA has acted as a paid consultant to a number of OVD manufacturers, including all of those whose products are referred to herein.

S. A. Arshinoff
York Finch Eye Associates, Humber River Regional Hospital, and The University of Toronto, Toronto, ON, Canada
e-mail: ifix2is@sympatico.ca

analyzed, it is understood that each sequential maneuver is the result of many years of painstaking research and trial and error, and consists of an initial subtask of stabilization of the surgical environment, followed by a specific surgical task in that environment. Ophthalmic viscosurgical devices (OVDs) have become the primary surgical tool of the ophthalmologists to create the environment needed to perform intraocular maneuvers in a controlled environment. When considering the effect of the smaller incisions on the use of OVD, all of the above must be reevaluated in all aspects.. Since the introduction of Healon® in 1979 [1], OVDs have proliferated and become essential tools in anterior segment surgery for space creation, balancing pressure in the anterior and posterior chambers, tissue stabilization and protection of the corneal endothelial cells from surgical trauma, free radicals, and other surgical hazards [2]. An understanding of the factors that need to be controlled in surgery, and the properties of the OVD tools available, allows the surgeon to perform at a higher level, and makes his/her surgery, in the created controlled environments optimized for each step, appear simpler and smoother than it really may be conceptually. The changes in phacoemulsification cataract surgery, over the past decade, have basically been a gradual movement toward more controlled environments and smaller incisions. Before addressing the specific spatial problems encountered in some difficult situations, and the method of dealing with them with smaller incisions, some understanding of the properties of the variety of OVDs available, and how they may integrate into modern cataract surgery, is important. The goal should always be to create an environment in which a given task can be performed easily, rather than learning to perform difficult and complex maneuvers to achieve the same goal in an uncontrolled environment.

6.4.1.1 The Nature of OVDs: Rheology

OVDs are pseudoplastic solutions of biopolymers. Pseudoplasticity means that when zero shear viscosity (the viscosity of the OVD at rest) is plotted against shear rate (a measure of the stress to which the viscoelastic is exposed in a standard rheometer), the viscosity of a pseudoplastic solution falls dramatically as the shear rate rises, but has a limiting value with declining shear rate. There are four types of behavior recognized for rheologic solutions when performing these measurements (Fig. 6.40). Newtonian fluids possess

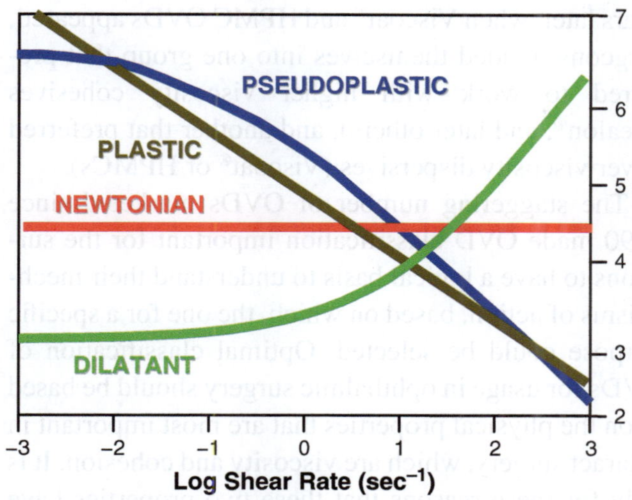

Fig. 6.40 Rheometric patterns of behavior of fluid viscosity in response to increasing rates of shear. The varying patterns of rheologic behavior of fluids

constant viscosity independent of shear rate. Plastics have a viscosity which increases to infinity with declining shear rate (thus making them behave as solids at zero or very low shear rates) whereas pseudoplastics have “pseudoplasticity curves” similar to plastics, but possess a limiting viscosity at low shear, above which viscosity does not increase as shear rate declines toward zero, thus remaining as fluids at very low shear rates, unlike plastics. The fourth type, dilatant fluids, have increasing viscosity as shear rates increase (the opposite of pseudoplastics). OVDs useful in ophthalmic surgery must have low viscosity at high shear rates in order to be deliverable through small bore cannulas, and should have high viscosity at low shear rates to maintain surgical spaces and stabilize the anterior chamber (AC), permitting delicate surgical maneuvers. All OVDs that have been found to be useful, to date, possess pseudoplastic rheologic behavior.

OVDs differ in their rheologically active polymeric substance(s) (hyaluronic acid, chondroitin sulfate and hydroxypropylmethylcellulose (HPMC) have been used to date), concentration(s), and chain length(s). These factors determine the viscosity, elasticity, and cohesion of the OVD, and so, significantly affect other physical and chemical properties [3].

6.4.1.2 The Classification of OVDs

The classification of OVDs is essential to develop surgical techniques which optimize their use. Initially, all cataract viscosurgery was done using Healon®. A few years later, when Viscoat® and HPMC OVDs appeared, surgeons divided themselves into one group that preferred to work with higher viscosity cohesives (Healon®, and later others), and another that preferred lower viscosity dispersives (Viscoat® or HPMCs).

The staggering number of OVDs marketed since 1990 made OVD classification important for the surgeons to have a logical basis to understand their mechanisms of action, based on which, the one for a specific purpose could be selected. Optimal classification of OVDs for usage in ophthalmic surgery should be based upon the physical properties that are most important in cataract surgery, which are viscosity and cohesion. It is only for these reasons that these two properties have been used to classify OVDs. There is a high degree of correlation between the zero shear viscosity of a hyaluronate-based OVD and it's cohesion. Most ophthalmic OVDs have hyaluronic acid as their rheologic polymer. Therefore the initial classifications of OVDs were based solely on zero shear viscosity.

After reviewing the various physical and chemical properties of OVDs, and assessing the most pertinent one to be used in ophthalmic surgery, Arshinoff devised a classification scheme based upon zero-shear viscosity, and noting the high correlation between zero-shear viscosity and the relative degree of cohesion or dispersion [4, 5]. Higher viscosity cohesives were excellent at creating spaces and sustaining pressure, whereas lower viscosity dispersives were capable of partitioning spaces and coating tissues. Each group was poor at performing the tasks in which the other group excelled, and so surgeons were forced to choose an OVD based on the type of complication they felt they might encounter in a particular case. The appearance of viscoadaptives in 1998 required expansion of the scheme (Table 6.1) [6], and the recent appearance of another new OVD, DisCoVisc™, which does not fit into the previous classification, required a further, more major, modification of the scheme, from a simple list to a two dimensional table (Table 6.2) [7].

6.4.1.3 Soft Shell and Ultimate Soft Shell Technique (SST & USST)

Since the evolution of the "viscoelastic dispersive-cohesive SST," and the "USST," it has been recognized that more physical effects can be achieved with two fluids of disparate properties than that can be achieved with any single fluid [8, 9]. Attempts are being made to design a single OVD that can replace multiple OVD techniques (e.g., DisCoVisc®), but, despite the success achieved for routine cataract cases, a single OVD can never replace the ability of SSTs to create physically different environments in adjacent spaces, separated only by the rheological characteristics of the two OVDs, for complicated cases. It can be argued that with progressively smaller incisions, the space creation role of OVDs can be, at least, partially replaced by pressurization of the AC with an irrigating hand piece, or that a lower viscosity OVD will tend to leak out of a smaller incision less than out of a larger incision, thus reducing the advantage of a higher viscosity cohesive OVD over a lower viscosity dispersive. Although this is true, it is easier to perform the surgery in an environment of low turbulence, but pressurized irrigation increases the turbulence. Lower viscosity OVDs will still leak out of smaller incisions, reducing AC stability for delicate maneuvers. Consequently, most OVD techniques designed to deal with difficult situations or complications are variations of the SST and USST and actually work with greater stability, with smaller incisions, and so should be modified only slightly for micro incisions as noted below.

Table 6.1 The classification of OVDs (Arshinoff 1990–2000) (primary parameter is zero shear viscosity)

OVD class	Zero shear viscosity	(mPaS)
■ Viscoadaptives	7- 24 x 10^6	(10Ms)
■ Higher viscosity cohesives	10^5 - 5 x10^6	
• Super viscous cohesive OVDs	1 - 5 x 10^6	(Ms)
• Viscous cohesive OVDs	10^5 - 10^6	(100Ks)
■ Lower viscosity dispersives	10^3 - 10^5	
• Medium viscosity dispersives	10^4 - 10^5	(10Ks)
• Very low viscosity dispersives	10^3 - 10^4	(Ks)

6.4.2 Routine, Special and complicated Cases

In routine phacoemulsification/PC IOL cases, in which complications do not occur, any marketed OVD will suffice. In conditions where, the patient is not squeezing, the AC is sufficiently deep, there is no posterior

Table 6.2 The classification of OVDs 2005

7–18 x 10^6 (ten millions) CDI H5 = 10–70 iVP = 9.6	**I. Pseudodispersive viscoadaptives** - *Healon5* - *iVisc (MicroVisc) Phaco* - *BD MultiVisc*	
1–5 x 10^6 (millions) CDI HealonGV = 72	**II. Higher viscosity cohesives** **A. Super viscous cohesives** - ***Healon GV*** - ***iVisc (MicroVisc, HyVisc) Plus*** - ***BD Visc***	**II. Higher viscosity dispersives** **A. Super viscous dispersives** - ***None***
10^5–10^6 (hundred thousands) CDI Healon = 37	**B. Viscous cohesives** - ***Healon*** - ***iVisc (MicroVisc, HyVisc)*** - ***Viscorneal Plus*** - ***Provisc*** - ***Opegan Hi*** - ***Viscorneal*** - ***Biolon Prime*** - ***Bilon*** - ***Amvisc Plus*** - ***Amvisc*** - ***Coese*** - ***Biocorneal***	**B. Viscous dispersives** - ***DisCoVisc*** CDI DisCoVisc = 12 CDI Viscoat = 3.2
10^4–10^5 (ten thousands)	**III. Lower viscosity cohesives** **A. Medium viscosity cohesives** - ***None***	**III. Lower viscosity dispersives** **A. Medium viscosity dispersives** - ***Viscoat*** - ***Biovisc*** - ***Opelead*** - ***Vitrax*** - ***Celoftal***
10^3–10^4 (thousands)	**B. Very low viscosity cohesives** - ***None***	**B. Very low viscosity dispersives** - ***Opegan*** - ***Occucoat, iCell, Ocuvis, Visilon, Hymecel, Adatocel, Celoftal (HPMCs)***

mPa.s milliPascal.seconds; *CDI* cohesion– dispersion index (%aspirated/mmHg)

pressure and the capsulorhexis does not run, the endothelial cell count and cellular morphology are excellent, and the zonules are complete and strong, there is no need to worry. SST and USST Techniques were designed to overcome any possible problem encountered in cataract surgery, and remain excellent choices for routine cases. However, many surgeons prefer to use only a single OVD for routine cases. This is a reasonable alternative as long as SST and USST OVDs are routinely available in the OR, on short notice, if a complication arises in routine cases. Newer OVDs are being designed that give reasonable zero-shear viscosity to overcome potential space creation and maintenance problems in routine cases, while at the same time being dispersive enough to protect the endothelial cells. DisCoVisc is an example of one of these efforts. The makeup of DisCoVisc is shown in Table 6.3, where it is compared to Viscoat. Alcon had to increase the zero shear viscosity of DisCoVisc in order to make it suitable to maintain spaces, while it remained dispersive. This was done by lowering the concentration and increasing the molecular weight of the NaHa in DisCoVisc, compared to Viscoat, while

Table 6.3 The nature of DisCoVisc

DisCoVisc™

- DisCoVisc™
  - 1.6% NaHa - MMW (1.7MD)
  - 4.0% CDS – 25KD
- Viscoat™
  - 3.0% NaHa – LMW (500KD)
  - 4.0% CDS – 25KD

SA

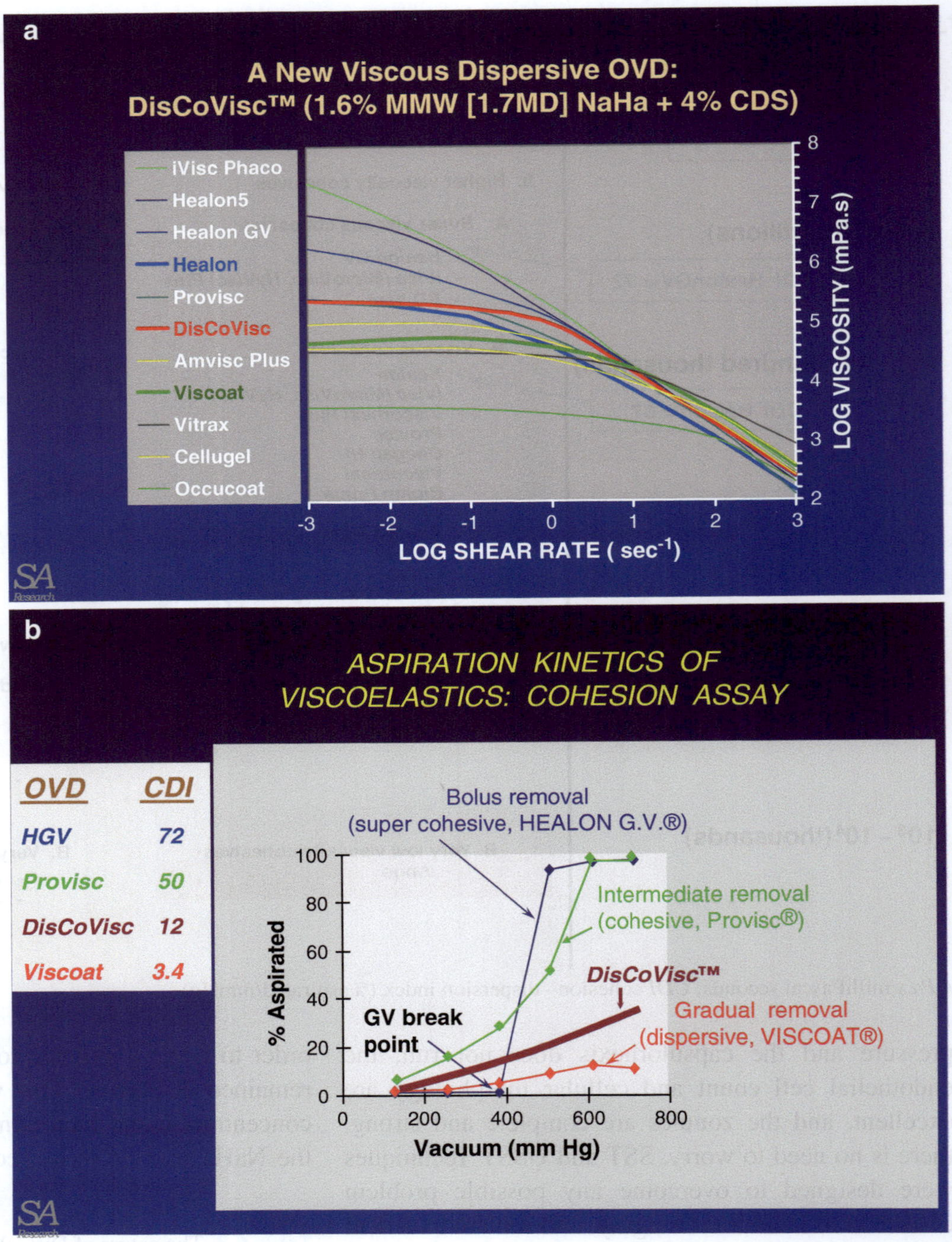

Fig. 6.41 The rheology of DisCoVisc. (**a**) Pseudoplasticity curves of DisCoVisc, showing zero-shear viscosity similar to Healon. (**b**) The Cohesion-Dispersion Index (CDI) of DisCoVisc is near Viscoat. The physical properties of DisCoVisc

the CDS concentration and molecular weight was kept the same. The result was an OVD with the zero shear viscosity of Healon, and the dispersive nature of Viscoat (Fig. 6.41a, b).

6.4.2.1 Phakic and Anterior Chamber IOLs

In recent years, special needs for OVDs have arisen. Two similar cases, as far as OVD selection goes, are phakic and AC IOLs. To implant an AC IOL, the surgeon needs a deep AC, despite an open incision, preferably with a flat iris, so that the iris is not snagged by the incoming IOL. Healon5 sounds terrific for this use, except that its removal is often problematic in AC IOL cases lacking an intact posterior capsule. Healon GV, the next most viscous and rigid OVD after Healon5, is a much better choice as it is easily fracturable by injecting BSS with a hockey stick cannula, thereby removing it easily. Similarly, many surgeons prefer HPMCs for phakic IOLs because the low turbulence needed for their removal reduces the likelihood of lens touch and possible cataract induction during this delicate maneuver.

6.4.2.2 Trabeculectomy and Phaotrabeculectomy

Another special use is the maintenance of the AC after phaco-trabeculectomy, or trabeculectomy alone. Lower viscosity OVDs disappear through the created filter in less than 24 h, thus creating a need for an alternate means to maintain a deep AC (suture, etc.). Healon5 can be used to fill the AC, and if left in place, will not induce elevated intraocular pressure, but will keep the AC formed for over 5 days, because it mixes so slowly with the aqueous.

6.4.2.3 Fuchs' Endothelial Dystrophy

Fuchs Endothelial Dystrophy cases are best handled with SST or USST variations. The idea is to first place a dispersive OVD on the lenticular surface, and then pressurize it up against the corneal endothelium by injecting a cohesive (SST) or viscoadaptive (USST) OVD below it. In USST, a further layer of BSS is then injected over the lenticular surface, below the OVDs. During phaco, the viscoadaptive layer can be preserved by a skilled surgeon experienced with USST, whereas the cohesive OVD (SST) will likely be aspirated. At the end of the case, residual viscoadaptive or cohesive OVD is removed, while the dispersive is left in the eye to protect the endothelium. The eye is best treated with a cholinergic ocular hypotensive agent, either intracameral carbachol (commercial preparation), or topical carbachol (0.2% topically) to prevent postoperative IOP spikes. If needed, a topical prostaglandin analogue may be added, but all the agents which reduce aqueous production by the ciliary body, delay OVD washout and are completely ineffective in reducing or preventing post op IOP spikes caused by OVDs [10].

6.4.2.4 Zonular Deficiency

It is not uncommon to encounter a post-traumatic situation, or a patient with Marfan's syndrome, or another reason to be missing a significant portion of the zonular ring. SSTs have greatly simplified these cases. First, the area of zonular deficiency is covered with a dispersive OVD. Then a cohesive (SST) or viscoadaptives (USST) is injected behind the dispersive to pressurize the AC and force most of the bulging vitreous, along with some dispersive OVD to return behind the cataractous lens. BSS is added on the lenticular surface (USST), and phaco is commenced. At the earliest sign of instability, a capsular tension ring, Cionni ring, or Ahmed segment is inserted and Grieshaber, or other hooks may be used as indicated. As there is no vitreous in the AC, these cases usually progress relatively routinely, with the capsular tension ring in place (Cionni variation or Ahmed segment may be needed in the presence of a larger zonular defect).

6.4.2.5 Capsular Staining for White & Black Cataracts

The first technique proposed for capsular staining with trypan blue, as described by Melles was simply to fill the AC with Vision Blue®, leave it in for 1 min, and then wash it out and continue the surgery with OVD injection followed by capsulorhexis.

Because of the concern for the amount of dye used in the Melles technique, many have used Vision Blue® under an air bubble, thus dramatically decreasing the amount needed, and endothelial contact with the dye.

Trypan blue, which dyes the anterior lens capsule beautifully, as it reduces its elasticity, has emerged as the leader among capsular dyes [11, 12]. Since the time the author first began using trypan blue (Vision Blue®) in late 1999, he also used a variation of the USST (below) and has addressed its use at many meetings [13]. Marques et al. published their three-step technique, which differs from the USST technique in that the last two steps are reversed. The author, however, still prefers the USST method. Trypan blue is listed as a carcinogen in the Merck Index. Yetil et al. [15] were able to successfully stain the anterior capsule with as little as 0.1 mL of 0.0125% trypan blue (1/4 commercial concentration), and the general trend is to use as little of any foreign substance as possible for capsular staining, since it may later prove to be hazardous, as in the case of ICG.

The ultimate soft shell capsular dye technique (USSCDT) is as follows:

1. The AC 80–90% should be filled with viscoadaptive OVD, being careful not to inject initially at the wound, which will blockade the incision and cause retention of aqueous behind the viscoadaptive blockade.
2. Trypan blue should be painted over the capsule, using only a tiny drop ejected onto the capsular surface through a 27 gauge hockey stick cannula, attached to a tuberculin syringe containing trypan blue (Fig. 6.42a). (Vision Blue® is now supplied in its own syringe. This syringe is considerably more difficult to use than a tuberculin syringe, but after a bit of practice, it

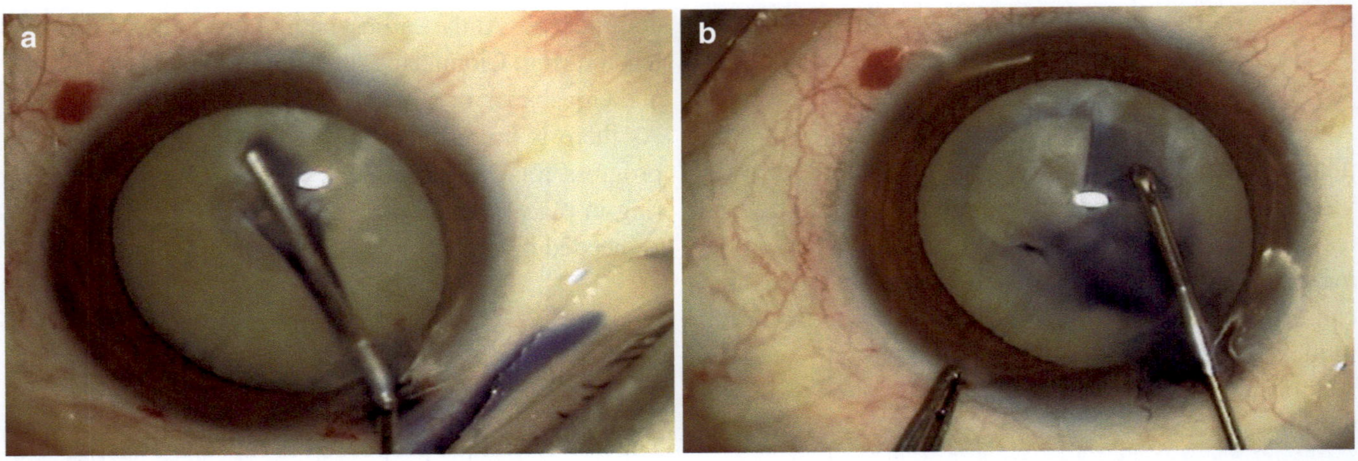

Fig. 6.42 The ultimate soft shell capsular dye technique (USSCDT). (a) After filling the AC 90% with viscoadaptives, trypan blue is painted over the anterior capsule, beneath the OVD. (b) The USSCDT provides extreme clarity for capsulorhexis in mature cataracts. Using Trypan Blue in the USSCDT

can be used. Alternatively, the syringe contents may be transferred to a tuberculin syringe.) The drop of trypan blue is then painted over the capsular surface using the distal "blade" of the hockey stick.

3. BSS should be slowly injected under the viscoadaptive onto the capsular surface, keeping the end of the injection cannula near the incision, using a 10 mL syringe and a 27 gauge hockey stick cannula, similar to the one used for the Vision Blue®. Slow injection will not move the overlying viscoadaptive mass, and will wash out any excess trypan blue. Then, the cannula should be moved distally across the AC, and the injection speed should be increased suddenly to a "pulse," injected away from the wound, with the cannula aperture positioned on the capsular surface near the remote pupil margin, remote from the incision, in the style of the USST. This will force the viscoadaptive upwards and backwards, toward the incision, to blockade the incision and pressurize the eye. Figure 6.42b illustrates the ensuing capsulorhexis, showing the crystal clear view of the capsule that ensues, greatly facilitating capsulorhexis.

6.4.2.6 Flomax® Intraoperative Floppy Iris Syndrome USST

Intraoperative floppy iris syndrome is an even more common problem due to the use of α-A1 antogonists, for benign prostatic hypertrophy, of which tamsulosin (Flomax) seems to be the worst, but it can occur with others and some psychiatric drugs as well. An OVD technique to manage IFIS has been described, which can be used alone, or in combination with iris hooks, a Malyugin ring, or alone, depending on the severity of the case [16].

The IFIS SST-USST is performed as follows (Fig. 6.43):

1. Preoperative dilation test: To determine in advance, the expected severity of IFIS during surgery, all patients on Flomax undergo a preoperative dilation test, 1 week prior to surgery: they are given Mydriacyl (tropicamide) 1% gtts × 2, 5 min apart, and Mydfrin (phenylephrine) 2.5% gtts × 1. After 20 min the pupils are measured. If the pupils exceed 6.5 mm, and especially if the patient has brown eyes, no particular difficulty is expected in surgery. 0.5 mL Intracameral phenylephrine (5 mL BSS mixed with 0.3 mL (all) of a phenylephrine 10% minim in a 6 mL syringe (diluted to 0.57%)) is injected into the AC after intracameral xylocaine, through the side port, and waited for 1 min before making the main incision and starting the surgery. IFIS SST-USST is used, but the flow rate is not generally reduced. If the pupils are about 6 mm, some difficulty will be encountered and the IFIS SST-USST is used in addition to intracameral phenylephrine, with lowered flow rates. If the pupils are less than 5.5 mm, and especially if the patient has blue irides, the intracameral phenylephrine and IFIS SST-USST is used with flow rates in the range of 15 mL/min, and a Malyugin ring is added
2. After making a 1 mm. side-port with the Arshinoff side-port diamond knife (Diamond Surgical Products, Thornville, OH), and firming up the eye with 1% nonpreserved isotonic lidocaine, the primary clear-corneal phaco incision is fashioned with the

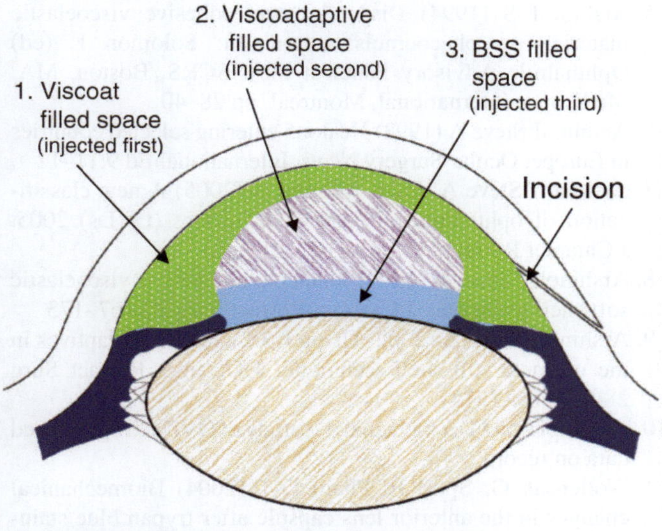

Fig. 6.43 Modified SST-USST for IFIS. The Flomax IFIS SST-USST

Arshinoff 2.7 mm soft-shoulder diamond knife (Diamond Surgical Products), trying to lengthen the tunnel such that the corneal internal entry is slightly central to the papillary margin. The width of the knife is significant in that both incisions are intentionally tight in order to prevent leakage and iris prolapse.

3. The AC is then filled, through the phaco incision, with Viscoat (Alcon Laboratories, Fort Worth, TX), until the AC is about 70% full. Healon5 is then injected onto the surface of the anterior lens capsule, in the center of the AC, and it proceeds, pushing the Viscoat upwards and outwards, until the pupil stops dilating. It is important that the boundary of the Healon5/Viscoat be at the pupillary margin. This will later serve as a fracture boundary, and will help to keep the iris stable, and the pupil dilated, throughout the surgery. At this point the AC should be, over 90%, full of OVD and the eye should feel slightly firm. This step is a variation of SST.
4. BSS, or some of the nonpreserved lidocaine or phenylephrine is then injected slowly under the Healon5 layer, on the surface of the lens capsule, with the cannula aperture placed at the very center of the lens surface, to elevate the OVD soft shell, which is created above, off the lens surface, and create a water pocket on the lenticular surface which is confined to the lenticular surface, and not spilling over the iris surface. This is a variation of USST.
5. A routine capsulorhexis is then performed using a bent needle, beginning at the center of the lens, and being sure to keep the diameter of the capsulorhexis smaller than the pupil diameter. This will later act to confine the fluid flow into an area smaller than the pupil, preventing turbulence from impacting the iris and the Viscoat layer, which would permit the pupil to constrict.
6. Hydrodissection is then performed with BSS on a 10 mL syringe with a 27 gauge hockey stick cannula, using small short pulses of BSS. As long as care is taken in performing the steps above, as well as in the placement of the BSS cannula, the BSS should be able to circulate around the lens and flow out of the eye, beneath the OVD shell, without disturbing the shell. If the OVD shell is disturbed in this step, and some OVD is lost, Healon5 is reinjected followed by BSS below it, before proceeding.
7. The Alcon Infiniti Phaco (or similar peristaltic) machine settings are adjusted to flow ≤20 mL/min, vacuum ≤250 mmHg, bottle height 75–80 cm above patient's eye, linear variable pulse mode. The procedure is performed using Phaco Slice & Separate or similar chopping technique, being sure to keep the Phaco tip at or below the capsulorhexis, and confining the fluid flow into the capsular bag [17]. All work is done in the capsular bag, and attempts to only engage the phaco into positions 1, 2 or 3 are made only with the phaco in the bag, and a piece of nucleus engaged. Unnecessary irrigation of the AC is avoided.

When the above steps are followed, paying careful attention to measuring the pupils preoperatively and creating tight incisions, Flomax cases become relatively routine procedures.

6.4.3 Discussion

Modern cataract surgery has brought modern challenges, due to new devices, methods, and patient medical status, and complicating systemic drugs. The recent move to smaller incision surgery, in the range of 2 mm, whether biaxial or coaxial, has changed our rheologic approach to phacoemulsification, but renewed attention is needed to understand what we are trying to do rheologically in different circumstances, and how the smaller incisions affect the rheological behavior of our OVDs, both in their surgical use and in later removal. A good understanding of rheological principles, however, in our new tighter environment, which in reality is changed only slightly from 3 mm incisions, can be used to create any physical environment that we can invent, limited only by our imaginations. Cataract surgery really is just the application of rheology. The only two factors that make a difference in phacoemulsification are phaco power modulations, and our manipulation of the flow parameters (rheology) of our surgery. Rheology is by general consensus, a difficult subject, but understanding it, and its applications, makes us much better cataract surgeons, in any incisional environment.

Take Home Pearls

- Smaller incisions make us less dependent upon high zero shear viscosity to maintain spaces, but once an instrument is inserted into the eye, lower viscosity dispersives begin to leak out, destabilizing the created surgical microenvironment.
- In special situations, with anticipated difficult OVD removal (phakic IOLs, AC IOLs), viscoadaptives are not the best choice of OVDs.
- Preoperative dilation test should be used for all Flomax cases. If the pupil dilates to > 6.5 mm, the case will not be difficult. If however, it dilates to <5.5 mm, difficulty can be anticipated and the IFIS SST-USST technique is used.
- Smaller incisions generally make OVD techniques more stable and easier to perform.

References

1. Balazs EA (1979) Ultrapure hyaloronic acid and the use thereof. US Patent No. 4.141.973
2. Arshinoff SA (1995) Dispersive and cohesive viscoelastic materials in phacoemulsification. Ophthalmic Pract 13:98–104
3. Arshinoff SA (1999) Dispersive-cohesive viscoelastic soft shell technique. J Cataract Refract Surg 25:167–173
4. Arshinoff SA (1989) Comparative physical properties of ophthalmic viscoelastic materials. Ophthalmic Pract 1:16–19; 36–37
5. Arshinoff S (1994) Dispersive and cohesive viscoelastic materials in phacoemulsification. In: Solomon L (ed) Ophthalmic Advisory Panel at the ASCRS, Boston, MA. Medicopea international, Montreal, pp 28–40
6. Arshinoff Steve A (1998) Healon5 entering selected countries in Europe. Ocular Surgery News, International Ed 9:11–12.
7. Arshinoff Steve A, Jafari Masoud A (2005) A new classification of ophthalmic viscosurgical devices (OVDs) 2005. J Cataract Refract Surg 31:2167–2171
8. Arshinoff Steve A (1999) Dispersive-cohesive viscoelastic soft shell technique. J Cataract Refract Surg 25:167–173
9. Arshinoff Steve A (2002) Using BSS with viscoadaptives in the ultimate soft-shell technique. J Cataract Refract Surg 28(9):1509–1514
10. Arshinof et al FDA metaanalysis study of OVDs. Unpublished data on record
11. Wollensak G, Spörl E, Pham D-T (2004) Biomechanical changes in the anterior lens capsule after trypan blue staining. J Cataract Refract Surg 30:1526–1530
12. Dick HB, Aliyeva SE, Hengerer F (2008) Effect of trypan blue on the elasticity of the human anterior leens capsule. J Cataract Refract Surg 34:1367–1373
13. Arshinoff Steve A (2005) Letter. Capsular dyes and the USST. J Cataract Refract Surg 31:259–260
14. Marques DM, Marques FF, Osher RH (2004) Three-step technique for staining the anterior lens capsule with indocyanine green or trypan blue. J Cataract Refract Surg 30(1):13–16
15. Yetil H, Devranoglu K, Ozkan S (2002) Determining the lowest trypan blue concentration that satisfactorily stains the anterior capsule. J Cataract Refract Surg 28(6):988–991
16. Arshinoff SA (2006) Modified SST–USST for tamsulosin-associated intraocular floppy-iris syndrome. J Cataract Refract Surg 32:559–561 (erratum, 32(7):1076)
17. Arshinoff Steve A (1999) Phaco slice and separate. J Cataract Refract Surg 4:474–478

6.5 Capsulorhexis

Mark Packer, I. Howard Fine, and Richard S. Hoffman

Core Messages

- Control is the key to a successful capsulorhexis.
- Maintaining the depth of the anterior chamber by utilizing a 1.4 mm clear corneal incision, which does not allow the egress of the viscoelastic, facilitates control.
- Exquisitely precise microforceps aid the surgeon in designing a superior capsulorhexis.

Enhanced control and increased flexibility constitute the two preferred reasons to initiate and complete the capsulorhexis through a 1.4 mm trapezoidal clear corneal incision with microforceps (e.g., 23 gauge curved Fine-Hoffman Capsulorhexis Forceps, Catalog # DFH-0002, Microsurgical Technologies, Redmond, WA). The micro incision capsulorhexis technique is started with radial paracentesis incisions in the superior and the inferior temporal quadrants, constructed with a trapezoidal diamond (e.g., Packer Bimanual Phaco Diamond Knife, Catalog # AE-8141, ASICO, Westmont, IL). These symmetric incisions measure 1.4 mm internally, precisely the size required for 20 gauge instrumentation such as the ones used for biaxial micro incision phacoemulsification. The trapezoidal shape of the incisions permits a wider range of intraocular motion without stretching the corneal tissue and prevents the wrinkling and folding of the cornea that impedes a clear view of the capsule.

We feel that the advantages of learning biaxial micro incision phaco outweigh any increased difficulty that may occur during a surgeon's early experience with the technique. These advantages include enhanced chamber stability due to a more perfectly closed system, better followability due to the separation of infusion and aspiration, access to 360° of the anterior segment with either infusion or aspiration (made possible by switching instruments from one hand to the other), the ability to use the flow of irrigation fluid as a tool to move material within the capsular bag or the anterior chamber (particularly from an open-ended irrigating chopper or manipulator), and significantly decreased chance of vitreous prolapse in the case of a posterior capsular tear or rupture due to the maintenance of a pressurized stream of irrigation from above.

In order to reap the benefit of these advantages, strict attention to detail is required. The first technique to master, is the construction of the incision; the second is the construction of the capsulorhexis. There is variability in the incision size among surgeons who employ biaxial phaco; 19 through 23 gauge instrumentation has been described. Twenty gauge is preferred here since it offers the right balance between control and efficiency. Because the outer diameter of the 20 gauge tip is approximately 0.9 mm and the circumference of the tip is 2.8 mm ($2\pi r = 2° \times 3.14° \times 0.45$), the incision should measure 1.4 mm. An incision smaller than 1.4 mm in width will stretch or tear, causing loss of self-sealability. These micro incisions are converted from a line to a circle by the introduction of the phaco tip and the irrigating chopper, and we want them to resume the configuration of a line when the tip is withdrawn. Compromise of the corneal collagen by stretching or tearing will reduce the likelihood that the incision will resume its native architecture at the end of the case. Diamond and metal knives specially designed for construction of these incisions are now available from a variety of manufacturers. It behooves the surgeon to purchase and learn to use this instrumentation, whether constructed of steel, diamond or other material.

Capsulorhexis construction represents the greatest hurdle in the biaxial surgery learning curve. This technique was initially begun with a bent-needle cystotome, and this continues to represent a viable approach. However, micro incision capsulorhexis forceps permit a greater degree of precision and control. The pinch type initiation of the capsulorhexis is particularly valuable in cases of zonular compromise since the forces acting on the capsule remain balanced (Fig. 6.44). Even with a severely wrinkling capsule due to traumatic zonular dialysis or pseudoexfoliation, these extraordinarily delicate forceps permit exquisite control of the capsulorhexis.

M. Packer (✉)
Oregon Health & Science University, Drs. Fine, Hoffman and Packer, 1550 Oak Street, Eugene, OR 97401, USA
e-mail: mpacker@finemd.com

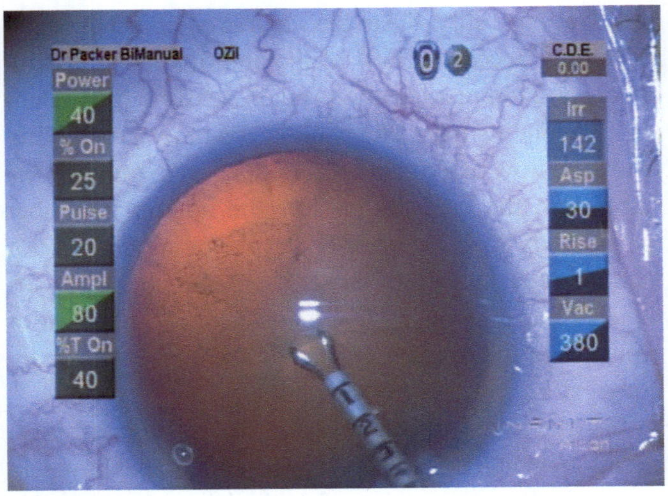

Fig. 6.44 The tips of the microforceps are touched to the anterior capsule surface with just enough pressure to cause slight dimpling; squeezing the handle tines then pinches the capsule and initiates the tear

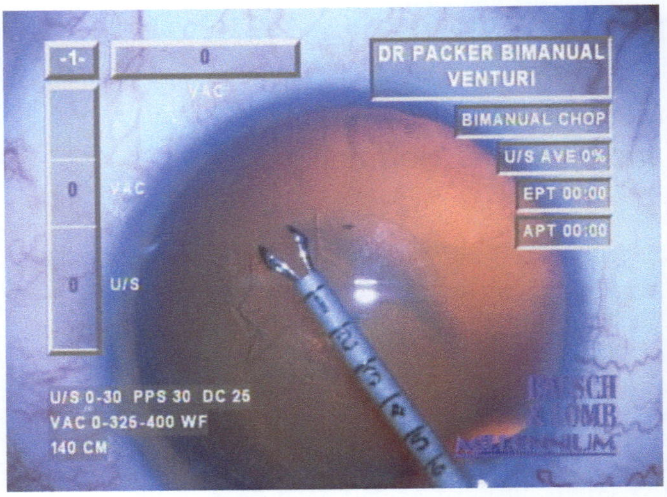

Fig. 6.45 In this large eye (axial length = 30.24 mm, horizontal white-to-white 12.50 mm, anterior chamber depth = 4.00 mm) with a widely dilated pupil, the Rhexis Ruler permits the control of the capsulorhexis size

Following incision construction and instillation of nonpreserved intracameral lidocaine, the anterior chamber is filled with a dispersive viscoelastic which will remain in the eye during high flow, high vacuum chopping techniques. The capsulorhexis is initiated centrally with a pinch and the flap is pulled in a counterclockwise motion. The fellow symmetric incision is always available, in case there is trouble and a need to switch hands, greatly increasing our surgical flexibility. The forceps is held and manipulated with the fingers and thumb like a pencil, in distinction to the wrist motion required for the handling of a standard Utrata forceps. The finger control enables greater precision and finer control of the instrument.

The micro incision forceps also allows excellent control of the capsulorhexis because of their firm grasp and additionally, the small corneal incisions facilitate the control of the capsulorhexis because the viscoelastic does not egress from the eye during intraocular maneuvers. The prevention of viscoelastic efflux means that the chamber remains stable. Pressure in the anterior chamber, on the anterior lens capsule, helps to control the capsulorhexis. It is well known that loss of chamber stability will cause the capsulorhexis to run out towards the periphery. One of the advantages of the micro incision technique is that the chamber remains stable during the completion of the capsulorhexis. This allows for a better control of the size, the diameter, and the position of capsulorhexis.

Newer technology IOLs, which prevent posterior capsular opacification with a square edge or facilitate accommodation with axial or translational movement, are dependent upon accurate sizing and the position of the capsulorhexis. In general, we desire a capsulorhexis which is smaller in diameter than the lens optic: 4.5 mm in the case of a 5.0 mm accommodative IOL or 5 mm in the case of a standard 6 mm multifocal or single vision lens.

The Seibel Rhexis Ruler (Catalog #DFH-0020, Microsurgical Technologies) offers a good alternative in large eyes with maximal pupillary dilation (Fig. 6.45). These myopic eyes have thin, friable capsules. The hugely dilated pupil removes the key customary landmark for sizing of the capsulorhexis, while the outsized anterior chamber defies adequate filling with OVD. In addition, constructing the rhexis through a standard 2.5 mm incision with Utrata forceps will allow the chamber to shallow, due to the efflux of viscoelastic. Without a solid chamber or any clear boundary, the rhexis will tend to run to the periphery before the surgeon can react. However, by employing a micro incision forceps technique, plenty of OVD and the Rhexis Ruler, this complication can be avoided.

The micro incision rhexis technique does not foreclose the option of standard coaxial phaco. In fact, this instrumentation should be viewed as an enhancement to any surgical strategy. One of the situations in which there is a particular advantage to the micro incision rhexis technique is the opaque mature or intumescent cataract. Of course, the use of a capsule stain such as trypan blue, greatly facilitates the rhexis,. However, the maintenance of pressure in the anterior chamber (again,

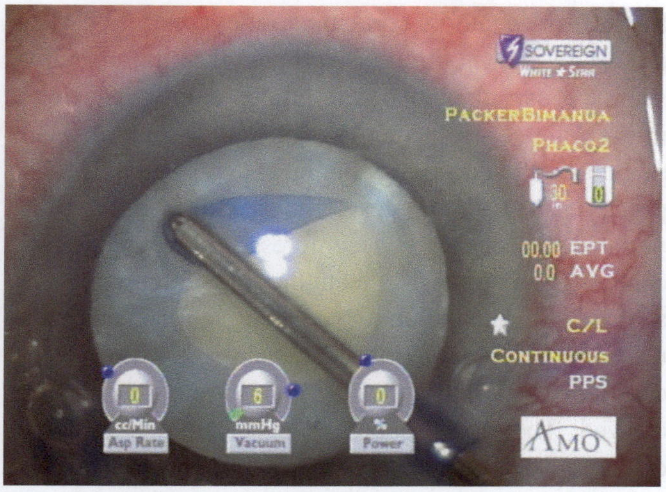

Fig. 6.46 The combination of trypan blue capsule staining and microforceps technique facilitates exquisite control of the capsulorhexis construction in this eye with an opaque cataract

because no OVD egresses through the micro incisions) together with the delicate, finely controlled application of the micro incision forceps improves visibility and control, preventing a tear out of the rhexis during construction (Fig. 6.46). The micro incision rhexis technique also facilitates rescue of the aberrant rhexis using Brian Little's rescue strategy [1]. The advantage of the routine use of micro incision forceps is that there is familiarity with their use while approaching a difficult and challenging situation in which they provide a particular advantage.

Take Home Pearls

- In difficult cases, or when the size and position of the capsulorhexis is of paramount importance (such as when the implantation of an accommodative intraocular lens is planned) the use of a microincision and microforceps is advantageous to the surgeon.
- Using a capsule dye as needed permits improved control, and should be considered whenever the anterior capsule is not clearly visible.

References

1. Little BC, Smith JH, Packer M (2006) Little capsulorhexis tear-out rescue. J Cataract Refract Surg 32(9):1420–1422

6.6 Hydrodissection and Hydrodelineation[1]

I. Howard Fine, Richard S. Hoffman, and Mark Packer

Core Messages

- Cortical cleaving hydrodissection:
- Cleaves the connections between the cortex and the lens capsule
- Facilitates mobilization and rotation of the lens within the capsule
- Facilitates cortical cleanup
- Adds safety to the procedure by reducing the incidence of capsule rupture occurring during cortical cleanup
- Hydrodelineation:
- Divides the nucleus into an endonucleus and an epinuclear shell
- Reduces the portion of the lens that has to be removed with ultrasound energy
- Provides a cushion, within which cracking, grooving, and chopping are contained
- Provides a protective cushion that keeps the capsule stretched and reduces the likelihood of capsule rupture during phacoemulsification

Hydrodissection of the nucleus in cataract surgery has traditionally been perceived as the injection of fluid into the cortical layer of the lens, under the lens capsule, to separate the lens nucleus from the cortex and the capsule [2]. With increased use of continuous curvilinear capsulorhexis and phacoemulsification in cataract surgery, hydrodissection became a very important step to mobilize the nucleus within the capsule for disassembly and removal [3–6]. Following nuclear

[1]This chapter is an update of the previously published by Fine et al. [1].

I. H. Fine (✉)
Oregon Health & Science University, Drs. Fine, Hoffman and Packer, 1550 Oak Street, Suite 5, Eugene, OR 97401, USA
e-mail: hfine@finemd.com

removal, cortical cleanup proceeded as a separate step, using an irrigation and aspiration handpiece.

Fine, first described cortical cleaving hydrodissection, which is a hydrodissection technique designed to cleave the cortex from the lens capsule and thus leave the cortex attached to the epinucleus [7]. Cortical cleaving hydrodissection usually eliminates the need for cortical cleanup as a separate step in cataract surgery, thereby eliminating the risk of capsular rupture during cortical cleanup.

A small capsulorhexis, 5–5.5-mm, optimizes the procedure. The large anterior capsular flap makes this type of hydrodissection easier to perform. The anterior capsular flap is elevated away from the cortical material with a 26-gauge blunt cannula (e.g., Katena Instruments No. K7–5150) prior to hydrodissection. The cannula maintains the anterior capsule in a tented-up position at the injection site, near the lens equator. Irrigation prior to elevation of the anterior capsule should be avoided because it will result in the transmission of a fluid wave circumferentially within the cortical layer thereby, hydrating the cortex and creating a path of least resistance that will disallow later cortical cleaving hydrodissection. Once the cannula is properly placed and the anterior capsule is elevated, gentle, continuous irrigation results in a fluid wave that passes circumferentially in the zone just under the capsule, cleaving the cortex from the posterior capsule in most locations (Fig. 6.47). When the fluid wave has passed around the posterior aspect of the lens, the entire lens bulges forward because the fluid is trapped by the firm equatorial cortical-capsular connections. The procedure creates, in effect, a temporary intraoperative version of capsular block syndrome as seen by an increase in the diameter of the capsulorhexis (Fig. 6.48). At this point, if fluid injection is continued, a portion of the lens prolapses through the capsulorhexis. However, if prior to prolapse, the capsule is decompressed by depressing the central portion of the lens with the side of the cannula, in a way that forces the fluid to come around the lens equator from behind, the cortical-capsular connections in the capsular fornix and under the anterior capsular flap are cleaved. The cleavage of the cortex from the capsule equatorially and anteriorly allows the fluid to exit from the capsular bag via the capsulorhexis, which constricts to its original size (Fig. 6.49), and mobilizes the lens in

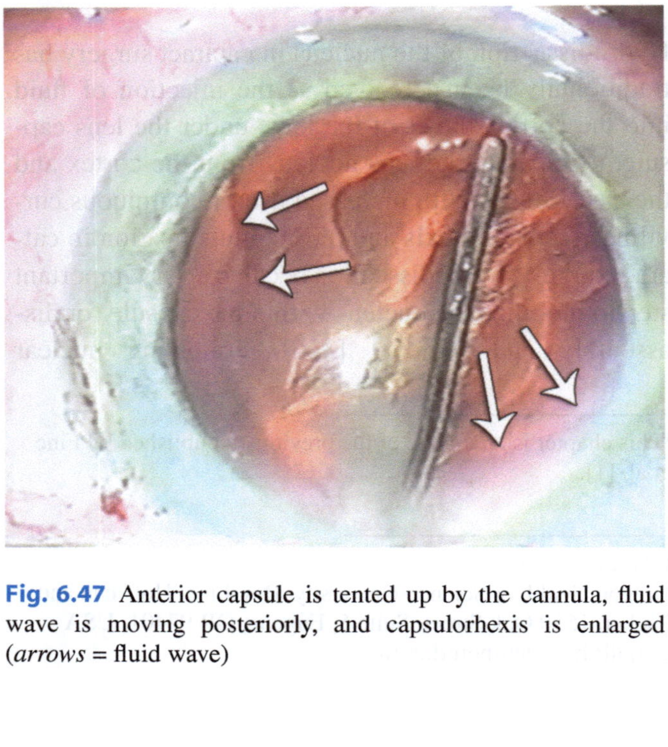

Fig. 6.47 Anterior capsule is tented up by the cannula, fluid wave is moving posteriorly, and capsulorhexis is enlarged (*arrows* = fluid wave)

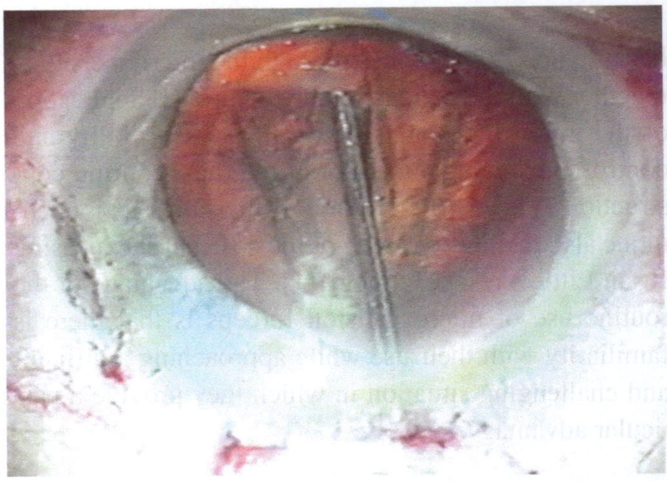

Fig. 6.48 Capsulorhexis is enlarged by the posterior loculated fluid pushing the lens forward

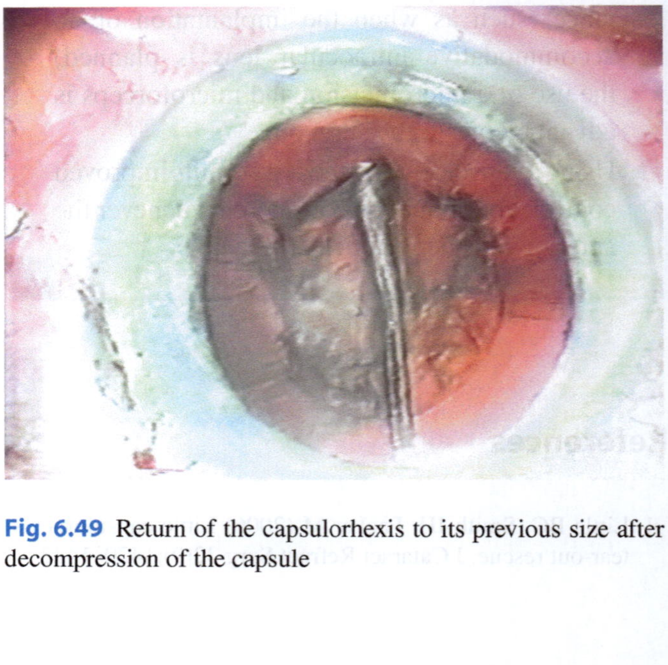

Fig. 6.49 Return of the capsulorhexis to its previous size after decompression of the capsule

such a way that it can spin freely within the capsular bag. Repeating the hydrodissection and capsular decompression, starting in the opposite distal quadrant may be helpful. Adequate hydrodissection at this point is demonstrable by the ease with which the nuclear-cortical complex can be rotated by the cannula.

Hydrodelineation is a term first used by Anis to describe the act of separating an outer epinuclear shell or multiple shells from the central compact mass of inner nuclear material, the endonucleus, by the forceful irrigation of fluid (balanced salt solution) into the mass of the nucleus [8].

The 26-gauge cannula is placed in the nucleus, off the center to either side, and directed at an angle, downward and forward towards the central plane of the nucleus. When the nucleus starts to move, the endonucleus has been reached. It is not penetrated by the cannula. At this point, the cannula is directed tangentially to the endonucleus, and a to-and-fro movement of the cannula is used to create a tract within the nucleus. The cannula is backed out of the tract approximately halfway, and a gentle but steady pressure on the syringe allows fluid to enter the distal tract without resistance. Driven by the hydraulic force of the syringe, the fluid will find the path of least resistance, which is the junction between the endonucleus and the epinucleus, and flow circumferentially in this contour. Most frequently, a circumferential golden ring will be seen outlining the cleavage between the epinucleus and the endonucleus (Fig. 6.50). Sometimes the ring will appear as a dark circle rather than a golden ring.

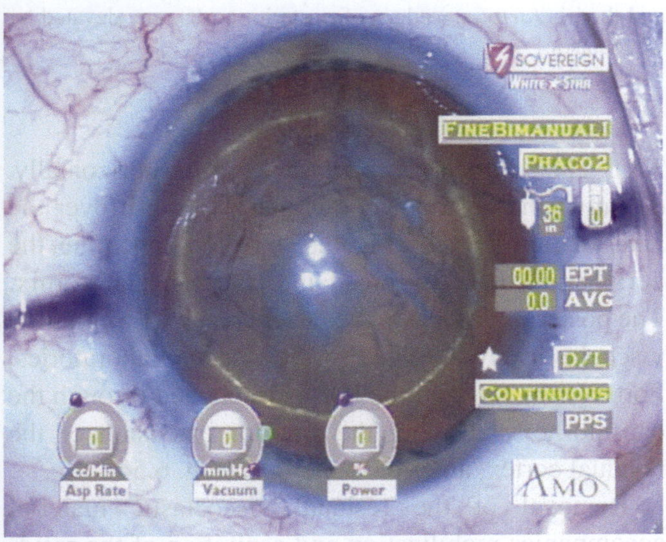

Fig. 6.50 The *golden ring* outlining the cleaving between the epinucleus and the endonucleus is clearly visible

Occasionally, an arc will result and surround approximately one quadrant of the endonucleus. In this instance, creating another tract of the same depth as the first, but ending at one end of the arc, and injecting into the middle of the second tract, will extend that arc (usually another full quadrant). This procedure can be repeated until a golden or dark ring verifies circumferential division of the nucleus.

For very soft nuclei, the placement of the cannula allows creation of an epinuclear shell of any thickness. The cannula may pass through the entire nucleus if it is soft enough and so, the placement of the tract and the location of the injection allow an epinuclear shell to be fashioned as desired. In very firm nuclei, one appears to be injecting into the cortex on the anterior surface of the nucleus, and the golden ring will not be seen. However, a thin, hard epinuclear shell is achieved even in the most brunescent nuclei. That shell will offer the same protection as a thicker epinucleus in a softer cataract.

Hydrodelineation circumferentially divides the nucleus and has many advantages. Circumferential division reduces the volume of the central portion of nucleus removed by phacoemulsification by up to 50%. This allows less deep and less peripheral grooving and smaller, more easily mobilized quadrants, after cracking or chopping. The epinucleus acts as a protective cushion within which all of the chopping, cracking and phacoemulsification forces can be confined. In addition, the epinucleus keeps the bag on stretch throughout the procedure, making it unlikely that a knuckle of capsule will come forward, occlude the phaco tip, and rupture.

Cortical cleanup is dramatically facilitated by cortical cleaving hydrodissection. After evacuation of all endonuclear material, the epinuclear rim is trimmed in each of the three quadrants, mobilizing cortex as well in the following way. As each quadrant of the epinuclear rim is rotated to the distal position in the capsule and trimmed, the cortex in the adjacent capsular fornix flows over the floor of the epinucleus and into the phaco tip. Then the floor is pushed back to keep the bag on stretch until three of the four quadrants of the epinuclear rim and forniceal cortex have been evacuated. It is important not to allow the epinucleus to flip too early, thus avoiding a large amount of residual cortex remaining after evacuation of the epinucleus.

The epinuclear rim of the fourth quadrant is then used as a handle to flip the epinucleus. As the remaining portion of the epinuclear floor and the rim is evacuated from the eye, 70% of the time, the entire cortex is

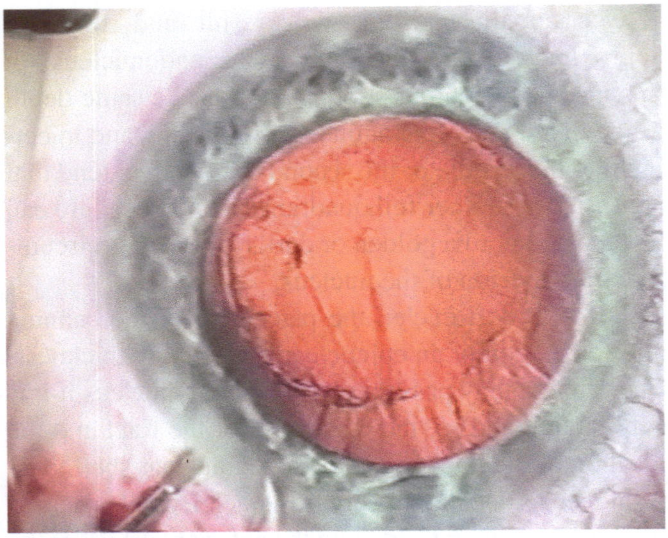

Fig. 6.51 Complete cortical envelope remains in the eye

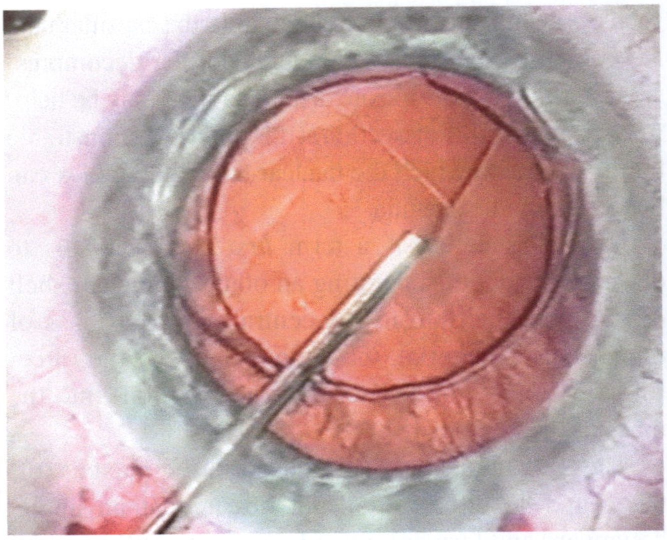

Fig. 6.52 Viscodissecting residual cortex

evacuated with it [9]. Downsized phaco tips with their increased resistance to flow are less capable of mobilizing the cortex because of the decreased minisurge accompanying the clearance of the tip, when going from foot position two to foot position three in the trimming of the epinucleus.

After the intraocular lens (IOL) is inserted, these strands, and any residual viscoelastic material, are removed using the irrigation and aspiration tips, leaving a clean capsular bag.

If the cortex is still remaining after the removal of the nucleus and the epinucleus (Fig. 6.51), there are three options to choose from. The phacoemulsification handpiece can be left high in the anterior chamber, while the second handpiece irrigates the cortex-filled capsular fornices. Often, this results in floating up of the cortical shell as a single piece and its exit through the phacoemulsification tip (in foot position two) because cortical cleaving hydrodissection has cleaved most of the cortical capsular adhesions.

Alternatively, if the surgeon wishes to complete the cortical cleanup with the irrigation and aspiration handpieces before lens implantation, the residual cortex can almost always be mobilized as a separate and discrete shell (reminiscent of the epinucleus) and removed without even turning the aspiration port down, to face the posterior capsule.

The third option is to viscodissect the residual cortex by injecting the viscoelastic through the posterior cortex onto the posterior capsule (Fig. 6.52). We prefer the dispersive viscoelastic device chondroitin sulfate-hyaluronate (Viscoat®, Alcon Laboratories, Fort Worth, TX). The viscoelastic material spreads horizontally, elevating the posterior cortex and draping it over the anterior capsular flap (Fig. 6.53). At the same time, the peripheral cortex is forced into the capsular fornix. The posterior capsule is then deepened with a cohesive viscoelastic device (e.g., Provisc®, Alcon Laboratories, Fort Worth, TX) and the IOL is implanted through the capsulorhexis, leaving the anterior extension of the residual cortex, anterior to the IOL (Fig. 6.54).

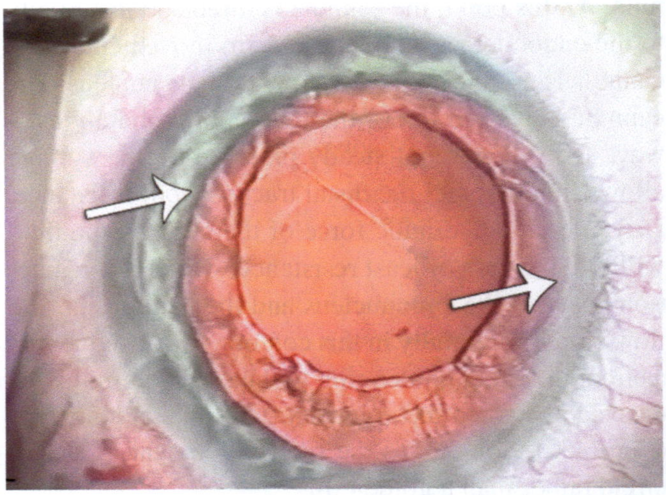

Fig. 6.53 Posterior cortex fully draped on top of the capsule and the iris (*arrows* = edges of posterior cortex are elevated by viscoelastic)

Removal of the residual viscoelastic material accompanies mobilization and aspiration of the residual cortex anterior to the IOL, which protects the posterior capsule, leaving a clean capsular bag.

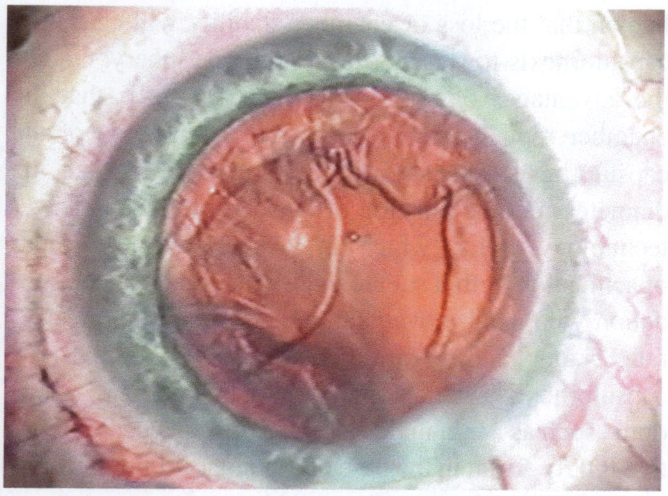

Fig. 6.54 Posterior cortex now draped back on *top* of the plate haptic IOL ready for mobilization

In summary, the lens can be divided into an epinuclear zone with most of the cortex attached and a more compact central nuclear mass. The central portion of the cataract can be removed by any endolenticular technique, after which the protective epinucleus is removed with all or most of the cortex attached. In most cases, irrigation and aspiration of the cortex as a separate step are not required, thereby eliminating that portion of the surgical procedure and its attendant risk of capsular disruption. Residual cortical cleanup may be accomplished in the presence of a posterior chamber IOL, which protects the posterior capsule by holding it remote from the aspiration port.

Take Home Pearls

- Cortical cleaving hydrodissection:
- Is an easy and atraumatic procedure;
- Provides safety and reduces surgical time;
- Provides for better cortical cleanup.
- Hydrodelineation:
- Circumferentially divides the nucleus;
- Provides a protective cushion;
- Reduces posterior capsule rupture during phacoemulsification.

References

1. Fine IH, Hoffman RS, Packer M Hydrodissection and hydrodelineation In: Colvard M (ed) Achieving excellence in cataract surgery: a step-by-step approach. SLACK, Thorofare, NJ (in conjunction with Advanced Medical Optics: Santa Ana, California. Reprinted with permission from Advanced Medical Optics)
2. Faust KJ (1984) Hydrodissection of soft nuclei. Am Intraocular Implant Soc J 10:75–77
3. Davison JA (1989) Bimodal capsular bag phacoemulsification: a serial cutting and suction ultrasonic nuclear dissection technique. J Cataract Refract Surg 15:272–282
4. Sheperd JR (1990) In situ fracture. J Cataract Refract Surg 16:436–440
5. Gimbel HV (1991) Divide and conquer nucleofractis phacoemulsification: development and variations. J Cataract Refract Surg 17:281–291
6. Fine IH (1991) The chip and flip phacoemulsification technique. J Cataract Refract Surg 17:366–371
7. Fine IH (1992) Cortical cleaving hydrodissection. J Cataract Refract Surg 18(5):508–512
8. Anis A (1991) Understanding hydrodelineation: the term and related procedures. Ocular Surg News 9:134–137
9. Fine IH (1998) The choo-choo chop and flip phacoemulsification technique. Oper Tech Cataract Refract Surg 1(2):61–65

6.7 Biaxial Microincision Cataract Surgery: Techniques and Sample Surgical Parameters

Mark Packer, I. Howard Fine, and Richard S. Hoffman

Core Messages

- Each step in cataract surgery builds on the preceding step.
- The clear corneal incision should be sized correctly for instrumentation.
- The capsulorhexis should be centered, round and slightly smaller than the optic of the intraocular lens to be implanted.
- Endo lenticular nucleofractis techniques protect both the capsule and the cornea.
- Separation of infusion and aspiration facilitates the removal of the lens material and has advantages in difficult and complicated cases.

To begin the bimanual vertical chop technique for a moderate 2+ nuclear sclerotic cataract in a patient with asteroid hyalosis, a paracentesis type of incision is made to the left, constructed with a trapezoidal diamond blade. This incision measures 1.2 mm internally, which is precisely the size required for 20 gauge instrumentation such as the one used for bimanual microincision phacoemulsification. The anterior chamber is filled with a dispersive viscoelastic which remain in the eye during the high flow, high vacuum chop technique. The capsulorhexis is initiated centrally with a pinch and pulled with a counterclockwise motion.

The microincision forceps (MST, Redmond, WA) allow excellent control of the capsulorhexis and in addition, the small incisions also facilitate the control of the capsulorhexis because the viscoelastic does not exit the eye. This means that the chamber remains stable. Pressure in the anterior chamber on the anterior lens capsule helps to control the capsulorhexis. It is well known that the loss of chamber stability will cause the capsulorhexis to run out towards the periphery. One of the advantages of microincision technique is that the chamber remains stable during the completion of the capsulorhexis. This allows better control of the size, the diameter, and the position of our capsulorhexis. Newer technology IOLs, which prevent posterior capsular opacification with a square edge or facilitate accommodation with axial movement, are dependent upon accurate sizing and position of the capsulorhexis. A capsulorhexis, which is smaller in diameter than the lens optic, such as 4 mm in the case of a 4.5 mm accommodative IOL or 5 mm in the case of a standard 6 mm multifocal or single vision lens, is needed.

Cortical cleaving hydrodissection is preformed by tenting up the anterior capsule and injecting the balanced salt solution under the rim of the capsule, and watching the fluid wave advance completely across the posterior capsule. The fluid wave is trapped temporarily between the lens and the posterior capsule, causing the lens to prolapse anteriorly. Repositioning the lens by pushing it posteriorly with the cannula in the center decompresses the fluid that is trapped, forcing it around the equator and lysing the corticocapsular connections. The lens is then rotated to make sure that it is free. Hydrodelineation can be carried out by embedding the tip of the cannula in the center of the lens and advancing it until the resistance of the endonucleus is encountered. A slight to and fro motion of the cannula will create a small space into which the balanced salt solution is injected. The fluid flows between the endonucleus and the epinucleus, forming the golden ring as seen in Fig. 6.55.

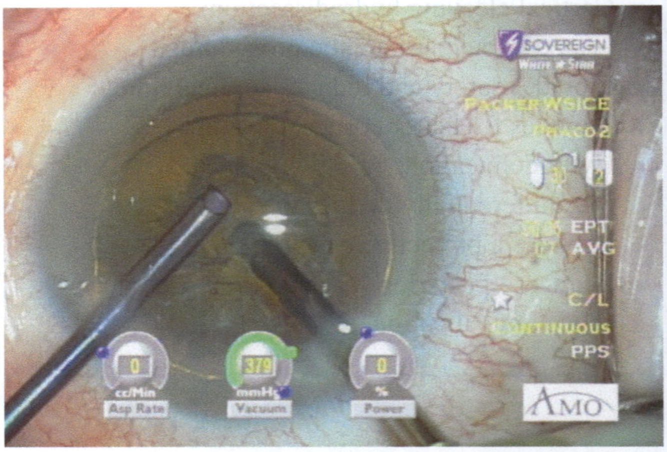

Fig. 6.55 The 20 gauge phaco needle is embedded in the endonucleus as the irrigating chopper is prepared to incise and split the lens

M. Packer (✉)
Oregon Health & Science University, Drs. Fine, Hoffman and Packer, 1550 Oak Street, Suite 5, Eugene, OR 97401, USA
e-mail: mpacker@finemind.com

The phaco needle is now embedded proximally with high vacuum and 40% power (Table 6.4). The vertical chopper, which will be used to split the nucleus into two, is held in the left hand. As vacuum builds to occlusion, the CASE software (Sovereign Phacoemulsification System; Advanced Medical Optics, Santa Ana, CA) enables a rapid rise time and the endonucleus is firmly grasped on the phaco needle. At the point where the occlusion is reached, the aspiration flow rate drops to zero. This is followed by the movement into foot position two so that a high vacuum is maintained and the power goes to zero (Fig. 6.55). The blade of the irrigating vertical chopper is brought down just distal to the phaco tip by slightly lifting up with the phaco needle. As a full thickness cleavage plane develops, which divides the nucleus into two, the surgeons separate

Table. 6.4 Dr.Packer AMO Sovereign "PACKER BIMANUAL WS ICE" Whitestar v6.1 Sov. ICE increased control efficiency

Phaco tip: gold straight 30 degree 20 ga. Cut-off yellow sleeve	Incision: Asico or para 0.7–1.2	NEVER CRUISE. Extra pole extender (2)

Start here, then to trim

Memory	Variable whitestar mem 1 (use for hard cats)	Chop phaco mem 2	Trim phaco mem 3	Flip phaco Mem 4	IA silicone curved tip	Viscoat removal silicone curved tip
Power	40	40	20	20		
Flow	30 Panel	30 Panel	22/16 Panel	24/16 Panel	22 Panel	40 Linear
Vacuum	500\380 [a]CASE panel	500\380 [a]CASE panel	200/50 Linear	200/80 Linear	500 Linear	500 Panel
Ramp (%)	30	30	30	30	85	85
Mode Unocclusion/ occlusion	Variable whitestar CN/CL/CF/CD 18%/20/33/43	Linear whitestar CL	Linear whitestar CL	Linear whitestar CL		
Other	ICE with 7% power kick	ICE with 7% power kick	Cont. irrig.	Cont. irrig.	Cont. irrig.	Cont. irrig.
Bottle ht	30 in.	30 in.	30 in.	30 in.	30 in.	30 in.

Use "PACKER BI-MANUAL WS ICE" program

Vitrectomy

#1 Oscillating Use blue wrapped	Flow 20	Vacuum 250	Cut rate 450	Bottle 20
#2 Guillotine; use disposable	Flow 20	Vacuum 250	Cut rate 400	Bottle 20

ICE increased control efficiency.

[a]Case – [replaces occlusion mode when selected] – (chamber stabilization environment)

Up threshold	70%
Down threshold	50%
Up time	500 ms

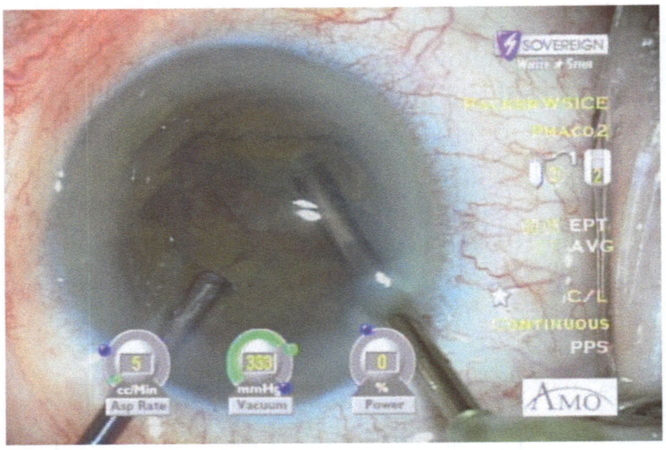

Fig. 6.56 The nucleus is divided to the right and the left. In this case, a posterior shelf has developed; it is particularly important to separate the instruments fully to insure a complete chop in this situation

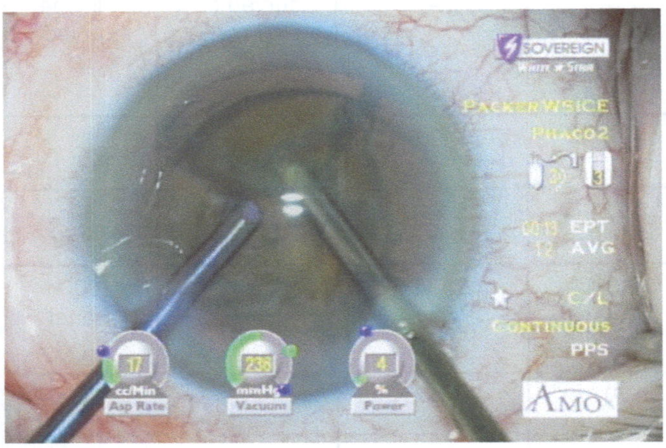

Fig. 6.57 After the second chop has divided one of the heminuclei, the first quadrant is mobilized

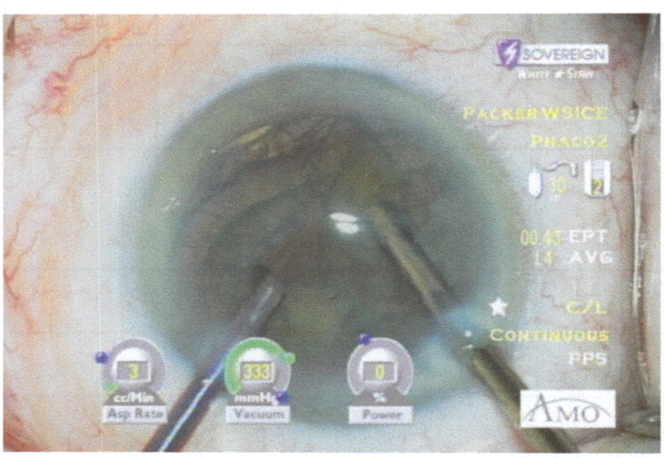

Fig. 6.58 The irrigating chopper is used to hold epinucleus back as another quadrant is aspirated

their hands to insure a complete chop (Fig. 6.56). In this case, the heminucleus to the left is larger and is therefore addressed first.

The lens can then be rotated with the irrigating chopper so that the first heminucleus can be chopped and consumed. If there is a disparity in size, the larger half is moved distally. The phaco needle is now embedded to the right using high vacuum and low levels of power. A quadrant size piece is chopped off and consumed (Fig. 6.57). The remaining quadrant of the first heminucleus is then impaled with the phaco tip and aspirated (Fig. 6.58). Total Effective Phaco Time (EPT) to this point is less than half a second. EPT is a useful parameter for surgeons to follow. It can not be compared across different machines made by different manufactures, however, when using one machine, it can be compared from one case to another case as a sign of surgical efficiency. EPT is the amount of time for which ultrasound would have been turned on if it had been running on 100% continuous power. This means that about half a second has been used, out of the maximum ultrasound power that the machine can produce, to remove half the nucleus. Continuous power can produce thermal energy, but using WhiteStar Technology, or micropulsed phaco, avoids any risk of wound burn. Despite the tightness of the incisions, minimal incisional outflow is present and has a cooling effect around the phaco needle.

To address the second half of the nucleus, it is first rotated with the irrigating chopper so that it is in the distal capsule. The phaco needle is embedded in the smaller heminucleus and it is subdivided with the irrigating chopper, again using high vacuum and low levels of power (Fig. 6.59). As the final quadrant is grasped and pulled centrally for aspiration, the sharp

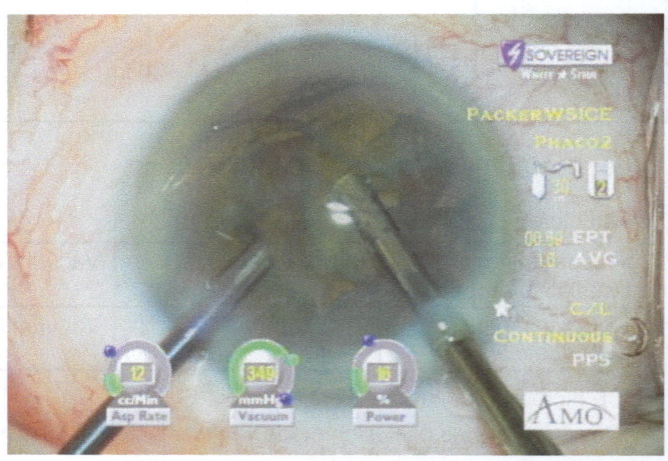

Fig. 6.59 A segment of the second heminucleus is aspirated

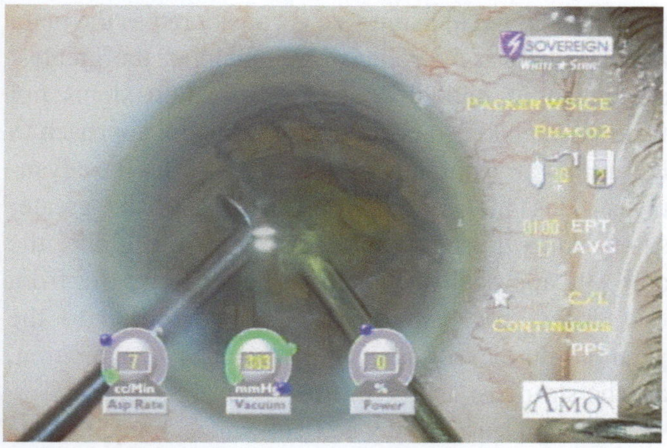

Fig. 6.60 As the final quadrant is aspirated, the chopper is turned sideways and the flow of the irrigation fluid is directed posteriorly to keep the posterior capsule at a safe distance

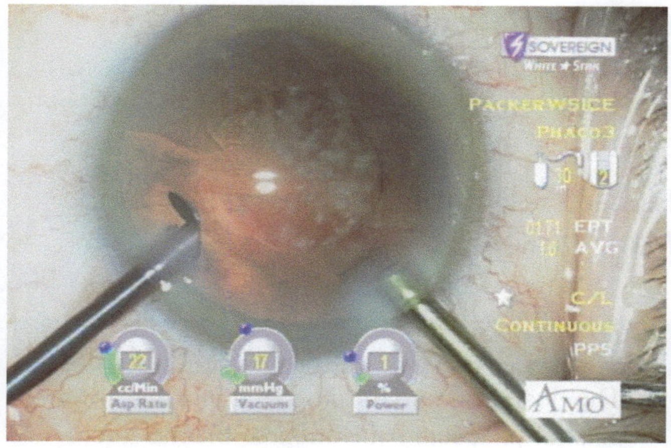

Fig. 6.62 The capsule is clean; asteroid hyalosis is visible in the vitreous cavity

blade of the irrigating chopper is turned sideways as a safety precaution (Fig. 6.60).

When addressing the epinucleus, the settings are reduced, the vacuum and flow rate are turned down and rim of the epinucleus is trimmed, disallowing the epinucleus from flipping into the phaco needle with the stream of irrigation fluid or the irrigating chopper itself. The advantage of the trimming procedure lies in the aspiration of cortical material from behind the epinuclear shell. In most cases this step eliminates the need for I/A prior to IOL insertion. Once three quadrants of the epinuclear shell have been rotated and trimmed, the final quadrant is used to flip the epinuclear bowl into the phaco needle (Fig. 6.61). Following aspiration of the epinucleus, the capsule is entirely free

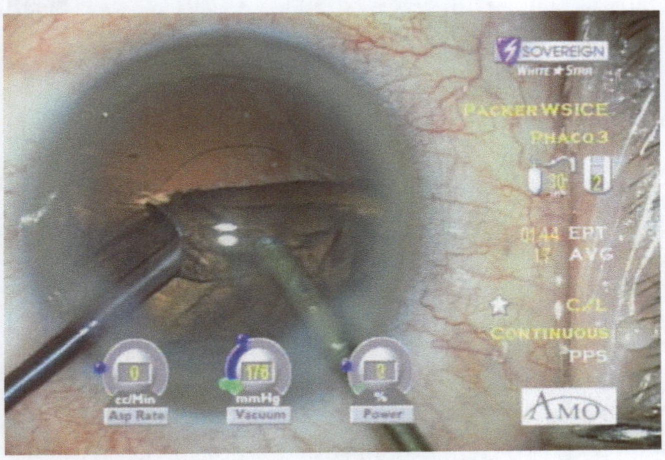

Fig. 6.61 The epinucleus is grasped with the phaco needle at reduced power, flow and vacuum and flipped

of cortex (Fig. 6.62). The asteroid hyalosis in the vitreous cavity is obvious.

The incision for the lens is constructed with the differentially beveled 3D Blade (Rhein Medical, Tampa, FL) which reproducibly creates a 2.5 mm incision at the shoulders. The relatively larger incision (approximately 2.5 mm) which is constructed for IOL insertion seals quite well because it has been only minimally disturbed. Stromal hydration is performed at all the incisions and Seidel test is performed at the conclusion of the case. Careful attention to sealing clear corneal incisions may be critical for the prevention of post operative infection.

Bimanual phaco with a vertical chop technique allows efficient lens extraction with rapid visual rehabilitation. This case demonstrates some of the tangible benefits of separating inflow from outflow such as enhanced cortical cleaving hydrodissection, use of irrigation fluid as an instrument to mobilize material, and reduced EPT.

Take Home Pearls

- Reduction of ultrasound energy improves the rapidity of postoperative visual rehabilitation.
- The stream of irrigation fluid from the irrigating chopper can be used as a gentle instrument in the eye to move material, keep the posterior capsule on stretch, and maintain the volume of the anterior chamber.
- Specific instrumentation for micro incision surgery has allowed the development of improved surgical technique.

6.8 Biaxial Microincision Phacoemulsification: Transition, Techniques, and Advantages

Richard S. Hoffman, I. Howard Fine, and Mark Packer

Core Messages

- The learning curve for the transition from coaxial phacoemulsification to biaxial microincision phacoemulsification is a relatively short and a safe one.
- The real benefits of biaxial microincision phacoemulsification stem from the ability to approach the lens from two different directions, rather than the benefits inherent in microincisions.
- Difficult and challenging cases such as pseudoexfoliation, subluxed, traumatic, mature, and posterior polar cataracts, are best addressed with a biaxial technique.
- The ability to maintain the infusion above the plane of the iris during phacoemulsification and the aspiration of the cortical material has allowed for better stabilization of the anterior chamber and less induced miosis in IFIS (intraoperative floppy iris syndrome) cases.

The idea of removing the cataractous lens through two microincisions is not a new concept and has been attempted with varying degrees of success and failure since the 1970s [1–3, 7–9]. With the development of new phacoemulsification technology and power modulations [5], we are now able to emulsify and fragment the lens material without the generation of significant levels of thermal energy. Thus, the removal of the cooling irrigation sleeve and the separation of infusion and emulsification/aspiration through two separate incisions is now a viable alternative to traditional coaxial phacoemulsification.

R. S. Hoffman
Oregon Health & Science University, Drs. Fine, Hoffman and Packer, 1550 Oak Street, Suite 5, Eugene, Oregon 97401, USA
e-mail: rshoffman@finemd.com

Although the incision size is considered as the main advantage for a microincision technique, the greatest advantage of biaxial phacoemulsification stems not from the incision size, but from the biaxial approach to lens removal. Although microincisions offer the advantages of less induced astigmatism and perhaps, greater safety following traumatic injuries to the globe, the ability to approach difficult and challenging cases from two different incision locations, in addition to the peculiar fluidics of biaxial irrigation and aspiration, are the strongest assets for this surgical technique.

Although learning any new surgical technique has its intimidating moments, the transition to biaxial microincision phacoemulsification is a relatively straightforward process with a short and a safe learning curve, and requires only a small investment in new surgical instrumentation.

6.8.1 Surgical Technique

The preoperative work-up and the preparation for surgery with regard to antibiotic prophylaxis and dilation drops are essentially the same for biaxial surgery and coaxial phacoemulsification. In this technique, a single 1.2 mm incision is created, 30–45° to the left of the temporal limbus using a 1.2 mm diamond or steel keratome (Fig. 6.63). A trapezoidal diamond keratome will create an incision configuration with an internal opening of

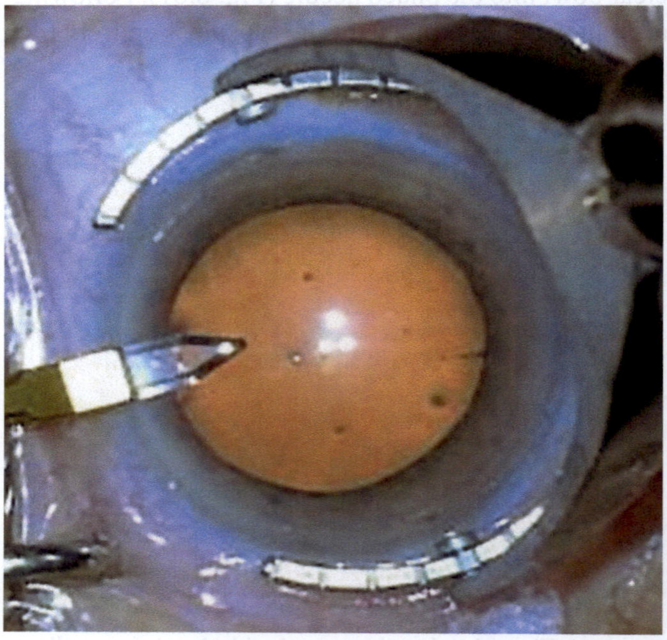

Fig. 6.63 1.2 mm microincision created to the left using a diamond keratome (Figure courtesy of Richard S. Hoffman)

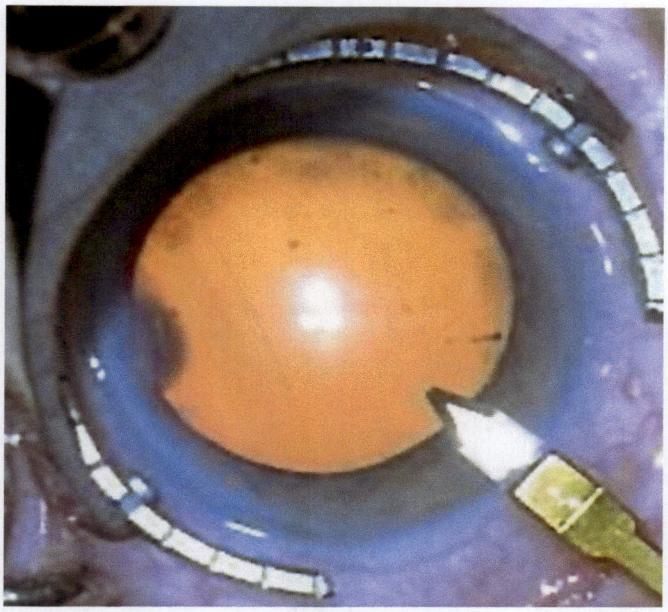

Fig. 6.64 Right-handed 1.2 mm microincision created after instillation of 1% lidocaine and OVD (Figure courtesy of Richard S. Hoffman)

1.0 mm and an external opening of 1.2 mm. This is followed by the instillation of 0.5 cc nonpreserved Lidocaine 1% and Viscoat. A second microincision is then created 90–120° from the left-sided incision (Fig. 6.64). Placing an OVD into the anterior chamber prior to creating the second microincision will repressurize the eye and insure a more accurate incision length.

The capsulorhexis can be started with a special forceps which is designed to function through a 1.2 mm incision. Most instrument companies are currently manufacturing microincision capsulorhexis forceps although there is a preference for the MST Fine/Hoffman microincision forceps (# DFH-0002, MicroSurgical Technology, Redmond, WA) (Fig. 6.65). The capsulorhexis is begun by puncturing the central lens capsule with the tips of the microincision capsulorhexis forceps. This is easily accomplished using a single blade of the forceps tip in the open configuration and then grasping the edge of the open capsule with the forceps in the closed configuration (Fig. 6.66). Following the completion of capsulorhexis, cortical cleaving hydrodissection and hydrodelineation are performed with a 26-gauge cannula. Rotation of the crystalline lens following hydrodissection, but prior to hydrodelineation will insure that both the endonucleus and the epinucleus are freely mobile. Once the lens is rotated, hydrodelineation can be performed to separate the epinucleus from the endonucleus and phacoemulsification can be commenced.

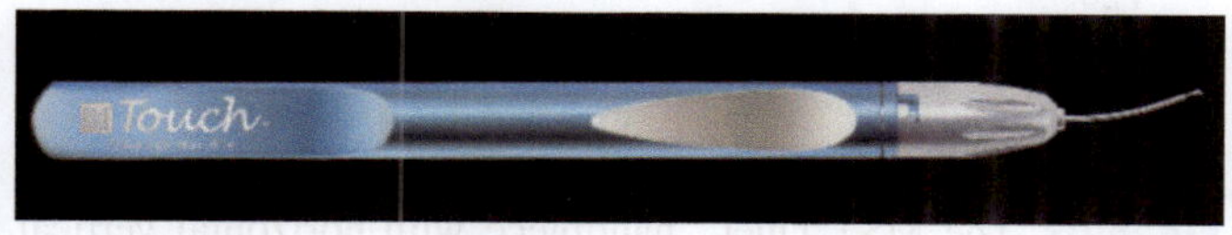

Fig. 6.65 Fine/Hoffman microincision capsulorhexis forceps on the MST Touch handle (Photo courtesy of MicroSurgical Technology)

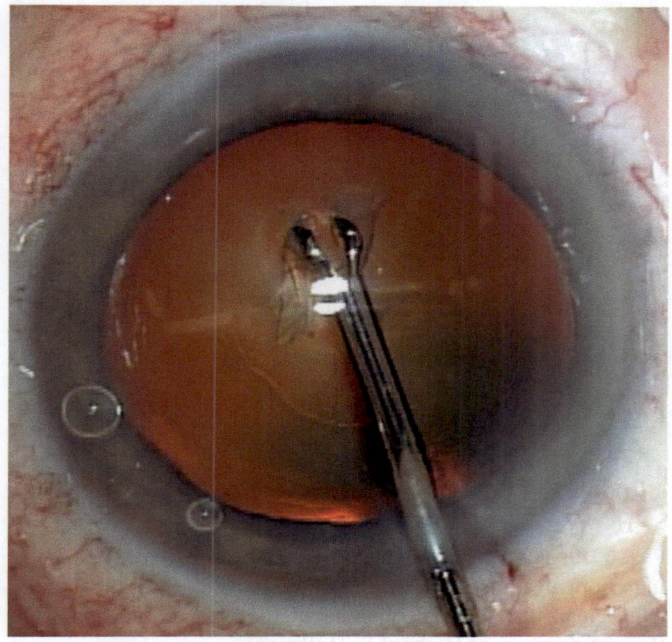

Fig. 6.66 Open configuration of MST (MicroSurgical Technology) Fine/Hoffman capsulorhexis forceps about to regrasp the anterior rhexis edge to continue and complete the capsulorhexis (Figure courtesy of Richard S. Hoffman)

Chopping is the preferred lens removal technique since it will allow for the lowest amounts of energy to be utilized and will lower any risk of incision burns. A 20-gauge irrigating chopper is inserted through the left-handed incision followed by the placement of the bare phacoemulsification needle (without an irrigation sleeve) through the right-handed incision. Microsurgical Technology's MST Duet System, which is available in both vertical and horizontal choppers, is currently preferred (Fig. 6.67). Insertion of the irrigating chopper is a maneuver that requires a short learning curve. It is best accomplished by inserting the vertical chopping element at the tip, parallel to the incision, until the distal aspect of the chopping segment clears the internal opening of the clear corneal incision (Fig. 6.68). Once the internal opening has been cleared, the handpiece can then be rotated to allow the remaining of the chopper to enter the eye.

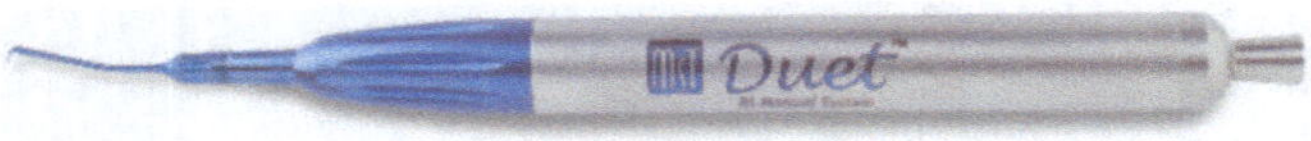

Fig. 6.67 The MST Duet™ handpiece with horizontal vertical chopper attached (Figure courtesy of MST MicroSurgical Technology)

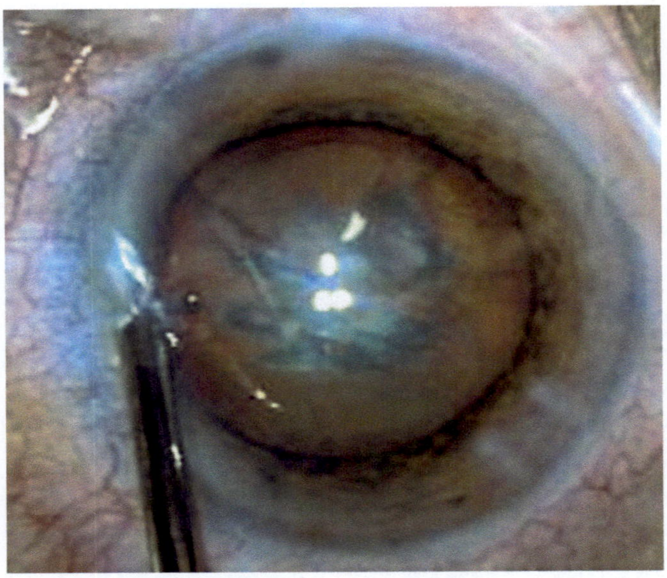

Fig. 6.68 The vertical element located on the tip of the irrigating chopper is inserted parallel to the incision until the leading edge clears the internal opening of the clear corneal incision (Figure courtesy of Richard S. Hoffman)

After trimming the anterior epinucleus with aspiration from the bare phaco needle, a horizontal chopper is placed at the distal golden ring and the phaco needle is buried proximally into the endonuclues to a depth of 50–60%. Horizontal chopping is then performed by bringing both instruments together and then pulling 90° away to create the first chop. The lens is then rotated 90° with either the chopper or the bare phaco needle and the second chop and segment removal is performed. Removal of the endonucleus is followed by trimming and flipping of the epinucleus, as previously described [4]. Rotating the vertical chopping element (located at the tip of the irrigating chopper), into a horizontal position during the removal of the last endonuclear segment and the removal of the epinucleus will decrease the chances of accidentally tearing the posterior capsule, if the capsule moves anteriorly, at this point in the procedure. If residual cortical material remains, it can be easily removed with the bimanual irrigation and aspiration handpieces (Fig. 6.69a, b).

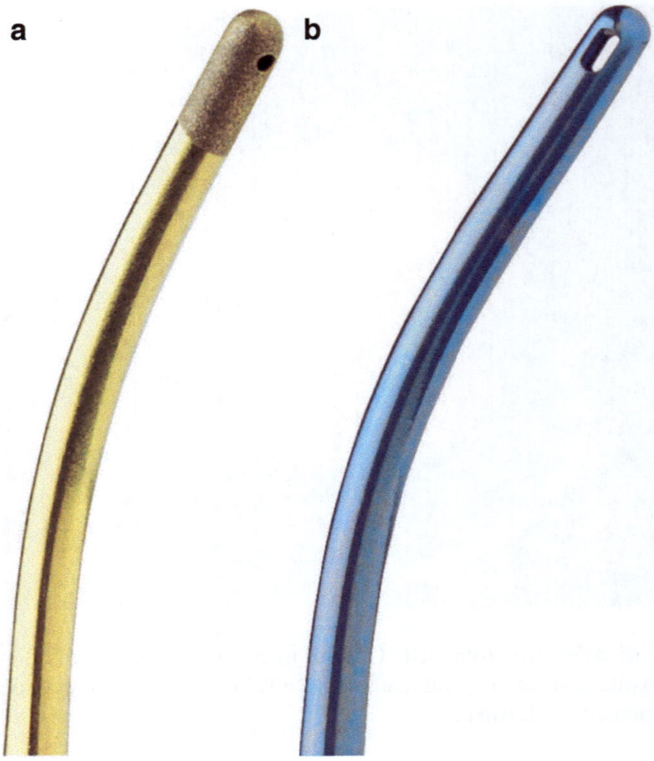

Fig. 6.69 (**a**) Magnified view of Duet™ aspiration tip and (**b**) irrigation tip utilized for bimanual I/A (Figure courtesy of MST MicroSurgical Technology)

6.8.2 Advantages

Why remove a lens through two 1.0–1.2 mm incisions rather than a 2.2–2.5 mm incision? While it is true that coaxial phaco is an excellent procedure with low amounts of induced astigmatism [6], biaxial phaco offers the potential for truly astigmatic neutral incisions. In addition, these microincisions should behave like a paracentesis incision with less likelihood for leakage and theoretically, a lower incidence of endophthalmitis.

The major advantage observed in biaxial microincisions is the improvement in the control of most of the steps involved in endocapsular surgery. Since OVDs do not leave the eye easily through these small incisions, the anterior chamber is more stable during capsulorhexis construction and there is much less likelihood for an errant rhexis to develop. A more controlled capsulorhexis has been extremely advantageous in cases of pseudoexfoliation, traumatic injury, lens subluxation, and mature cataracts. Also, hydrodelineation and hydrodissection can be performed more efficiently by virtue of a higher level of pressure building in the anterior chamber, prior to the eventual prolapse of the OVD through the microincisions.

In addition, separation of irrigation from aspiration allows for improved followability by avoiding competing currents at the tip of the phaco needle. In some instances, the irrigation flow from the irrigating handpiece can be used as an adjunctive surgical device – flushing nuclear pieces from the angle or loosening epinuclear or cortical material from the capsular bag. In the same respect, it is important to avoid directing the fluid flow from the irrigating handpiece to the tip of the phaco needle since this will dislodge nuclear fragments from the tip and actually worsen the followability.

The fluidics of separate infusion and aspiration have been extremely advantageous in intraoperative floppy iris syndrome (IFIS). Much of the billowing of floppy irides and the resultant miosis appears to stem from the infusion of the fluid behind the iris plane. With a coaxial technique, the infusion fluid is placed behind the iris plane during lens grooving and virtually all aspects of in situ phacoemulsification unless the lens nucleus is brought up to the anterior chamber for phacoemulsification. Similarly, aspiration of the cortex with a coaxial handpiece creates the same infusion currents behind the iris plane. With a biaxial technique, the infusion can be placed high in the anterior chamber, in front of the iris plane during phacoemulsification, and the aspiration of the cortex has been found to create a much stabler anterior chamber in IFIS cases with less likelihood for iris billowing and subsequent miosis.

Perhaps, the greatest advantage of the biaxial technique lies in its ability to switch handpieces between the similarly sized microincisions located 90° away from each other. The ability to approach the lens from two different directions has been invaluable in cases with compromised zonules and posterior polar cataracts. Directing aspiration forceps away from areas of enhanced zonular integrity, rather than from areas of zonular weakness creates a scenario, that is much less likely to extend zonular dialyses or worsen lens subluxation. The ability to switch the irrigating chopper and the phaco needle between the two incisions is also helpful when lens material cannot be rotated to the distal location for efficient aspiration and phacoemulsification. In posterior polar cataracts, the ability to approach and aspirate all the lens material without rotating the endonucleus or epinucleus, minimizes the chances of placing undue stress on the fragile or compromised posterior capsule, which would result in posterior capsule rupture and vitreous loss. This capacity to switch handpieces during I&A of the cortex has simplified cortical clean-up, allowing for easy access to 360° of the capsular fornices and lowering the chances for capsular aspiration and tears during the removal of the subincisional cortex (Fig. 6.70).

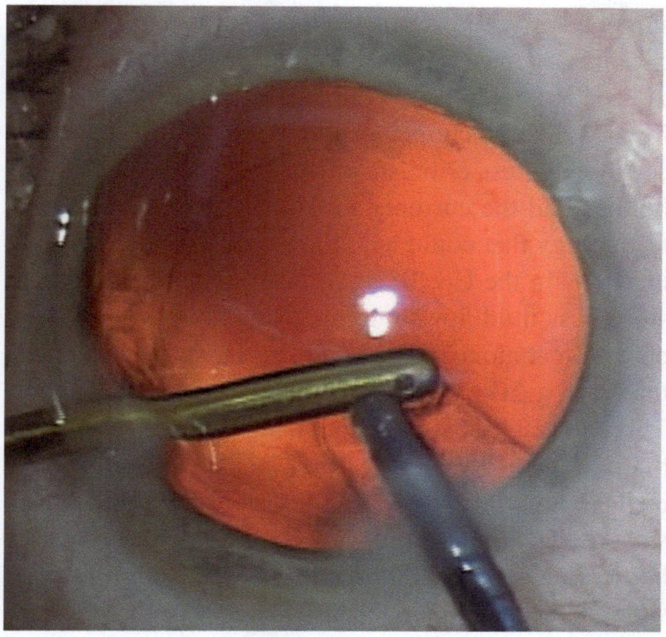

Fig. 6.70 Removal of subincisional cortex utilizing bimanual irrigation/aspiration system (Figure courtesy of Richard S. Hoffman)

6.8.3 Disadvantages

The disadvantages of biaxial microincision phacoemusification are real but easy to overcome. Maneuvering through 1.2 mm incisions can be awkward, early in the learning curve. Capsulorhexis construction requires the use of a bent capsulotomy needle or specially fashioned microincision forceps that have been designed to perform through these small incisions. Microincision capsulorhexis forceps is the best instrument for performing capsulorhexis and requires a small financial investment in the instrumentation. Although more time is initially required to learn to perform a capsulorhexis with these forceps, with experience, the maneuvers become a routine.

Also, additional equipment is necessary in the form of small incision keratomes, irrigating choppers and bimanual I/A handpieces. All of the major instrument companies are currently designing irrigating choppers and other microincision adjunctive devices such as capsulorhexis forceps. For the divide-and-conquer surgeon, irrigation can be accomplished with the bimanual irrigation handpiece that can also function as the second "side-port" instrument negating the need for an irrigating chopper.

The greatest criticism of biaxial phaco lies in the fluidics and the current limitations in intraocular lens technology that could be utilized through these micro-incisions in the US. Because of the size of these incisions, less fluid flows into the eye than what occurs in coaxial techniques. Most, current irrigating choppers integrate a 20-gauge lumen that limits fluid inflow. This can result in significant chamber instability when high vacuum levels are utilized and occlusion from nuclear material at the phaco tip is cleared. Thus, infusion needs to be maximized by placing the infusion bottle on a separate IV pole that is set as high as possible. Also, vacuum levels usually need to be lowered below 350 mmHg to avoid significant surge flow, although newer phacoemulsification machines continue to improve the ability to raise vacuum and maintain a stable anterior chamber.

6.8.4 Final Thoughts

Ultimately, the surgeons and the marketplace forces will dictate how cataract surgical technique will evolve. The hazards and the prolonged recovery time of large incision intra- and extracapsular surgery eventually spurred the acceptance of phacoemulsification, despite the difficult learning curve. Surgeons comfortable with their extracapsular skills disparaged phaco until the advantages were too powerful to ignore. Similar inertia has been evident in transitioning to foldable IOLs, clear corneal incisions, and topical anesthesia and the use of these practices is increasing every year. The future lens procedure of choice will eventually be decided by its potential advantages over traditional methods and by the collaboration of surgeons and industry to deliver a safe and effective technology. Biaxial microincision phacoemulsification is the next step in the evolution of phacoemulsification.

Take Home Pearls

- The capsulorhexis can be started using the sharp tip of a single blade of the rhexis forceps in the open position and then completed by grasping the edge of the rhexis in a standard fashion.
- It should be ensured that the leading tip of the chopping element is past the internal incision opening prior to rotating the chopper handpiece and inserting the remainder of the irrigating chopper.
- Cortical cleaving hydrodissection should be performed and the lens should be rotated prior to performing hydrodelineation. This will insure that both the endonucleus and the epinucleus are freely mobile. Free mobility of both the epinucleus and the endonucleus will greatly facilitate lens removal with a biaxial method.
- The vertical chopping element of the chopper should be rotated counter-clockwise into a horizontal position when aspirating the epinucleus, to lessen the likelihood of tearing the posterior capsule with the chopper.
- Biaxial I&A facilitates cortex removal by allowing easy access to 360° of the capsular fornices. This lessens the chances for capsule tearing during the removal of subincisional cortex.

References

1. Agarwal A, Agarwal A, Agarwal S et al (2001) Phakonit: phacoemulsification through a 0.9 mm corneal incision. J Cataract Refract Surg 27:1548–1552
2. Shock JP (1972) Removal of cataracts with ultrasonic fragmentation and continuous irrigation. Trans Pac Coast Otoophthalmol Soc Annu Meet 53:139–144
3. Girard LJ (1978) Ultrasonic fragmentation for cataract extraction and cataract complications. Adv Ophthalmol 37:127–135
4. Fine IH (1998) The choo-choo chop and flip phacoemulsification technique. In: Elander R (ed) Operative techniques in cataract and refractive surgery. W.B. Saunders, Philadelphia, PA, pp 61–65
5. Fine IH, Packer M, Hoffman RS (2001) The use of power modulations in phacoemulsification: choo choo chop and flip phacoemulsification. J Cataract Refract Surg 27: 188–197

6. Masket S, Tennen DG (1996) Astigmatic stabilization of 3.0 mm temporal clear corneal cataract incisions. J Cataract Refract Surg 22:1451–1455
7. Shearing SP, Relyea RL, Loaiza A, Shearing RL (1985) Routine phacoemulsification through a one-millimeter non-sutured incision. Cataract 2:6–10
8. Tsuneoka H, Shiba T, Takahashi Y (2001) Feasibility of ultrasound cataract surgery with a 1.4 mm incision. J Cataract Refract Surg 27:934–940
9. Tsuneoka H, Shiba T, Takahashi Y (2002) Ultrasonic phacoemulsification using a 1.4 mm incision: clinical results. J Cataract Refract Surg 28:81–86

6.9 BiMICS vs. CoMICS: Our Actual Technique (Bimanual Micro Cataract Surgery vs. Coaxial Micro Cataract Surgery)

Jerome Bovet

Core Messages

- Reduction of the incision size is one of the goals of microincision cataract surgery in order to avoid induced astigmatism.
- A balance between irrigation and aspiration is the key element to avoid complications in phacoemulsification by microincision.
- The inflow of the fluid inside the anterior chamber is as important as the outflow.

6.9.1 Introduction

Bimanual and coaxial microincision cataract surgery are not two conflicting surgical techniques, but rather, they are the products of a common goal to control better, and reduce induced astigmatism during cataract surgery [12] (Fig. 6.71). The 3 mm incision has already become obsolete, just as that of the 12 mm and subsequently, the 6 mm incisions [4, 14]. The decrease in the size of cataract incisions will reduce, if not eliminate, induced astigmatism, thus bringing the surgery under better control of the surgeon [9]. Likewise, it opens the door to refractive lens surgery (as an application of bioptics to cataract surgery), combining both phacoemulsification and intraocular lens (IOL) implantation with LASIK during presby surgery.

J. Bovet
clinique de l'oeil, 15 bois de la chapelle, 1213 Onex, Geneva, Switzerland
e-mail: jbovet@vision.tv

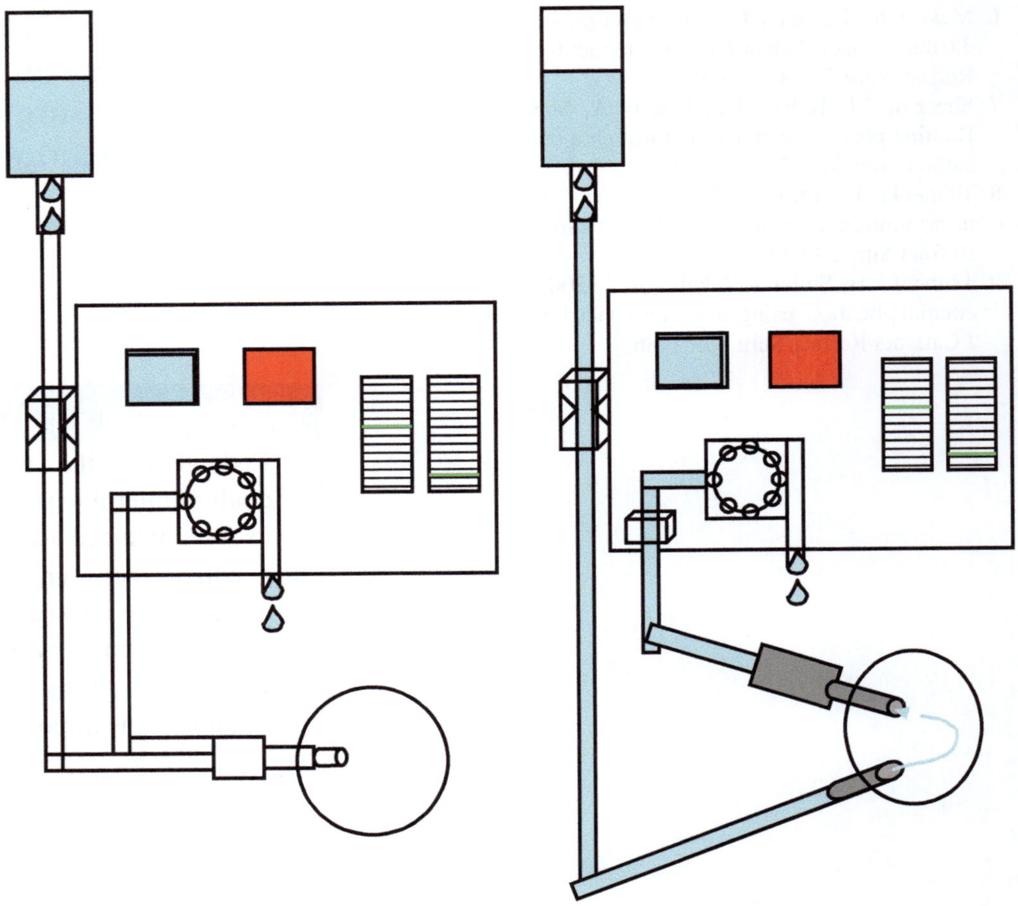

Fig. 6.71 Set up CoMics vs. BiMics

6.9.2 Historical Background

Biaxial and coaxial microincision cataract surgeries are complementary and, as Olson [16] says, are likely to dominate lens surgical techniques in the very near future.

6.9.3 BiMICS. BiManual MicroIncision Cataract Surgery

6.9.3.1 Introduction

BiMICS (Fig. 6.72) is a surgical technique performed through two microincisions, one for irrigation and the other for aspiration, of reduced sizes, usually under 1 mm [1, 2, 6, 13.

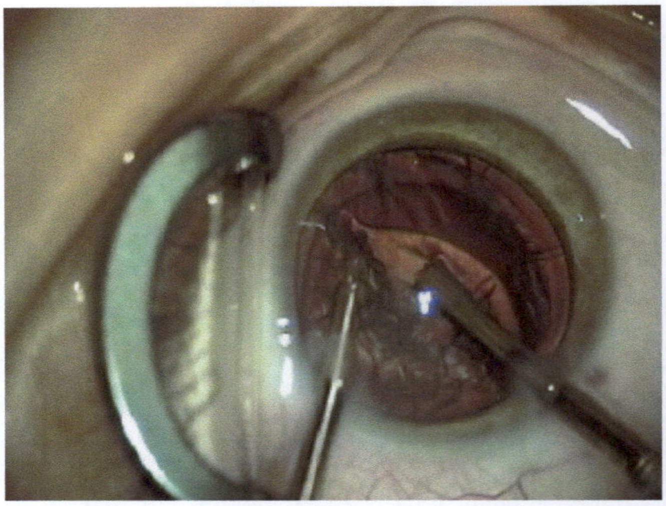

Fig. 6.72 BiMics technique

6.9.3.2 Instrumentation

The instruments for BiMICS (Fig. 6.73) present only slight changes from conventional phaco instruments. However, particular attention will have to be given to microphacodynamics, as well as to the incisions made, which have to be chosen and tested meticulously.

6.9.3.3 Microphacodynamics [3, 5, 8]

The incoming flow should be superior to the outgoing flow. Using the Poiseuille's law (Fig. 6.74), it is

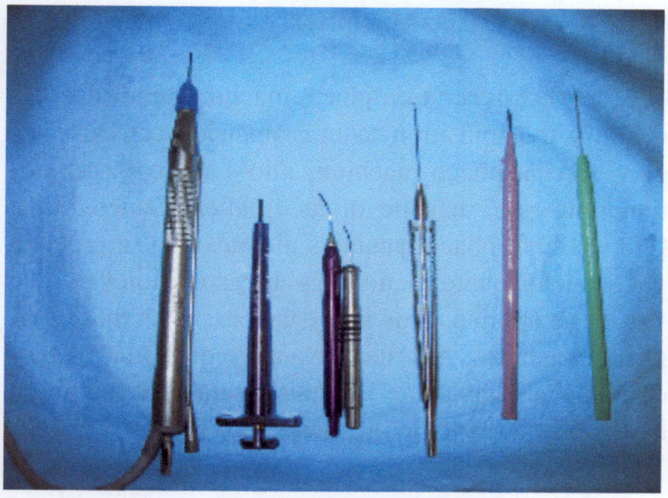

Fig. 6.73 Material for the Bimanual phaco technique

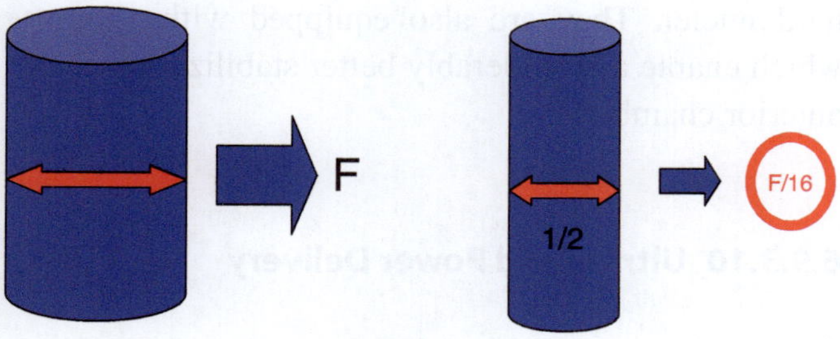

Fig. 6.74 Law from Poiseuille-Hagen

possible to increase the flow significantly without modifying the intraocular pressure, by using only slightly increased internal tubing diameter.

The choice of the irrigation instrument is very important in order to produce the fluid dynamics. The internal diameter of the irrigation tube must be of a superior gauge than that of the aspiration tube, in order to compensate for fluid losses, diminish intraocular pressure, and to avoid anterior chamber instability.

6.9.3.4 Irrigation-aspiration [10] (Fig. 6.75)

In bimanual phaco, for an aspiration instrument with an internal diameter of 20 G, an irrigation instrument with an internal diameter of 19 G [5] should be used, and for an aspiration instrument with an internal diameter of 21 G [16, 17], an irrigation instrument with an internal diameter of 20 G should be used. A slightly larger diameter of the irrigation instrument compensates for surge and reduces intraocular pressure as well. The instruments for irrigation and aspiration of the MST Duet® Bimanual System (MicroSurgical Technology Inc., Redmond, WA) offer an optimal relationship between the internal and external diameters of these instruments.

While using BiMICS technique, the irrigator manipulator with the irrigation at the tip of the instrument should be used in order to avoid the a surge while switching back to the manipulator.

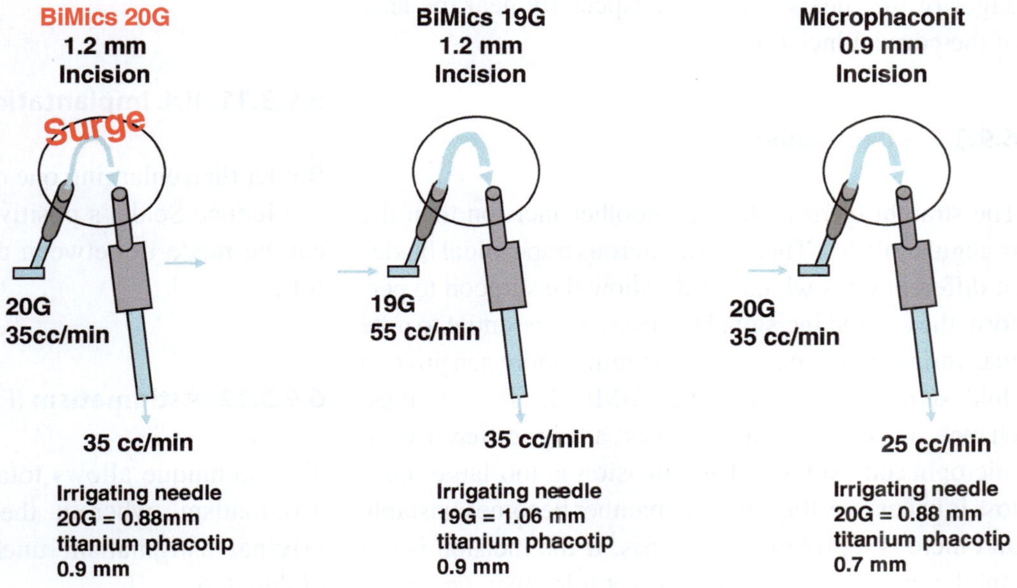

Fig. 6.75 Microphacodynamics BiMics

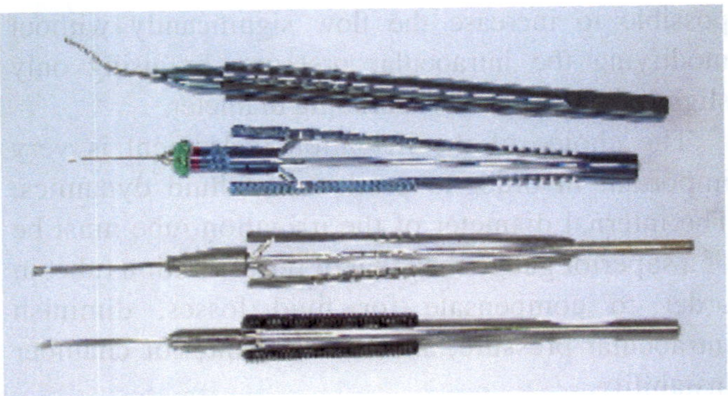

Fig. 6.76 Capsulorhexis forceps

6.9.3.5 Phacotips

The phacotips are usually equipped with an external diameter of 21 G (0.9 mm). It is important to control the internal diameter of these tips also in order to avoid surge. The tip is straight with a 30° bevel.

6.9.3.6 Capsulorhexis

The needle is the simplest way to create a capsulorhexis through a microincision (Fig. 6.76). It can be easily performed with a viscoelastic gel such as methylcellulose. The microinstrument for capsulorhexis is a bit more complex. Furthermore, using vitrectomy forceps is also not a simple task.

The capsulorhexis forceps should have a smaller diameter than the incision, with a distal opening mechanism that can be maneuvered without creating much movement of the body of the instrument. It should also be curved on both sides in order to permit grasping the edges of the rhexis with ease, especially near the area of the corneal incision.

6.9.3.7 Phaco Knives

The straight blades allow a smoother incision than the triangular blades. There are numerous trapezoidal blades of different sizes which would allow the surgeon to perform the desired incision. However, it is essential to note that variation in incision sizes is much more sensitive to fluid dynamics when using BiMICS. The slightest change in incision size makes a big difference in microphacodynamics. If the incision is too large, fluid loss is excessive, the anterior chamber becomes unstable and there is a prolapse of the iris. If the incision is too small, corneal burns and Descemet folds may occur.

6.9.3.8 The Phaco Machines

The newest generation phaco machines considerably simplify the transition to microincision cataract surgery. Recent phaco machines allow sufficient aspiration flow rate, in spite of its smaller diameter tips. Conventional phacodynamics dictates that in order to obtain an adequate suction, greater aspiration flow rate should be applied. This is not the case with these new phaco machines. Another advantage of the latest generation phaco machines is that it regulates heat emitted by the phaco tip at the incision site.

6.9.3.9 Phaco Pumps

The newer phaco pumps combine the benefits of both the peristaltic and venturi systems. They allow for more flexibility and are more effective in the presence of hard nuclei. They are also equipped with systems, which enable a considerably better stabilization of the anterior chamber.

6.9.3.10 Ultrasound Power Delivery

The most recent machines have notably reduced thermal energy due to power modulation that includes pulses and bursts with microsecond duration. However, even with the old phaco machines, it is possible to reduce the thermal energy using the foot pedal during the short interval, reducing the phaco power time.

6.9.3.11 IOL Implantation (Fig. 6.77)

Rather than enlarging one of the microincisions, which can induce Seidel's positive incisions, a third incision can be made in between the first two, to implant the IOL.

6.9.3.12 Astigmatism (Fig. 6.78)

This technique allows total neutralization of induced astigmatism, wherein the microincisions leave the original astigmatism unchanged, if not eliminated (Table 6.5).

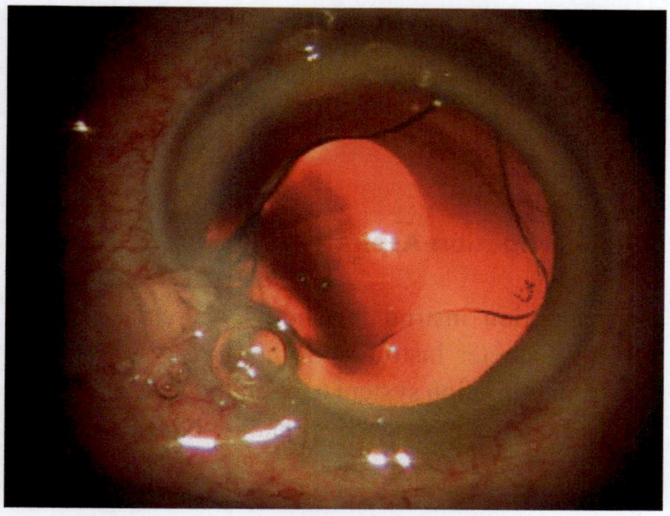

Fig. 6.77 Insertion of an Acri Smart 36 A the catridge stay outside

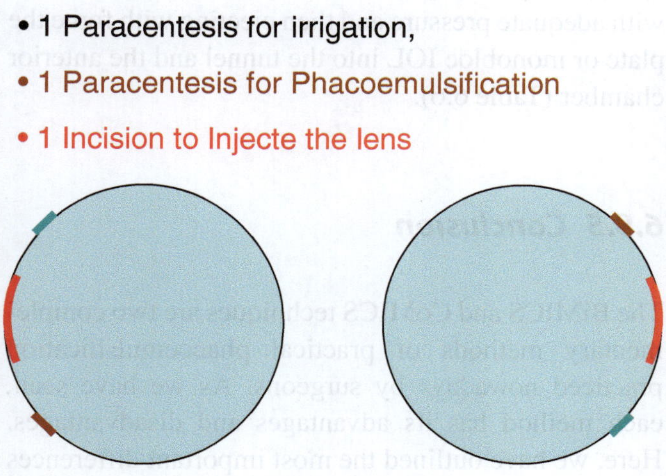

Fig. 6.78 BiMics incision

6.9.4 CoMICS: Coaxial MicroIncision Cataract Surgery [12, 15, 18] (Figs. 6.79 and 6.80)

CoMICS surgical technique was developed after BiMICS surgical technique, to lessen the learning curve and the difficulties encountered with the BiMICS technique. CoMICS was the perfect choice for the implantation of a lens at 2.2 mm incision width without changing much of the conventional phacoemulsification technique. At that size, there is no risk of inducing anterior chamber instability, as well as producing corneal burns. Likewise, there is no need to change all the instruments, thus making this technique more cost-effective than BiMICS.

Table 6.5 Advantages/disadvantages of BiMics

Advantages of BiMICS	Disadvantages of BiMICS
Two microincisions, down to 0.9 mm in width	Steep learning curve
Implantation of an IOL through an incision below 2.2 mm wide	A precise setting of the parameters for irrigation and aspiration flow is mandatory
No induced astigmatism, which allows precise control of astigmatism	Sensitive phacodynamics
Separate irrigation flow allowing minimum turbulence during aspiration	Specific instrumentation required
Most appropriate technique for small pupils or in cases of floppy iris syndrome	

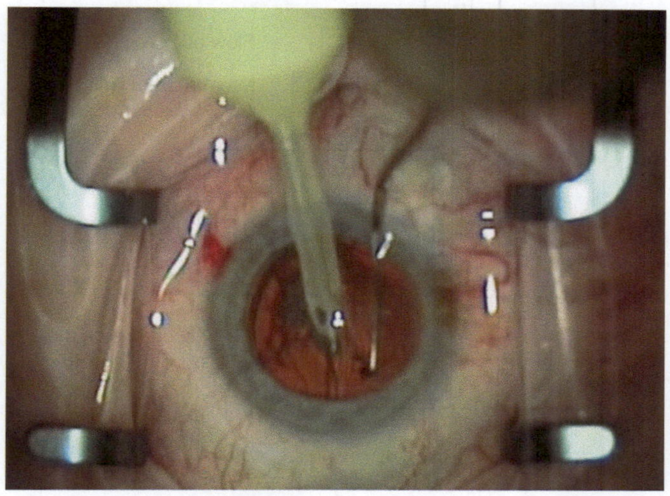

Fig. 6.79 CoMics technique

6.9.4.1 Capsulorhexis

Most of the fine capsulorhexis forceps can be used through a 2.2 mm incision. It becomes necessary to use a capsulorhexis forceps that has a distal opening mechanism for incisions smaller than this size.

6.9.4.2 Phacotips

Two sizes of phacotips with external diameter sizes of 0.9–1.1 mm are used. Both have an angle of 30 or 45°.

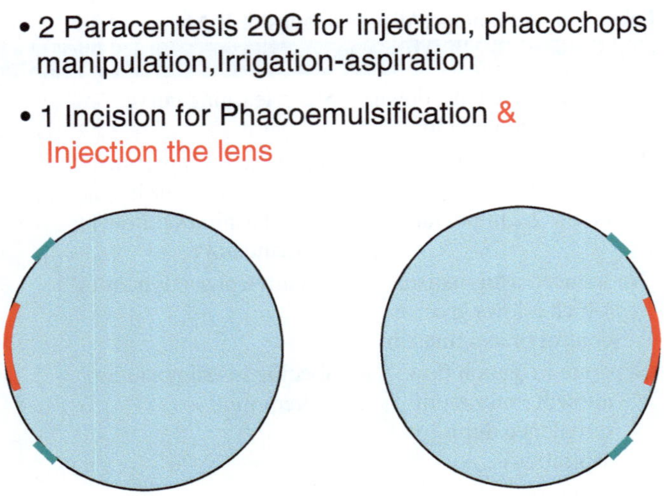

Fig. 6.80 CoMics incision

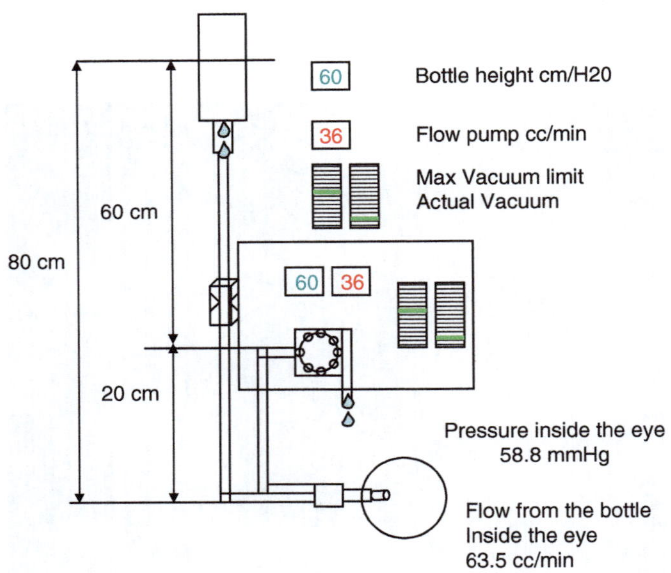

Fig. 6.81 Real pressure and flow with the CoMics

6.9.4.3 The Phaco Machines (Fig. 6.81)

The level of the irrigation bottle should be between 80 and 100 cm. The aspiration flow rate used is 25 mL/min. The aspiration pressure is set at 400 mmHg. It is imperative to set the irrigation bottle sufficiently high in order to maintain adequate fluid inflow, thereby avoiding corneal burns which can be produced by the phaco tip.

6.9.4.4 Phaco Pumps

It is easier to use a machine combining peristaltic and venturi pumps.

6.9.4.5 Ultrasound Power Delivery

Any phaco machine with the surgeon's desired phaco setting can be used with CoMICS.

6.9.4.6 Irrigation-Aspiration

The aspiration instrument should be replaced by a 2.2 mm diameter instrument when using a bimanual irrigation aspiration system to maintain water tightness so that the anterior chamber remains stable.

6.9.4.7 Incision-Assisted IOL Implantation

Most IOLs can be injected through a 2.2 mm incision by applying the injector directly against the incision with adequate pressure and then ejecting with force the plate or monobloc IOL into the tunnel and the anterior chamber (Table 6.6).

6.9.5 Conclusion

The BiMICS and CoMICS techniques are two complementary methods of practical phacoemulsification practiced nowadays by surgeons. As we have seen, each method has its advantages and disadvantages. Here, we have outlined the most important differences that would enable a surgeon to choose one method over the other.

It is easier to transition from the classic phacoemulsification technique to the CoMICS technique as only the parameters of the machine being used need to be changed. The learning curve in the CoMICS technique is less steep than in the BiMICS technique. In addition, improper planning of the incisions for both irrigation and aspiration in BiMICS can lead to anterior chamber instability and consequently lead to complications.

On the other hand, the BiMICS technique has an advantage of allowing a wider room for movement inside the anterior chamber, as both the functions of irrigation and aspiration are separated. Any complications experienced during the operation are easier to manage using the BiMICS technique.

These two technical differences can help the surgeon to choose one surgical technique over the other.

Table 6.6 Advantages/disadvantages of CoMics

Advantages of CoMICS	Disadvantages of CoMICS
No learning curve	The width of the incision is limited to 1.6 mm
Increased water tightness of the incision	Management of posterior capsular rupture is more problematic than with BiMICS
The setting for the phacomachine is comparable to the 3 mm incision technique	Small pupils are more difficult to deal with than with BiMICS
IOLs and injectors are well adapted to a 2.2 mm incision	

However, if we consider the visual outcomes of the patient, it is important to note the following aspects. First, the incision length of CoMICS, which at the minimum is 1.6 mm, cannot be reduced due to the limitations of the instrument. This, in addition to implanting the IOL in the same site instead of at the periphery, can lead to induced astigmatism.

In contrast, BiMICS allows reduction of the incision sizes up to 0.7 mm. The incision for the IOL implantation can be performed at another site, different from the first two incisions. This allows the incision to be exactly the size of the implant. It also allows a more precise positioning of the incision in relation to the patient's preexisting astigmatism. The introduction of toric implants presents an important development and is the only real technique for fine correction of astigmatism. BiMICS will therefore, be the method of the future for allowing neutrality of astigmatism.

Take Home Pearls

- If one wants to shift from conventional phacoemulsification to microincision cataract surgery, it is safer and more secure to start with CoMICS.
- Understanding the phacodynamics during MICS is the key element to any successful surgery.
- If one would like to use the newer generation IOLs, namely, the toric, multifocal and aspheric IOLs, it is best to use BiMICS.

References

1. Agarwal A, Agarwal A, Agarwal S et al (2001) Phakonit: phacoemulsification through a 0.9 mm corneal incision. J Cataract Refract Surg 27:1548–1552
2. Agarwal A, Agarwal S, Agarwal A (2003) Phakonit with an AcriTec IOL. J Cataract Refract Surg 29:854–855
3. Barret G (1995) Maxi-flow phaco needle. ASCRS-ASOA Film Festival
4. Bovet JJ, Baumgartner JM, Bruckner JC et al (1997) Chirurgie de la cataracte en topique intracamérulaire, Abstract SSO-SOG
5. Bovet J (2006) 19 G Bimanual MicroPhaco. ASCRS-ASOA, Abstract
6. Bovet J Achard O, Baumgartner JM et al (2004) Bimanual phaco trick and track. ASCRS-ASOA Film, San Diego
7. Bovet J Achard O, Baumgartner JM et al (2003) 0.9 mm Incision bimanual phaco and IOL insertion through a 1.7 mm incision. In: Symposium on Cataract, IOL and Refractive Surgery. Abstract ASCRS-ASOA, San Francisco
8. Bovet J (2007) Phacodynamics: bimanual microphaco. In: Ashok G, Fine H, Alio JL et al (eds) Mastering the phacodynamics (tools, technology and innovations). Jaypee Brothers, India
9. Bovet J (2007) Break the phaco barrier. In: Garg, A, Fine, H, Alio, JL, et al (eds) Mastering the phacodynamics (tools, technology and innovations) Jaypee Brothers, India
10. Brauweiler P (1996) Bimanual irrigation/aspiration. J Cataract Refract Surg 22:1013–1016
11. Dogru M, Honda R, Omoto M et al (2004) Early visual results with the rollable ThinOptX intraocular lens. J Cataract Refract Surg 30:558–565
12. Cavallini GM, Campi C Masini C et al (2007) Bimanual microphacoemulsification versus coaxial miniphacoemulsification: prospective study. J Cataract Refract Surg 33:387–392
13. Garg A, Fine I, Chang D et al. (eds) (2005) Mastering the art of bimanual microincision phaco. Jaypee Brothers, India
14. Kelman CD (1967) Phacoemulsification and aspiration: a new technique of cataract extraction. Am J Ophthal 64:23
15. Buratto L Werner L, Zanini M et al (2003) Phacoemulsification: principles and techniques, 2nd edn. Slack, Thorofare
16. Olson RJ (2004) Clinical experience with 21 gauge manual microphacoemulsification using Sovereign WhiteStar technology in eyes with dense cataract. J Cataract Refract Surg 30:168–172
17. Sharing SP, Releya RL, Loiza A et al (1985) Routine phacoemulsification through a one-millimeter non sutured incision Cataract 2:6–10
18. Tsuneoka H, Shiba T, Takahashi Y (2001) Feasibility of ultrasound cataract surgery with a 1.4 mm incision. J Cataract Refract Surg 27:934–940
19. Wong VWY Lai TYY Lee GKY et al (2007) Safety and efficacy of micro-incisional cataract surgery with bimanual phacoemulsification for white mature cataract. Ophthalmologica 221:24–28

6.10 Endophthalmitis Prevention

Ayman Naseri and David F. Chang

Core Messages

- Antibiotic administration and wound construction are important factors in endophthalmitis prevention.
- Many factors can affect the antibiotic selection for the prophylaxis of endophthalmitis, including efficacy, safety, patient compliance, and cost.
- Regardless of the wound size and the location, one must be prepared to suture a cataract incision if it is not sufficiently watertight.

Continuing advances in cataract surgery technique and technology have raised expectations for both patients and surgeons alike. Cataract surgery is expected to be a relatively painless and quick procedure that achieves outstanding visual results within days after the procedure. With excellent outcomes becoming the norm, cases of acute, postoperative endophthalmitis (POE) are particularly devastating. Since even prompt treatment may not prevent significant morbidity and visual loss, much attention has been focused on POE prevention.

Worrisome trends regarding POE rates following cataract surgery have been reported in the past several years, causing ophthalmologists to reconsider both, the method of antibiotic prophylaxis and the safety of the phaco incision. A study of the US Medicare population revealed a surprisingly high rate of endophthalmitis from the years 1994 to 2001 (1). This study also concluded that the rate of infection had increased over the course of this period, which is of even greater concern. From 1998 to 2001, the rate of endophthalmitis was as high as 0.262% with an average of 0.249%, corresponding to approximately 1 in 400 cases. The authors hypothesize that this increase in the rate of POE may be related to the adoption of sutureless, clear corneal incisions. However, a close look at the data from that study revealed that there was a stepwise increase in the rate of endophthalmitis between the years 1997 and 1998, when the rate increased by 46% from 1.73 to 2.53, with a relative plateau in POE rate from 1998 to 2001 (1).

Taban et al. published a meta-analysis which also suggested that the rate of POE may be increasing. In their systematic review of peer-reviewed English language studies, they documented a disturbingly high rate of POE (2). They determined that the average rate of POE had risen to 0.265% between 2000 and 2003, which also corresponded temporally to the period when sutureless, clear corneal incisions had reached a wider adoption. The relative risk of endophthalmitis in that study was 2.55 times greater for clear corneal incisions compared to that of scleral tunnel wounds. Notably, limbal wounds were also found to be protective against POE when compared to clear corneal incisions. It is not clear if limbal incisions in this study were placed beneath the conjunctival insertion, or if they were a variant in the construction of clear corneal incisions with a more posterior external wound. It is also not clear as to how often the sutures were used in each group.

Other researchers did not report any statistically significant increase in the rate of endophthalmitis over the same time period at their institutions (3–6). These reports specifically did not find a statistical link between clear corneal incisions and POE. Instead, some of these studies suggested that the route of antibiotic administration may be one of the most important factors in preventing POE. Incision size may be another potential risk factor. By minimizing the incision size, surgeons may be able to decrease the risk of bacterial contamination and POE.

Because of the concern over the increasing rates of POE, we will review two major factors in the risk of infection: antibiotic prophylaxis and wound construction.

6.10.1 Antibiotic Prophylaxis

There are several potential routes of antibiotic administration for the prophylaxis of POE. Instead of systemic routes, ophthalmologists are able to employ topical, subconjunctival, and intracameral methods of antibiotic delivery to the surgical site. Because of the low rate of surgical infection, it is difficult to conduct prospective, randomized trials that are large enough to prove the efficacy of any method.

A. Naseri
Department of Ophthalmology, University of California, San Francisco, CA, USA
e-mail: Ayman.Naseri@va.gov

Table 6.7 Use of prophylactic antibiotics reported by 1,312 respondents from the 2007 ASCRS Endophthalmitis Survey [26]

	Use (%)	Don't Use (%)
Peri-op topical antibiotics	91	9
Post-op antibiotics	88	12
Intracameral antibiotics –	30	70
Antibiotics at the conclusion of surgery	90	10
Post-op antibiotics	98	2

This problem is certainly true with respect to using topical antibiotics for the prevention of POE (7). Nonetheless, this method of prophylaxis is universally used in the US. In a recent survey of members of the American Society of Cataract and Refractive Surgery (ASCRS), 91% of respondents stated that they used topical antibiotics perioperatively, while 98% used topical antibiotics postoperatively (Table 6.7) (8). 93% of those using perioperative topical antibiotics employed fluoroquinolones, with 81% using either gatifloxacin or moxifloxacin. Methods of prophylaxis in other countries may be quite different. In a survey of the ophthalmologists in the United Kingdom conducted in 2008, subconjunctival and intracameral cefuroxime were used predominantly, while the most common topical preparation was a combination steroid/neomycin drop (9). It should be noted that neither gatifloxacin nor moxifloxacin are available in the United Kingdom.

The rationale for using topical antibiotics is supported by several types of indirect evidence, including studies of experimental endophthalmitis, measurements of aqueous penetration of topical antibiotics, consideration of the spectrum of anti-bacterial activity, and clinical experience (10–15). To our knowledge, there is only one large retrospective clinical study reporting the rate of endophthalmitis, while using the latest generation fluoroquinolones preferred by most of the respondents who took the ASCRS survey in 2007 (16). Unfortunately, that study was designed to exclude any patient that had an intraoperative complication or a wound leak either before or after the surgery. Since these two exclusion criteria are known risk factors for the development of POE, and since they cannot be predicted preoperatively, this study does not adequately address the efficacy of the latest generation topical fluoroquinolones. Therefore, despite their widespread popularity, the efficacy or superiority of gatifloxacin or moxifloxacin over other agents in the prophylaxis of POE has not been proven.

Subconjunctival injection is another common route of antibiotic administration, although only 13% of the respondents employed this method in the ASCRS survey conducted in 2007 (Table 6.8) (8). This suggests that the use subconjunctival antibiotics has decreased since 1996, when they were used by 46% of ASCRS members surveyed, and this trend could be explained by the shift to topical anesthesia (17). Although there are no prospective, randomized studies to support the use of subconjunctival antibiotics, there is some peer-reviewed clinical evidence suggesting its efficacy in preventing POE. In a study of Canadian patients, Colleaux et al. found that the rate of POE was significantly lower in patients receiving subconjunctival antibiotics (0.011 vs. 0.179%, $p = 0.009$) (18). Notably, this study did not find a statistically significant association of POE with clear corneal incisions. A second retrospective study from the UK also found that subconjunctival antibiotics were of statistical benefit in the prevention of POE (19).

Finally, in their large, retrospective case control study, Ng and et al. also found that subconjunctival antibiotics and preoperative antisepsis were associated with a significant reduction in the risk of POE (6). Because most of the surgeons used topical antibiotics and did not use intracameral antibiotics, there was insufficient statistical power to assess the benefit of either of these methods of antibiotic prophylaxis. In the same study, however, clear corneal wounds were not associated with an increased risk of POE compared to other wound types.

Although the direct intracameral injection of antibiotics for the prevention of POE has recently become a frequent and fiercely debated topic, the clinical evidence supporting its use dates back to over three decades. During cataract surgery camps in South India

Table 6.8 Preferred routes of antibiotic prophylaxis immediately following surgery as per 2007 ASCRS Endophthalmitis Survey [26]

How do you Administer Antibiotics at the Conclusion of the Surgery	Percentage
Topical application	83
Intracameral injection	15
Subconjunctival injection	13
Collagen shield	3

Percentages total more than 100 because respondents could indicate multiple methods from 1961 to 1975, Peyman et al. demonstrated a reduction in the rate of endophthalmitis from 3.6 to 0.37%, in a study of over 50,000 patients (20). In the era of large incisions and intracapsular cataract surgery, this remarkable result was achieved with a direct prophylactic intracameral injection of gentamicin. In the phacoemulsification era, Gimbel et al. reported their early experience with intracameral gentamicin and vancomycin. They did not find any case of endophthalmitis in 11,748 patients, which is suggestive of the relative safety of their technique as reflected by the endothelial cell counts (21).

More recent studies have focused on the use of intracameral cephalosporins. In the year 2002, Montan et al. reported the early Swedish experience with direct intracameral cefuroxime injections (22). In their retrospective study of over 32,000 cases, they discovered an endophthalmitis rate of 0.06%, which was significantly lower that the US published rates over a similar period. Of the 13 cases of culture-positive endophthalmitis, 12 infections occurred from organisms resistant to cefuroxime, suggesting that the intracameral route of administration was highly effective against organisms sensitive to cefuroxime (12).

The use of intracameral cephalosporins as prophylaxis against POE has not been limited to cefuroxime. In two retrospective studies from Spain, patients who received an intracameral injection of cefazolin had more than a tenfold lower rate of endophthalmitis than those that did not receive intracameral antibiotics (23, 24). In each of those reports, the rate of endophthalmitis was determined in one group of patients that received intracameral cefazolin, and in another group that did not. In each study, there was more than a tenfold reduction in the rate of endophthalmitis in the group that received intracameral cefazolin.

More recently in a prospective study conducted in Sweden, the outcomes of more than 225,000 cataract extractions, in which patients received an intracameral injection of cefuroxime, revealed an endophthalmitis rate of less than 0.05% (25). Remarkably, this was achieved despite the fact that less than 10% of the patients in that study received any topical antibiotics whatsoever. The strongest evidence of the efficacy of intracameral cephalosporin injections was the prospective, randomized, multi-center trial on the prophylaxis of POE by the European Society of Cataract and Refractive Surgery Surgeons (ESCRS) (26). Although that study was designed for the intended recruitment of 32,000 patients, the study management team and the data monitoring committee (DMC) determined that the study should be unmasked when approximately half that number had been enrolled. At that time the DMC "advised that it would be unethical to withhold the use of prophylactic intracameral cefuroxime from the two groups who did not receive it." The rates of culture proven endophthalmitis in the two groups that did not receive intracameral cefuroxime injections were 0.226 and 0.176%, compared to that of 0.050 and 0.025% in the two groups that did receive intracameral cefuroxime. Because endophthalmitis caused by Streptococcus species often leads to severe visual loss (27), it is important to note that there was no Streptococcal endophthalmitis in the two groups receiving intracameral cefuroxime injections (26).

The ASCRS survey conducted in 2007 showed that despite the conclusions of the ESCRS prospective, randomized study, 77% of the respondents were still not using a direct intracameral injection of the antibiotic for prophylaxis (Table 6.8) (8). There are two likely reasons for this outcome, though they are only speculations. First, unavailability of commercial antibiotic preparation that is approved for intraocular use, and fear of risk of using intracameral injections. Forty five percent of those not using intracameral injections were concerned about the risk. Eighty two percent indicated that they might use an intracameral antibiotic injection if it were commercially available at a reasonable cost. Second, the ESCRS study control group did not reflect the most common topical antibiotic regimens, in which most respondents were using topical gatifloxacin or moxifloxacin (81%), and starting topical prophylaxis at least 1 day preoperatively (78%) and immediately postoperatively (66%). Therefore, the ESCRS study did not address whether intracameral cefuroxime was equal to, superior to, or of adjunctive benefit to the most commonly used topical antibiotic protocols.

The ideal antibiotic for direct intracameral injection is not known. Some authors have suggested that if intracameral antibiotics are to be used, latest generation fluoroquinolones may be a better choice. Although there is some preliminary data supporting the safety of intracameral injection of this class of antibiotics (28–30), the clinical efficacy of these antibiotics are yet to be determined in large clinical studies. The majority of large clinical studies advocate the use of cefuroxime intracamerally, but the intracameral injection of cefazolin, vancomycin, and gentamicin has also been reported. Montan et al. studied the safety and pharmacokinetics

Table 6.9 Antibiotics preferred by those using an intracameral route (direct injection or placement in the irrigating bottle) from the 2007 ASCRS Endophthalmitis Survey [26]

Intracameral antibiotics	Percentage
Vancomycin	61 (37% inject, 63% bottle)
Cephalosporin	23
Quinolone	22
Other antibiotics	12

of intracameral cefuroxime (31), while Gimbel et al. published their experience with intracameral vancomycin (21). Finally, Murphy et al. used serial aqueous taps postoperatively to show that a single intracameral injection of 0.1 mg vancomycin still provided an aqueous level that was four times the minimum inhibitory concentration (MIC) for most gram positive bacteria, 26 h later (32). Table 6.9 shows the preferred antibiotic choices for intracameral injection among ASCRS members surveyed in 2007 (8).

In summary, the majority of peer-reviewed clinical evidence, both retrospective and prospective, seems to support the prophylactic efficacy of an intracameral level of antibiotic, although the ideal agent is not known. While the evidence of efficacy is the strongest for a direct intracameral antibiotic injection (33), there are also retrospective clinical studies supporting the use of subconjunctival antibiotics, which presumably also achieve an intracameral level of a drug. Although there is no direct evidence that topical antibiotics are efficacious, the improved intracameral penetration of newer generation topical fluoroquinolones at least provides some rationale for their popularity and use (7).

6.10.2 Wound Construction

Modern phacoemulsification incisions also play an important role in the prevention of POE. Regardless of the incision type, any postoperative wound leak would increase the risk of endophthalmitis. In fact, Wallin et al. found that a wound leak on postoperative day one was associated with a 44-fold increase in the risk of POE (34). Most of the debate about wound construction has centered on the relative risk of scleral tunnel vs. sutureless clear corneal incisions. In their prospective randomized study of over 12,000 cataract surgeries, Nagaki et al. found an increased risk of POE in patients who had temporal corneal incisions (35). The findings of this study supported the observations found in other retrospective, case–control studies (36, 37). Taban et al. further postulated that the overall increase in the rate of POE observed since 1992 is related to the introduction and the adoption of clear corneal incisions (2).

Several studies have offered a hypothesis to determine the role of clear corneal incisions in increasing the risk of POE. These studies have suggested that postoperative fluctuation in intraocular pressure or external manipulation could lead to wound gaping and inflow of surface fluid into the anterior chamber. In a laboratory model using human globes, four of seven eyes demonstrated ingress of India ink into the eye through 3 mm clear corneal incisions (38). The ingress of blood-tinged tear fluid has also been observed in a clinical study of eight patients, when a cannula was used to apply external pressure to the posterior side of clear corneal incisions (39). Other studies have suggested that postoperative fluctuation in intraocular pressure and hypotony may lead to wound incompetence and ingress of extraocular surface fluid, although stepped incisions may be more resistant to this phenomenon (40–42).

An important consideration, however, is the significant variability in how clear corneal incisions are constructed. These wounds can vary in width, radial length, depth, location, angle, anterior and posterior thicknesses, shape, and entry point. There is also variance in the types of blades used for wound construction. Even if surgeons could consistently produce the same incision architecture every time, other variables, such as wound manipulation during cataract surgery can vary. Most of the large retrospective studies that have implicated clear corneal incisions as a risk factor for endophthalmitis have not characterized or commented on their architecture.

Increased scrutiny of clear corneal incisions has allowed some surgeons to identify the features that may influence the risk of endophthalmitis. Investigators from the Bascom Palmer Eye Institute in Miami observed that 86% of the cases of POE at their institution occurred in right eyes with incisions located inferotemporally (8). One hypothesis might be that wounds in this location are in closer proximity to the inferior lid margin and tear meniscus. Others suggested that the shape of the incision is more important to its self-sealing properties. They suggested that square incisions are superior to rectangular ones, because the former are more stable and therefore resistant to early postoperative hypotony and leakage (43). Tam et al. reported another potential flaw in wound construction and closure. The clear corneal tongue may be associated with postoperative wound leak even when a suture is used to reinforce wound closure (44).

Other studies suggested that there is no increased risk of POE with sutureless clear corneal incisions. In a retrospective study of POE from 2000 to 2004, Miller et al. found a relatively low overall rate of POE and no statistically significant risk from clear corneal incisions (3). In another large retrospective report from the United Kingdom, no significant increase in the rate of POE was identified from 1996 to 2004, a period when there was a transition from scleral tunnel to clear corneal incisions (4). As mentioned previously, Ng et al. found no relationship between wound type and POE (6). The largest study looking at the endophthalmitis risk of clear corneal incisions was conducted as part of the National Cataract Registry in Sweden (25). In that prospective study of 225,471 cataract surgeries, there was a slightly higher rate of POE in eyes with clear corneal incisions (0.053%) compared to scleral incisions (0.036%), but that difference did not reach statistical significance ($p = 0.14$). Notably, 99% of the patients in that study received an intracameral cefuroxime injection, while less than 5% received postoperative topical antibiotics (25).

One rationale cited for using micro-coaxial or microbiaxial phacoemulsification is the possibility that smaller incisions might reduce the risk of POE. As with prophylactic antibiotics, the low incidence of infection makes it very difficult to prove the superiority of one incision size over the other in a prospective study. Furthermore, improperly constructed incisions or those that are stretched by instrumentation can always leak, regardless of their width. Nonetheless, a smaller incision should be more watertight if all other variables are the same. Finally, there is a general agreement that a suture should be placed if the incision is not watertight at the conclusion of surgery (45).

6.10.3 Summary

Because of the low incidence of POE, it is difficult to conduct clinical trials of sufficient size to prove or compare the efficacy of different preventive measures. Overall, evidence-based literature supports the notion that delivering a large intracameral level of antibiotic immediately postoperatively is beneficial in preventing infection. The majority of clinical evidence suggests that this can be achieved very effectively using an intracameral injection of antibiotic at the end of the case. Other methods, such as subconjunctival injection or topical administration, may also be able to achieve a high level of intracameral antibiotic. Although there is less clinical evidence demonstrating efficacy, the experimental rationale, ease of use, commercial availability, and track record of safety likely underpin the widespread use of topical antibiotics in some countries.

Incision integrity is another important factor in the rate of POE. Poor wound construction, regardless of the size, type, and location, undoubtedly increases the risk. Because of their shorter radial length, clear corneal incisions are likely to be less forgiving for faulty wound architecture or distortion by instrumentation. Regardless of its size and location, one must be prepared to suture the incision if it is not sufficiently watertight.

Take Home Pearls

- Retrospective, clinical studies suggest that subconjunctival antibiotics may be protective against endophthalmitis.
- Although the ideal antibiotic choice for endophthalmitis prevention is not known, fluoroquinolones are the commonly used topical agents, while cefuroxime and vancomycin are the most common intracameral choices.
- There is no consensus on the ideal mode of antibiotic administration, but there is significant clinical evidence supporting the direct intracameral injection of antibiotic.

References

1. West ES, Behrens A, McDonnell PJ et al (2005) The incidence of endophthalmitis after cataract surgery among the U.S. medicare population increased between 1994 and 2001. Ophthalmology 112:1388–1394
2. Taban M, Behrens A, Newcomb RL et al (2005) Acute endophthalmitis following cataract surgery: a systematic review of the literature. Arch Ophthalmol 123:613–620
3. Miller JJ, Scott IU, Flynn HW et al (2005) Acute-onset endophthalmitis after cataract surgery (2000–2004): incidence, clinical settings, and visual acuity outcomes after treatment. Am J Ophthalmol 139:983–987
4. Mollan SP, Gao A, Lockwood A et al (2007) Postcataract endophthalmitis: incidence and microbial isolates in a

United Kingdom region from 1996 through 2004. J Cataract Refract Surg 33:265–268
5. McCulley JP (2005) Low acute endophthalmitis rate: possible explanations. J Cataract Refract Surg 31:1074–1075
6. Ng JQ, Morlet N, Bulsara MK, Semmens JB (2007) Reducing the risk for endophthalmitis after cataract surgery: population-based nested case-control study. J Cataract Refract Surg 33:269–280
7. Schein OD (2007) Prevention of endophthalmitis after cataract surgery: making the most of the evidence. Ophthalmology 114:831–832
8. Chang DF, Braga-Mele R, Mamalis N et al (2007) ASCRS Cataract Clinical Committee. Prophylaxis of postoperative endophthalmitis after cataract surgery: results of the 2007 ASCRS member survey. J Cataract Refract Surg 33:1801–1805
9. Gordon-Bennett P, Karas A, Flanagan D et al (2008) A survey of measures used for the prevention of postoperative endophthalmitits after cataract surgery in the United Kingdom. Eye 22:620–627
10. Solomon R, Donnenfeld ED, Perry HD et al (2005) Penetration of topically applied gatifloxacin 0.3%, moxifloxacin 0.5%, and ciprofloxacin 0.3% into the aqueous humor. Ophthalmology 112:466–469
11. Levine JM, Noecker RJ, Lane LC et al (2004) Comparative penetration of moxifloxacin and gatifloxacin in rabbit aqueous humor after topical dosing. J Cataract Refract Surg 30:2177–2182
12. McCulley JP, Caudle D, Aronowicz JD, Shine WE (2006) Fourth-generation fluoroquinolone penetration into the aqueous humor in humans. Ophthalmology 113:955–959
13. Kim DH, Stark WJ, O'Brien TP, Dick JD (2005) Aqueous penetration and biological activity of moxifloxacin 0.5% ophthalmic solution and gatifloxacin 0.3% solution in cataract surgery patients. Ophthalmology 112:1992–1996
14. Price FW Jr, Dobbins K, Zeh W (2002) Penetration of topically administered ofloxacin and trimethoprim into aqueous humor. J Ocular Pharmacol Ther 18:445–453
15. Kowalski RP, Romanowski EG, Mah FS et al (2004) Topical prophylaxis with moxifloxacin prevents endophthalmitis in a rabbit model. Am J Ophthalmol 138:33–37
16. Moshirfar M, Feiz V, Vitale AT et al (2007) Endophthalmitis after uncomplicated cataract surgery with the use of fourth-generation fluoroquinolones: a retrospective observational case series Ophthalmology 114:686–691
17. Leaming DV (1997) Practice styles and preferences of ASCRS members - 1996 survey. J Cataract Refract Surg 23:527–535
18. Colleaux KM, Hamilton WK (2000) Effect of prophylactic antibiotics and incision type on the incidence of endophthalmitis after cataract surgery. Can J Ophthalmol 35:373–378
19. Kamalarajahl S, Ling R, Silvestri G et al (2007) Presumed infectious endophthalmitis following cataract surgery in the UK: a case–control study of risk factors. Eye 21:580–586
20. Peyman GA, Sathar ML, May DR (1977) Intraocular gentamicin as intraoperative prophylaxis in South India eye camps. Br J Ophthalmol 67:260–262
21. Gimbel GV, Sun R, DeBrof BM (1994) Prophylactic intracameral antibiotics during cataract surgery: the incidence of endophthalmitis and corneal endothelial cell loss. Eur J Implant Ref Surg 6:280–285
22. Montan PG, Wejde G, Koranyi G, Rylander M (2002) Prophylactic intracameral cefuroxime. Efficacy in preventing endophthalmitis after cataract surgery. J Cataract Refract Surg 28:977–981
23. Garat M, Moser CL, Alonso-Tarrés C et al (2005) Intracameral cefazolin to prevent endophthalmitis in cataract surgery: 3-year retrospective study. J Cataract Refract Surg 31(11):2230–2234
24. Romero P, Méndez I, Salvat M et al (2006) Intracameral cefazolin as prophylaxis against endophthalmitis in cataract surgery. J Cataract Refract Surg 32:438–441
25. Lundström M, Wejde G, Stenevi U et al (2007) Endophthalmitis after cataract surgery: a nationwide prospective study evaluating incidence in relation to incision type and location. Ophthalmology 114:866–870
26. Endophthalmitis Study Group (2007) European Society of Cataract & Refractive Surgeons. Prophylaxis of postoperative endophthalmitis following cataract surgery: results of the ESCRS multicenter study and identification of risk factors. J Cataract Refract Surg 33:978–988
27. Lalwani GA, Flynn HW, Scott IU et al (2008) Acute-onset endophthalmitis after clear corneal cataract surgery (1996–2005): clinical features, causative organisms, and visual acuity outcomes. Ophthalmology 115:473–476
28. Espiritu CRG, Caparas VL, Bolinao JG (2007) Safety of prophylactic intracameral moxifloxacin 0.5% ophthalmic solution in cataract surgery patients. J Cataract Refract Surg 33:63–68
29. O'Brien TP, Arshinoff SA, Mah FS (2007) Perspectives on antibiotics for postoperative endophthalmitis prophylaxis: potential role of moxifloxacin. J Cataract Refract Surg 33:1790–1800
30. Donnenfeld ED (2007) Based upon the ESCRS randomized study, should I use intracameral antibiotics? Curbside Consultation in Cataract Surgery. Chang DF (ed) Slack Inc
31. Montan PG, Wejde G, Setterqust H et al. (2002) Prophylactic intracameral cefuroxime: evaluation of safety and kinetics in cataract surgery. J Cataract Refract Surg 28:982–987
32. Murphy CC, Nicholson S, Quah SA et al (2007) Pharmacokinetics of vancomycin following intracameral bolus injection in patients undergoing phacoemulsification cataract surgery. Br J Ophthalmol 91:1350–1353
33. Yu-Wai-Man P, Morgan SJ, Hildreth AJ et al (2008) Efficacy of intracameral and subconjunctival cefuroxime in preventing endophthalmitis after cataract surgery. J Cataract Refract Surg 34:447–451
34. Wallin T, Parker J, Jin Y et al. (2005) Cohort study of 27 cases of endophthalmitis at a single institution. J Cataract Refract Surg 31:735–741
35. Nagaki Y, Hayasaka S, Kadoi C et al (2003) Bacterial endophthalmitis after small-incision cataract surgery. Effect of incision placement and intraocular lens type. J Cataract Refract Surg 29:20–22
36. Cooper BA, Holekamp NM, Bohigian G, Thompson PA (2003) Case-control study of endophthalmitis after cataract surgery comparing scleral tunnel and clear corneal wounds. Am J Ophthalmol 136:300–305
37. Lertsumitkul S, Myers PC, O'Rourke MT, Chandra J (2001) Endophthalmitis in the western Sydney region: a case-control study. Clin Exp Ophthalmol 29:400–405

38. Sarayba MA, Taban M, Ignacio TS et al (2004) Inflow of ocular surface fluid through clear corneal cataract incisions: a laboratory model. Am J Ophthalmol 138:206–210
39. Herretes S, Stark WJ, Pirouzmanesh A et al (2005) Inflow of ocular surface fluid into the anterior chamber after phacoemulsification through sutureless corneal cataract wounds. Am J Ophthalmol 140:737–740
40. McDonnell PJ, Taban M, Sarayba M et al (2003) Dynamic morphology of clear corneal cataract incisions. Ophthalmology 110:2342–2348
41. Shingleton BJ, MD, Rosenberg RB, Teixeira R, O'Donoghue MW (2007) Evaluation of intraocular pressure in the immediate postoperative period after phacoemulsification. J Cataract Refract Surg 33:1953–1957
42. May W, Castro-Combs J, Camacho W et al (2008) Analysis of clear corneal incision integrity in an ex vivo model. J Cataract Refract Surg 34:1013–1018
43. Masket S, Belani S (2007) Proper wound construction to prevent short-term ocular hypotony after clear corneal incision cataract surgery. J Cataract Refract Surg 33:383–386
44. Tam DY, Vagefi MR, Naseri A (2007) The clear corneal tongue: a mechanism for wound incompetence after phacoemulsification. Am J Ophthalmol 143:526–528
45. Nichamin LD, Chang DF, Johnson SH et al (2006) American Society of Cataract and Refractive Surgery Cataract Clinical Committee. ASCRS White Paper: what is the association between clear corneal cataract incisions and postoperative endophthalmitis? J Cataract Refract Surg 32:1556–1559

Biaxial Microincision Phacoemulsification for Difficult and Challenging Cases[1]

7

I. Howard Fine, Jorge L. Alió, Richard S. Hoffman, and Mark Packer

Core Message

- The advantages of biaxial microincision phacoemulsification have been elaborated in a variety of papers in the literature [2–10]. This technique is believed to have distinct fluidic advantages.
- The separation of inflow from aspiration and phaco allows the fluid to come in through one side of the eye and exit through the opposite side.
- Competing currents are absent at the phaco tip.
- It is easier to achieve a nearly closed system.
- Cases that are extremely challenging or even impossible with coaxial phaco are easily accomplished by biaxial microincision phaco.

7.1 High Myopia

In highly myopic eyes, a situation in which the anterior chamber is maintained in a completely stable configuration without trampolining the vitreous face can be achieved by keeping the irrigating handpiece in the eye throughout the case. Chopping takes place in the usual manner. With the completion of chopping and mobilization of the segments and the epinucleus,the irrigating chopper should be kept in the eye and the phaco needle should be removed. Then after removing the residual cortex, the viscoelastic Viscoat® (Alcon Laboratories, Fort Worth, Texas) should be infused for the implantation of the intraocular lens (IOL), without shallowing the anterior chamber. It is believed that eventually there may be a documented decreased incidence of retinal detachment in high myopia as a result of nontrampolining of the vitreous face during phaco, and the implantation of IOLs that fill the capsule, such as dual-optic IOLs or IOLs that arch posteriorly, as does the Crystalens.

7.2 Posterior Polar Cataract (Fig. 7.1)

In cases of posterior polar cataracts, 35% have defective posterior capsules [11, 12] and almost all have weakened capsules, and so, it is very important not to overpressurize the eye and perhaps, force nuclear material through the defective posterior capsule. By the same token, it is important not to shallow the chamber and have the nucleus come forward, and possibly open the defect in the posterior capsule. These cases are advantageously done with biaxial microincision phacoemulsification, because of the anterior chamber stability [13].

Hydrodelineation is done,without hydrodissection, and then the endonucleus is carefully chopped into

[1]This chapter is an update of the previously published Fine et al. [1]. Reprinted with permission from Jaypee Brothers, New Delhi, India

I. H. Fine
Oregon Health & Science University, Drs. Fine, Hoffman and Packer, 1550 Oak Street, Suite 5, Eugene, OR 97401, USA
e-mail: hfine@finemd.com

J. L. Alió, I. H. Fine (eds.), *Minimizing Incisions and Maximizing Outcomes in Cataract Surgery*,
DOI: 10.1007/978-3-642-02862-5_7, © Springer-Verlag Berlin Heidelberg 2010

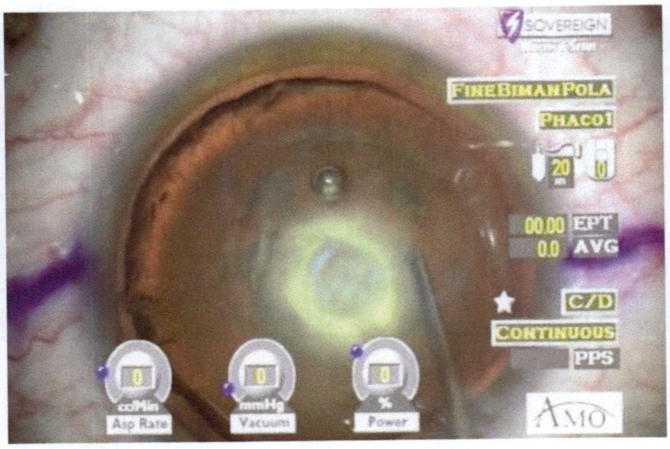

Fig. 7.1 Hydrodelineation of a posterior polar cataract

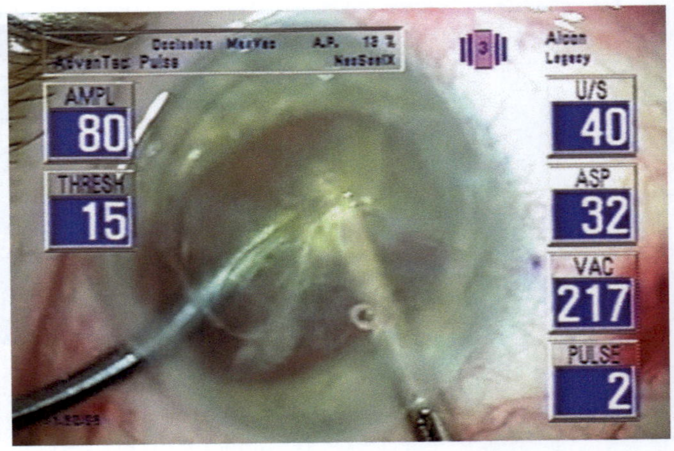

Fig. 7.2 Phacoemulsification of a subluxed cataract in the anterior chamber

pie-shaped segments and evacuated from the eye. Once the endonucleus is removed, the epinucleus is viscodissected from its position against the cortex without removing the irrigating chopper. In this way, there is a layer of cortex and Viscoat® under the epinucleus at the time of evacuation, so that, even if the the capsule opens, it is less likely for the lens material to spill into the vitreous. Once the epinucleus is gone, we leave the irrigation system in the eye, remove the phaco needle, and add Viscoat®. We viscodissect the cortex up into the plain of the capsulorhexis, in the same way and remove it while having a thick layer of viscoelastic on top of the fragile posterior capsule. We never polish the posterior segment of the capsule prior to the IOL implantation, but would rely on YAG laser if there were visually significant opacities within the visual axis, post-operatively

7.3 Posterior Subluxed Cataracts (Fig. 7.2)

For posterior subluxed cataracts, which are hinged to a small zone of attached zonules, a pars plana incision is made and the lens is prolapsed in its capsule, up into the anterior chamber, and the Viscoat® is added under the lens. The lens is then phacoed with biaxial micro-incision instrumentation utilizing an irrigating cannula in the left hand and a phaco needle in the right, keeping the irrigation on top of the Viscoat® but below the cataract. Disassembling these cataracts is not attempted, but they are phacoed from the outside, in. In general, with irrigation under the nuclear material, there is a system in which there is fluid circulating in a circuitous pattern on top of the Viscoat® and the chips that are liberated from the mass of the nucleus tend to circulate entirely within the anterior segment and do not get deposited into the vitreous. After the removal of the cataract, a partial anterior vitrectomy is done and a foldable IOL is implanted through a 2.5-mm incision, with the haptics under the iris and the optic on top. This allows the haptics to indent the undersurface of the iris and be easily identifiable. The haptics are then sutured to the iris and the optic is nudged beneath the pupillary margin. There had been a great success with this technique.

7.4 Mature Cataract with Zonular Dialysis (Fig. 7.3)

In cases in which there is a dialysis of the zonular apparatus during phacoemulsification, as in a case of unrecognized pseudoexfoliation in the presence of a dense cataract, the nucleus is held with the phaco tip and the irrigating chopper is removed. The Viscoat® is then placed under the lens, and then is put the irrigating handpiece without a chopper, under the lens and the lens is again phacoed entirely within the plain of the capsulorhexis. Nuclear material can be mobilized from the posterior chamber with an unsleeved phaco tip because there is no irrigation going along with the phaco tip, as in coaxial phaco, which would force the nuclear material into the vitreous cavity. This is not

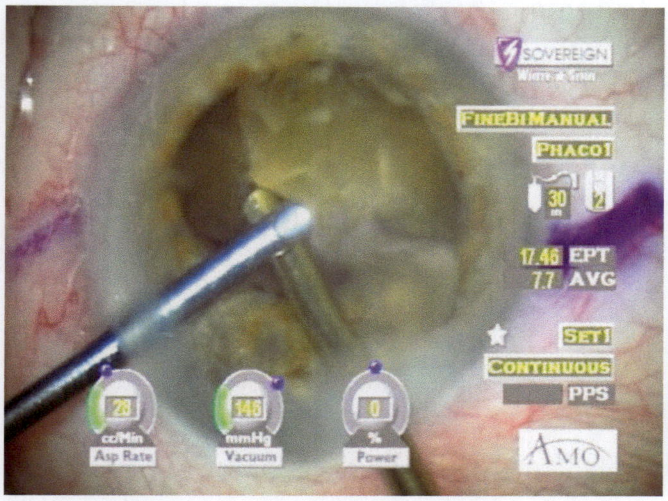

Fig. 7.3 Bringing nuclear material out of the posterior chamber with an unsleeved phaco tip in the presence of zonular dialysis

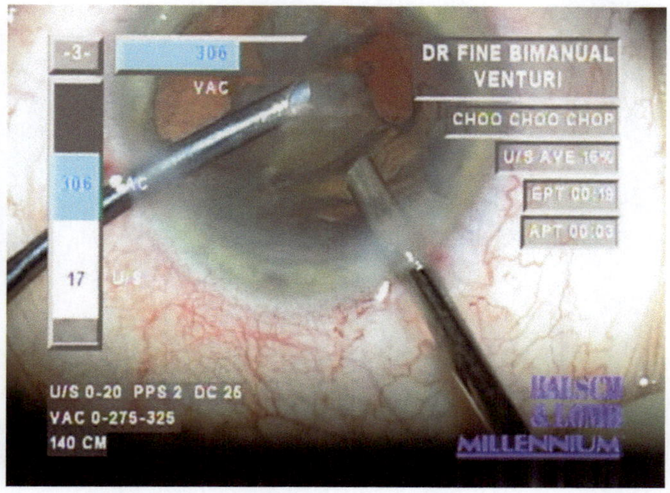

Fig. 7.4 Completing phacoemulsification in the presence of a punctured posterior capsule

possible with a coaxial phaco tip. In these cases, chips that circulate in the fluid above the Viscoat® which is sitting on top of the vitreous are seen, but chips that move posteriorly are not seen. Once this has been completed, a biaxial microincision partial anterior vitrectomy, or a pars plana 25 gauge transcleral microincision vitrectomy is done, and an anterior chamber lens is implanted or a posterior chamber lens is implanted, and sutured to the iris.

7.5 Punctured Posterior Capsule (Fig. 7.4)

In the case where the capsule is punctured during the course of phacoemulsification, irrigation can be continued high in the anterior chamber and the endolenticular space can be reentered with the unsleeved phaco tip, and the phacoemulsification is completed without further enlarging the puncture in the posterior capsule. The cortex is removed without removing the irrigator, and more Viscoat® is instilled. The lens is then implanted into the capsular bag or into the ciliary sulcus. Residual Viscoat® is removed with a vitrector to avoid the possibility of bringing vitreous to the wound. This procedure would be impossible with a coaxial phaco tip because a continuously changing fluid wave from the phaco sleeve would enlarge, or extend, the capsular tear out to the periphery of the capsule, with the loss of lens material into the vitreous.

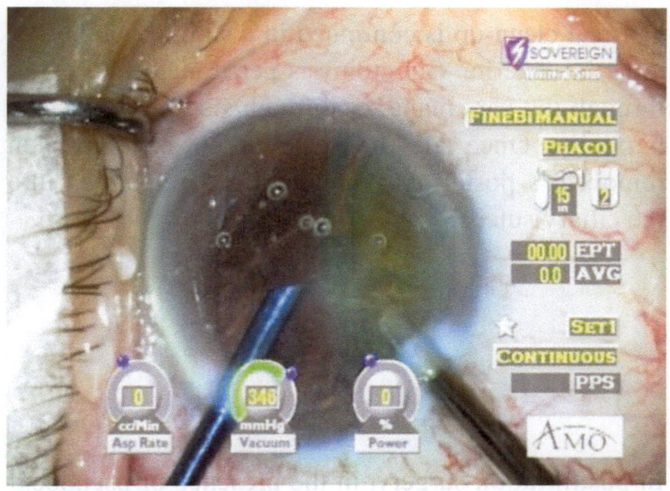

Fig. 7.5 Holding the Nucleus with an unsleeved phaco tip prior to removing the chopper and adding Viscoat® under the nucleus in the presence of a large posterior capsule rupture

7.6 Posterior Capsule Rupture (Figs. 7.5 and 7.6)

In an extensive posterior capsule rupture, the entire endonucleus is brought up into the anterior chamber by holding it with the phaco tip. Very little fluid leaks out of the incision while removing the irrigating chopper. Viscoat® is placed under the nucleus, and the irrigator is placed under the lens. Phacoemulsification is continued in the plain of the capsulorhexis or in the anterior chamber, with the irrigator beneath the nucleus and it is carouselled, or phacoed, from outside in.

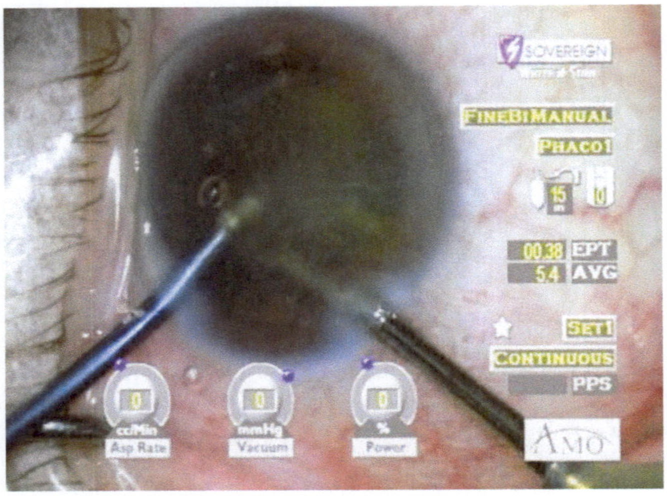

Fig. 7.6 Irrigating below the cataract in the presence of a capsule rupture

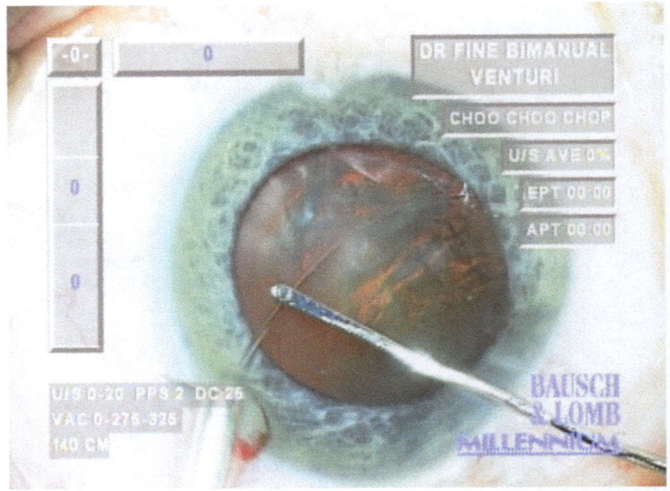

Fig. 7.7 Injection of a capsule tension ring through a microincision controlled by a Lester hook in the right hand

Cortical clean-up is continued in a similar manner, or a partial anterior vitrectomy is performed first, either through the pars plana, or through side-port incisions biaxially. Once all the residual cortex has been removed, a posterior chamber lens is implanted into the ciliary sulcus.

7.7 Pseudoexfoliation (Fig. 7.7)

In postfiltration surgery, in the presence of pseudoexfoliation, an endocapsular tension ring that can be introduced through a side-port with an injector is used, following gentle cortical cleaving hydrodissection. The injector doesn't enter the incision and is just held against the incision, and the forces on the capsule, as the endocapsular tension ring is being inserted, are contained by the use of a Lester hook in the opposite hand (Fig. 7.7). Biaxial microincision horizontal chopping of the lens is then performed so as not to add any downward force on the lens which might stress the residual zonules. Cortical clean-up is facilitated in the presence of an endocapsular tension ring, by performing gentle cortical cleaving hydrodissection prior to the implantation of the ring. The lens is then implanted into the capsular bag through an incision between the two side-port incisions, which is a routine method for IOL implantation in the presence of two 1.1 mm phacoemulsification incisions.

7.8 Rock-Hard Nuclei (Fig. 7.8)

Rock-hard nuclei can be phacoemulsified with the same facility and ease with which biaxial microincision phacoemulsification of softer nuclei is carried out, and usually ends up with an average phaco power under 10% and effective phaco time under 10 seconds, in spite of the density of these nuclei. This is an enormous advantage in terms of corneal endothelial protection because of the great stability of the anterior chamber. A 30° phacoemulsification tip is used with the bevel down. This allows the achievement of vacuum once the tip touches the endonucleus. A bevel-up tip must go deeply into the nucleus before occlusion

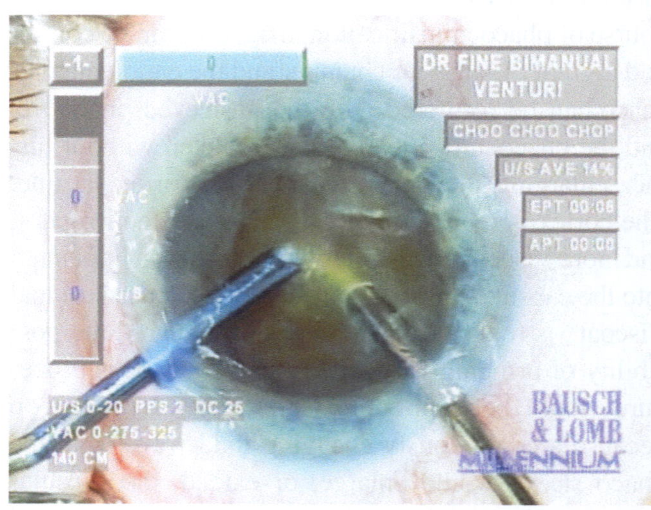

Fig. 7.8 Chopping a rock hard nucleus

and vacuum are achieved. With a bevel-down tip, all of the energy is directed toward the nucleus and none toward the corneal endothelium or trabecular meshwork. Finally, pie-shaped segments can be mobilized from the level of the capsulorhexis, up, rather than having to go deeply into the endolenticular space to achieve occlusion to mobilize these segments, as with that of a bevel-up configuration.

7.9 Switching Hands (Fig. 7.9)

In cases of zonular dialysis, another advantage of biaxial microincision phacoemulsification is that the phaco tip can be used with either hand. After inserting an endocapsular tension ring through one of the microincisions, the lens should be hydroexpressed into the plain of the capsulorhexis and then the phaco tip should be utilized in either the right or left hand, depending on the location of the zonular dialysis. For dialyses that are on the operating surgeon's right side, the phaco tip should be used in the right hand, drawing material in the anterior chamber toward the area of weakened zonules, rather than away from it, which would stress the intact zonules. For dialyses that are on the left-hand side, the phaco tip should be used in the left hand and the irrigating chopper in the right, to remove the nucleus, thereby closing the zonular dialysis with the activation of flow and vacuum toward the left side.

7.10 Microcornea or Microphthalmos (Fig. 7.10)

For very small eyes, the use of biaxial phacoemulsification is an enormous advantage because the smaller size of the instruments avoids creasing of the cornea, which compromises visualization of intraocular structures. A coaxial tip, which is much larger in size, would indent the cornea while being manipulated and partially obscure the visualization of the intraocular structures. This has turned out to be especially advantageous in cases with a microcornea or a microphthalmic eye, in the presence of an unusually large lens.

7.11 Large Iridodialysis and Zonular Defects (Fig. 7.11)

In cases where there are large iris defects and missing zonules, the area is straddled with the microchopper and the phaco tip and the anterior chamber is fractionated with Healon 5 to keep the vitreous back and proceeded in the usual manner. This has been very efficacious and has not resulted in bringing vitreous out of the posterior segment. This is exemplified in the case of a woman who had 100° of ciliary body and iris, except for the pupillary margin, excised in the management of a choroidal/ciliary body malignant melanoma, resulting additionally in fragile and atrophic sclera and conjunctiva at the tumor site.

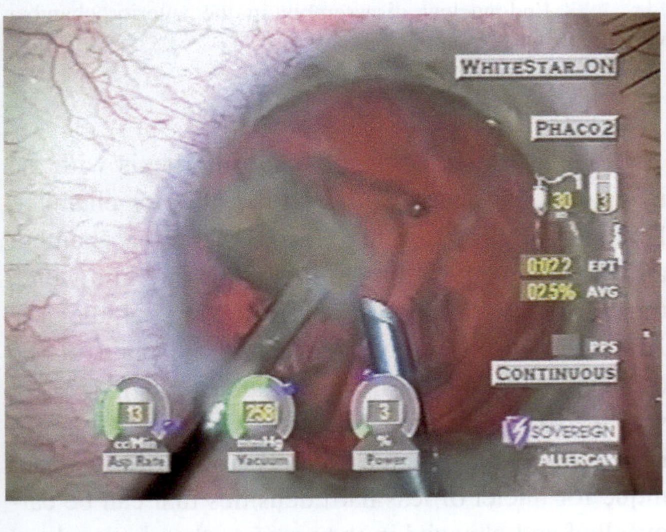

Fig. 7.9 Phacoemulsification tip in the left hand in the presence of zonular dialysis (surgeon's perspective)

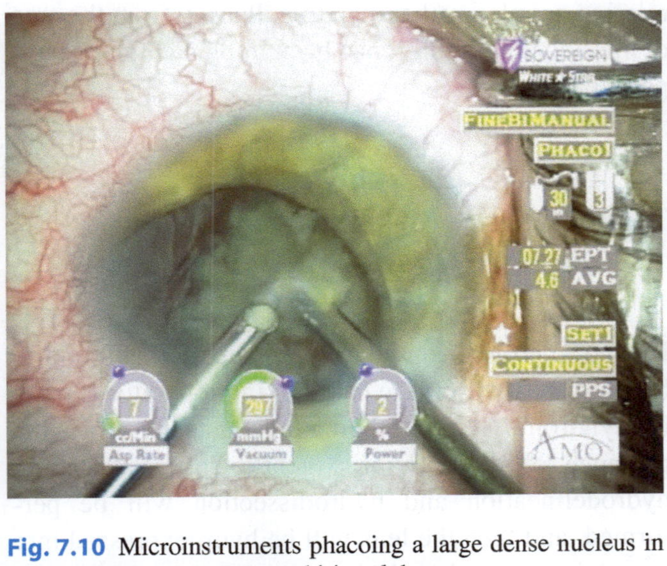

Fig. 7.10 Microinstruments phacoing a large dense nucleus in an eye with micro cornea and iris coloboma

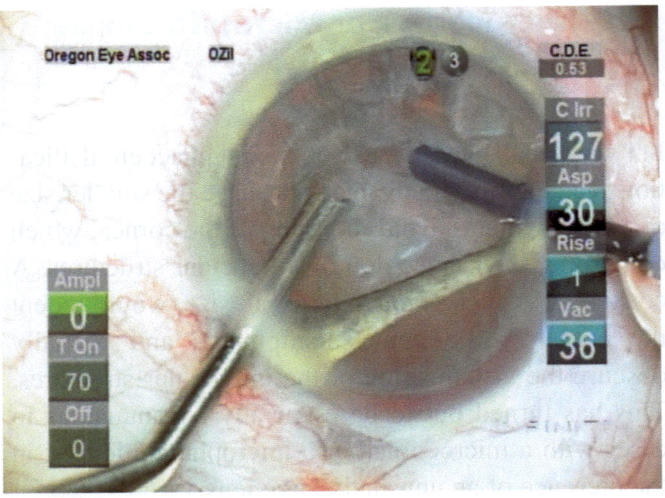

Fig. 7.11 Initial chop of the cataract post 100° ciliary body excision for malignant melanoma

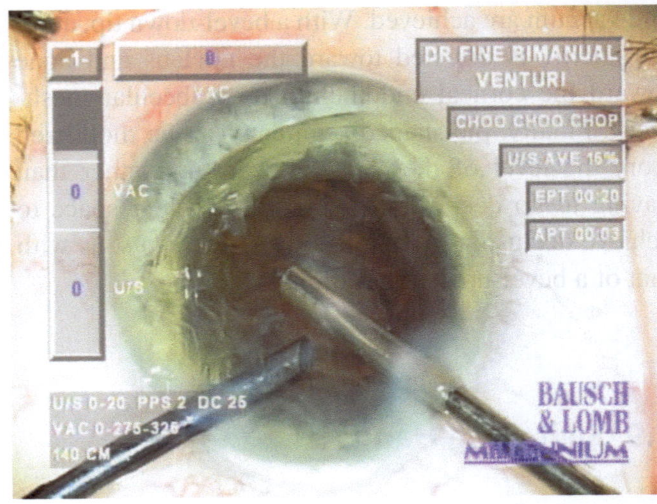

Fig. 7.12 Epinucleus holding the iris back after carouselling the endonucleus in the presence of intraoperative floppy iris syndrome (IFIS)

In this case, it was possible to perform biaxial microincision phacoemulsification through two microincisions on each side of the 100° of atrophic sclera and conjunctiva, and missing ciliary body and iris. The advantage here was that with the vitreous face open to the anterior chamber, the material could be drawn toward the area of missing zonules, after sequestering the vitreous in that area with Healon 5 (Advanced Medical Optics, Santa Ana, California). Phacoemulsification performed through an incision in other locations would bring vitreous to the phaco tip and provide a much more challenging situation. The IOL was implanted nasally over the intact zonules to force the lens to push against the capsular fornix in the area of missing zonules, rather than to pull away from the area of missing zonules, if it had been implanted in the temporal periphery.

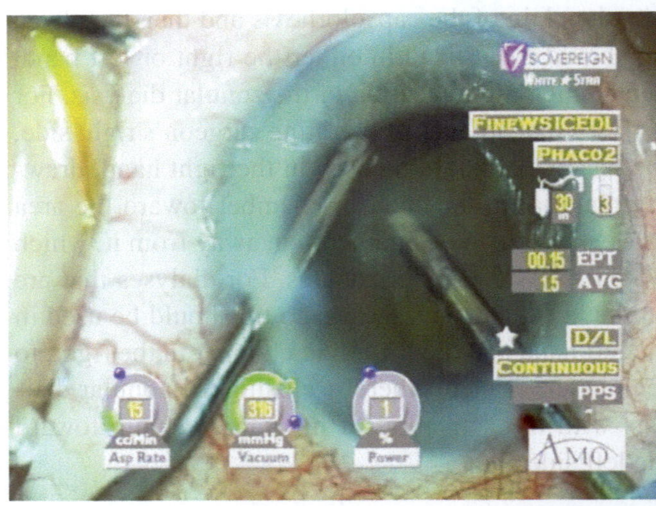

Fig. 7.13 Endonuclear disassembly in the anterior chamber with the irrigator tamponading the iris

7.12 Intraoperative Floppy Iris Syndrome (IFIS) (Figs. 7.12–7.16)

Biaxial microincision phacoemulsification is found to be enormously useful in cases of intraoperative floppy iris syndrome (IFIS). If there is adequate dilation in the presence of a floppy iris, gentle cortical cleaving hydrodelineation and hydrodissection will be performed, and then the lens will be hydroexpressed into the plain of the iris. The endonucleus will then be carouselled in the plain of the capsulorhexis with the irrigating cannula held high in the anterior chamber. Holding the irrigator high in the anterior chamber allows for a tamponading of the iris by the fluid which then disallows floppiness, or billowing, of the iris. After removing the endonucleus in the plain of the capsulorhexis, a fully intact epinuclear shell is seen, which had been sitting on top of the iris, helping to hold it back. This is an extremely advantageous technique for nuclei of less hard densities that can be carouselled and phacoed in the anterior chamber without threatening the corneal endothelium.

For harder cataracts, and in the presence of pupils that will not dilate well, the pupil is dilated with Healon 5, and a rather large capsulorhexis is done followed by an endolenticular chop. The irrigating chopper high is kept in the anterior chamber and with the unsleeved phaco tip, nuclear material is brought up to the chopper held high in the anterior chamber for further disassembly. This allows, once again, a tamponading of the iris and prevention of billowing or floppiness. The phaco needle is kept occluded and in foot position two or three, but with a clearance of occlusion, foot position one is reached in order to minimize evacuation of Healon 5, which is holding the pupil open.

After removing the endonucleus in this way, the epinucleus is removed. Since it is harder to keep the tip occluded with epinuclear trimming and flipping, there tends to be evacuation of Healon 5 and a reduction of the size of the pupil, although because of the irrigator held high in the anterior chamber, it does not billow. Healon 5 is then re-instilled to expand the bag and redilate the pupil prior to cortical clean-up. Then, once again, holding the irrigator high in the anterior chamber, the aspirating microincision handpiece is kept occluded by going circumferentially around the capsulorhexis, with the port facing the capsule fornix, removing the cortical material from only the fornix of the capsule, letting it sit as a cluster in the central portion of the capsule. After all of the cortex has been mobilized from the capsular fornix, the residual cortex is removed from the eye. In this way, Healon 5 is kept in the eye and miosis of the pupil is disallowed until the case is complete.

In some cases, the pupil is intractably small and won't respond to Healon 5 expansion. In these cases, a pupil expander ring (Morcher Pupil Expander Ring, Type 5S, FCI Ophthalmics, Marshfield Hills, MA; or a Malyugin Ring, Catalog #MAL-0001, MicroSurgical Technology, Redmond, WA) is used. These are implanted through a 2.5-mm clear corneal incision to enlarge the pupil (Fig. 7.14), after which biaxial phacoemulsification is performed through the two side-port incisions, and the larger incision remains sealed during the operation because of its self-sealing construction and architecture. The pupil expander rings are advantageous because the pupil can be moved away from the incisions just by pushing on the ring.

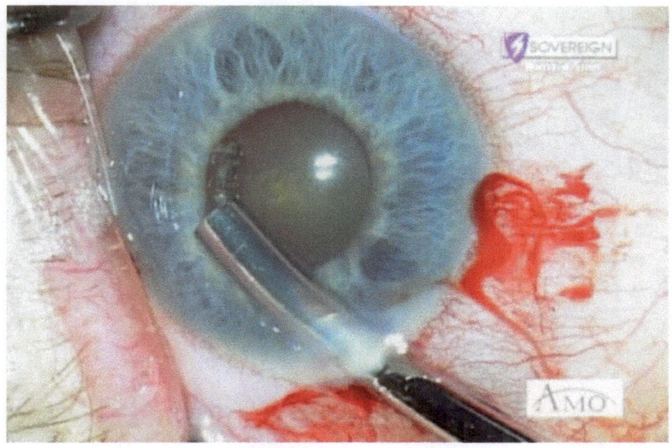

Fig. 7.14 A Morcher Pupil Expander Ring (Type 5S, FCI Ophthalmics, Marshfield Hills, MA) is injected through a 2.5-mm clear corneal incision

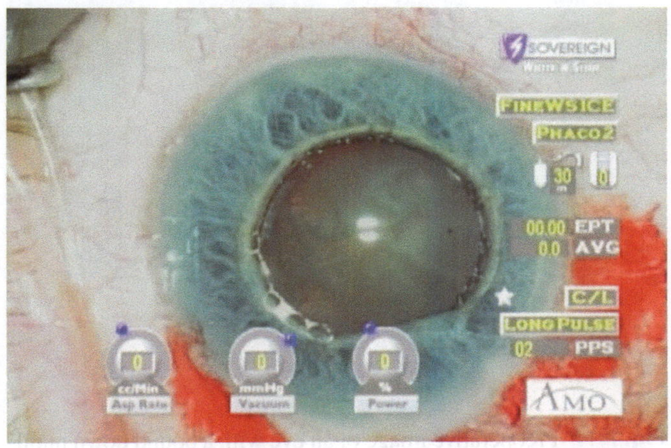

Fig. 7.15 The Morcher Pupil Expander Ring in place

With the ring in place (Fig. 7.15), it was found in some cases that it is not possible to adequately perform hydrodissection or hydrodelineation. When it is not possible to perform the hydrosteps because of the tendency of the pupil to extrude, a bevel-down phaco tip is used to bowl out the center of the cataract, and then an inside-out hydrodelineation is done, as described by Abhay Vasavada [14]. The residual endonucleus is then chopped in the usual fashion, and then the epinucleus is removed.

In some cases, subincisional cortical removal may be performed by using a coaxial irrigation handpiece in the 2.5 mm incision to hold the iris back, while going to a distal location through a microincision with a 0.2-mm port aspirator to remove the subincisional cortex (Fig. 7.16). This has been very efficacious.

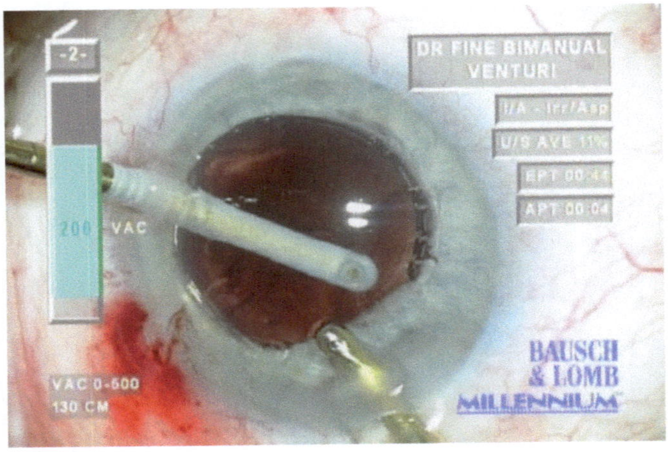

Fig. 7.16 The use of a coaxial irrigation handpiece with a micro aspirator to remove subincisional cortex

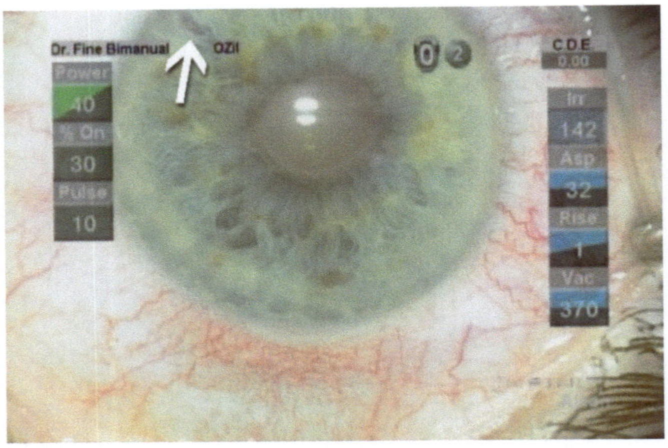

Fig. 7.17 Preoperative image of an eye with a bound down pupillary membrane. *Arrow* indicates small, peripheral iridotomy

7.13 Every Small Pupil Must Be Viewed as a Potential IFIS

Every small pupil must be viewed as a potential floppy iris case because multiple drugs and neutraceuticals that have antialpha-1A properties which create an intraoperative floppy iris syndrome, have been identified . Small pupils are not stretched because if they become IFIS cases, the floppiness would get exacerbated by the disruption of the only portion of the iris (the pupil) which retains structural integrity. The only exceptions to that are the pupils that are bound down by inflammatory pupillary membranes, or that have a long history of exposure to miotic drops, and a clear absence of medications that might produce a floppy iris.

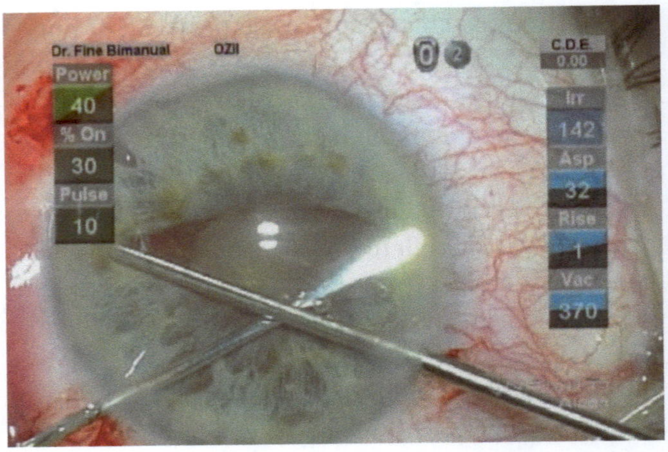

Fig. 7.18 Stretching the pupillary membrane in one direction and the iris just distal to the pupillary membrane in the opposite direction in the same meridian

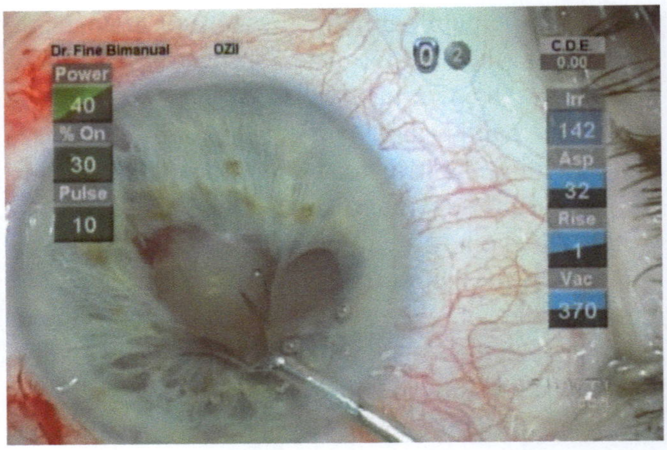

Fig. 7.19 Stripping the pupillary membrane

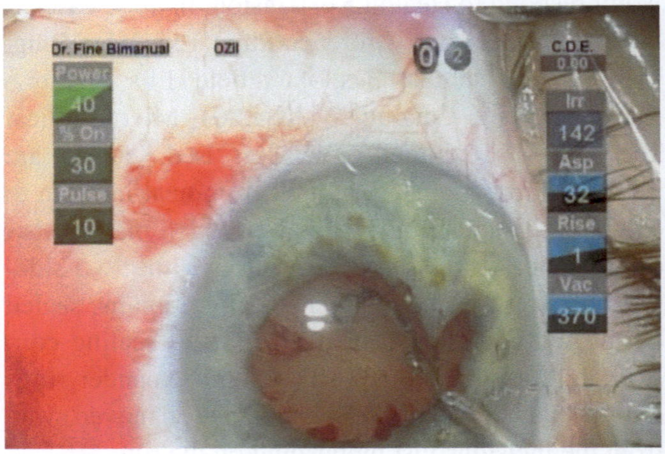

Fig. 7.20 Releasing the last adhesion of the pupillary membrane

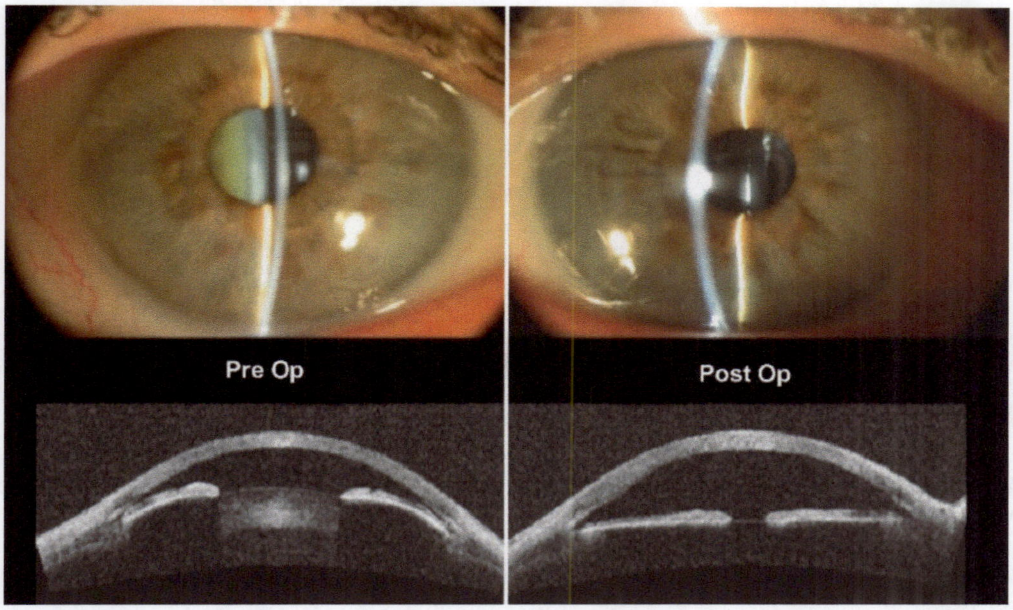

Fig. 7.21 Preoperative slit-lamp and optical coherence tomography (OCT) images of a very shallow anterior chamber. The postoperative images demonstrate the increase in anterior chamber depth due to the 25 gauge transcleral pars plana vitrectomy

7.14 Iris Bombé (Figs. 7.17–7.20)

For pupils that are completely bound down by a pupillary membrane, biaxial phacoemulsification is used. It is commenced with a small iridotomy peripherally, close to one of the microincisions (Fig. 7.17). Viscoat® is used to elevate the iris and its cannula to sweep the pupillary membrane from the anterior lens capsule. The pupillary membrane is then stretched in one direction and the iris is stretched just distal to the pupillary membrane in the opposite direction in the same meridian (Fig. 7.18). This results in a lysing of the pupillary membrane for several clock hours from the pupil itself, and allows the surgeon to go back and, using tangential forces with a microincision capsulorhexis forceps, strip the pupillary membrane from the pupil (Figs. 7.19 and 7.20). Following this, Healon 5 allows for maximum dilation of the pupil and the process is proceeded with in the usual manner.

7.15 Very Shallow Anterior Chambers (Fig. 7.21)

For very shallow anterior chambers biaxial phacoemulsification is also a great advantage because the instruments are indeed smaller and fit more readily in the eye; however, if the anterior chambers are too shallow (Fig. 7.21), a 25-gauge transcleral pars plana vitrectomy is performed, before proceeding with biaxial phacoemulsification. It is very important to use these microvitrectors in order to use a finger of the nondominant hand to maintain tactile contact with the eye, so that the eye is not over-softened. These vitrectors are capable of, between 1,200 and 1,500 cuts/min. In spite of their small gauge, unless care is taken, the eye could be excessively softened, retroplacing the lens and creating new difficulties and challenges.

7.16 Refractive Lens Exchange (Figs. 7.22–7.25)

Refractive lens exchange can be done very easily, and safely, with biaxial microincision phacoemulsification. Cortical cleaving hydrodissection is performed instead of hydrodelineation. The lens is then hydroexpressed into the plain of the capsulorhexis, and carouselled, without any phacoemulsification energy for soft lenses, usually encountered in refractive lens exchange (Figs. 7.22 and 7.23). An entirely fluidic-based extraction is done and then, because of cortical cleaving hydrodissection, the cortex is evacuated by just tilting the phaco tip back into the posterior chamber where it jumps into the phaco tip as a single piece (Figs. 7.24 and 7.25).

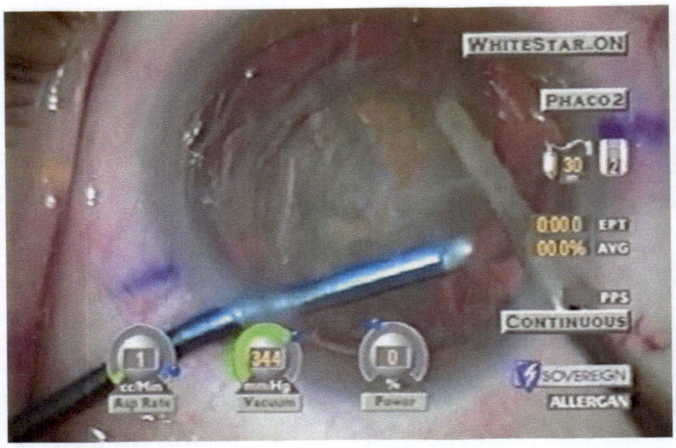

Fig. 7.22 Carouselling the nucleus in refractive lens exchange without using any phacoemulsification energy

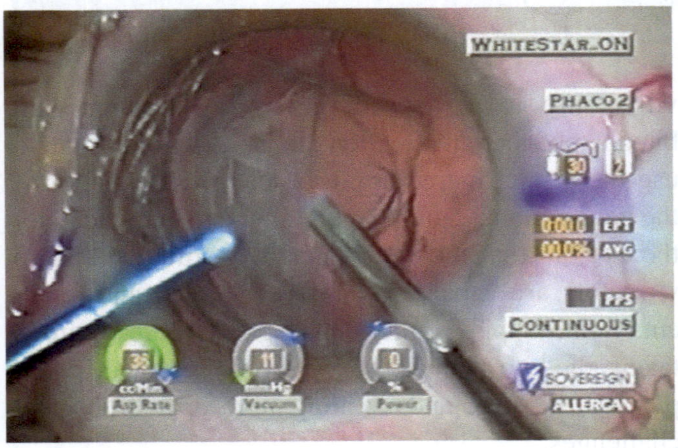

Fig. 7.23 Endonucleus removal complete with only cortex remaining. No phacoemulsification energy was used to remove the endonucleus

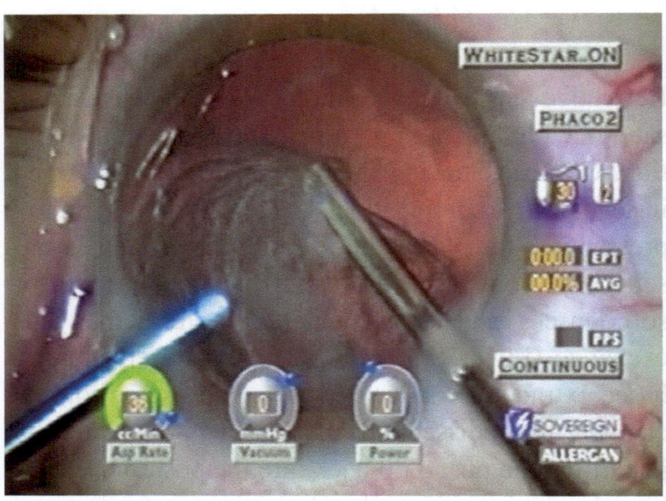

Fig. 7.24 Removing cortex in refractive lens exchange by tilting the phaco tip back into the posterior chamber

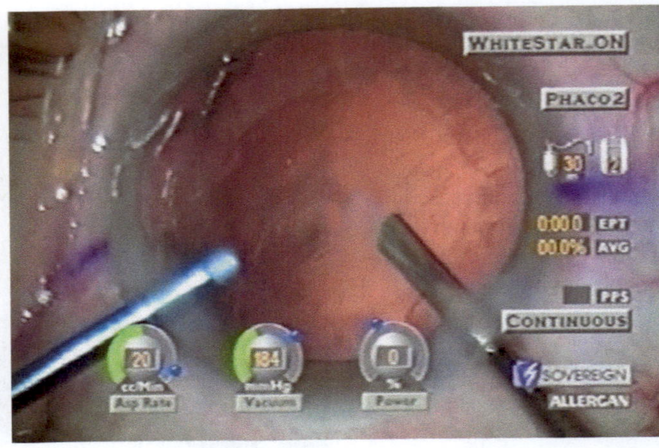

Fig. 7.25 Cortex completely removed

7.17 Refractive Lens Exchange in Post Radial Keratotomy (RK) (Fig. 7.26)

In cases where previous radial keratotomy (RK) has been performed, biaxial microincision clear lens or cataract removal is done by going between two previously placed radials, making it much less likely that the radial incisions are ruptured during the course of the lens extraction. An incision is then made between two microincisions for implantation of the IOL, but in the presence of previous RK, it is made through the posterior limbus for the implantation of the IOL.

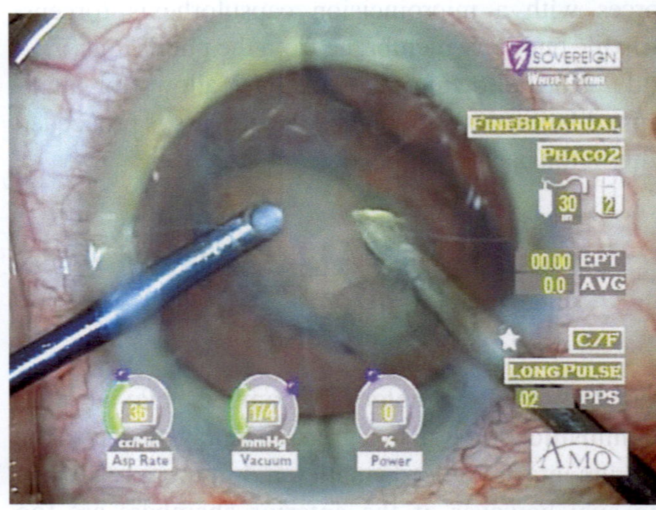

Fig. 7.26 Bimanual microincision phacoemulsification of a cataract between RK incisions

7.18 Intraocular Cautery (Fig. 7.27)

It has been found that biaxial microincision instruments allow intraocular cautery by using an irrigating cannula in one of the microincisions and a microincision bipolar cautery in the other. Pinching of the irrigation tubing leads to bleeding, clearly identifying the point source because the eye softens and the bleeding points start to ooze. They are precisely cauterized with the bipolar cautery, and therefore trauma to intraocular structures is minimized by avoiding more cautery than is necessary [15].

7.19 Biaxial Microincision Instruments (Figs. 7.28 and 7.29)

There are a number of other instruments that have been developed for use through 1.1 mm microincisions. Iris reconstruction is very much easier utilizing intraocular forceps that stabilize the iris for suturing. New intraocular needle holders are also usable through a 1.0-mm incision. In this way, very fragile and atrophic irides can be sutured without putting excessive stress on the iris tissue. The knots are tied with a Seipser external tying mechanism [16] and the knots are cut with an intraocular microincision scissors, that is also admissible through a 1.0-mm incision.

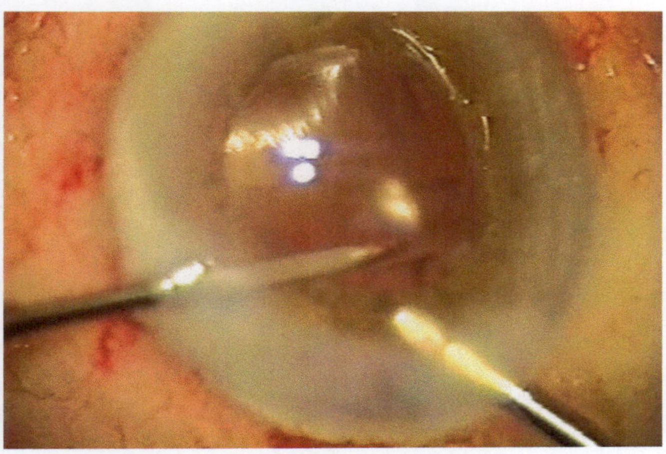

Fig. 7.27 Bipolar intraocular microcauterization with easy identification of the bleeding point by pinching the infusion tubing

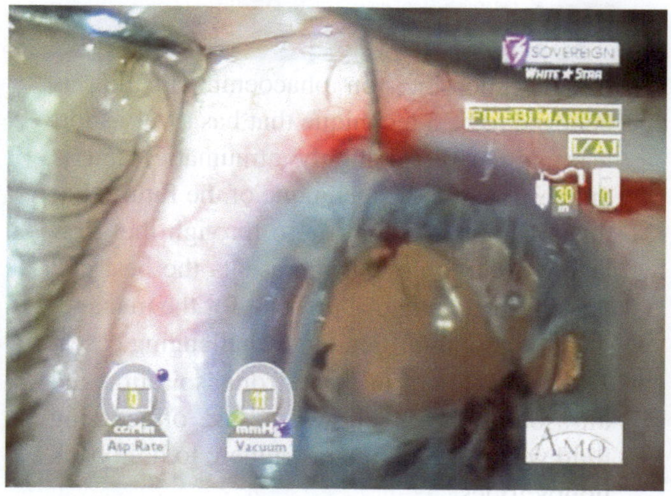

Fig. 7.28 Suturing of atrophic iris using microincision intraocular forceps

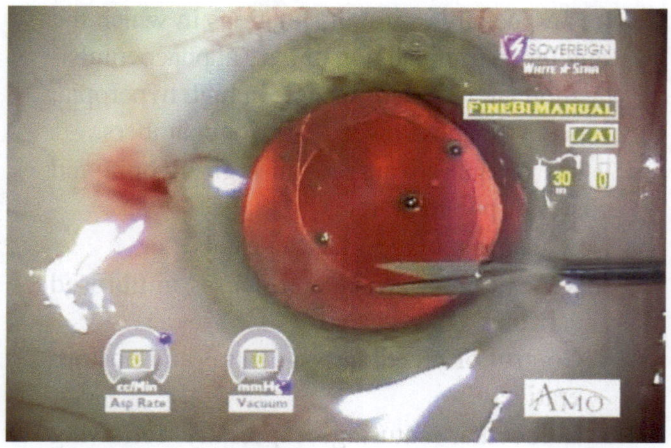

Fig. 7.29 Nicking the capsulorhexis with microincision scissors prior to enlarging the capsulorhexis

For late reopening of capsular bags to recenter IOLs, a capsulorhexis is enlarged in the late postoperative period by nicking the rhexis with a microincision intraocular scissors, and then tearing a larger opening with a microincision capsulorhexis forceps. Viscodissection of the lens [17] within the capsular bag, can be accomplished through microincisions which also allow for repositioning of IOLs without the need to make larger incisions to manipulate them intraocularly. There are currently additional microincision instruments under a state of development, including microincision Collibri forceps, microincision iris graspers, and microincision IOL holders and cutters.

Take Home Pearls

- Biaxial microincision phacoemulsification is believed to be a technique that has a very short learning curve, is highly atraumatic, and is unquestionably the technique of the future. For those who are willing to go through the short learning curve now, it represents the best and the safest technique at present, for the management of certain difficult and challenging cases.
- The separation of infusion from aspiration and ultrasound energy allows the use ofincoming fluid wave as a unique instrument to hold back floppy irides.
- The anterior segment can be sequestered from the posterior segment in cases of ruptured capsules and zonular dialyses.
- It is especially useful in situations in which the smaller instrumentation of biaxial phacoemulsification are required, such as in high hyperopia, small eyes, and crowded anterior chambers.
- It has unique advantages in high myopia and posterior polar cataracts.
- New instrumentation facilitates:
  - Repositioning decentered lenses in fibrosed capsules
  - Control of bleeding pre-, intra- and postoperatively
  - Intraocular suturing, especially following iris trauma

References

1. Fine IH, Hoffman RS, Packer M (2008) Use of bimanual microincision phacoemulsification for difficult and challenging cases. In: Garg A, Fine IH, Alió JL, Chang DF, Weinstock RJ, Mehta KR, Bovet JJ, Tsuneoka H, Malyugin B, Pinelli R, Pajic B, Mehta CK (eds) Mastering the techniques of advanced phaco surgery. Jaypee Brothers, New Delhi, India
2. Girard LJ (1978) Ultrasonic fragmentation for cataract extraction and cataract complications. Adv Ophthalmol 37:127–135
3. Shearing SP, Relyea RL, Loaiza A, Shearing RL (1985) Routine phacoemulsification through a one-millimeter non-sutured incision. Cataract 2:6–10
4. Hara T, Hara T (1989) Endocapsular phacoemulsification and aspiration (ECPEA) – recent surgical technique and clinical results. Ophthalmic Surg 20(7):469–475
5. Tsuneoka H, Shiba T, Takahashi Y (2001) Feasibility of ultrasound cataract surgery with a 1.4 mm incision. J Cataract Refract Surg 27:934–940
6. Agarwal A, Agarwal A, Agarwal S, Narang P, Narang S (2001) Phakonit: phacoemulsification through a 0.9 mm corneal incision. J Cataract Refract Surg 27(10): 1548–1552
7. Tsuneoka H, Shiba T, Takahashi Y (2002) Ultrasonic phacoemulsification using a 1.4 mm incision: clinical results. J Cataract Refract Surg 28:81–86
8. Tsuneoka H, Hayama A, Takahama M (2003) Ultrasmall-incision bimanual phacoemulsification and AcrySof SA30AL implantation through a 2.2 mm incision. J Cataract Refract Surg 29(6):1070–1076
9. Fine IH, Packer M, Hoffman RS (2004) Power modulations in new technology: improved outcomes. J Cataract Refract Surg 30:1014–1019
10. Fine IH, Hoffman RS, Packer M (2004) Optimizing refractive lens exchange with bimanual microincision phacoemulsification. J Cataract Refract Surg 30:550–554
11. Osher RH, Yu BC-Y, Koch, DD (1990) Posterior polar cataracts: a predisposition to intraoperative posterior capsule rupture. J Cataract Refract Surg 16:157–162
12. Vasavada AR, Sing R (1999)Phacoemulsification in posterior polar developmental cataracts. In: Lu LW, Fine IH (eds) Phacoemulsification in difficult and challenging cases. Thieme, New York, NY, pp 121–128
13. Aravind H, Aravind S, Vadi K, Natchair G (2006) Bimanual microphaco for posterior polar cataracts. J Cataract Refract Surg 32(6):914–917
14. Vasavada AR, Raj SM (2004) Inside-out delineation. J Cataract Refract Surg 30(6):1167–1169
15. Fine IH, Hoffman RS, Packer M (2004) Bimanual bipolar diathermy for recurrent hyphema following anterior segment intraocular surgery. J Cataract Refract Surg 30(9): 2017–2020
16. Seipser SB (1994) The closed chamber slipping suture technique for iris repair. Ann Ophththal 26(3):71–72
17. Fine IH, Hoffman RS (1997) Late reopening of fibrosed capsular bags to reposition decentered intraocular lenses. J Cataract Refract Surg 23:990–994

7.1 MICS in Special Cases: Incomplete Capsulorhexis

Arturo Pérez-Arteaga

Core Messages

- While performing Cataract Surgery with MICS, the surgeon has a better potential to solve problems related to an incomplete capsulorhexis.
- Capsulectomy with micro-scissors in the dominant hand, while holding the eye with the non-dominant hand is an important maneuver to direct the course of a failed capsulorhexis and is also very helpfulin cases of zonular weakening.
- If the surgeon is unsure of the completion of capsulorhexis, special care should be taken and the case should be proceeded with assuming that it is incomplete, to avoid further complications.
- The key to the management of an incomplete capsulorhexis case is to work at the iris plane, avoiding applying forces to the capsular bag and the zonular ligament.
- The prechop maneuvers can be easily done with MICS at the iris plane. The "lens salute technique" is a good maneuver for MICS surgeons to use in these particular cases.

7.1.1 Introduction

To deal with an incomplete capsulorhexis is a situation, which directly affects the knowledge and the skills of the ophthalmic surgeon. Every surgeon who has faced this stressful situation knows about the significant complications that can occur, if an appropriate management is not done. In fact, it is a particular situation that predisposes to other complications. It is better termed as a particular event or feature occurring during the start of lens extraction. With proper management, the surgeon may avoid most of the potential complications such as vitreous loss, nuclear, and epinuclear fragments dislocated to the vitreous, complete luxation of the nucleus to the vitreous cavity, and problems in intraocular lens (IOL) placement that can range from decentration to a complete dislocation. This is the interesting feature of this situation. It is almost a complication, but not a complete one. The proper management of this situation will help the surgeon avoid dealing with true complications.

It is also a situation that cannot be defined in one single term. "Incomplete Capsulorhexis" can include a wide variety of situations, ranging from a single accidental tear occurring in the anterior capsule that can be corrected by performing a wider capsulorhexis, to a bigger tear involving the posterior capsule that will change the entire management of the case. This is what is interesting about this situation.

In the past years, the biaxial approach has proved to be more advantageous in managing an anterior capsule tear than the coaxial approach, not only in routine microcapsulorrhexis, but also in the management of surgical complications that can occur during this step (Fig. 7.30). This chapter will first discuss the correct way to perform biaxial microcapsulorrhexis in order to decrease the rate of complications. Then, the different types of "incomplete capsulorrhexis" that can occur and their management using the biaxial approach will be described. Finally, some variations in the technique of phacoemulsification that should be done in these particular cases will be discussed, emphasizing the advantages of biaxial phaco over coaxial phaco, and therefore, encouraging more surgeons worldwide to adopt this technique for their patients' benefit.

Many techniques described here regarding coaxial and biaxial cataract surgery and their differences, have been part of several publications. Some are part of instructional courses of MICS presented at international meetings (AAO, ASCRS, ESCRS). Finally some of the techniques

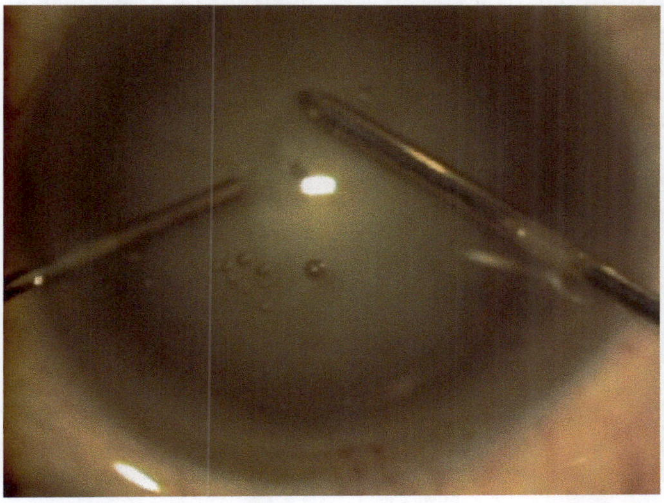

Fig. 7.30 Performing Microcapsulorhexis in Biaxial Approach

belong to the authors' personal experience in the operating room. Science is always changing. With the passing of time, improvements in the technique will come. At this moment, this is the best, we ophthalmologists have.

7.1.2 Avoiding Complications While Constructing Your Microcapsulorhexis

The biaxial surgeon has many advantages in comparison with the coaxial surgeon in constructing a capsulorrhexis:

1. The incisions are smaller and so, both the anterior chamber depth and positive intraocular pressure are maintained, because of minimal leakage at the incision sites (Fig. 7.30).
2. The microcapsulorrhexis forceps does not have the "opening mechanism" at the incision site unlike conventional capsulorrhexis forceps, decreasing in this manner, the trauma to the corneal tissue and possible leakage (Fig. 7.31).
3. The nondominant hand is holding the eye through the side incision. It helps in decreasing the movement of the eye while performing the capsulorrhexis. It also helps to reposition the eye for better visualization of the capsule, capsular reflex and the red reflex during this step (Fig. 7.30).
4. It may be helpful if the instrument held in the nondominant hand is a viscoelastic cannula, so that the surgeon can inject the viscoelastic, if needed, maintaining a positive IOP during the entire step, and thereby eliminating the need for changing instruments (Fig. 7.30).
5. The surgeon can have two (and sometimes three) angles to approach the capsulorrhexis,so that he can switch to either incision site to insert the forceps depending on the particular case or situation.

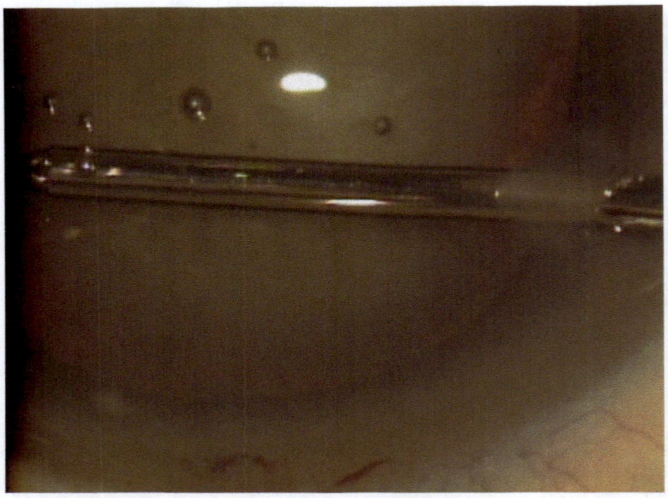

Fig. 7.31 Microcapsulorhexis forceps. Notice the stability of the chamber and the incision

These advantages of the biaxial technique during capsulorrhexis will be of particular benefit in avoiding complications, and this is more important in the management of an incomplete capsulorhexis. So the biaxial surgeon must try to perform each and every capsulorrhexis under these conditions.

A step-by-step guide on how to avoid an incomplete capsulorrhexis during cataract surgery will be described in the succeeding paragraphs. Other possible surgical maneuvers and/or devices such as capsular rings and capsular staining will not be discussed, because the focus of the authors is the biaxial approach of managing a complicated capsulorrhexis:

(a) *Initial Capsule Puncture*: Before performing the first puncture in the anterior capsule (with coaxial forceps or with cystotome), the anterior chamber should be completely filled with the viscoelastic. Otherwise, if low IOP is present during this first step, the rhexis can run easily to the periphery. Complete visualization of what is being done is essential. The nondominant hand can aid the surgeon to fixate the eye in the position where he can have the best view of his surgical field. During the puncture, the elasticity of the capsule can be felt. If it is too fibrotic, the surgical plan can be changed. The same is true if there is movement of the entire crystalline lens. Weak zonules (e.g., pseudoexfoliation syndrome, high myopia) should be noted at this time. The initial puncture is the perfect time to obtain invaluable information regarding the capsule, the zonules and the density of the cataract (Fig. 7.32).

(b) *Cutting instead of pulling the capsule for cases with weak zonules*: If a fibrotic capsule is present or if there is excessivemovement in the lens, avoid, pulling the anterior capsule, as much as possible. "To cut the capsule" (micro-capsulectomy) is the recommended technique, which avoids the transmission of forces to the capsular bag and to the zonules. The biaxial approach can be performed by taking advantage of the bimanual stabilization of

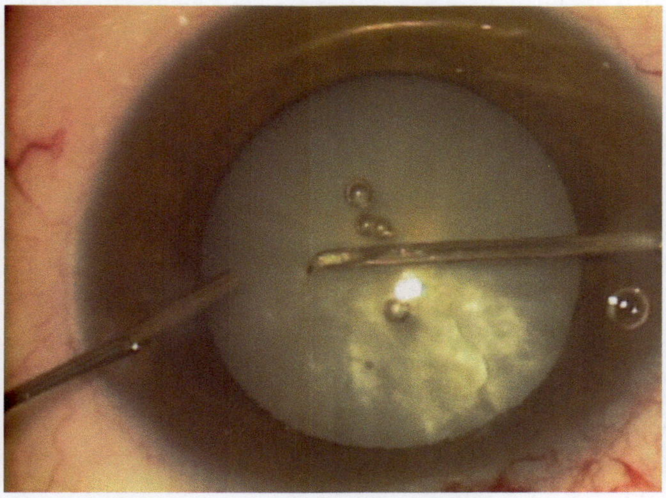

Fig. 7.32 Initial capsular punctura with cystotome in a biaxial approach

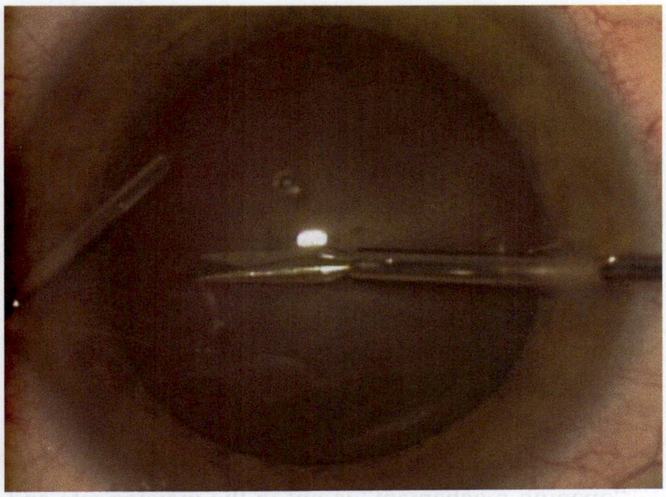

Fig. 7.33 Biaxial Micro-capsulectomy. Notice he micro-scissors in biaxial approach

the eye (Fig. 7.33.). The viscoelastic cannula is held with the nondominant hand and maintained inside the wound to fixate the eye. Then a micro-scissors on the dominant hand is inserted through the main incision. The capsule is cut with the micro-scissors as far as it can be reached to advance the CCC. Once this has been done, it is possible to change to the micro-capsulorrhexis forceps to complete the CCC as planned. With this maneuver, the initial capsular pull is avoided and less transmission of forces against the capsule occurs. Although capsular tension rings are always useful for these situations, rin this chapter, the advantage of the biaxial capsular maneuver in order to decrease complications is emphasized.

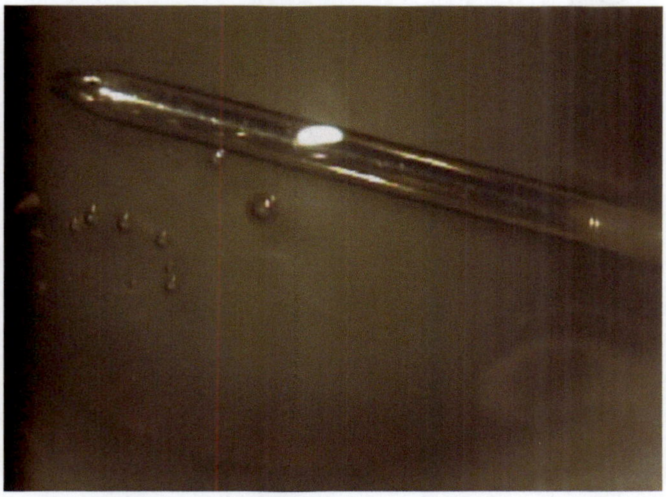

Fig. 7.34 Pulling the capsule for CCC creation

(c) *Pulling towards the meridian of the forceps insertion* (Fig. 7.34): By pulling, instead of pushing towards the meridian of the forceps insertion during the initial creation of the capsulorrhexis, the surgeon can control the eye with the nondominant hand, counteracting the movement of the eye to the opposite meridian. Also, one can decrease with this maneuver, the transmission of forces to the capsular bag and zonules. Initiating the capsulorrhexis too peripheral should be avoided. In fact, after the completion of capsulorrhexis 360° and after passing through the starting point, if the size of the rhexis is not adequate enough, the rhexis can be enlarged by extending more peripherally. If it is started para-centrally, there will be more space to enlarge the rhexis, and enough time to stop, in case a peripheral tear starts. In these cases, stop for a whilefill the anterior chamber again with the viscoelastic, and then proceed to continue with the CCC once or twice. If the peripheral tear can be controlled by pulling the anterior capsule toward the same meridian,

(d) *Pulling to the opposite side* (Fig. 7.35): What is to be avoided, when a capsular tear has started, is further complications of letting it run to the periphery. So, if by trying to pull the same capsule flap, an even larger tear is created, the surgeon should leave this first capsular flap and start a second one. The surgeon should grasp the anterior capsule at the site of first puncture and perform the capsulorrhexis going to the opposite direction. Since every precaution was made not to start the initial flap at the periphery, this second capsulorrhexis can be moved far away from the initial flap. The eye should be stabilized

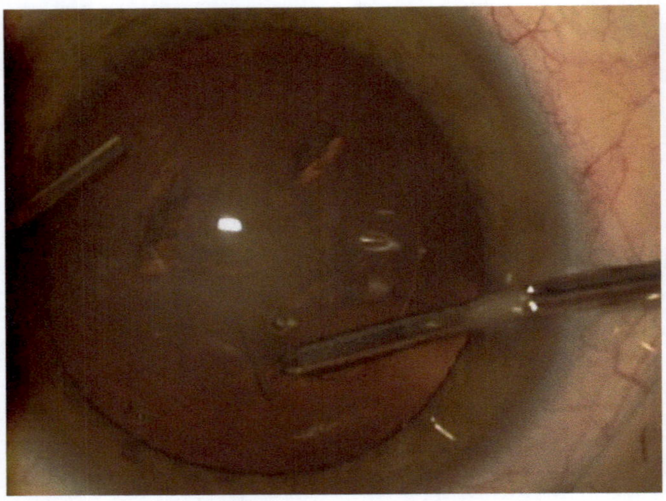

Fig. 7.35 Performing CCC in the opposite direction that it starts; the initial point will be covered by the CCC

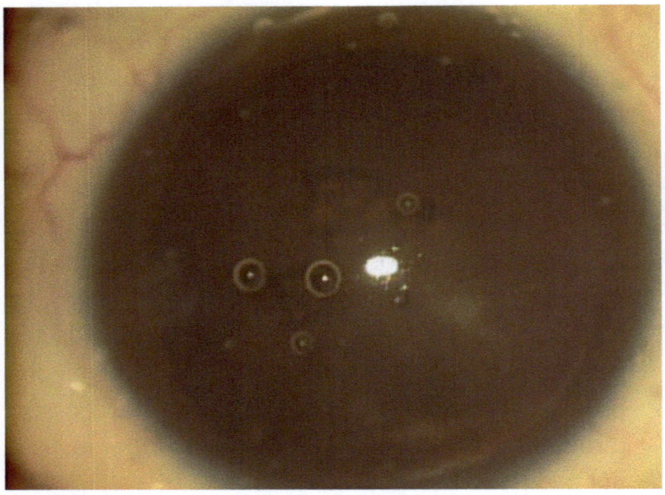

Fig. 7.36 Two differents points of start CCC were done in the anterior capsule

with the viscoelastic cannula through the incision site on the nondominant hand. If needed, the surgeon should fill the anterior chamber with viscoelastic at all times. This biaxial approach makes it possible to perform this maneuver with ease.

(e) *Performing a new puncture* (Fig. 7.36): Sometimes it is difficult to create a new tear in the same site. Pulling the flap several times as one tries to salvage the capsulorrhexis may not be possible and so it is better not to attempt any furtheras there is a high risk of a peripheral tear while trying to pull to the opposite meridian. In such cases, stay calm, fill the anterior chamber with the viscoelastic, and forget about the first capsular puncture, and create a new puncture in another meridian of the anterior capsule. This new site should be easily accessible and be visualized very well. The nondominant hand should always be used to stabilize the eye and provide better visualization.

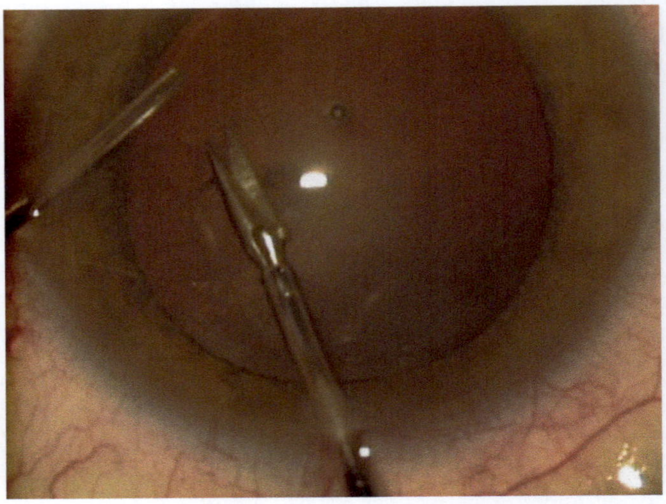

Fig. 7.37 Micro-scissors entering at a new angle to create a new capsular flap

(f) *Microcapsulectomy to redirect capsulorhexis* (Fig. 7.37): Since the surgeon is working with both hands in the biaxial approach, he may use micro-scissors whenever required. . Sometimes, if there is a failure in creating a good capsular flap, it is best to direct the new flap in another area of the anterior capsule with capsular scissors. This maneuver is possible only in a biaxial approach, because the micro-scissors can go inside the eye through a 0.7-mm incision. The "opening mechanism" is not in the incision site and the maintenance of a well formed AC is guaranteed, because the surgeon can perform the maneuvers without any leakage. Hence, the surgeon should perform an initial flap with scissors, and then move to the micro-forceps to continue the creation of CCC.

(g) *Multiple capsulectomies* (Fig. 7.38): If there is still some difficulty in controlling the anterior capsule and the possibility of a peripheral tear exists, the surgeon can use the micro-scissors to cut the capsule in a continuous curvilinear manner. The surgeon can perform one or two clear corneal incisions in other meridians for this purpose, to help redirect the capsule while he is advancing the CCC. For this maneuver, it is very useful to always keep the eye stable with the use of the cannula in his nondominant hand. It is sometimes difficult to perform, particularly for the beginning biaxial surgeon, but it is the safest way to control the size and direction of the CCC.

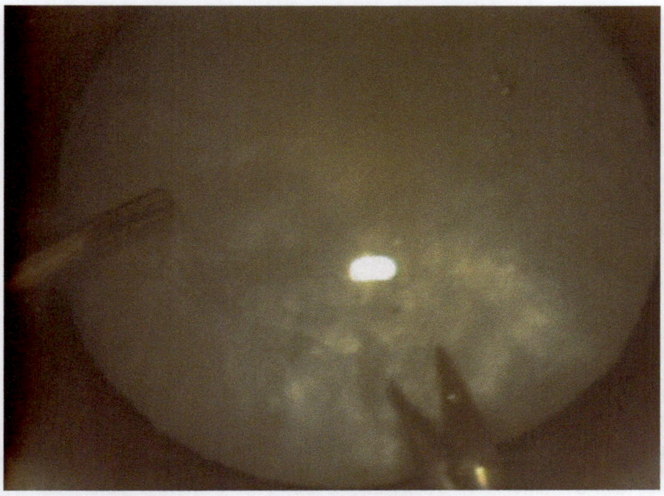

Fig. 7.38 Using micro-scissors to save the rhexis

(h) *Multiple capsular punctures or capsular relaxing incisions as the final option* (Fig. 7.39): When everything has failed and a capsular tear has occurred (or perhaps, the surgeon is uncertain that there is, but is highly suspicious that it has happened), perform multiple punctures or multiple relaxing incisions, either with cystotome or with scissors. If tears are already present, perform relaxing capsular incisions to the opposite side of the tear and to many meridians as possible, in order to redistribute the forces that may cause extension of the tears to the lens equator. This is the final option when everything has failed. It will not be a nice and round CCC, but the possibility of a tear transmitted to the posterior capsule will be less.

7.1.3 Avoiding Complications During Biaxial Phaco with an Incomplete Capsulorhexis

Once the surgeon is sure that he has an incomplete capsulorrhexis and doesn't know exactly if the tear has extended to the posterior capsule, the golden rule is, *to avoid transmission of forces to the capsular bag*. It must be an "in the air surgery," meaning, performing the whole procedure at the iris plane.

Some years ago, Prof. Keiki Mehta from Mumbai, India, described what he called, "*The Lens Salute Technique*," that consists of a hemi-luxation of the nucleus to the iris plane, during hydrodissection and hydrodelineation (Fig. 7.40). The authors have found that during their surgical practice, this maneuver helps to decrease the transmission of forces to the capsular bag and to the zonula, even in noncomplicated cases (which means completed cases with nice, round capsulorrhexis). In cases of incomplete capsulorrhexis, this maneuver can be a safer way of performing a noncomplicated phacoemulsification. The key is to work at the iris plane.

(a) *Performing gentle hydrodissection* (Fig. 7.41): Because in many cases the surgeon cannot know exactly the state of the capsular bag when a capsulorrhexis is incomplete, added precaution should be taken when performing hydrodissection and hydrodelineation. The surgeon has to perform soft and slow maneuvers inside the capsular bag, separating only the layers adjacent to the anterior capsule

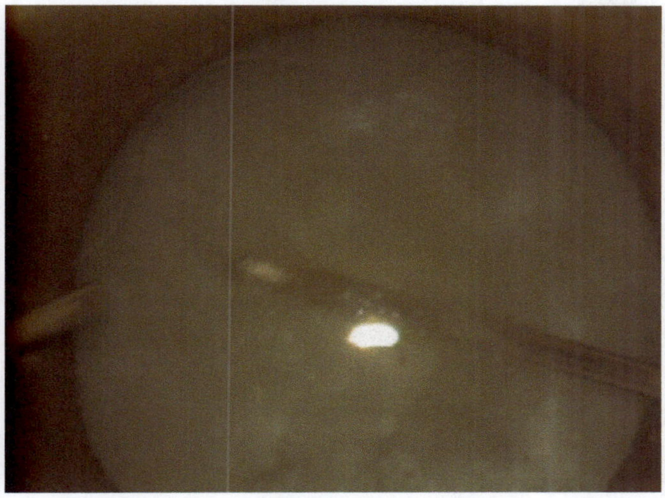

Fig. 7.39 Multiple capsulotomies as a final option

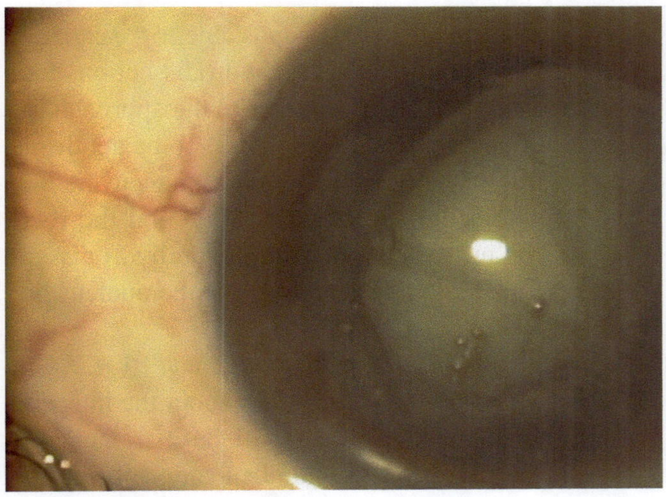

Fig. 7.40 Nucleus placed in lens salute position

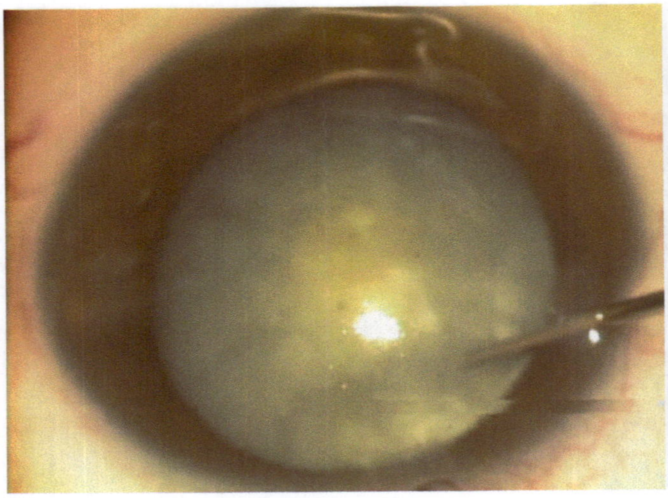

Fig. 7.41 Gentle hydrosurgery

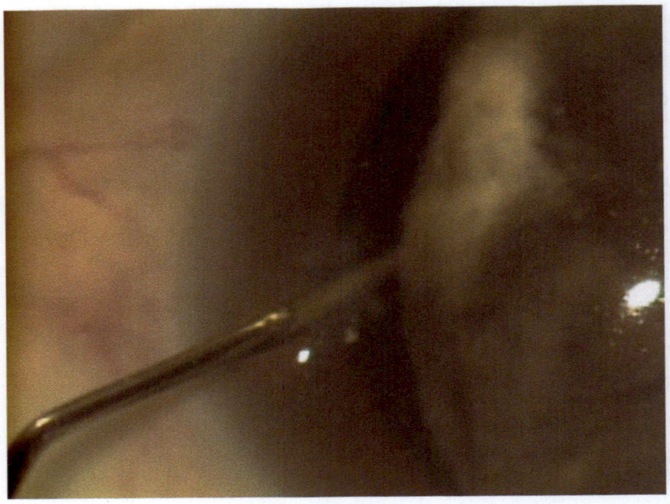

Fig. 7.42 Taking the nucleus to a lens salute position with hydrodisection cannula

in the meridians, where it is possible to visualize it well. This maneuvers of hydrodissection and hydrodelineation is very similar to the approach for cases of Posterior Polar Cataracts. "To be gentle" is the key for this surgical step. Avoid maneuvers like vigorous injection of irrigating fluid and the rotation of the nucleus. Even with gentle hydrodissection, the goal should still be to take the nucleus out of the capsular bag.

(b) *Searching for an easy "Lens Salute Position"* (Fig. 7.42): Because the surgeon is uncertain about the integrity of the posterior capsule, it will be a tremendous mistake to perform phacoemulsification inside the capsular bag. Maneuvers like prechop, vigorous chopping and stop and chop in the bag, must be avoided. The key factor for phacoemulsification is to work outside the capsular bag. In these cases, the surgeon can apply the concept of "the safest place to work for a cataract surgeon is at the iris plane" Once the nucleus is at the iris plane, the transmission of forces to the "incomplete" capsular bag, posterior capsule and zonules should be avoided. Furthermore, while working in a biaxial approach, the irrigating cannula (or irrigating chopper) can be placed behind the nucleus (Fig. 7.43). Irrigation from the irrigating chopper helps separate the nucleus from the posterior capsule or in such cases, from the hyaloid face. If the surgeon is working in a coaxial approach, it is impossible because there is no irrigation available at his nondominant hand and worst, the coaxial irrigation pushes the nucleus back to the incomplete capsular bag. The main concept that must be learned in these cases is that the surgeon has to believe that the posterior capsule is broken, even if he has signs that it is not, with the goal to avoid initial or subsequent damage. There are two ways to take the nucleus outside the capsular bag:

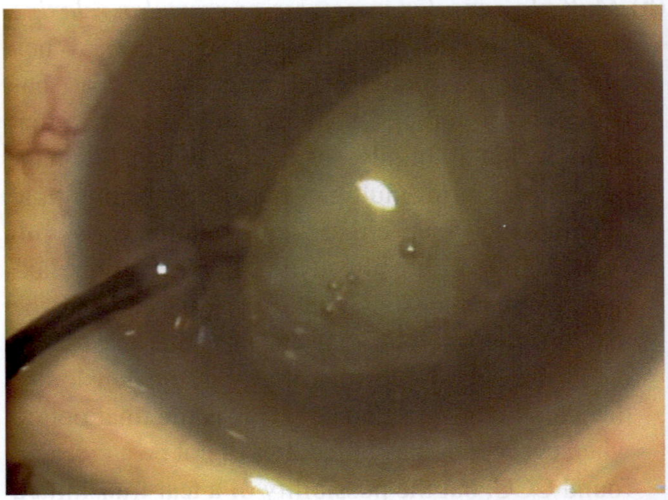

Fig. 7.43 Irrigating cannula behind the nucleus

- Perform the "Lens Salute Technique" during the hydroprocedures (Fig. 7.42): If the surgeon is uncertain about the integrity of the posterior capsule and he has to be gentle during the hydrodissection without rotating the nucleus, a small amount of solution can be injected behind the anterior capsule in a place where he can best visualize it. While injecting, gently press down the equator of the nucleus in this same position. Do not press the nucleus in the center or in the mid-periphery. It has to be pressed at the extreme periphery; otherwise, the nucleus might get pushed into the vitreous. While injecting and at the same time pressing the equator, the solution will run behind the nucleus to the opposite side, creating a posterior fluid wave that pushes the nucleus forward. This fluid wave moves between the nucleus and the posterior capsule. Even if the posterior capsule is absent, the wave will move between the nucleus and the hyaloid face, pushing the nucleus forward. This is why this maneuver will not work if the surgeon pushes the nucleus in another location, different from the extreme periphery. Disastrous consequences may occur if this maneuver is not performed properly. Remember that the aim of this maneuver is for the nucleus to reach its final position, which is, the "tilt" position, a plane of inclination that will allow the surgeon to place his irrigating chopper or cannula behind the nucleus (Fig. 7.43) as it reaches the iris plane. The key factor is to move the nucleus out of the capsular bag. The nucleus will tilt forward easily because of the absence of a small CCC that can keep it in the capsular bag.

– If the surgeon does not have enough skills, or is afraid to perform hydroprocedure in a possible broken capsular bag, there is one technique that can help move the nucleus from the capsular bag. Gentle and soft hydrodissection without nuclear rotation can be performed, followed by the insertion of the irrigating chopper (or cannula) and the phaco needle to the anterior chamber (Fig. 7.44a). There should be enough fluid (active or passive infusion according to the gauge of preference) to avoid surge and high vacuum (according to the phaco needle and the phaco-machine parameters). Start the irrigation and impale the phaco needle with a small amount of ultrasonic power into the center of the nucleus (Fig. 7.44b). Avoid pushing the nucleus during this maneuver. Once the phaco needle is deep enough in the nucleus, stop the ultrasonic force but not the vacuum. The surgeon should avoid performing a groove, remember that he needs to work outside the capsular bag, and keep the vacuum active. Do not lose the nucleus, and keep itkept in place with only the vacuum force firmly holding it. In a single swift, but gentle movement, the surgeon should pull the phaco needle-nucleus outside the capsular bag. This maneuver is similar to that of intracapsular surgery, when the unit, cryo probe-cataract are moved in a single but gentle movement, to remove the cataract from the eye (Fig. 7.44c). In this case, the movement is just to put the nucleus at the iris plane. Once the surgeon is at the iris plane, vacuum should not be stopped. As the nucleus is held firmly by the phaco needle, the irrigating chopper (or cannula) on the nondominant hand is slipped behind the nucleus. This instrument has irrigation, so it is easy to know that it is placed properly behind the nucleus. This irrigation, acting as the surgeon's third hand in this situation cannot be obtained in a coaxial approach. Once the irrigating device is behind the nucleus keep it firmly held with the vacuum, and simply move the irrigating device to cut the nucleus (Fig. 7.44d). With sustained vacuum at the iris plane, from the rear to the front, the surgeon will obtain a nice division of the nucleus in two halves at the iris plane, far away from the corneal endothelium and from the possible damaged capsular bag (Fig. 7.44e).

(c) *Maintaining a positive IOP with irrigation*: Because the aim is to work at the iris plane, the maintenance of wide spaces in the anterior and posterior chambers plays an essential role. If the surge is present, the damage to the intraocular structures is possible. Surge can cause damage to the posterior capsule, ultimately causing nuclear material to lodge in the vitreous cavity. More importantly, it can decrease the speed of recovery of a patient suffering from corneal edema because of endothelial touch. Enough fluid to work with, will help the surgeon create space to maneuver inside the eye, thereby, avoiding touch of intraocular structures. Moreover, this fluid-filled space can support high vacuum levels during phaco. As a general rule, while using an irrigating device of 19G or wider, passive infusion (gravity force) can be utilized. But when using diameters of 20G or smaller, avoid the risk of surge . Use forced infusion, whether internal or external because it assures the surgeon success in these complicated cases.

(d) *Biaxial prechop technique at the iris plane (with lens salute or with "pull the nucleus technique")*: Whichever way the nucleus is placed at the iris plane, a mechanical fracture of the nucleus performed between the phaco needle (placed in the front part of the nucleus) and irrigating device, either chopper or cannula (placed in the rear part of

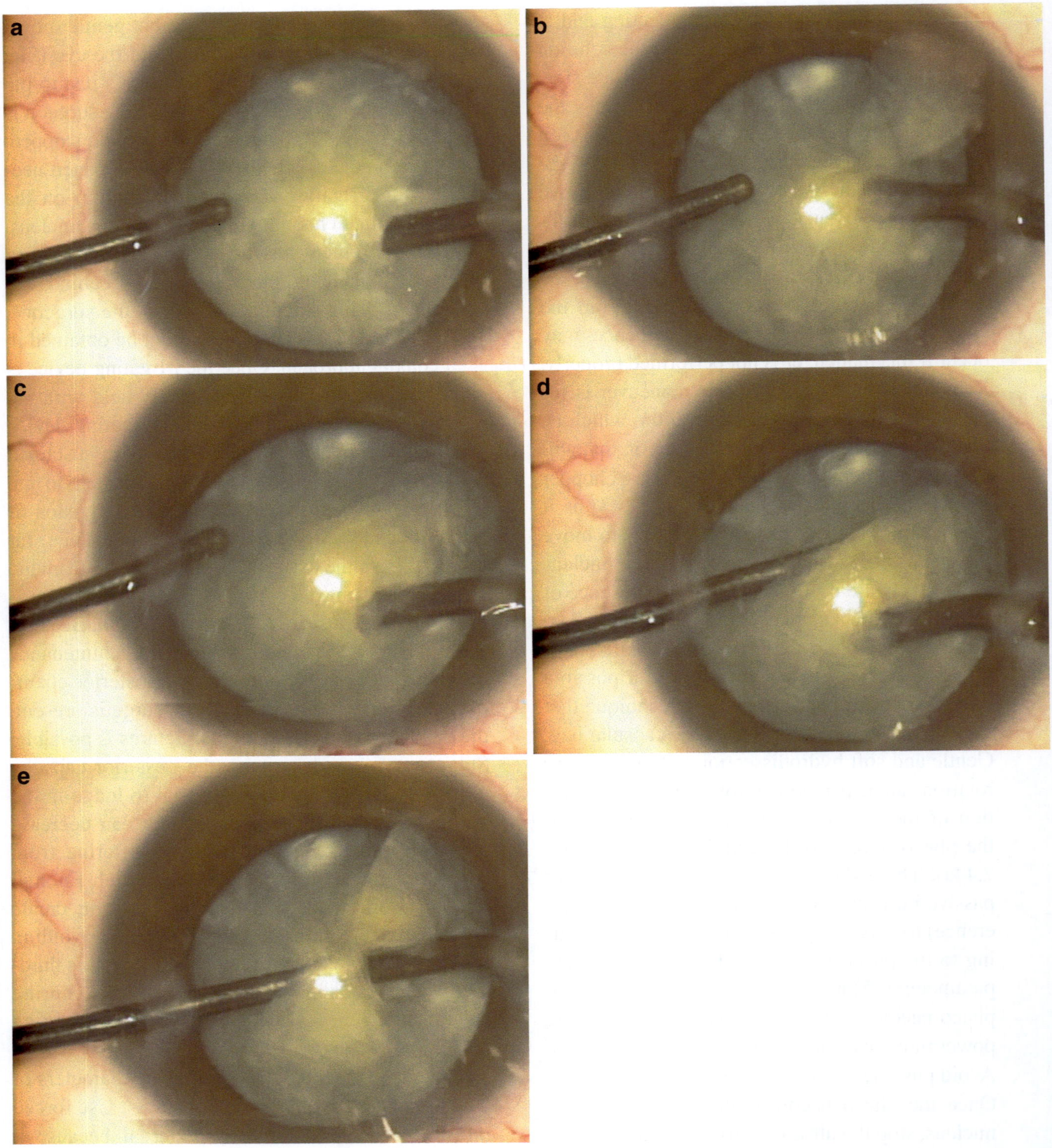

Fig. 7.44 (**a**) Starting Bi-Axial Phaco. (**b**) Entering the nucleus with slow ultrasonic power. Be careful not to groove. (**c**) Pulling the nucleus outside the capsular bag with vacuum. (**d**) Mechanical fragmentation of the nucleus at the iris plane. (**e**) Nuclear division in two pieces at the iris plane

the nucleus), is the key to success (Fig. 7.45). The surgeon now has the following advantages:

- Now, the surgeon works outside the capsular bag.
- There is an irrigating force separating the nucleus from the posterior chamber structures, although he is not certain of the integrity of the posterior capsule.
- It is possible to emulsify all the nuclear strands from the front to the rear, so an incomplete chop is almost difficult to occur, unless he loses vacuum force.
- Because the surgeon is firmly holding the nucleus with vacuum, it functions as a unit, as a single piece that can be managed in single movements.

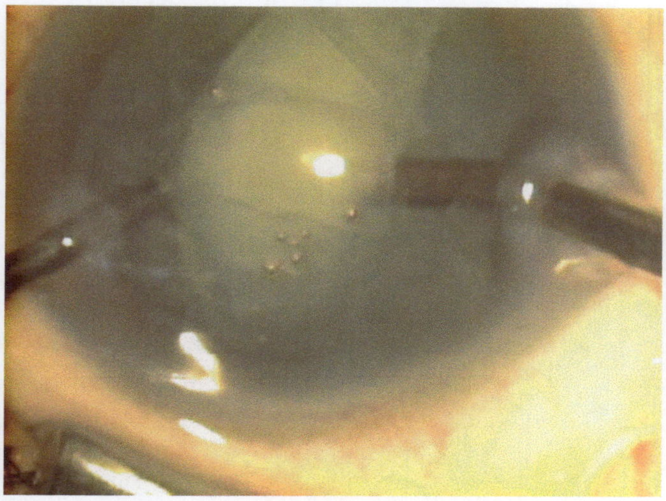

Fig. 7.45 Biaxial Prechop

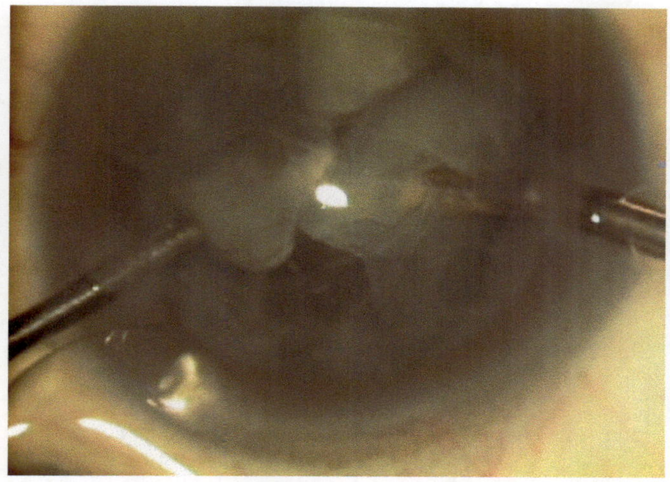

Fig. 7.46 Mechanical fragmentation at the iris plane

- iHe has irrigation posterior to the nucleus, and hence, the pieces are pushed forward, and never to the posterior chamber.

Avoid the use of prechopper forceps, prechopping inside the capsular bag, coaxial irrigation, stop and chop techniques, and all the techniques that will take the surgery again to the posterior chamber. Extra precaution should be taken not to touch the corneal endothelium. Work at the iris plane and not at the anterior chamber. Fragment the nucleus into pieces as much as possible at the iris plane. Divide the nucleus several times with the same technique; apply vacuum force to the nucleus and vertical chop at the same time from the rear to the front.

(e) *Avoiding work at the capsular bag. pulling the fragments to the iris plane* (Fig. 7.46): Because of the uncertainty of the integrity of the posterior capsule, placing the irrigation behind the nucleus is the key. The surgeon has a third hand in helping to keep the nuclear fragments at the iris plane and maintaining the broken posterior capsule or the vitreous body away from the surgical space. Nevertheless, some surgeons recently have pointed out the benefits of placing a mechanical device behind the nucleus in order to have a safe phacoemulsification, when there is a damaged posterior capsule (artificial posterior capsule). The future will tell us about their real benefits and possible complications. They, however, share with us the same way of thinking, that is, in cases of phacoemulsification performed with an incomplete capsulorrhexis, the working space must be at the iris plane. Some physical force (either fluid or mechanical) must be inserted or instilled behind the nucleus to avoid loss of nuclear fragments to the vitreous cavity, and eventually to avoid more damage to the structures located in the posterior chamber.

(f) *Maintaining a positive IOP while switching to I/A mode:* Because the surgeon is working in a biaxial approach, it is possible to switch from phaco mode to Irritagion/Aspiration mode, without the need to stop irrigation. In a coaxial approach, this is not possible. Once the surgeon has finished the emulsification of the nucleus, he has to switch from one handpiece to another. Irrigation is stopped between the steps, unless viscoelastic material is injected through a second incision to maintain a stable anterior and posterior chamber. If this is the case, the surgeon is very near to being converted from a coaxial to a biaxial surgeon. With the biaxial approach, the surgeon only needs to switch from the phaco probe to the aspirating cannula with the dominant hand, and with the help of his assistant holding the irrigating handpiece on the nondominant hand and keeping the eye stable, thereby maintaining the anterior and posterior chambers wide open, and the damaged capsule, hyaloid face or vitreous body far away from the incisions. It is a tremendous advantage of a micro-incisional surgery in a biaxial approach (Fig. 7.47a–c).

(g) *Biaxial I/A*: After switching instrumentation, I/A is performed in the usual manner. In this particular step, it is possible to review the integrity of your the capsular bag and also the presence of the vitreous, the Because of the separation between irrigation

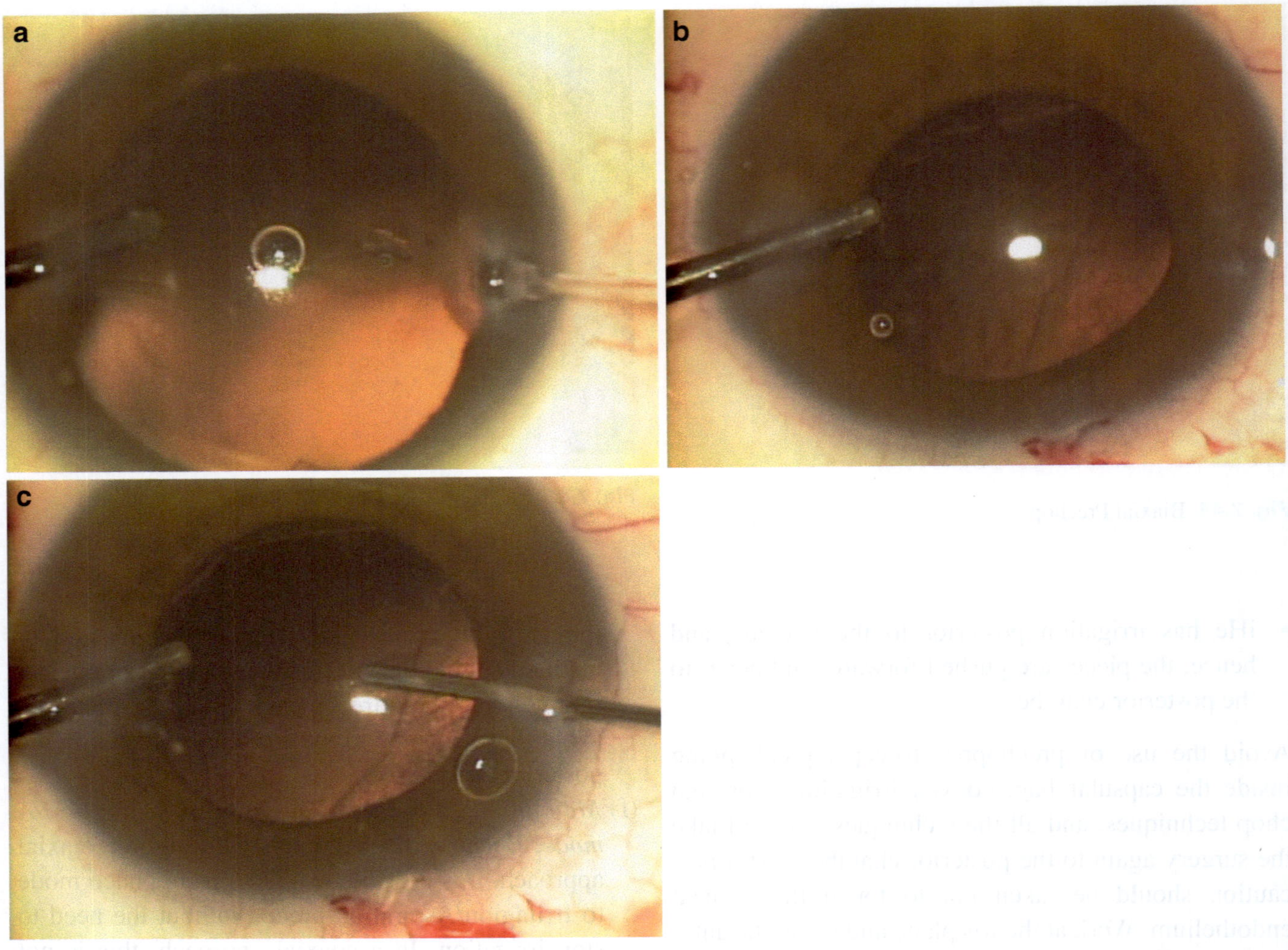

Fig. 7.47 (**a**) Maintaining the irrigation on. Notice the filtration through the incision with possitive IOP. (**b**) Notice the hydrostatic pressure maintaining the hyaloid face in a case of posterior capsule rupture. (**c**) With positive IOP viscoelastic is applied and no vitreous loss is present

and aspiration, the surgeon has the advantage of a wide chamber and a closed system to have a good view of the structures and easy recovery of the cortical material (Fig. 7.48).

(h) *Biaxial anterior vitrectomy if needed* (Fig. 7.49): If vitreous is present because of a rupture in the anterior hyaloid face, perform biaxial irrigation aspiration. Do not withdraw the irrigating device, and continue active irrigation, but decrease the irrigation force (active or passive). Change the aspirating cannula on the dominant hand to a posterior vitrector. This maneuver helps the surgeon to maintain a deep and stable anterior chamber and likewise maintain positive pressure. As much as possible, avoid vitreous leakage into the anterior chamber,

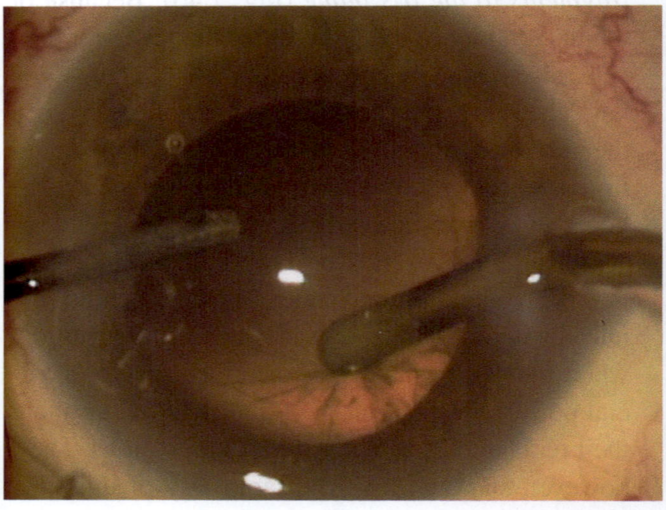

Fig. 7.48 Posterior capsule pulling during biaxial IA

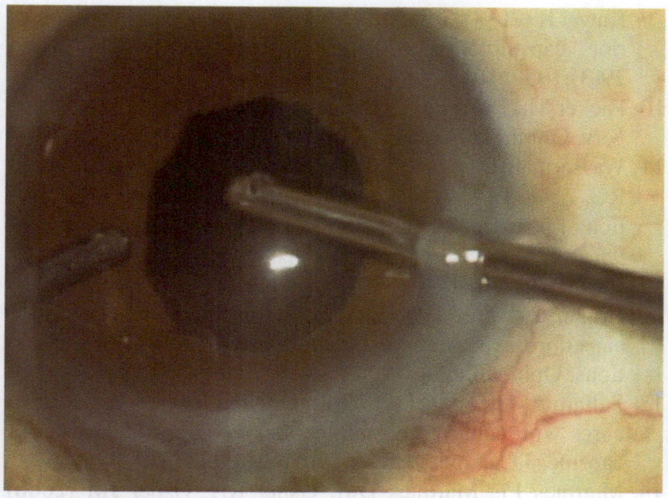

Fig. 7.49 Performing biaxial anterior vitrectomy in a sealed chamber

Fig. 7.50 A 3 pieces silicon IOL implanted in the bag, in a case of incomplete capsulorhexis

maintaining it behind the iris plane. Avoid possible surges. If a vitrector is not available or if the surgeon wants to have an immediate complete visualization of the intraocular structures before removing the irrigating device, he should change his aspirating cannula to a viscoelastic syringe using his dominant hand, and inject viscoelastic before removing the irrigating cannula (Fig. 7.47c). Once the eye is filled completely with the viscoelastic and there is enough positive pressure, irrigation should be stopped and the irrigating cannula should be removed. Now anterior chamber is completely formed with the viscoelastic, without surge or negative pressure induced to the eye. Now, the current state of the intraocular tissues can be reviewed calmly by the surgeon.

7.1.4 Avoiding Complications During IOL Insertion with an Incomplete Capsulorhexis

IOL implantation in cases of incomplete capsulorrhexis is only mentioned briefly because it is something that should be evaluated depending on each case, either coaxial or biaxial, when a lack of posterior capsular integrity is highly suspected. It is not the aim of this chapter to make an analysis of each these steps. It is sufficient to mention the decisions to be taken by the surgeon at the end of each case of incomplete capsulorhexis:

1. Perform an adequate re-evaluation of integrity of capsular bag
2. Decide on the best IOL based on the particular circumstance (absence or presence of posterior capsule)
3. Be careful with injectors in the absence of the posterior capsule; consider the use of forceps when inserting the IOL.
4. Decide on the use of a helping device such as a capsular tension ring.
5. Decide on the technique for IOL fixation (e.g., iris suture, sulcus fixation, glue implantation) according to the situation and surgical experience (Fig. 7.50).

7.1.5 Conclusions

Many advantages have been observed when performing biaxial lens surgery in the management of complicated capsular case. These advantages can be noted from the first steps wh the surgeon starts to feel the capsular tissue and to the maneuvers that can be performed in order to avoid a more complicated case. But furthermore, these advantages are more evident during the management of the chop maneuvers, phacoemulsification, I/A and biaxial anterior vitrectomy when needed. It is completely true that MICS is not only a matter of incision size. It is a whole new perspective on the utilization of new tools, new maneuvers, new forces, new fluidics inside the eye, which helps the surgeon to decrease the possible complications of cataract surgery. But of even great importance is its value in solving complex and challenging cases like that, which was presented in this chapter.

Remember to avoid applying force to the residual capsular bag and the zonular ligament if the surgeon is unsure that the capsulorhexis is complete.

Take Home Pearls

- MICS surgery has distinct advantages over coaxial techniques in the management of incomplete capsulorhexis cases.
- The irrigation handpiece in the nondominant hand becomes a powerful tool in maintaining a positive intraocular pressure. Moreover, it keeps the nuclear fragments away from the endothelium and from the residual posterior capsule (or even the vitreous body).
- With MICS, it becomes easier for the surgeon to work safely at the iris plane in these particular cases.

References

1. Sacu S, Menapace R, Findl O (2006) Effect of optic material and haptic design on anterior capsule opacification and capsulorrhexis contraction. Am J Ophthalmol 141(3):488–493
2. Jacobs DS, Cox TA, Wagoner MD, Ariyasu RG, Karp CL (2006) Capsule staining as an adjunt to cataract surgery: a report from the american academy of ophthalmology. Ophthalmology 113(4):707–713
3. Alió J, Rodríguez-Prats JL, Galal A, Ramzy M (2005) Outcomes of microincision cataract surgery versus coaxial phacoemulsification. Ophthalmology 112(11):1997–2003
4. Garg A (2007) Dinamics of capsulorrhexis. In: Pinelli R, Fazio P (eds) Mastering the phacodynamics (tools, technology and innovations), Chapter 12. Jaypee Brothers Medical Publishers, India
5. Kurz S, Krummenauer F, Gabriel P, Pfeiffer N, Dick HB (2006) Biaxial microincision versus coaxial small-incision clear cornea cataract surgery. Ophthalmology 113(10):1818–1826
6. Brar N, Cremers SL (2007) Assessing surgery skills. Ophthalmology 114(8):1587–1587
7. Muqit MM, Menage MJ (2006) Intraoperative floppy Iris syndrome. Ophthalmology 113(10):1885–1886
8. Kawai K, Suzuki T, Hayakawa K (2005) The 23 gauge capsulorrhexis forceps having a cystotome function. Tokai J Exp Clin Med 30(1):11–13
9. Kawai K (2004) Comparison of 23 gauge and 25 gauge anterior capsulotomy forceps. Tokai J Exp Clin Med 29(3):105–110
10. Packer M., Hoffmann R., Fine H (2006) Refractive lens surgery. Ophthalmol Clin North Am 19(1):77–88
11. Wasserman D, Apple DJ, Castaneda VE, Tsai JC, Morgan RC, Assia EI (1991) Anterior capsular tears and loop fixation of posterior chamber intraocular lenses. Ophthalmology 98(4):425–431
12. Castaneda VE, Legler UF, Tsai JC, Hoggatt JP, Assia EI, Hogan C, Apple DJ (1992) Posterior continuos curvilinear capsulorrhexis. An experimental study with clinical applications. Ophthalmology 99(1):45–50
13. Sallam A, Sherafat H (2007) Intraocular lens implantation in cases with anterior capsule tears extending to the posterior capsule. J Cataract Refract Surg 33(6):938–939
14. Marques FF, Marques DM, Osher RH, Osher JM (2006) Fate of anterior capsular tears during cataract surgery. J Cataract Refract Surg 32(10):1638–1642
15. Fishkind WJ, Discussion paper by Gimbel HV, Sun R. Ferensowics M (2001) Intraoperative management of capsular tears in phacoemulsification and intraocular lens implantation. Ophthalmology 108:2190–2192
16. Gimbel HV, Teuhann T (1990) Development, advantages and methods of continuos curvilinear capsulorhexis technique. J Cataract Refract Surg 16:31–37
17. Assia EI, Apple DJ, Tsai JC, Morgan RC (1991) Mechanism of radial tear formation after anterior capsulectomy. Ophthalmology 98:432–437
18. Vajpayee RB, Sharma N, Dada T, Gupta V, Kumar A, Dada VK (2001) Management of posterior capsule tears. Surv Ophthalmol 45(6):473–488
19. Gimbel HV, Sun R, Ferensowicz M, Anderson Penno E, Kamal A (2001) Intraoperative management of posterior capsule tears in phacoemulsification and intraocular lens implantation. Ophthalmology 108(12):2186–2189; discussion 2190–2192
20. Assia EI, Apple DJ, Barden A, Tsai JC, Castaneda VE, Hoggatt JS (1991) An experimental study comparing various anterior capsulectomy techniques. Arch Ophthalmol 109(5):642–647
21. Hettlich HJ, El-Hifnawi ES (1997) Scanning electron microssopy studies of he human lens after capsulorhexis. Ophthalmologe 94(4):300–302
22. Hamada S, Low S, Walters BC, Nischal KK (2006) Five-year experience of the 2.incision push-pull technique for anterior and posterior capsulorhexis in pediatric cataract surgery. Ophthalmology 113(8):1309–1314
23. Oner FH, Durak I, Soylev M, Ergin M (2001) Long term results of various anterior capsulotomies and radial tears on intraocular lens centration. Ophthalmic Surg Lasers 32(2):118–123
24. Sallam A, Sherafat H (2007) Intraocular lens implantation in cases with anterior capsule tears extending to he posterior capsule. J Cataract Refract Surg 33(6):938–939; author reply 939–940
25. Osher RH (2007) Reply: inraocular lens implantation in cases with anterior capsule tears extending to he posterior capsule. J Cataract Refract Surg 33(6):939–940
26. Wilson ME (2004) Anterior lens capsule management in pediatric cataract surgery. Trans Am Ophthalmol Soc 102:391–422

27. Kwartz J (1996) Implantation of foldable intraocular lenses in the presence of anterior capsular tears. Eye 10(Pt 4): 529–530
28. Perez-Arteaga A (2008) Step by step to biaxial lens surgery. Jaypee Brothers Medical Publishers, New Delhi, India

7.2 MICS in Special Cases (on CD): Vitreous Loss

Jerome Bovet

Core Messages

- As soon as the surgeon recognizes the presence of a posterior capsule rupture and vitreous loss, it is best to remove all the instruments from the eye with care.
- Triamcinolone may be injected inside the anterior chamber to visualize the vitreous.
- Bimanual anterior vitrectomy or sutureless pars plana bimanual vitrectomy can be performed.
- Both the techniques result in faster visual rehabilitation and better visual outcomes in patients with posterior capsule rupture and vitreous loss during MICS.

7.2.1 Introduction (Fig. 7.51)

MICS surgery has been the preferred method of cataract extraction during the last décade [1, 2]. A major advancement in the management of cataracts is early surgery, when the nucleus is still soft and before it becomes more dense. However, there are patients who already have mature cataracts at the time of the first examination. This obviously creates difficulties during surgery. Other ocular conditions that may present alone or in combination with cataracts are pseudoexfoliation syndrome (PEX), iridodonesis-phacodonesis, zonulolysis, lens subluxation, and posterior polar cataracts. All of these may be addressed as the precursors of a probable intraoperative complication along with the mature white cataracts [3–5].

Vitreous loss is probably the most frequent serious complication encountered by cataract surgeons. A vitreous loss may increase the risk of cystoid macular

J. Bovet
Clinique de l'oeil, 15 bois de la chapelle,
1213 Onex /Geneva, Switzerland
e-mail: jbovet@vision.tv

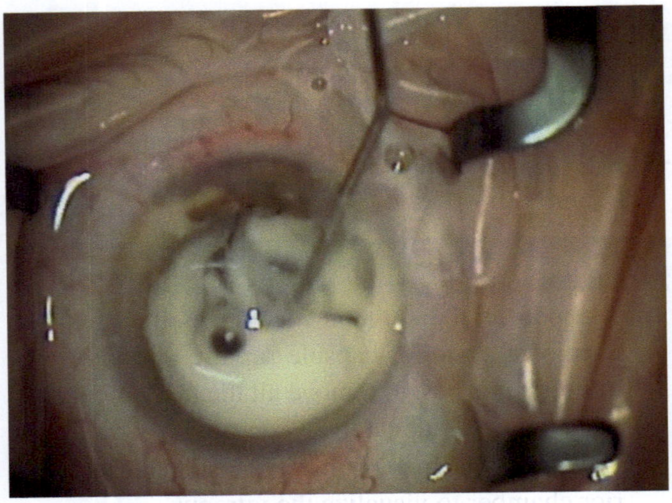

Fig. 7.51 Triamcilonone acetonide anterior chamber injection

edema and retinal detachment [6]. Luxation of the nucleus material is not a rare complication of phacoemulsification procedures (0.3–1.1%), and it often requires vitreoretinal surgical intervention [7–9].

As soon as the surgeon recognizes the presence of a posterior capsule tear or a zonulysis, he should immediately change some parameters on the phaco machine and inject triamcinolone acetonide inside the anterior chamber to localize the vitreous strands [10–12].

Fluidics inside the chamber should be kept to a minimum so that the lens material and possibly the capsule are not aspirated too quickly, offering the surgeon more precise control of the complication and more time to think and react. As this is being done by the surgeon, the assistant should already prepare the bimanual gauge 23 vitrector. [13, 14]. Even when a vitreous loss occurs, proper management of this complication can facilitate IOL implantation in the sulcus or even in the capsular bag and therefore can provide an excellent visual outcome [15].

7.2.2 Posterior Capsule Tears and Vitreous Prolapse *(Figs. 7.52–7.54)*

When vitreous loss through a capsular tear is present, the early detection of vitreous prolapse is the key to a successful outcome. The goals should be to maintain capsular support for a posterior chamber implant, and to limit the risk of retinal complications [16]. The likelihood of achieving these goals decreases with increased manipulation of the vitreous.

When a posterior capsule break is identified, the first maneuver should be to determine the presence or the absence of the vitreous. A vitreous prolapse should be suspected in the absence of a visible posterior capsule break if there are indirect signs of vitreous traction. Careful inspection of the anterior segment will establish vitreous prolapse if there is any abnormal peaking or configuration of the pupil margin or the margin of the capsular break. If there is suspicion of vitreous prolapse, the first maneuver is to inject *0.5 mL triamcinolone acetonide on a solution of 4 mg/mL* to the anterior chamber. Triamcinolone is then washed carefully with BSS, which will stain all the vitreous strands in the anterior chamber, white. All the old maneuvers such as sweeping of the anterior chamber with a cyclodialysis spatula or the weck-cel at the wound margin should be avoided [17]. Special care should be taken not to pull on the vitreous, which can enlarge the capsule tears.

If the presence of the vitreous material is confirmed, any further manipulations should be deferred until the vitreous has been completely removed. Inadequate removal of vitreous from the anterior chamber and corneal wound increases the likelihood of immediate and long-term complications. If a vitreous traction stays around the pupil margin postoperatively, it will increase the chance of cystoid macular edema (Irvine-Gass syndrome) [18].

Newer 23 gauge bimanual vitrectomy techniques with single-use air vitrector and irrigation cannula are more efficient than the old magnetic vitrectors. The 23 gauge vitrector and the 20 gauge irrigation cannula are placed into the anterior chamber through the same enlarged paracentesis that is done at the beginning of the MICS procedure for irrigation-aspiration. The irrigation cannula is directed away from MICS incision site in order to achieve a stable anterior chamber, constant intraocular pressure, and prevent hydration of the vitreous. Continuous infusion and aspiration through the anterior vitrectomy cutter and corneal incision increase vitreous prolapse into the corneal wound. For this reason, the cutting rate should be relatively high, while the irrigation, aspiration, and vacuum levels should be maintained at a minimum [19–22]. (Figs. 7.55 and 7.56). Furthermore, it tends to hydrate the vitreous and exerts more traction on the peripheral vitreous, which then increases the risk for postoperative retinal detachment [23].

Vitrectomy done through the pars plana approach on the other hand, is a better alternative. When the vitrectomy is performed via the pars plana, the vitreous is

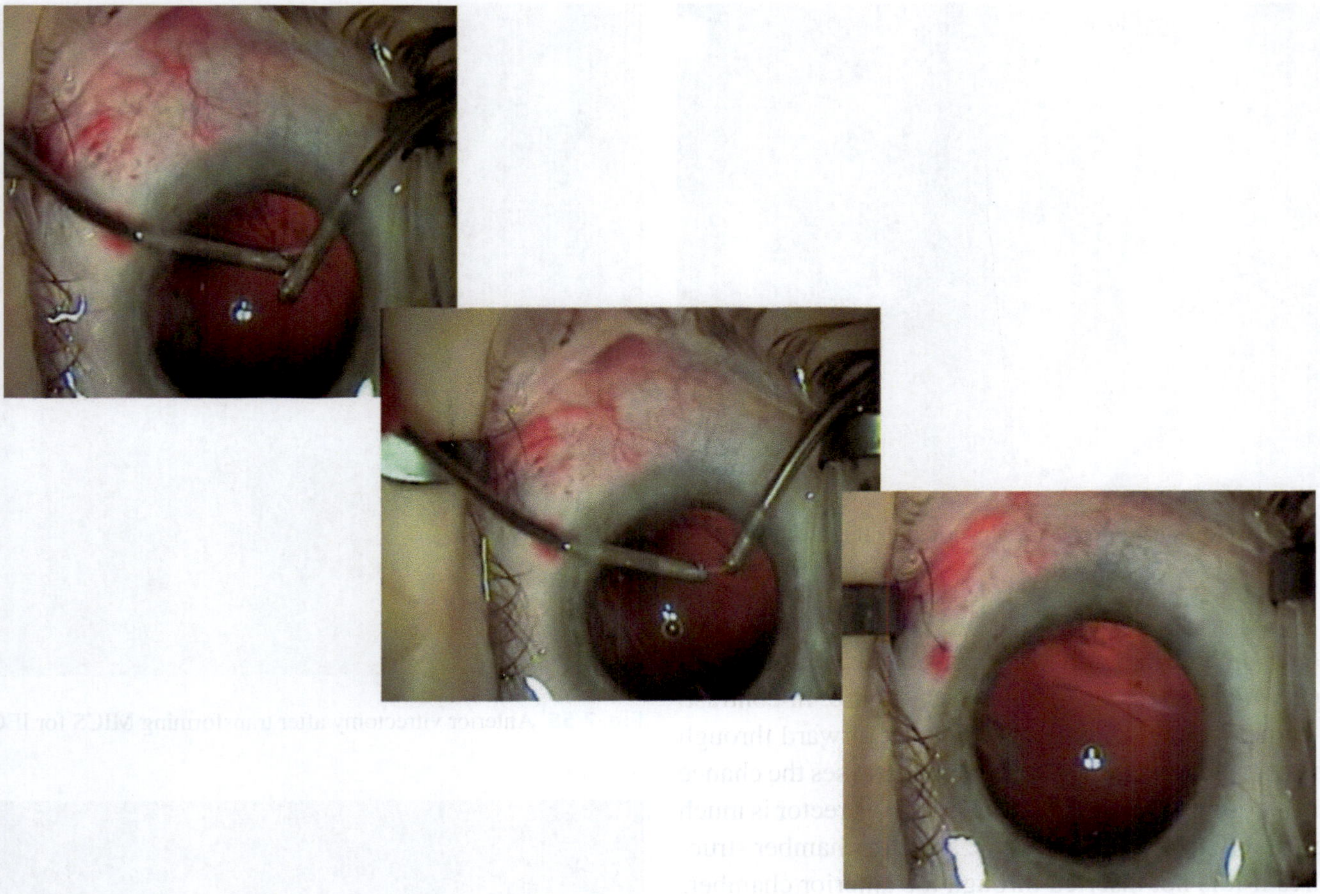

Fig. 7.52 With attention you could know when you have break up the capsule

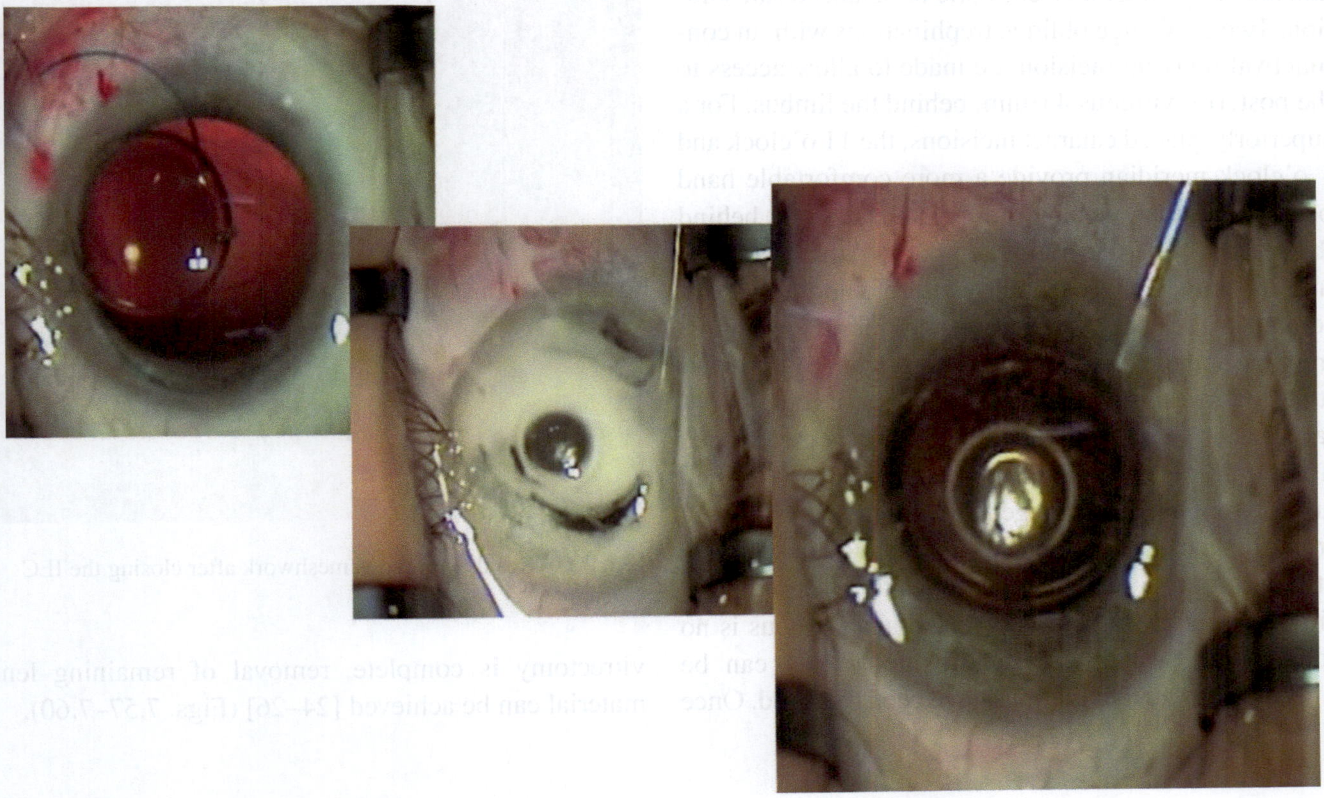

Fig. 7.53 When you have a posterior capsule break always check vitreous at the end with triamcinolone

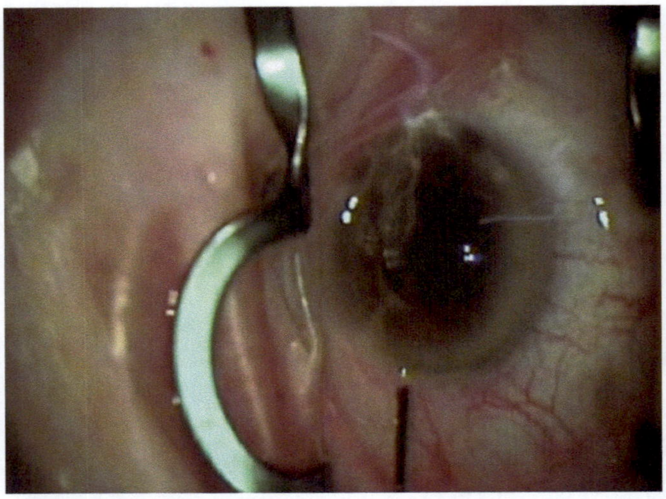

Fig. 7.54 Residual vitreous meshwork after IOLXchange

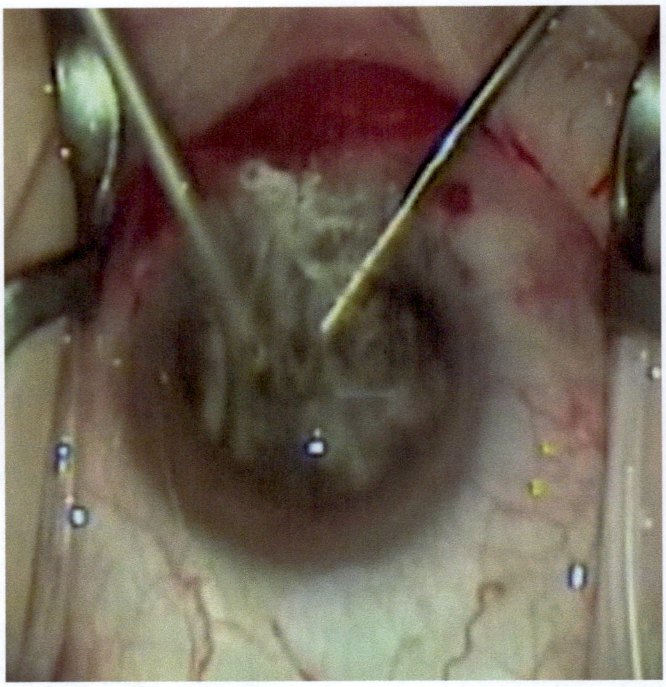

Fig. 7.55 Anterior vitrectomy after transforming MICS for IEC

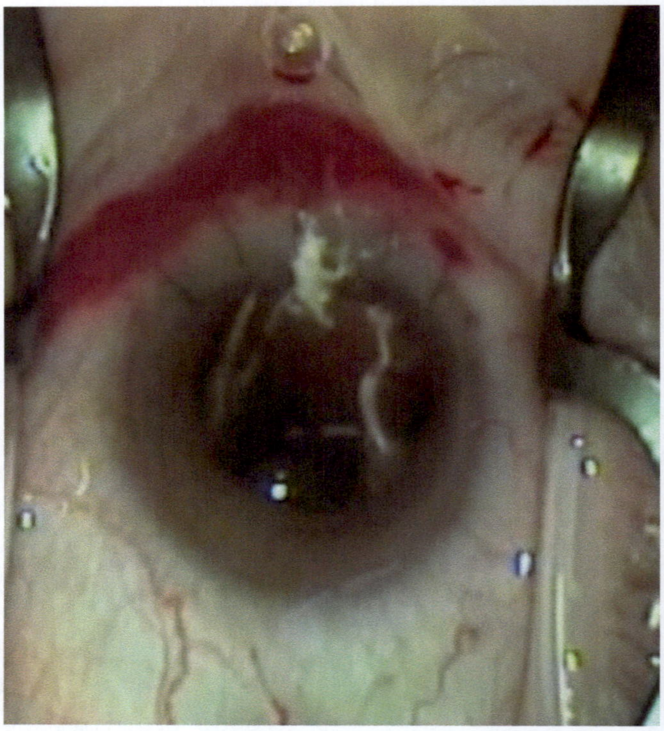

Fig. 7.56 Residual vitreous meshwork after closing the IEC

being drawn out of the anterior chamber space, thus applying less tension on the vitreous base. In contrast, a corneal approach pulls the vitreous forward through the tear, creating more tension and increases the chance of enlarging the tear. Additionally, the vitrector is much less likely to disturb any of the anterior chamber structures if it is not inserted through the anterior chamber.

The pars plana vitrectomy in this situation begins by removing all instruments from the anterior chamber and injecting either a viscoelastic or balanced salt solution. Two 20-Gauge oblique trephinations without conjunctival relaxing incision are made to allow access to the posterior vitreous 4.0 mm, behind the limbus. For a superiorly-placed cataract incisions, the 11 o'clock and 1 o'clock meridian provide a more comfortable hand positioning, than placing the incisions directly behind the wound. When operating temporally, the pars plana incision may be placed slightly inferotemporal. A sclerotomy is created with a 20-Gauge microvitreoretinal trephine and the tip is visualized through the pupil after it has passed through the tutor cannula into the pupillary space. The 23 gauge vitrectomy tip is then placed a few millimeters behind the posterior capsular tear, and the foot pedal is engaged, drawing the vitreous out from the tear. The handpiece should be held relatively still with only a few slow movements. Once no anterior segment movement is detected and vitreous is no longer present, more triamcinolone acetate can be injected until all the tractions have been removed. Once vitrectomy is complete, removal of remaining lens material can be achieved [24–26] (Figs. 7.57–7.60).

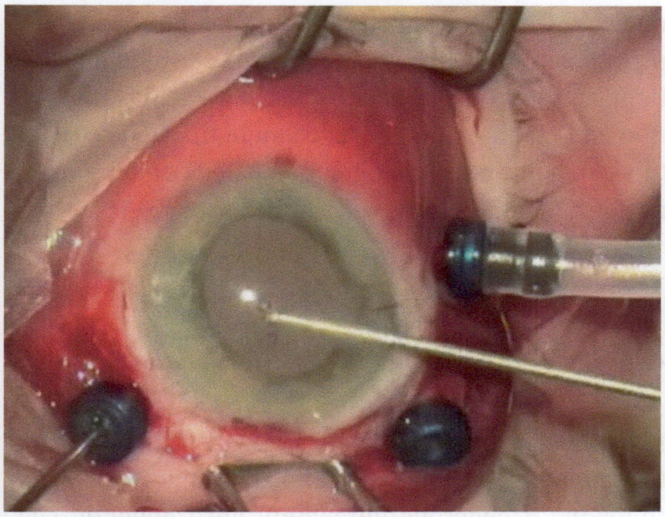

Fig. 7.57 23-Gauge vitrectomy

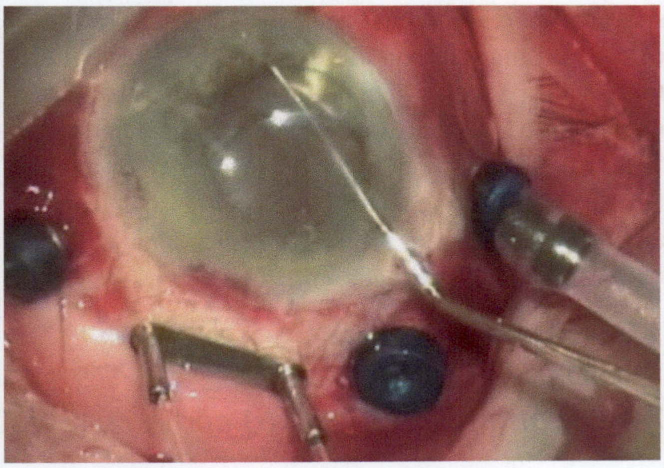

Fig. 7.58 23-Gauge vitrectomy & IOL in sulcus position

7.2.3 Vitreous and the Epinucleus or Cortex

Before any manipulation, the surgeon has to inject triamcinolone acetate inside the anterior chamber to assess the gravity of the problem and to plan the next step. If vitreous prolapse is already present and the nuclear fragments are admixed in the vitreous, then the vitreous should be addressed first.

Particular attention must be paid to limit the borders of the tear and to aspirate the cortex carefully. A gentle, low-flow automated irrigation aspiration may be used with caution stripping the cortex under the viscoelastic from the equator toward the tear, avoiding any stress which may extend the tear.

It is also possible to use the new air-vitrector to aspirate the cortex without cutting through the tear. If the tear is small and central, it may be possible for the surgeon to carefully convert the tear into a continuous posterior capsulorhexis [27–31].

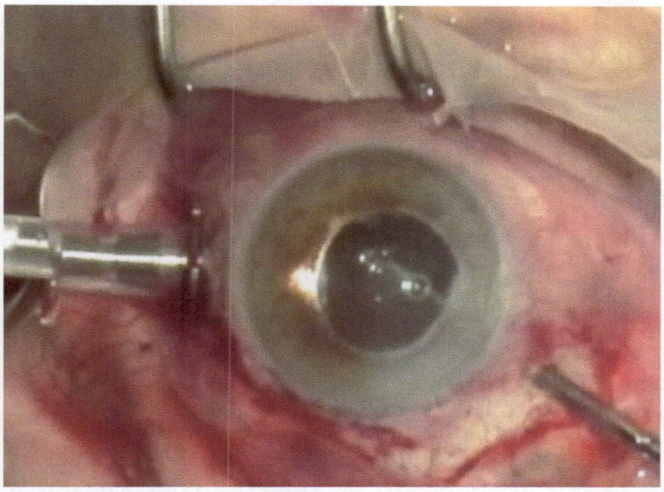

Fig. 7.59 Pars plana vitrectomy

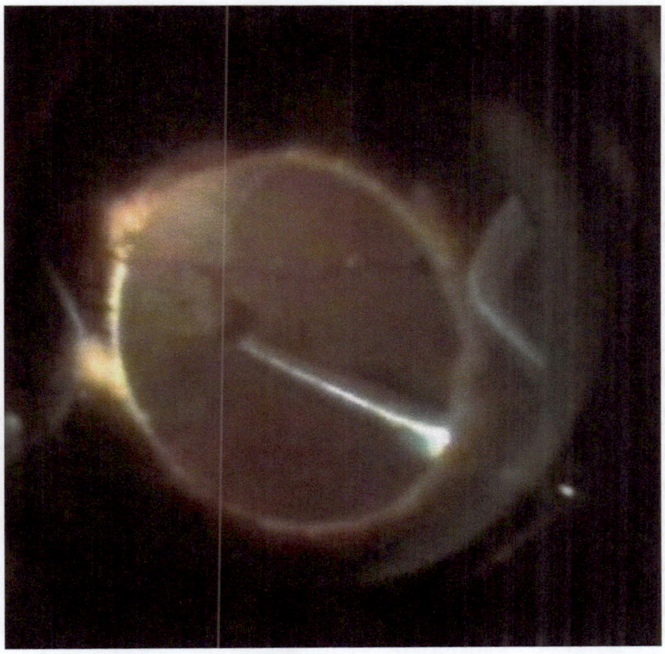

Fig. 7.60 Vitrectomy with phacofragmentation

7.2.4 Different Techniques Other than Pars Plana Vitrectomy for Nuclear Loss in Vitreous

If nuclear material remains, it should be removed either with phacoemulsification or by converting to an extracapsular procedure. Converting to an extracapsular technique is suited for cases in which one or two large pieces remain. If the surgeon chooses to enlarge the wound, it must be large enough to remove the largest fragment in one piece.

Viscoelastic should be placed under the nuclear fragments, which are retrieved by a lens loop. Attempted nuclear expression will likely result in more vitreous prolapse and increases the risk of posterior dislocation of the nuclear material.

Converting MICS to a larger, extracapsular wound is challenging. First, a groove should be extended to the maximum length of the intended enlarged incision, while maintaining a triplanar incision. When closing the wound, care should likewise be taken to prevent a leakage particularly at the main MICS incision.

When the anterior hyaloid face has been ruptured but the nuclear material has not yet luxated into the vitreous, it is recommended to convert to conventional ECCE. Elevating the nucleus with an instrument inserted through the phaco incision is often difficult because of the steep and anterior angle of the approach [43–45]. If total zonulolysis more than 180° is noticed, it will be useful to convert the MICS phaco technique to the old efficient IEC, using dispersive sodium hyaluronate to protect the endothelium.

The posterior assisted levitation (PAL) technique may prevent many complications of a dropped nucleus. It may also prevent the need for three-port pars plana vitrectomy to remove posteriorly dislocated lens fragments. PAL consists of inserting a spatula downward via the pars plana with its tip inclined to the posterior pole of the eye, placing it underneath the nucleus. The spatula then lifts the partially dropped nucleus forward into the anterior chamber. Surgery is completed by extending the wound and expressing the nucleus or by phacoemulsification with a sheet glide behind the nucleus fragments to protect it from falling into the vitreous. A modified PAL technique using sodium hyaluronate 3.0% – chondroitin sulfate 4.0% (Viscoat, Alcon Inc., Fort Worth) was described. The Viscoat PAL may be performed for a partially descended nucleus after posterior capsule rupture. Following pars plana sclerotomy, the nucleus can be elevated by combining posteriorly directed Viscoat viscoelastic injection and manipulation of its cannula tip. If successful, this can help prevent a retained nucleus or subsequent posterior segment surgery to retrieve it [46–48].

7.2.5 Pars Plana Vitrectomy

If the nuclear material has dislocated posteriorly into the vitreous cavity, attempts to float the nucleus upward following a generous vitrectomy are frequently successful. However, there are cases in which it may be best to temporarily leave the lost nucleus behind, clean up the prolapsed vitreous, remove the cortex, and implant an intraocular lens. Consultation with a retina specialist is recommended for the secondary removal of the lens material via a three-port pars plana vitrectomy with phacofragmentation, and it can be scheduled in the early postoperative period. Heroic efforts to "catch" a falling nucleus or retrieve a fallen nucleus from the anterior segment have been associated with an increased risk of retinal complications and ultimately, poorer visual outcomes.

7.2.6 Zonulolysis *(Figs. 7.61 and 7.62)*

Zonulolysis is the most challenging complication that an anterior surgeon can encounter. It may be present naturally, prior to surgery, either as a result of trauma or in association with Marfan Syndrome, Weil-Marchesani Syndrome, or homocystinuria, phacodonesis and iridodonesis. Vitreous in the anterior chamber or visibility of the lens equator may provide important clues to zonular instability. Exfoliation syndrome also results in weakened zonules. Zonulolysis also occurs from intraocular manipulations during surgery. Prompt recognition and avoidance of further trauma is the best initial management.

The capsulorhexis may be more difficult when loose zonules are present and slow movements assisted by a viscoelastic are recommended. The capsular bag can be locally stabilized in the meridian of dehiscence by placing flexible iris retractors around the capsulorhexis

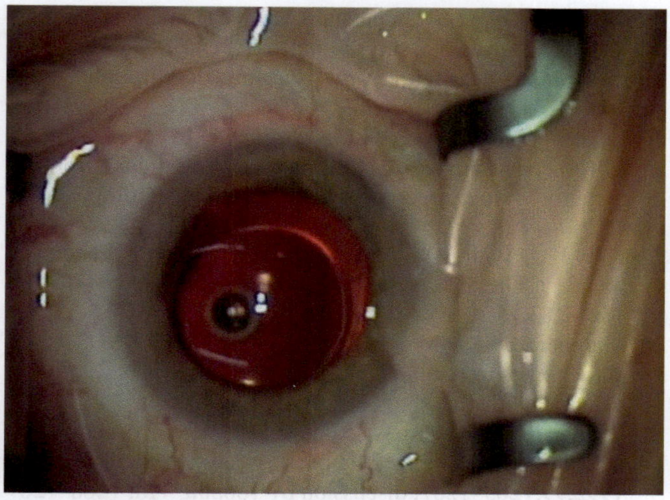

Fig. 7.61 Zonulolysis

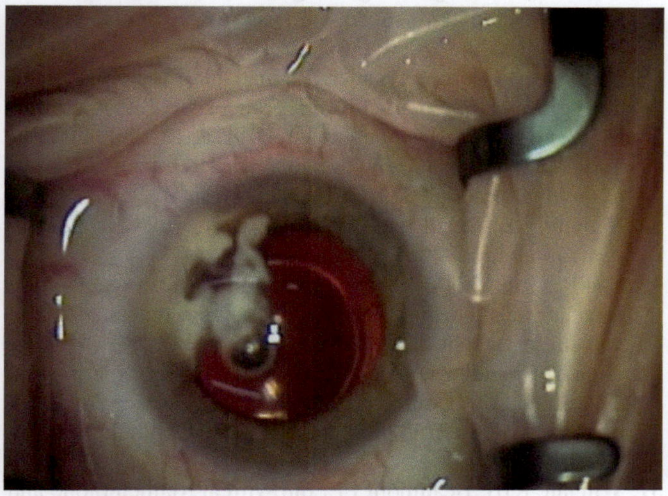

Fig. 7.62 Zonulolysis, vitreous meshwork

margin or placing the Malugin ring [32–34]. The chop phacoemulsification technique will usually allow safe removal of the nucleus.

A highly retentive viscoelastic agent may tamponade the hyaloid face, helping to prevent vitreous prolapse into the anterior chamber. A low bottle height will limit the tendency towards vitreous overhydration. Also, low aspiration settings may help prevent chamber fluctuations, vitreous prolapse, and unintentional traction on the remaining zonules. When zonulolysis is present, cortical aspiration should be performed by gentle irrigation and aspiration with the aid of a viscoelastic, directing all forces tangentially. A capsular tension ring keeps the capsular bag open and evenly distributes the forces on the zonules, making implantation of an intraocular lens into the capsular bag possible [35].

After implanting the lens, the surgeons inject triamcinolone acetate inside the anterior chamber to visualize any vitreous meshwork. If there remains any, an anterior bimanual vitrectomy is recommended.

Take Home Pearls

- Early identification, and successful management of intraoperative complications are the keys to the success of the surgery.
- The triamcinolone stain provides a direct observation of the vitreous and assists surgeons in identifying and completely removing vitreous in the anterior segment, intraoperatively.
- Vitreous visualization by using triamcinolone is useful in minimally invasive surgical techniques to clear the vitreous and to avoid excessive surgical intervention during the management of posterior capsule rupture. However, visualizing the vitreous body using triamcinolone has a potential risk for postoperative steroid-related complications such as glaucoma and infection [36–39].
- The 23 gauge anterior bimanual vitrector is useful to cut a few vitreous strands, but the pars plana sutureless vitrectomy is far more superior in managing vitreous loss after posterior capsular rupture during phacoemulsification [40–42].

References

1. Alio JL. What does MICS require? The transition to microincisional surgery. In: Alio JL, Rodriguez-Prats JL, Galal A (eds), MICS: micro-incision cataract surgery. El Dorado, Republic of Panama, Highlights of Ophthalmology International 2004;1–4
2. Agarwal A, Agarwal A, Agarwal S, et al Phakonit: phacoemulsi-fication through a 0.9 mm corneal incision. J Cataract Refract Surg 2001;27:1548–1552
3. Fine IH, Packer M, Hoffman RS. Management of posterior polar cataract. J Cataract Refract Surg 2003;29:16–19
4. Hyams M, Mathalone N, Herskovitz M, et al Intraoperative complications of phacoemulsification in eyes with and without pseudoexfoliation. J Cataract Refract Surg 2005;31:1002–1005
5. Lifshitz T, Levy J. Posterior assisted levitation: long-term follow-up data. J Cataract Refract Surg 2005;31:499–502

6. Snyder ME, et al Management of intraoperative complication. In: Gills JP (ed), Cataract Surgery: the state of the art. 1998
7. Chitkara DK, Smerdon DL. Risk factors, complications, and results in extracapsular cataract extraction. J Cataract Refract Surg 1997;23:570–574
8. Drolsum L, Haaskjold E. Causes of decreased visual acuity after cataract extraction. J Cataract Refract Surg 1995;21:59–63
9. Ionides A, Minassian D, Tuft S. Visual outcome following posterior capsule rupture during cataract surgery. Br J Ophthalmol 2001;85:222–224
10. Peyman GA, Cheema R, Conway MD, Fang T. Triamcinolone acetonide as an aid to visualization of the vitreous and the posterior hyaloid during pars plana vitrectomy. Retina 2000;20:554–555
11. Burk SE, Da Mata AP, Snyder ME, et al Visualizing vitreous using Kenalog suspension. J Cataract Refract Surg 2003;29:645–651
12. Yamakiri K, Uchino E, Kimura K, Sakamoto T. Intracameral triamcinolone helps to visualize and remove the vitreous body in anterior chamber in cataract surgery. Am J Ophthalmol 2004;138:650–652
13. Hansson L-J, Larsson J. Vitrectomy for retained lens fragments in the vitreous after phacoemulsification. J Cataract Refract Surg 2002;28:1007–1011
14. Chalam KV, Shah VA. Successful management of cataract surgery associated vitreous loss with sutureless small-gauge pars plana vitrectomy. Am J Ophthalmol 2004;138: 79–84
15. Jaffe N. Cataract surgery and its complications. 3rd ed. St.Louis, CV Mosby, 1981; 576–79
16. Luther L. Fry cataract surgical problem: october consultation #10. J Cataract Refract Surg 2005;31:1864–1865
17. Sonoda K-H, Sakamoto T, Enaida H, et al Residual vitreous cortex after surgical posterior vitreous separation visualized by intravitreous triamcinolone acetonide. Ophthalmology 2004;111:226–230
18. Schepens CL, Avila MP, Jalkh AE, et al Role of the vitreous in cystoid macular edema. J Cataract Refract Surg 1984;28: 499–504
19. Berger BB, Zweig KO, Peyman GA. Vitreous loss managed by anterior vitrectomy; long-term follow-up of 59 cases. Arch Ophthalmol 1980;98:1245–1247
20. Li KK, Carl G, Wong D. Management of traumatic posterior capsular rupture: corneal approach with high speed vitrector. J Cataract Refract Surg 2005;31:1666–1668
21. Chang C-J, Chang Y-H, Chiang S-Y, Lin L-T. Comparison of clear corneal phacoemulsification combined with 25-gauge transconjunctival sutureless vitrectomy and standard 20-gauge vitrectomy for patients with cataract and vitreoretinal diseases. J Cataract Refract Surg 2005;31:1198–1207
22. Brauweiler P. Bimanual irrigation/aspiration. J Cataract Refract Surg 1996;22(8):1013–6
23. Moore JK, Scott IU, Flynn HW Jr, et al Retinal detachment in eyes undergoing pars plana vitrectomy for removal of retained lens fragments. Ophthalmology 2003;110:709–713; discussion by Aaberg TM Jr, 713–714
24. Chalam KV, Gupta SK, Vinjamaram S, Shah VA. Small-gauge, sutureless pars plana vitrectomy to manage vitreous loss during phacoemulsification. J Cataract Refract Surg 2003;29:1482–1486
25. Shah VA, Gupta SK, Chalam KV. Management of vitreous loss during cataract surgery under topical anesthesia with transconjunctival vitrectomy system. Eur J Ophthalmol 2003;13:693–696
26. Lakhanpal RR, Humayun MS, de Juan E Jr, et al Outcomes of 140 consecutive cases of 25-gauge transconjunctival surgery for posterior segment disease. Ophthalmology 2005; 112:817–824
27. Kim JE, Flynn HW Jr, Smiddy WE, et al Retained lens fragments after phacoemulsification. Ophthalmology 1994;101: 1827–1832
28. Margherio RR, Margherio AR, Pendergast SD, et al Vitrectomy for retained lens fragments after phacoemulsification. Ophthalmology 1997;104:1426–1432
29. Gilliland GD, Hutton WL, Fuller DG. Retained intravitreal lens frag-ments after cataract surgery. Ophthalmology 1992;99:1263–1267; discussion by Topping TM, 1268–1269
30. Borne MJ, Tasman W, Regillo C, et al Outcomes of vitrectomy for retained lens fragments. Ophthalmology 1996; 103:971–976
31. Jonas JB, Kreissig I, Degenring RF. Intravitreal triamcinolone acetonide for pseudophakic cystoid macular edema. Am J Ophthalmol 2003;136:384–386
32. Graether JF. Pupil expander for managing the small pupil during surgery. J Cataract Refract Surg 1996;22(5):530–5
33. McCuen BW II, Hickenbotham D, Tsai M, deJuan E Jr. Temporary iris fixation with a micro-iris retractor. Archives of Ophthalmology 1989;107(6):925–7
34. Malyugin B. Small pupil phaco surgery: a new technique. Ann Ophthalmol 2007;39:185–193
35. Sun R, Gimbel HV. In vitro evaluation of the efficacy of the capsular tension ring for managing zonular dialysis in cataract surgery. Ophthalmic Surg Lasers 1998;29:502–5
36. Hida T, Chandler D, Arena JE, Machemer R. Experimental and clinical observations of the intraocular toxicity of commercial corticosteroid preparations. Am J Ophthalmol 1986; 101:190–195
37. Wingate RJB, Beaumont PE. Intravitreal triamcinolone and elevated intraocular pressure. Aust NZ J Ophthalmol 1999; 27:431–432
38. Jonas JB, Degenring RF, Kreissig I, et al Intraocular pressure elevation after intravitreal triamcinolone acetonide injection. Ophthalmology 2005;112:593–598
39. Sakamoto T, Enaida H, Kubota T, et al Incidence of acute endophthalmitis after triamcinolone-assisted pars plana vitrectomy. Am J Ophthalmol 2004;138:137–138
40. Leaming DV. Practice styles and preferences of ASCRS members – 2003 survey. J Cataract Refract Surg 2004;30:892–900
41. Yap EY, Heng W-J. Visual outcome and complications after posterior capsule rupture during phacoemulsification surgery. Int Ophthalmol 1999–2000;23:57–60
42. Ng DT, Rowe NA, Francis IC, et al Intraoperative complications of 1000 phacoemulsification procedures: a prospective study. J Cataract Refract Surg 1998;24:1390–1395
43. Ah-Fat FG, Sharma MK, Majid MA, Yang YC. Vitreous loss during conversion from conventional extracapsular cataract extraction to phacoemulsification. J Cataract Refract Surg 1998;24:801–805
44. Akura J, Hatta S, Kaneda S, et al Management of posterior capsule rupture during phacoemulsification using the dry technique. J Cataract Refract Surg 2000;27:982–989

45. Rao SK, Chan W-M, Leung ATS, Lam DSC. Impending dropped nucleus during phacoemulsification [letter]. J Cataract Refract Surg 1999;25:1311–1312
46. Packard RB, Kelman C. Posterior capsular rupture: PAL technique. Video J Cataract Refract Surg 1996;12:30
47. Teichmann KD. Posterior assisted levitation [letter]. Surv Ophthalmol 2002;47:78
48. Chang DF, Packard RB. Posterior assisted levitation for nucleus retrieval using viscoat after posterior capsule rupture. J Cataract Refract Surg 2003;29:1860–1865

7.3 How to Deal with Very Hard and Intumescent Cataracts

L. Felipe Vejarano

Core Messages

- Hard and intumescent cataracts are challenging and difficult cases for the surgeon and so special care must always be taken.
- It is essential to know the size of each instrument that will be used, and to plan the incision size carefully so as to avoid too tight incisions that would compromise maneuvrability, or too large incisions that would cause leakage and anterior chamber instability.
- During capsulorhexis, it is recommended to stain the anterior capsule with a dye in order to best visualize it and then minimize the tension within the capsular bag by extracting the milky cortical substance.
- Hydrodissection is an important step that should be done carefully in order to avoid "Capsular Block syndrome."
- Knowledge of the fluidics of the machine and proper instrumentation is essential to perform phacoemulsification in these cases.

7.3.1 Introduction

Any kind of cataract should pose as a challenge to all cataract surgeons, because there is no one case exactly alike. This is particularly true with very hard and intumescent cataracts, because they are always challenging cases in coaxial phaco, more so in biaxial microincision phacoemulsification.

In this chapter, techniques on how to deal with very hard cataracts will be explained. Beginning with incision

L. F. Vejarano
Department of Ophthalmology, Universidad del Cauca, Popayán, Colombia
e-mail: felipev@fov.com.co

up to phacoemulsification, a step-by-step approach to manage hard cataracts and those with absorbed cortex will be elaborated. The advantages of biaxial and microbiaxial techniques over the coaxial technique will be emphasized.

7.3.2 Types of Cataracts

As a review, cataracts can now be classified based on the lens opacities classification III (LOCS III) (Fig. 7.63). It involves grading four features of the cataract by comparing features seen against a set of transparencies. These four parameters are:

1. Nuclear color (NC)
2. Nuclear opalescence (N)
3. Cortical cataract (C)
4. Posterior subcapsular (P)

Based on this classification, hard and intumescent cataracts can be graded as NO5 to NO6 with NC4 to NC6.

7.3.3 Management of Hard Cataracts Through Biaxial Technique

The Biaxial (less than 1.5 mm) or MicroBiaxial (less than 1 mm) technique which separates the two functions in phacoemulsification (irrigation/manipulation from the aspiration/ emulsification) offers more than just the advantage of incision size in these types of cataracts. Starting with capsulorrhexis, smaller incision sizes prevent the evacuation of the viscoelastic (OVD) during this step, thereby diminishing the risk of the anterior capsular tear. Furthermore, it provides better and safer manipulation of the capsule and an easier hydrodissection. Also, depending upon the fluidics, the stability of the anterior chamber during emulsification is maintained, guaranteeing less risk of posterior capsule rupture, less endothelial cell and uveal trauma and consequently, a faster recovery time for the patient.

7.3.4 Incision

The side port incision must be watertight when the instrument (irrigating chopper) is in place, without compromising its maneuverability. This is a very important aspect, since in biaxial phaco, this is the instrument that makes most of the movements necessary to emulsify the nucleus. For this reason, the authors suggest the use of a trapezoidal-shaped knife to create the side port incision. This means internally, the incision is narrower which makes it watertight, and externally it is wider to provide more room for the movement of the instrument. If the surgeon finds maneuvering of the instrument through this incision difficult, it is a

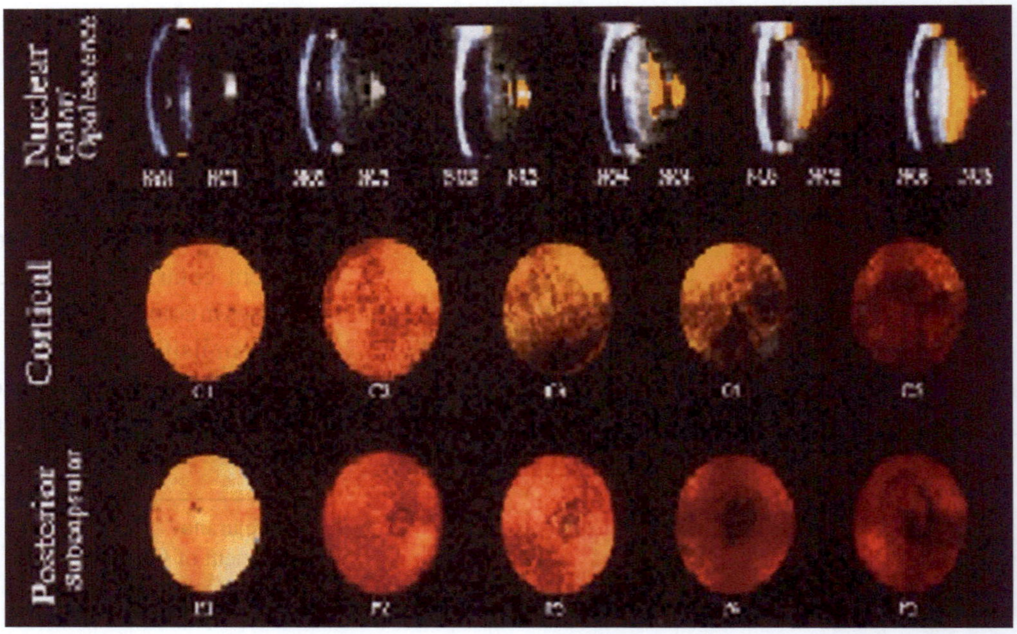

Fig. 7.63 The lens opacities classification system III (LOCS III)

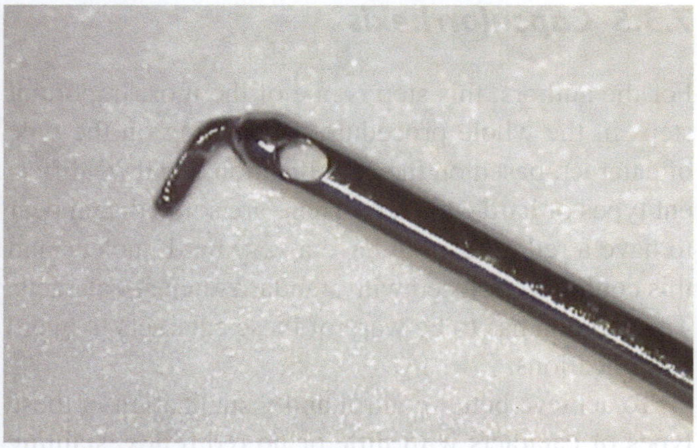

Fig. 7.64 Vejarano's irrigating chopper 20 guage. with oval lateral holes

good idea to apply a small amount of viscoelastic on the chopper to make its movement easier.

The authors have found that for performing a trapezoidal 0.9/1.3 mm (inner/outer size) incision, Vejarano's irrigating chopper® (AC7340, Accutome, Malvern) (Fig. 7.64) can be used.

It has a 20 gauge tip (approximately 0.9 mm diameter), and fits snugly into the incision, thus there is no leakage from the site. It also provides very good maneuverability which is suitable for the biaxial approach. To achieve a good wound architecture, the authors, likewise, suggest the use of a 0.9/1.3 mm diamond knife (Accutome, Malvern) (Fig. 7.65) to create this incision is suggested. An alternative is to use 20 gauge vitreoretinal blades (Fig. 7.66) or 1.2/1.4 mm steel blades (MicroSurgical Technology – MST, Redmond) (Fig. 7.67).

When performing the main incision, a 1.2 mm diamond lancet or the same 0.9/1.3 mm diamond knife can be used to avoid additional expense (Both Accutome, Malvern). When using a 20-gauge Phaco Microtip, it is not necessary for the main incision to be trapezoidal in shape because in the biaxial approach, the phaco needle does not move considerably. Mainly, the movements of the phaco tip are restricted to forward and backward movements only to look for the fragmented nucleus, then return back to the center to emulsify them, and bring the fragments near the internal lip of the incision to unocclude the tip. It also serves to reduce the excessive movements of the second instrument thus preventing additional damage or deformation of the sideport incision.

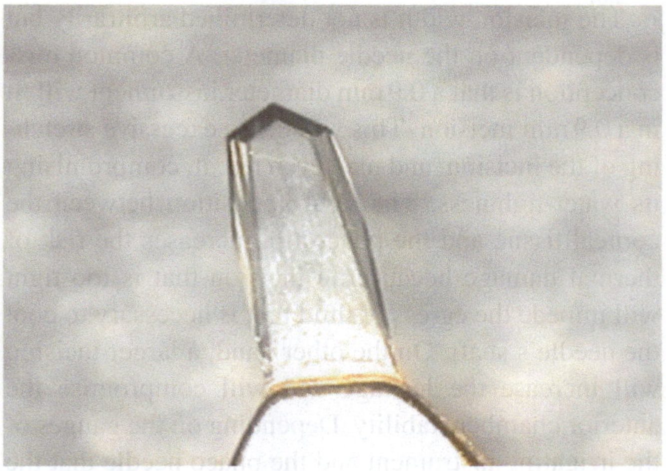

Fig. 7.65 Diamond blade for side port incision

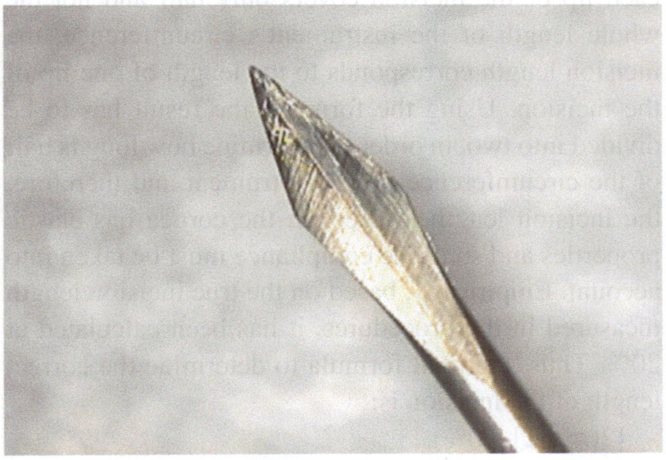

Fig. 7.66 MVR blade 20 guage

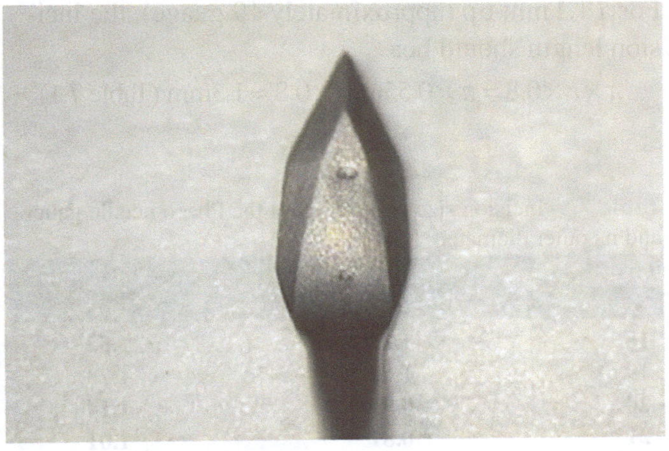

Fig. 7.67 Trapezoidal metal blade

The incision width is not determined arbitrarily but is dependent on the needle diameter. A common misconception is that a 0.9 mm diameter instrument will fit in a 0.9 mm incision. This will cause excessive stretching of the incision, and may even tear it, compromising its water-tightness. The tight apposition between the corneal tissue and the phaco tip, increases the risk of thermal damage because an incision that is too tight will impede the egress of fluid that is necessary to cool the needle's shaft. On the other hand, a larger incision will increase the leakage and will compromise the anterior chamber stability. Depending on the gauges of the irrigating instrument and the phaco needle that the surgeon used, he can determine the proper size of the incisions. He can calculate the circumference length of the instrument using the formula $[2(\pi \times r)]$, where "r" means the radius of the instrument in mm. Then, since each lip of the incision covers only half and not the whole length of the instrument's circumference, the incision length corresponds to the length of one lip of the incision. Using the formula, the result has to be divided into two, in order to determine how long is half of the circumference of the instrument and therefore, the incision length. Moreover, the cornea has elastic properties and so tissue compliance must be taken into account. Empirically, based on the true incision length measured in the procedures, it has been calculated at 20%. Thus, the final formula to determine the correct length of the incision is:

$[2(\pi r / 2]–20\%)$.

This may be simplified as:

$\pi \times r \times 0.8$.

For instance, for a 0.9 mm tip (approximately 20 guage), the incision length should be:

$\pi \times r \times 0.8 = \pi \times 0.45\text{mm} \times 0.8 \approx 1.1\text{mm}$.

For a 1.1 mm tip (approximately 19 guage), the incision length should be:

$\pi \times r \times 0.8 = \pi \times 0.55\text{mm} \times 0.8 \approx 1.3\text{mm}$ (Table 7.1).

Table 7.1 Incision size depending on the Phaco needle gauge and its outer diameter [1–4]

Gauge	Milimeters	Incision (mm)
18	**1.22**	**1.53**
19	1.02	1.28
20	**0.91**	**1.14**
21	**0.81**	**1.01**
22	**0.71**	**0.89**

7.3.5 Capsulorrhexis

For the authors, this step is one of the most important steps in the whole procedure. Depending on the type of cataract, based on the classification, we have different types of hard cataracts. There are some that appear to have a red reflex, but have a very hard nucleus and this could be confused with standard nuclear cataracts. The surgeon has to be wary of these cataracts to avoid complications.

To achieve better control and visualization in these types of cataracts with little or no red reflex, staining the anterior capsule is suggested to ensure a complete curvilinear capsulorrhexis. Staining also avoids undue zonular stress in cases of difficult capsulorhexis because most of these cataracts have weak zonules.

Depending on whether the surgeon is dealing with intumescent cataracts or hard ones with absorbed cortex, the capsulorrhexis is different for each type of cataract.

Intumescent Cataracts: As mentioned before, when the lens become swollen by absorbing water in cases of intumescent cataracts, the whole capsular bag is tense because of the liquid that fills the bag. When the anterior capsule is punctured to initiate the capsulorrhexis and release the tension inside, there is a big chance for the tear to extend into the periphery. There are many ways to avoid this. One is taking a photograph of the anterior chamber using the Pentacam preoperatively with dilated pupil, and measuring the anterior chamber and nuclear thickness [5] to be sure that it is a real intumescent cataract or just a milky one.

To determining whether it is a real intumescent cataract, it is recommended to fill the anterior chamber with the dye of preference. Trypan Blue can be used, diluting the commercially available 0.1% solution to a 0.05% solution for contrast and visualization of the anterior capsule. It perfectly stains the anterior capsule even if diluted. The dye is left to stain the capsule for at least 30 s and is removed with the viscoelastic. The best kind of viscoelastic for this purpose, due to its rheological properties, is the cohesive one. This is due to the fact that cohesive OVD's do not seep out from the small incision and it maintains the anterior capsule flat and deep enough to avoid any unexpected tear.

The next step is to make a puncture in the anterior capsule and release the tension inside. There are many ways to do this as well. First, with a needle engaged in a syringe and inserted inside the bag, the milky

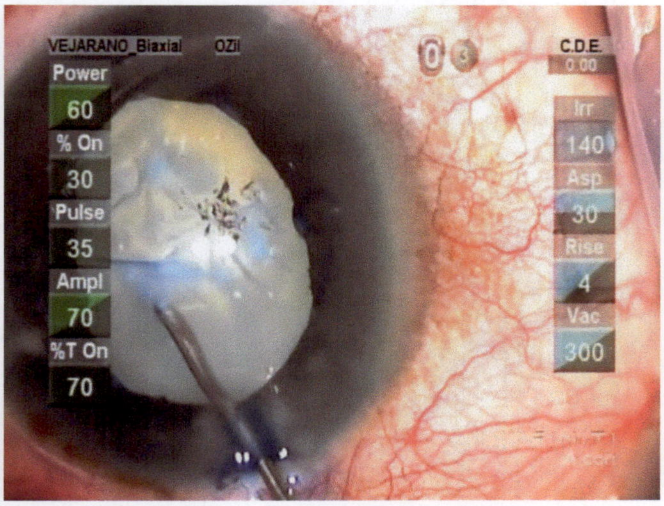

Fig. 7.68 Needle puncture of the anterior capsule to release the tension inside the capsular bag

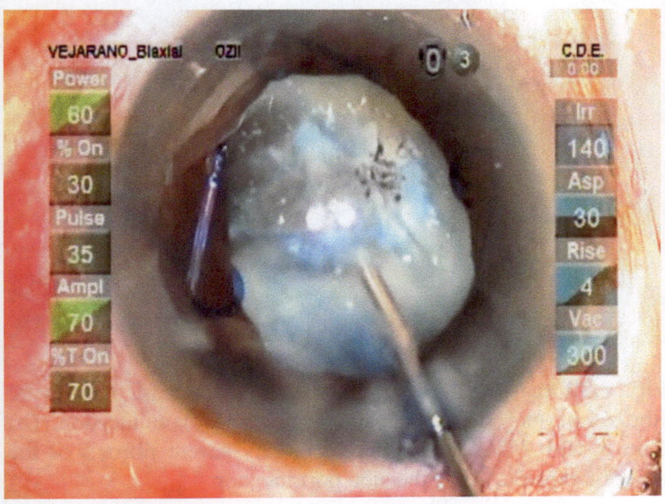

Fig. 7.69 Filling the capsular bag with viscoelastic after aspiration of the milky substance

substance is aspirated through the needle or the cannula (Fig. 7.68).

After this, the MicroUtrata forceps (MicroSurgical Technology – MST) is inserted and the rhexis is done. Depending on the amount of the milky substance that was removed and the size of the nucleus, the bag can be filled with a Viscoelastic to separate both capsules and to reshape the bag thereby, improving the rhexis (Fig. 7.69).

Another maneuver is also to make a small central tear with one of the tips of the microutrata (Fig. 7.70a) (MicroSurgical Technology – MST) and immediately lift up a flap of the anterior capsule and begin the rhexis tear. The milky liquid is released out of the bag,

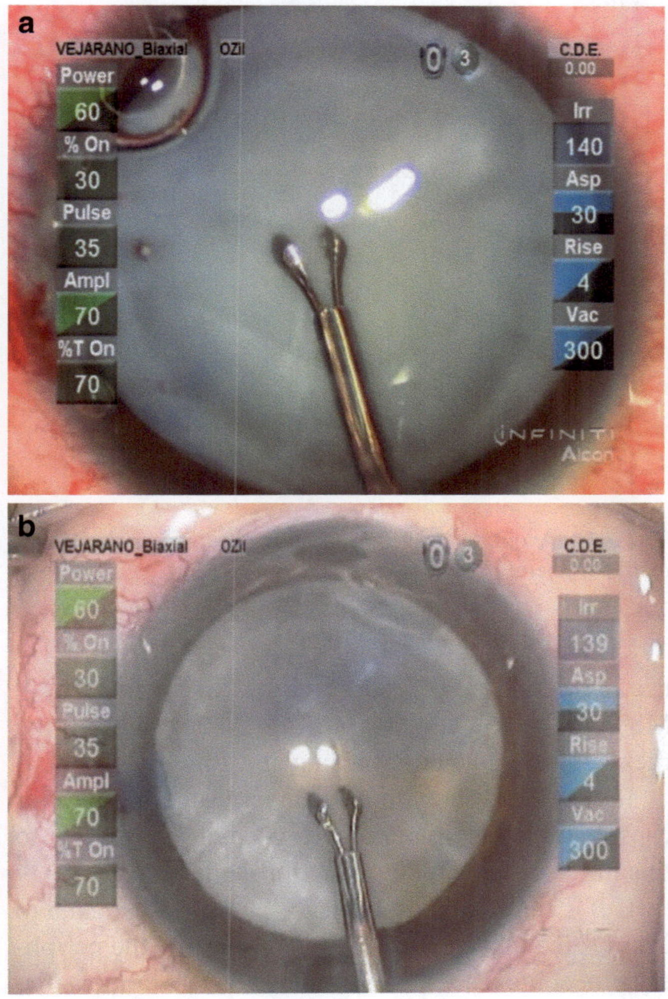

Fig. 7.70 (**a**) Begin the tear directly with the tip of the Microutrata, and lift the flap to initiate the Rhexis. (**b**) Begin the tear directly with the tip of the Microutrata, and lift the flap to initiate the Rhexis

causing forward pressure over the posterior lip of the incision to force out some Viscoelastic mixed with the cataract substance. Refill the anterior chamber with clear Viscoelastic and continue the rhexis.

The other maneuver is the introduction of the phaco needle bevel down, to aspirate the anterior capsule just at the center and the release of a short burst of Ultrasound to open the anterior capsule in a circular shape. Immediately aspirate some material to decrease the tension and facilitate the rhexis.

Hard Cataract with Reabsorbed Cortex: Almost all of these cataracts don't have any cortex material, but compared with intumescent cataracts, there is a greater zonular traction and stress because of the fibrosis or retraction of the anterior capsule. After staining and flattening the capsule, the surgeon can

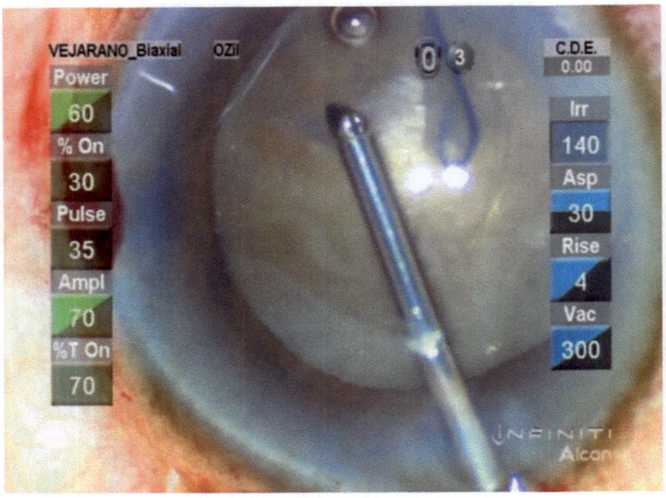

Fig. 7.71 Avoid the subcapsular fibrosis making the rhexis more peripheral

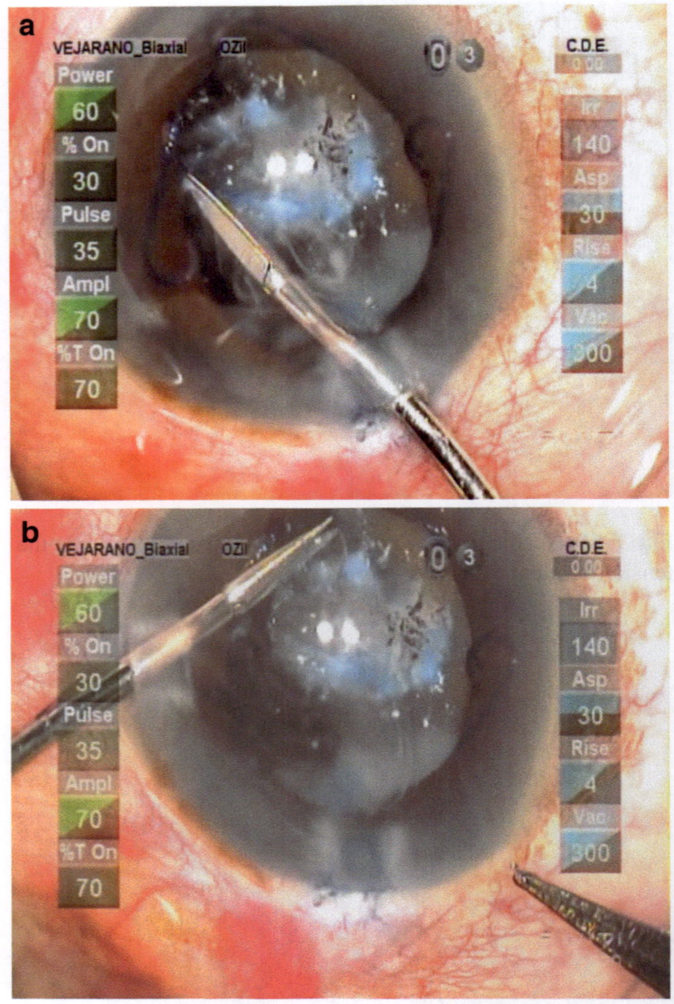

Fig. 7.72 (**a**) Rhexis with Microscissors because the severe fibrosis of the anterior capsule, using the main incision. (**b**) Rhexis with Microscissors because they severe fibrosis of the anterior capsule, using the side port incision

use a MicroUtrata tip (MicroSurgical Technology – MST) to create a central tear (Fig. 7.70b) and start the rhexis in slow manner avoiding any zonular tension.

If there is some fibrosis underneath the anterior capsule, it is recommended to go more peripheral to this fibrosis and avoid passing through it (Fig. 7.71).

If it is impossible to avoid it, care must be taken to avoid force that can direct the tear towards the periphery. In some cases, the fibrosis covers almost the whole anterior capsule preventing a normal rhexis with the Microutrata. For this purpose, Microscissors (MicroSurgical Technology – MST) can be used to cut the fibrosis and continue the rhexis. However, there are some cataracts with severe fibrosis and the whole rhexis needs to be performed with microscissors (MicroSurgical Technology – MST) using both incisions (main and sideport) to achieve a complete continuous Capsulorhexis (Fig. 7.72a, b).

When the surgeon starts the capsulorrhexis, he should always lift it up and fold it over to have control of the tear. Grasp the flap as many times as needed. The size of the rhexis is very important in these cases. Even if it is recommended to create a 5.5–6.0 mm capsulorrhexis to avoid posterior capsule opacification in order to prevent the contact of both the capsules with the anterior capsule over the optic zone of the IOL, a larger rhexis is needed. This facilitates the removal of the pieces of the nucleus that are very large, rigid and adherent to the bag. It also prevents any zonular traction, tension and forces against the zonular fibers, thereby avoiding zonular dialysis.

7.3.6 Hydrodissection

This is another surgical step that is very important, especially in these kinds of cataracts. One has to be certain that the nucleus is free from adherences to the bag, mainly from the equator and also from the posterior capsule plaque.

Unlike the coaxial Phaco, in biaxial phaco, the incision is very small and tight. To prevent any sudden rise of the IOP that can cause backward distension of the zonula, before injecting BSS into the bag, some of the Viscoelastic must be extracted from the anterior chamber. Always use a blunt cannula. Begin with an anhydric dissection, which means that the anterior capsule in its edge is lifted, separating the anterior surface of the nucleus from the posterior surface of the anterior capsule. In hard cataracts with reabsorbed cortex, where the space between the two is very tight, this technique helps to create some space that allows the surgeon to introduce the cannula and the fluid. In intumescent cataracts, the surgeon aspirates the cortex, most of the time, the nucleus is already loose and it is not necessary to perform hydrodissection.

A stream of BSS is injected in a controlled and continuous fashion. Since it is impossible to see the wave underneath the nucleus, the surgeon needs to be aware of the time when the nucleus moves up and forward against the edges of the rhexis, and at that precise moment stop injecting BSS. The nucleus is pushed away 180° from the injection site to avoid bag distension that can cause rupture of the posterior capsule and nucleus drop by blocking the egress of BSS (*capsular block syndrome*). The nucleus is also pushed back to allow the fluid, retained underneath the hard cataract, to escape thereby releasing the nucleus from its adherences, to the equator and facilitating its rotation.

The surgeon has to be sure that the nucleus is free of all its attachments to the capsule by rotating it carefully bimanually with two hooks (Sinskey, Lester or Kuglen) with viscoelastic or with a curved blunt cannula, irrigating continuously to avoid zonular stress, because in most of the cases of hard cataracts, its zonules are weak.

7.3.7 Phacoemulsification

When performing Biaxial or MicroBiaxial microincision Phacoemulsification surgery, knowledge and management of fluidics are crucial [1, 2, 6, 7]. The issue of an unstable anterior chamber during the procedure, mentioned by several authors [8, 9], like Tsuneoka et al. [10], is basically due to the fact that more fluid is going out of the eye than the amount that is entering into the anterior chamber in a given moment. Although smaller-incision surgery provides a more tightly closed and stable anterior chamber, the equilibrium between inflow and outflow is still critical. This has been one of the biggest problems for surgeons learning Biaxial or MicroBiaxial Phaco, since the rate of irrigation in this technique is usually less than in standard Coaxial Phacoemulsification (Table 7.2).

The factors that influence the fluid balance in Biaxial or MicroBiaxial microincision Phacoemulsification are the following:

Table 7.2 Comparative Inflow between coaxial and most of the irrigating choppers in the Market

Irrigating chopper	Gravity 2 extenders (mL/min)	IOP 100 mmHg (mL/min)	AVGFI 120 mmHg (mL/min)
Coaxial	114	142	131
Tsuneoka	74	88	75
Olson I – II	73	81	77
Nagahara	74	84	75
Braga-mele	**60**	**68**	**61**
Vejarano hor.	**57**	**66**	**60**
Vejarano inf.	**44**	**55**	**45**
Vejarano 22 ga	**44**	**55**	**54**
Irrig. 20 GA	58	67	64
Irrig. 22 GA	46	58	53

Table 7.3 Relative flow depends on the phaco needle diameter based on Poiseuille's law (courtesy Uday Devgan, M.D.)

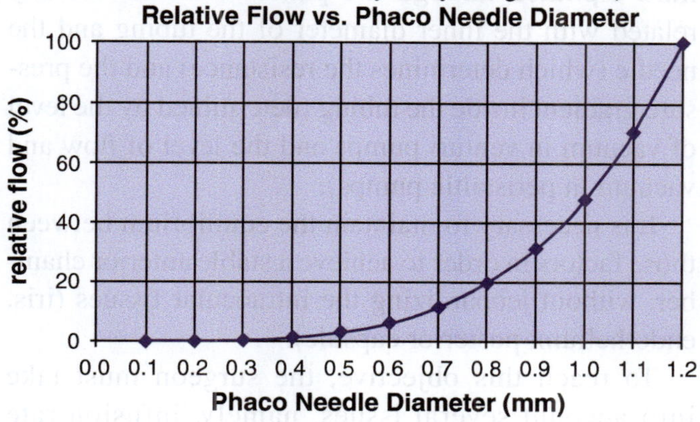

- *The infusion rate of the irrigating instruments*: This is determined by the fluidic resistance of the irrigating line and the instruments (determined by the inner diameter of tubing and instruments – chopper – and the irrigating port size) and the pressure of the fluid (bottle height or amount of positive pressure applied to the bottle by any active system).

The flow of the fluid may be calculated using the Poiseuille's equation (Table 7.3):

$$F = \Delta P \cdot \pi r^4 / 8\eta L,$$

where F: flow; ΔP: pressure gradient; π: 3.1416; r^4: radius of the tube at fourth power; η: viscosity of fluid; L: length of the tube. So inflow is directly proportional to the radius of the tube or instrument's hollow shaft and the pressure gradient of the fluid (determined by gravity according to bottle height, or the amount of positive pressure applied to the bottle by any active system), and inversely proportional to the length of the tube and the viscosity of the fluid. In clinical settings, usually the first two factors may be modified easily. The last two usually, are rather constant.

- *The amount of leakage through the incisions*: This is determined by the relation between the outer diameter of the instruments (Phaco needle and irrigating chopper) and the incisions' architecture (shape, size and presence of an inner valve).
- *The amount of fluid aspirated through the phaco needle:* This is determined by the resistance of the aspirating line (the inner diameter of tubing, needle and tubing compliance) and the level of the vacuum in venturi pumps and the level of the flow and the vacuum in peristaltic pumps.

This may be calculated again using the Poiseuille's equation (Table 7.3), which states that the amount of fluid aspirated through the phaco needle is directly related with the inner diameter of the tubing and the needle (which determines the resistance) and the pressure gradient inside the tubing (determined by the level of vacuum in venturi pumps and the level of flow and vacuum in peristaltic pumps).

It is necessary to maintain the equilibrium between those factors in order to achieve a stable anterior chamber, without jeopardizing the intraocular tissues (iris, endothelium, posterior capsule).

To reach this objective, the surgeon must take into account several issues, namely, infusion rate of the irrigating instruments, amount of leakage through the incisions, and amount of fluid aspirated through the phaco needle.

In Biaxial or MicroBiaxial phaco, it is not possible to have the same high vacuum levels that the surgeon was used to, because the inflow that he got through an irrigating chopper would never be like the one that could be obtained through coaxial irrigation in standard phacoemulsification (Table 7.2). It is, however, very similar with the new Microcoaxial Phacoemulsification with the Ultrasleeve. The Inflow in Biaxial with the Vejarano's Irrigating chopper 20 guage (AC7340, Accutome, Malvern) (Fig. 7.73) is 49% of the Coaxial and 84% of the Microcoaxial. The Inflow in MicroBiaxial with the Vejarano's Irrigating Chopper 22 guage (MicroSurgical Technology – MST) (Fig. 7.74) is 41% of the Coaxial and 70% of the Microcoaxial, and the Microcoaxial is 58% of the standard Coaxial Phaco (Table 7.4). It is recommended that the surgeon change and adapt the parameters depending on the irrigating chopper that he is going to use. For example, if the irrigation is located in front, he has to reduce the parameters to 65%, if it has inferior irrigation, to 58%, and if the irrigation is at the lateral side to 50% (based on the data of the Table 7.2 comparing with a Coaxial Inflow).

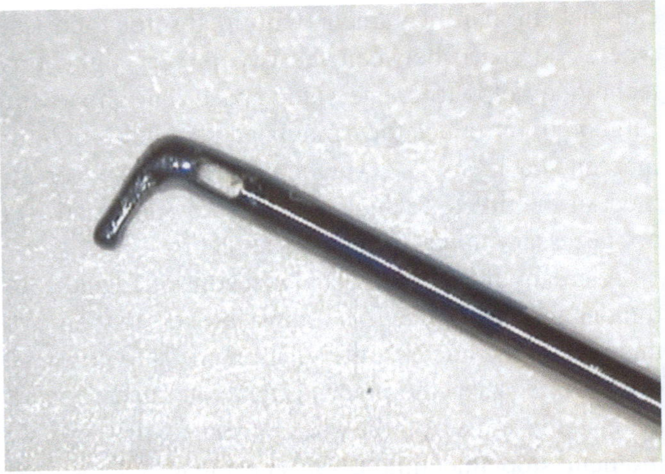

Fig. 7.73 Vejarano's irrigating chopper 22 guage. with rectangular lateral holes

Also the aspiration flow has to be adjusted in order to avoid surpassing levels above 25–30 mL/min, using the fluidic control software of the phaco machine with bimodal or linear aspiration. This reduces the rise time and makes the events inside the anterior chamber more controllable [11–13].

Since the goal of the surgery is not solely to maintain the anterior chamber depth, but also to permit the emulsification of the nucleus, it is necessary to use levels of vacuum which would allow the surgeon to achieve a good hold of the nucleus and its fragments, and likewise, perform an effective chopping procedure. In peristaltic machines, it is necessary to use standard flow levels between 25 and 30 mL/min and vacuum levels of 250–300 mmHg. In venturi machines, a vacuum level of 120–160 mmHg would suffice.

Table 7.4 Comparative Inflow depending on the phaco tip, sleeve and incision size in coaxial and microcoaxial phacoemulsification (courtesy Armando Crema, M.D.)

Irrig / min (mL)	Percentage of Irrig	Tip	Incision (mm)
136	**100**	**1.1 Flared**	**2.75**
106	78	1.1 Flared mini/tape	2.75
95	**69**	**1.1 Flared**	**2–2.2**
79	**58**	**Tapered or mini-flared**	**2–2.2**

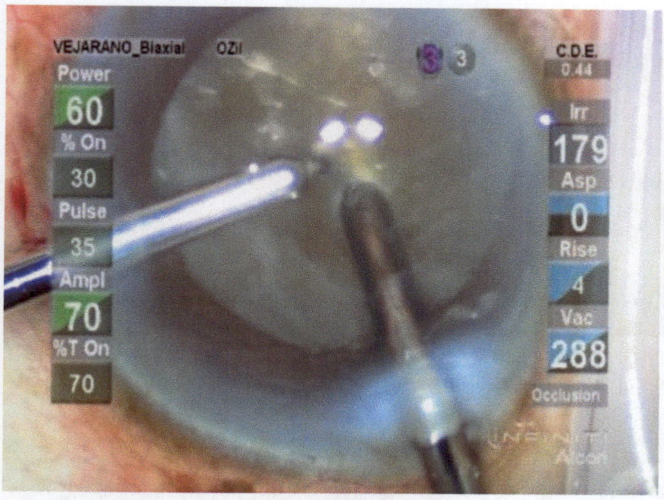

Fig. 7.74 Impaling the nucleus with the phaco tip bevel down, before the chopping maneuver

Poiseuille's equation states that with a smaller diameter of the needle, the flow will be less (Table 7.3). This means that the vacuum needs to be increased to be comparable with the holding power of needles with larger diameters.

In Biaxial phacoemulsification, although any technique can be used to emulsify the nucleus such as divide and conquer, nucleus disassembly or nucleus fracture, these are not recommended in hypermature cataracts due to its bare tip, less maneuverability and tight incisions which makes it more difficult for these maneuvers.

For this reason, in these hypermature cataracts, it is better to use chopping techniques that the surgeon is familiar with. However, the authors recommend the Vejarano's safe chop [14–24].

Briefly described, the phaco tip, with its bevel down after aspirating the anterior cortex and epinucleus, is placed in the proximal portion of the nucleus, and pulsed or preferably applied with burst ultrasound energy, so that it penetrates deep into the nuclear core (Fig. 7.74).

When the tip is impaled into the nucleus, the foot pedal is switched to position two. At this moment, the irrigating chopper is lightly rotated horizontally, tilted, so that the longest length of the tip is against the space between the CCC edge and the lens material (space that, in brunescent and very hard cataracts is very small, or even absent). The tilted chopper is slid beneath the anterior capsule, 180° from the side port incision (Fig. 7.75). This maneuver is much easier to perform,

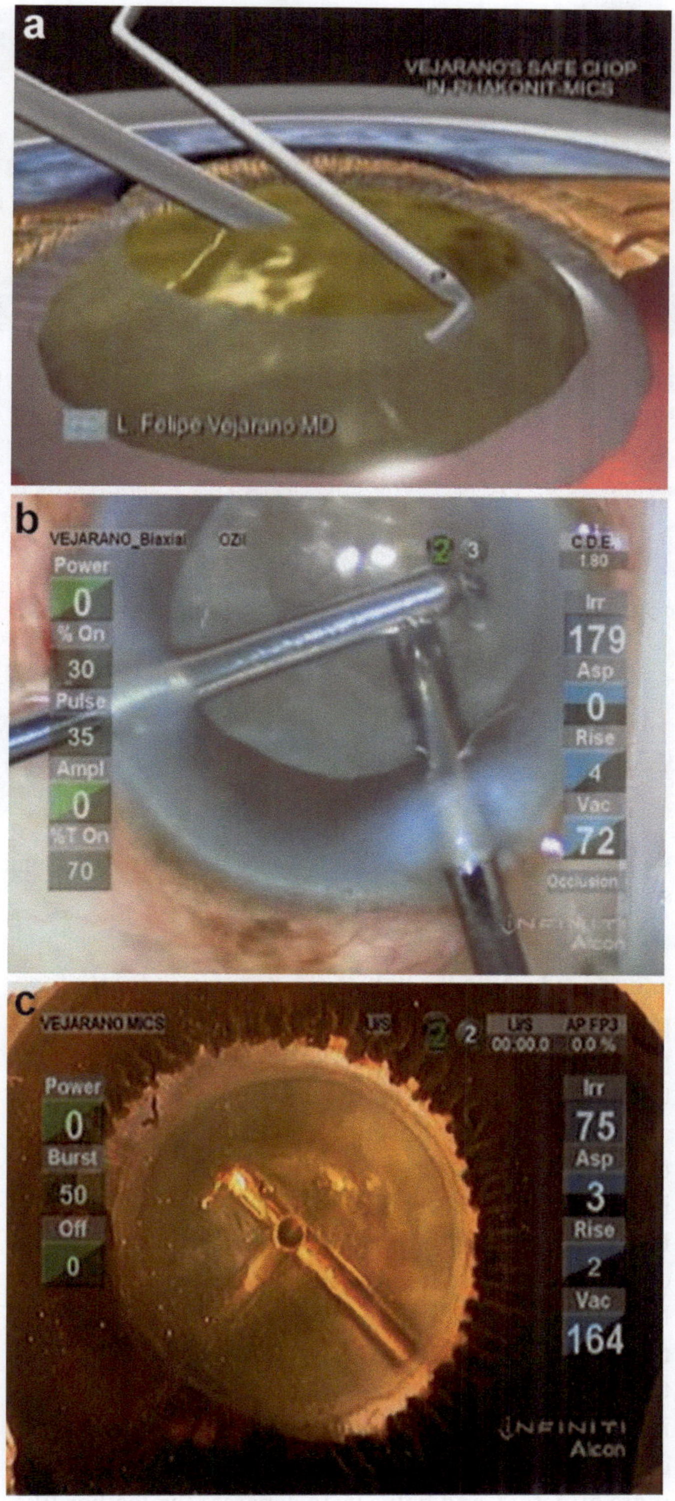

Fig. 7.75 Irrigating chopper tilted, sliding underneath anterior capsule avoiding its damage, going to equator capsular bag previous to its rotation; (**a**) 3D animation, (**b**) surgeon view, (**c**) Miyake view

than trying to slide it under the anterior capsule, just in front of the phaco tip. Afterwards, when reaching the equator of the nucleus, the chopper is rotated vertically

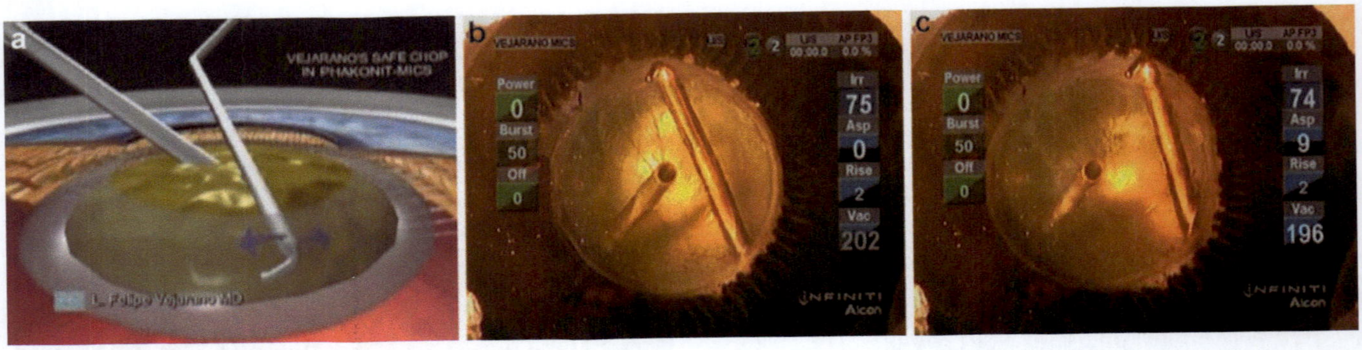

Fig. 7.76 Irrigating Chopper underneath anterior capsule inside the capsular bag rotating until inferior part of the nucleus; (**a**) 3D animation, (**b**, **c**) Miyake view

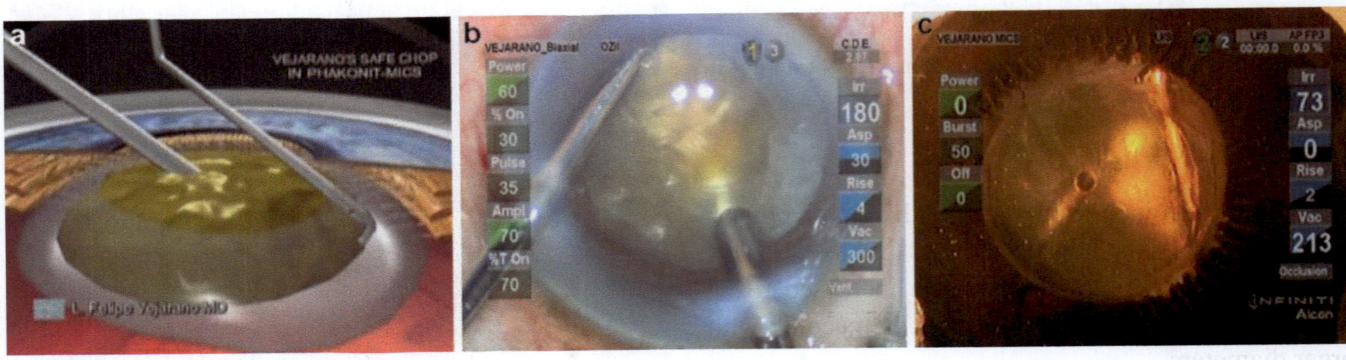

Fig. 7.77 Irrigating Chopper is in position to make the chopping maneuver at inferior equator of the nucleus; (**a**) 3D animation, (**b**) surgeon view, (**c**) Miyake view

and moved inside the bag, to the position in front of the phaco tip (Fig. 7.76). The chopping maneuver takes place. In hard cataracts the nucleus is held between the two instruments for a moment, and a small amount of additional pulsed ultrasound energy is applied, so that the tip penetrates deeper in the nuclear material improving the holding power (Fig. 7.77). This allows to gain improved control of the whole nucleus during the chopping process, since it doesn't become easily dislodged, as long as the high vacuum and the deep position of the tip maintain a tight occlusion seal around the tip. One very important advantage of this technique is that with this very good purchase of the nucleus, especially in hard cataracts, the chopping process is more effective, and helps us to separate the leather-like very hard posterior layers of those cataracts, that often present a challenge to the surgeon.

After dividing the nucleus into halves, it is rotated 45° to try to get the first piece of the heminucleus. The technique to avoid damaging the CCC while chopping the nuclear fragments, is to insert the irrigation chopper vertically and along the fracture lines of the nucleus (Fig. 7.78), where there is more room for the chopper. It is moved to reach its chopping position again only when it is already at the lens' equator, inside the capsular bag, thereby, making this step completely SAFE (thus the name of the technique). It is repeated as many times as necessary to remove the first piece (Fig. 7.79).

The features of the fluidics and the design of the Vejarano's irrigating chopper (AC7340, Accutome, Malvern – MicroSurgical Technology – MST), with lateral oval irrigating ports and olive-tip at its end makes it easier to slide the chopper's tip inside the bag, since it inflates the bag (Fig. 7.76a), and also protects the posterior capsule from accidental puncture.

The subsequent fragments are managed in the same way. When several nuclear fragments have been emulsified, the amount of remaining nuclear material is less and there is more room in the center, so that it is not usually necessary to go beneath the anterior CCC in order to chop them.

The epinucleus, if present, is aspirated using a flip technique. The posterior capsule is protected with the irrigation chopper that is used like a barrier, to avoid damaging the tissues. Bimanual Irrigation/Aspiration of cortical remnants using bimanual handpieces and, if necessary, posterior capsule polishing are done.

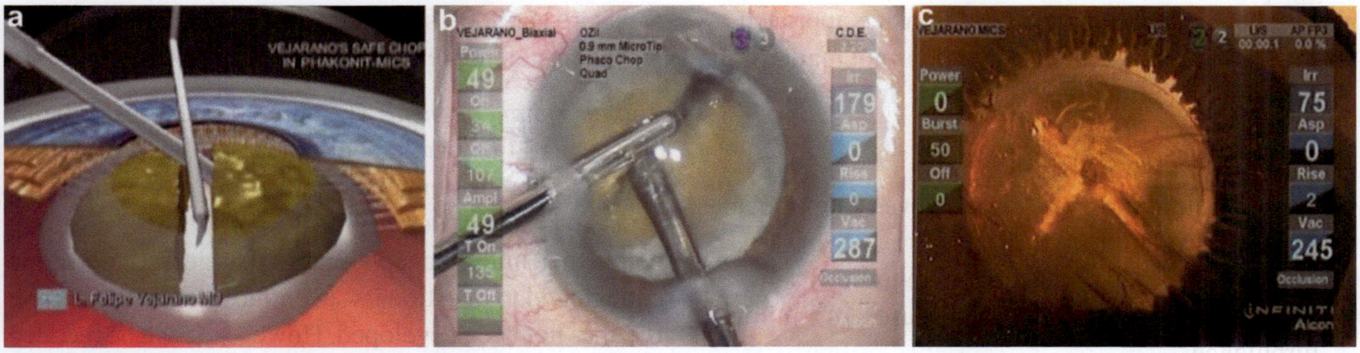

Fig. 7.78 Irrigating Chopper is introduced along the fracture line avoiding any damage of the anterior capsule and giving it the SAFE position inside the capsular bag to rotate it again; (**a**) 3D animation, (**b**) surgeon view, (**c**) Miyake view

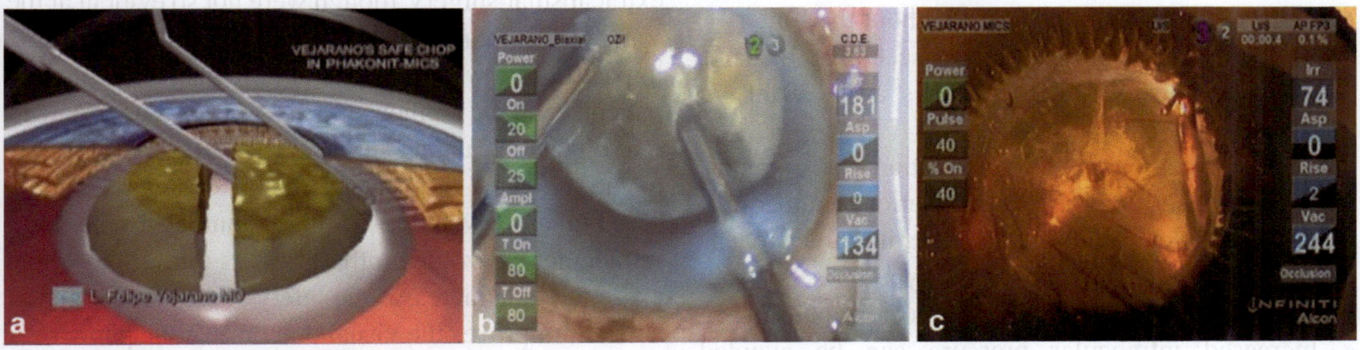

Fig. 7.79 The SAFE maneuver is repeated as many times as is necessary, rotating the Irrigating Chopper close to the equator until inferior nucleus and making the chop to obtain nuclear pieces to emulsify them at the center; (**a**) 3D animation, (**b**) surgeon view, (**c**) Miyake view

The use of capsular tension rings (CTR) depends if the nucleus is subluxated because of the capsular retraction or if the zonular support is felt to be very weak.

The decision of the IOL is still a point of discussion, if you have to enlarge the main incision or if you make a new one between your two incisions, only to insert your IOL.

7.3.8 Conclusion

The author had been doing Biaxial since October 2002 and MicroBiaxial since November 2005 and in December 2005, switched entirely to Microincision and stopped performing Coaxial. This means that any kind of cataract, be it the hypermature type, could be extracted by Phacoemulsification through Microincision with Biaxial or MicroBiaxial technique.

These techniques are very reliable and safe, if one understands the fluidics more than just the power modulation, because with only the pulse mode, it is possible to perform this technique. There is not a single case reported with corneal burn with Biaxial. This technique does not need the obligatory power modulation software in the machine. Of course, it would be better if it is available, however, if the surgeon can control solely the fluidics, he can avoid the instability of the anterior chamber thus causing less endothelial and uveal trauma. There will be no turbulence, and the followability and the holding power remain identical. It should not be forgotten that the hypermature cataracts are different from any of the regular cataracts. The red reflex is absent, the anterior capsule is very thin and fragile and there is that great chance of producing a peripheral tear. A large capsulorhexis is recommended to supply enough room to remove the pieces from the bag, to the iris plane to emulsify them. Most of the zonular support is weak. The hardness of the cataract and its adherence to the posterior capsule are potential difficulties, which can increase the energy delivered, and the surgical time.

It is possible to overcome these difficulties with the MicroBiaxial technique because of the following reasons:

- Smaller incisions mean a less invasive approach
- True anastigmatic incisions. It does not matter if the position is temporal or superior. It is possible to induce only 0.06 D
- True water-tight incisions
- Less possibility of iris extrusion even in intraocular floppy iris syndrome (IFIS)
- Higher resistance to postoperative trauma
- Minimum uveal trauma because of minimal turbulence
- Less amount of endothelial cell loss because of minimal turbulence and low U/S emission
- Corneal stability and faster visual recovery
- Deep anterior chamber all throughout the surgery
- Less BSS consumption in each case. Only 60–80 mL of BSS is used in regular cases and 120 mL in hypermature cataracts
- Less fluctuation and mobilization of vitreous, because of the stability of the anterior chamber during the whole procedure. It is better in refractive lens exchange (high myopes and hyperopes) and in patients with previous retinal tears or retinal surgery
- Increased intraocular pressure can be avoided depending on the high In-flow in coaxial, thus can be used in glaucoma patients. It also keeps a safe range of retinal irrigation, that is, 3 min at 70 mmHg. Outside this range, one can cause retinal damage. With the biaxial technique, one can obtain between 20 and 30 mmHg during the surgery. In Coaxial, it can rise to 60 mmHg or more, so the risk of retinal and optic nerve damage is greater
- Better maintenance of the anterior chamber with viscoelastic during the capsulorhexis, when introducing a CTR and when managing cases with small pupils
- the capsulorhexis can be made from both incisions
- The hands can be easily switched in Phaco
- It is possible to perform this technique with any machine
- Hyperpulses is not a necessity
- Easier removal of subincisional cortex
- The irrigation is a third instrument
- The main incision helps to mobilize fragments
- Theoretically less incidence of endophthalmitis
- Indicated in cases of previous PKP, RK or Seton devices
- Better control in uveal effusion
- Better management of complications
- Easier to teach in right and left handed Residents or fellows
- There are good softwares and new machines which can hasten the learning curve

Author's final comment: The author hopes that with this chapter and this whole book, more and more surgeons will take the challenge and make this next step in the future of cataract surgery. It is so easy to fall in false belief that microincision cataract surgery is not good enough and to question its' usefulness when the perfect IOL has not been developed. However, it can be recalled that in the beginning of phacoemulsification when only rigid IOL's existed, incisions were likewise enlarged. But still, many surgeons believed that its' benefits over extracapsular surgery, though were not so evident at the start, were a hundred-fold and that, in the future, its' impact on the way the ophthalmologists treat cataract patients will be immense. This is true likewise with microincision cataract surgery. The IOL technology, as of the moment, is not a plus factor of this technique. The biggest advantage of this technique is the calm intraocular environment that it offers during the whole procedure that increases the safety of the surgery and as a result, improves the visual outcome of the patient.

Take Home Pearls

- Hypermature cataracts are more difficult and challenging. Special care has to be taken. Regarding the incision, precalibrated knifes should be used to obtain more anterior chamber stability, to avoid leakage.
- During capsulorhexis, it always helps to stain the capsule even if it has some red reflex. This gives the surgeon more control and safety during this step.
- The major goal in intumescent cataracts is to decrease the intracapsular pressure to avoid peripheral tears and to avoid any subcapsular fibrosis and peripheral traction in hard ones without cortex.
- Hydrodissection is mandatory to mobilize the nucleus in hard cataracts. Though in intumescent cataracts, it is seldom necessary, it always helps to be sure that the nucleus is free from adherences before starting phacoemulsification.
- Finally during phaco, one can use any technique, however the "safe chop" is the recommended one in these cases.

References

1. Vejarano L. Felipe, Tello Alejandro (2004) Chapter 4: Fluidics in bimanual phaco. In: Agarwal A (ed) Bimanual phaco: mastering the phakonit/MICS technique. Slack, Thorofare
2. Vejarano L. Felipe, Vejarano Alberto, Tello Alejandro (2005) Chapter 17: Fluidics in phakonit. In: Ashok Garg (ed) Mastering the art of bimanual microincision phaco (phakonit/MICS). Jaypee Brothers, New Delhi, India
3. http://www.bplastic.de/Deutsch/WebShopLinkdateien/Chart_ british_imperial_and_us_gauge_to_mm.pdf
4. http://www.inoxidable.com/tablas_utiles.htm
5. Virgilio Centurion (2006) Ocul Surg News (Latin America Edition) 1–3
6. Vejarano L. Felipe, Vejarano Alberto, Tello Alejandro (2007) Chapter 41: Fluidics in phakonit and microphakonit. In: Ashok Garg (ed) Mastering the phacodynamics (tools, technology and innovations). Jaypee Brothers, New Delhi, India
7. Vejarano L. Felipe, Vejarano Alberto, Tello Alejandro, Bovet Jerome (2008) Chapter 5: Fluidics in biaxial lens surgery. In: Arturo Perez-Arteaga (ed) Step by step biaxial lens surgery. Jaypee Brothers, New Delhi, India
8. Blumenthal M, Assia E (1994) Using an anterior chamber maintainer to control intraocular pressure during phacoemulsification. J Cataract Refract Surg 20:93–96
9. Agarwal A, Agarwal S, Agarwal A (2002) Antichamber collapser (letter). J Cataract Refract Surg 28:1085
10. Tsuneoka H, Shiba T, Takahashi Y (2002) Ultrasonic phacoemulsification using a 1.4 mm incision: clinical results. J Cataract Refract Surg 28:81–86
11. Vejarano L. Felipe, Tello Alejandro (2006) Chapter 18: Facoemulsificación: Equipos y Sistemas. In: Virgilio Centurion (ed) El libro del cristalino de las Américas. Editorial Santos, Säo Paulo, Brasil
12. Vejarano L. Felipe, Olivella Manuel Julian, Tello Alejandro (2008) Chapter 5: Phacoemulsification: equipments and systems. In: Ashok Garg (ed) Mastering the techniques of advanced phaco surgery. Jaypee Brothers, New Delhi, India
13. Vejarano L. Felipe, Olivella Manuel Julian, Tello Alejandro, Bovet Jerome (2008) Chapter 4: Phacoemulsification machines and systems for biaxial lens surgery. In: Arturo Perez-Arteaga (ed) Step by step biaxial lens surgery. Jaypee Brothers, New Delhi, India
14. Vejarano L. Felipe, Tello Alejandro, Vejarano Alberto, Vejarano Manuel (2004) The safer and most effective techniques in cataract surgery. Highlights Ophthalmol (International English Edition) 32(2):10–16
15. Vejarano L. Felipe. Preliminary results on phakonit, the new era for phaco surgery. Ophthalmology Times
16. Vejarano L. Felipe, Tello Alejandro (2005) Vejarano SAFE CHOP makes transition to chopping easier. Ocul Surg News 23(5):10–11
17. Vejarano L. Felipe, Tello Alejandro (2005) Vejarano SAFE CHOP, makes transition to Chopping easier. Ocul Surg News (Europe/Asia-pacific Edition) 16(5):19–22
18. Vejarano L. Felipe, Tello Alejandro (2005) Vejarano's safe chop technique: a safer chopping. Tech Ophthalmol 3(3):109–115
19. Vejarano L. Felipe, Vejarano Alberto (2004) Chapter 14: Safe chopping in bimanual phaco. In: Amar Agarwal (ed) Bimanual phaco: mastering the phakonit/MICS technique. Slack, Thorofare, USA
20. Vejarano L. Felipe, Vejarano Alberto, Tello Alejandro (2005) Chapter 21: Implantation techniques in microphaco: Vejarano's safe chop in phakonit. In: Ashok Garg (ed) Mastering the art of bimanual microincision phaco (phakonit/MICS). Jaypee Brothers, New Delhi, India
21. Vejarano L. Felipe, Tello Alejandro, Vejarano Alberto (2005) Chapter 6: Safe chop: a safer technique in phaco chop. In: Boyd S, Dodick J (eds) Highlights collection, vol I: New outcomes in cataract surgery. Highlights of Ophthalmology, Ciudad de Panamá, Panamá
22. Vejarano L. Felipe, Tello Alejandro (2006) Chapter 5: Using safe horizontal chopping to prevent ruptures. In: Amar Agarwal (ed) Phaco nightmares. Slack, Thorofare, USA
23. Vejarano L. Felipe, Tello Alejandro (2006) Chapter 48: Phakonit and microphakonit. In: Virgilio Centurion (ed) El libro del cristalino de las Américas. Editorial Santos, Säo Paulo, Brasil
24. Perez-Arteaga Arturo, Vejarano Luis Felipe, Tello Alejandro, Bovet Jerome (2008) Chapter 22: Biaxial cataract surgery: personal techniques. In: Arturo Perez-Arteaga (ed) Step by step biaxial lens surgery. Jaypee Brothers, New Delhi, India

IOL Types and Implantation Techniques

8

8.1 MICS Intraocular Lenses

Jorge L. Alió and Pawel Klonowski

Core Messages

- All micro-incisional cataract surgery (MICS) lenses can be injected through 1.5–1.8 mm incision or less
- Only one lens – ThinOptX MICS intraocular lens (IOL) – can be injected through 1.1 mm incision
- Optical quality of MICS IOLs are equal to or better than standard surgery IOLs
- Clinical data suggest that MICS with MICS IOLs can improve refractive result and optical quality of the eye, thanks to the improved quality of the corneal optics obtained with MICS.

8.1.1 *Introduction*

Modern innovations in cataract surgery take all the ideas from the Kelman idea of the phacoemulsification lens removal technique and intraocular lens (IOL). Thanks to foldable lenses in the mid-1990s, the incision could be diminished to 2.75 mm. At the end of the twentieth century, new surgical techniques were invented which diminished the incision to 1.5 mm. Today micro-incisional cataract surgery (MICS) can diminish the incision size to 0.7 mm. To achieve these incisions, new surgical tools were used and the system of the lens fragmentation and the active use of fluidics were changed. Foldable lenses have to be adapted for such a small incision. Surgery today is feasible through sub-1 mm incision. However, MICS currently uses an incision size of 1.7 mm due to the limitations caused by the evolution of the lenses. The minimization of incision is the consequence of a natural evolution of the cataract surgery technique. MICS IOLs should accomplish the following conditions in order to fit adequately into modern cataract surgery:

- Be implantable through a sub-1.5–1.7 mm incision or less
- Not suffer any structural or optical changes after folding, injecting and unfolding
- Not induce additional optical phenomenon: halo, glare, aberrations
- Have high in-the-bag stability
- Have high biocompatibility index
- Not induce posterior capsule opacification (PCO)

J. L. Alió (✉)
Department of Research and Development, Vissum-Instituto Oftalmologico de Alicante, Avda de Denia s/n, Edificio Vissum, 03016 Alicante, Spain
e-mail: jlalio@vissum.com

J. L. Alió, I. H. Fine (eds.), *Minimizing Incisions and Maximizing Outcomes in Cataract Surgery*,
DOI: 10.1007/978-3-642-02862-5_8, © Springer-Verlag Berlin Heidelberg 2010

- Not induce corneal endothelial decompensation
- Be compatible with other materials, e.g., silicon oil
- Improve optical quality of the operated eye

The design of the optics, the index of the refraction and the deformability factor all determine the incision size. The optic of the lens is difficult to fold, compress and shift inside the cartridge. Higher-order aberrations can decrease the quality of vision as much as lower-order aberrations and cannot be corrected by spectacle lenses after the cataract surgery. However, aspheric IOLs can be used to correct most of the optical problems after surgery; moreover, the IOL asphericity is the way to reduce the lens width [1]. The high refractive index and proper Abbey factor of the IOL material is the key to reduce the thickness of the lenses. New intraocular lenses will have the high refractive index and the elasticity of silicone or of new hybrid polymers which allow them to be provided through small corneal incision. Reducing the lens width and lens optic diameter is also one way to diminish the incision size. Haptics must keep proper position of the lens after unfolding and stabilize the lens. Modern lenses should have lower inflammation levels and improved biocompatibility gradient. The material and the shape of the lens should diminish the PCO rate and the anterior capsular fibrosis. Most of the MICS lances are one-piece lenses. These types of lenses are well verified in MICS [2, 3]. Only a few lenses comply with the conditions above. Table 8.1 shows the list of these lenses [25].

Table 8.1 List of commercially available MICS lenses

Name of the lens	Company
Zeiss – Acri.Tec MICS IOLs Family	Zeiss – Acri.Tec, Berlin, Germany
ThinOptX MICS IOLs	ThinOptX, Abingdon, VA
Akreos AO Micro Incision MI60	Bausch & Lomb, Rochester, NY
IOLtech MICS lens	IOLtech, La Rochelle, France and Carl Zeiss Meditec, Stuttgard, Germany
TetraFlex KH-3500 and ZR-1000	Lenstec, St. Petersburg, FL
MicroSlim, Slimflex IOL	PhysIOL, Liège, Belgium
CareFlex IOL	W20 Medizintechnik AG, Bruchal, Germany
AcriFlex MICS 46CSE IOL	Acrimed GmbH, Berlin, Germany
Hoya Y-60H	Hoya Corporation, Tokyo, Japan
Miniflex IOL	Mediphacos Ltda., Minas Gerais, Brasil

8.1.2 Lenses

8.1.2.1 Zeiss – Acri.Tec MICS IOLs (Zeiss – Acri.Tec Berlin, Germany)

This is a group of IOLs that cover all aspects of modern IOL technology in which all of them are implanted through a sub-2 mm incision. They are all one-piece, foldable, hydrophilic, acrylate lenses, containing 25% of water and they have a square edged optic and haptic with UV-absorber. The total diameter of the all lenses is 11 mm. They differ in diameter and type of the optics. The haptic angulation is 0^0.

Acri.Smart 46S: This is a lens with a 6 mm optic diameter and has an equiconvex optic design. The range of diopters is from +16.0 to +27.0 D.

Acri.Smart 36A: This lens has an optic diameter of 6 mm. The optic is equiconvex and aspheric. Acri. Smart 36A is available from 0.0 to +32.0 D.

Acri.Smart 46LC: This lens has a 6 mm optic diameter. The range of diopters is from 0.0 to +32.0 D. Refractive index for this lens is 1.51 dry and 1.46 after hydration.

Acri.Smart 48S: The optic diameter is 5.5 mm. The optic design is equiconvex. Available diopters are from +10.0 to +30.0 D.

Acri.Comfort 646 TLC: The optic diameter for this lens is 6.0 mm. It has a square edged optic and haptic lens. The optic design is bitoric, biconvex and aspheric. The range of available spherical diopters is from −10.0 to +32.0 D. The range of cylinder diopters is from +1.0 to +12.0 D.

Acri.Lisa Toric 466TD: The optic diameter is 6 mm. The total diameter of the lens is 11 mm. The optic design has a toric anterior surface and its posterior surface is bifocal with aberration-free technology and smooth micro phase technology. Optical addition of this lens is +3.75 D. The material is a foldable acrylate with 25% water content with a hydrophobic surface. Spherical diopters range is: −10.0 to +32.0 D and the cylinder diopters range is: +1.0 to +12.0 D (Fig. 8.1).

Acri.Lisa 366D: The optic diameter of this lens is 6 mm. The optic design is bifocal, biconvex, optimized aspheric, and corrects optical system SMP. This lens combines diffractive and refractive optics. Illuminance refractive distance focus is 65% and the illuminance diffractive near focus 35%. The lens has +3.75 D power in addition to the near focus. This lens helps to

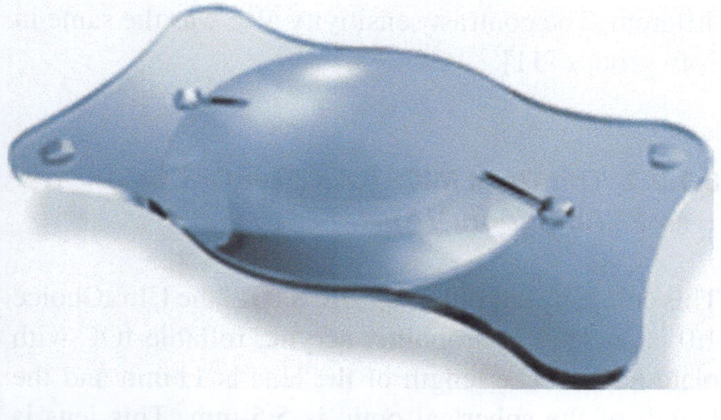

Fig. 8.1 Acri.Lisa Toric 466TD lens

achieve good near and far vision in different lighting conditions and in different pupil sizes. The range of diopters is from 0.0 to +40.0 D.

Acri.Shooter A2-2000 and Acri.Smart Cartridge injector system is recommended for these lenses. This injector enables the lens to pass through the incision size of about 1.7 mm (Table 8.2).

There is no statistical difference in retinal image quality between conventional IOL AcrySof MA60BM and MICS IOL: Acri.Smart 48S and UltraChoice 1.0. The 0.5 modulation transfer function (MTF) statistical difference for these lenses was not significant. AcrySof and UltraChoice 1.0 ($U = 38$; $p = 0.825$) or for the AcrySof and Acri.Smart 48S ($U = 20$; $p = 0.070$). Also, the 0.1 MTF values were not statistically significant for AcrySof and UltraChoice ($U = 40$; $p = 0.965$) or AcrySof and Acri.Smart ($U = 21$, $p = 0.085$). Thin optics, lens injection, lens folding and unfolding under the injector pressure can damage optics. In this study, MICS lenses show excellent MTF performance which are presented after the implantation in the eye through 1.5 mm incision [3].

Other investigations proved that there were no statistical changes in corneal aberrations after MICS with Acri.Smart 48S lens. They demonstrated that the total RMS can slightly decrease from 2.15μm ± 2.51 (SD) preoperative to 1.96 ± 2.01 μm postoperatively and the corneal astigmatism also decreases from preoperative −0.80 ± 0.76 D to postoperatively −0.63 ± 0.62 D after this type of surgery. The use of Acri.Smart lens and cataract surgery through incisions smaller than 1.5 mm do not affect the cornea and they can improve optical quality of the eye [4].

Wehner et al. presented and evaluated the position of the Acri.Smart 46S lens after 1½ years of implantation in 43 eyes in 37 patients. The lenses were implanted through a 1.4-mm microincision. The results indicated that there was no lens decentration during this period and the position of those lenses remained stable. First multi center study of the Acri.Smart 48S lens was carried out by Wehner. He injected these lenses by a 1.7–2.0 mm tunnel. He did not observe decentration or dislocation and none of the lens surfaces were damaged. The PCO was observed in two eyes out of 100 [5].

Lubinski et al. did MICS with Acri.Smart 48S lens. The mean incision size was 1.56 ± 0.07 mm. One month after surgery, the preoperative UCVA was 0.49 ± 0.33; and postoperative UCVA was 0.97 ± 0.11. The change was statistically significant $p < 0.001$. BCVA was also changed. Preoperative was 0.68 ± 0.3 and postoperatively 1.0 ($p < 0.001$). BCVA for near vision was improved from preoperative 5.27 ± 3.30 to postoperatively 2.91 ± 1.48 ($p = 0.002$). Authors argue that MICS with Acri.Smart 48S lens implantation is a safe and effective procedure [6].

Table 8.2 Zeiss – Acri.Tec MICS IOLs

Lens	Optic mm	Angulation	Range of diopters (D)	Material	Optic characteristic
Acri.Smart 36A	6	0	0.0 to +32.0	Acrylate	Spheric
Acri.Smart 46S	6	0	0.0 to +32.0	Acrylate	Aspheric
Acri.Smart 46LC	6	0	0.0 to +32.0	Acrylate	Aspheric
Acri.Smart 48S	5.5	0	+10.0 to +30.0	Acrylate	Aspheric
Acri.Comfort 646 TLC	6	0	spherical −10.0 to +32.0 cylinder +1.0 to +12.0	Acrylate	Bitoric, biconvex and aspheric
Acri.Lisa Toric 466TD	6	0	spherical:−10.0 to +32.0 cylinder: +1.0 to +12.0	Acrylate	Anterior surface toric, posterior surface bifocal with aberration-free technology
Acri.Lisa 366D	6	0	0.0 to +32.0	Acrylate	Diffractive and refractive. Light distribution 65:35

Mencucci et al. evaluated Acri.Smart and UltraChoice 1.0 lenses in the electron microscopy. In this study the authors did not find any lens damage after unfolding, which could be connected to the mechanical injury during injection process. They also did not notice post injector surface modification. They confirmed good system injection and excellent material quality of the lenses. They demonstrated only the OVD sediment on the surface of the lens. The conclusion of this investigation demonstrates that MICS lenses have a very good structure and acceptable surface properties after injecting through MICS incision [7].

Synder et al. evaluated Acri.Smart lenses after MICS. They did the mean incision size about 1.7 mm. They concluded that MICS is a safe method allowing for minimization of corneal incision. The IOLs were very well centered in all cases [8].

We evaluated implantation of the Acri.Smart 48S lens in 45 eyes. The mean corneal incision size was 1.46 ± 0.19 mm. The UCDVA before surgery was 0.2 ± 0.2 and 0.7 ± 0.3 after surgery. This difference was statistically significant 6 months after surgery. The BCDVA before surgery was 0.4 ± 0.2 and 0.9 ± 0.2 after surgery. The difference was statistically significant 6 months after surgery. The UCNVA was 0.6 in 60% of the patients and the BCNVA was 0.8 in 90% of the cases 6 months after surgery. The residual sphere was ±1.25D in 81.1% of eyes and residual cylinder was −1.25D in 62.2% of eyes. The spherical equivalent in 42.8% of the eyes was within ±1.25D of the desired correction, and in 30.5% cases it was between −1.25 and −2.0 D. Mean addition for near vision was +1.5D or less in 70% of cases. The IOL position did not change in any of the cases during 6 months [9].

Cavallini et al. evaluated Acri.Smart 46S IOL in aspect of the use in vitreoretinal surgery. In all cases, the fundus of the eye was excellent, even when up to the extreme periphery, without glare or reflections. This lens allows the surgeon to comfortably perform vitrectomy of the vitreous base and laser retinopexy up to extreme periphery without complications [10].

Kurz et al. investigated the possibility to compensate the positive spherical aberration of the cornea. The Acri.Smart 46S IOL and Acri.Smart 36A IOL 8 weeks after surgery did not differ in baseline characteristics. Implantation of both IOL types resulted in a negative spherical aberration Z_4^0, which was significantly different between two groups. The postoperative visual acuity and pupil size were not statistically different. The contrast sensitivity also was the same in both groups [11].

8.1.2.2 ThinOptX MICS IOLs (ThinOptX, Abingdon, VA)

This company has only one MICS IOL: the UltraChoice 1.0 is an 18% hydrophilic, acrylic, rollable IOL with plate-haptic. The length of the lens is 11 mm and the length of the spherical optic is 5.5-mm. This lens is very thin, central optical zone is only 350 μm thick and the haptic is 50 μm thick. This lens can be rolled and inserted through an incision less than 1.5 mm. The optic has a refractive–diffractive design. The central optical zone has five concentric diffractive segments of the posterior surface. The rings can create single focused images, because they are independent optical units. However, when they act together they may create focused image (Fig. 8.2).

Thin-Roller Injector is a single-use injector. It consists of a loading chamber and a tip with an injector. This lens can be injected also by the Geuder Cartridge (Geuder Instruments, Germany) [12].

In a clinical study in which we evaluated different MICS IOLs, we demonstrated that there were no statistical differences in retinal image quality between conventional IOL AcrySof MA60BM and MICS IOL: Acri.Smart 48S and UltraChoice 1.0. This study shows excellent optic attribute of this MICS lenses after injecting and unfolding [3].

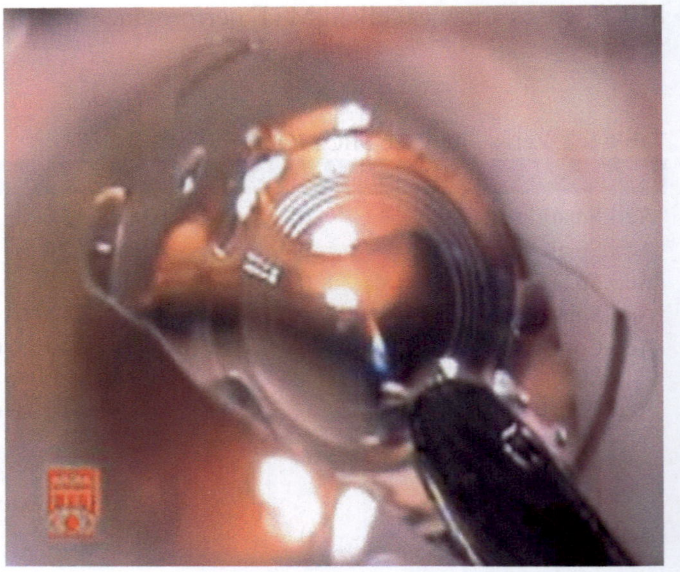

Fig. 8.2 ThinOptX MICS IOLs

Mencucci at al. analyzed electron microscopic scans of this lens and did not notice post injector surface damage [7]. Many authors confirm that UltraChoice 1.0 lens has the perfect characteristics. This lens can be easily inserted through incisions smaller than 1.5 mm. The perfect flexibility and ability to retain the original memory indicate that the lens can easily adapt to capsule [13].

Dogru et al. published visual results 6 months after the implantation of ThinOptix OIL. They compared this lens with AcrySof IOL (MA60BM). They did not notice any post operated statistical significant difference between these lenses in visual acuity, IOP, endothelial cell density and opacification changes. They found a significant change in intermediate and low-contrast charts. The mean contrast visual acuity scores were higher in the intermediate and low-contrast charts in the ThinOptiX group than in the AcrySof group [12].

Kaya et al. compared 1 year follow-up of UltraChoice 1.0 and Acrysof lenses (MA30AC). They noticed statistically significant lower visual acuity and higher PCO scores in the ThinOptix OILs group. The contrast sensitivity was also lower in the ThinOptix IOLs group [14].

Cinhuseyinoglu at al. evaluated ThinOptiX lens with MICS in a large group of 85 patients. They found that 92.22% of the patients had BSCVA equal to or better than 0.8 when evaluated 6 months after surgery. They concluded that MICS and the ThinOptiX rollable IOL implantation could be the future of cataract refractive surgical procedures [15].

Prakash et al. inserted ThinOptiX lens through a clear corneal 1.7 mm incision. They confirmed good visual acuity after surgery in their patients. However, they noticed a higher rate of POC in some cases of this lens implantation. The PCO rate was 16.12% at 15 months after surgery [16].

During the live surgery session at Alicante Refractiva Internacional (ARI 2006 Alicante, Spain), it was also demonstrated that the UltraChoice 1.0 IOL is implantable through incisions of 1.1 mm.

8.1.2.3 Akreos MI60 AO Micro Incision IOL (Bausch & Lomb, Rochester, NY)

This is a single-piece lens consisting of central optic and four flexible haptics. This biconvex, aspheric lens is made of 26% hydrophilic acrylic material with UV-absorber. Its lens has a 6 mm optic diameter and the angulation is 10^0. The lens has the posterior ridge to prevent PCO. The lens is available in three diameters – 10.5, 10.7 and 11.0 mm. The power of the lens ranges from +10.0 to +30.0D. This lens can be implanted through incisions less than 1.8 mm. Akreos MI60 can be injected with LP604350 single-use injector Viscoject™ Injector and 1.8 Viscoglide cartridge (Medicel, Widnau, Switzerland) (Fig. 8.3).

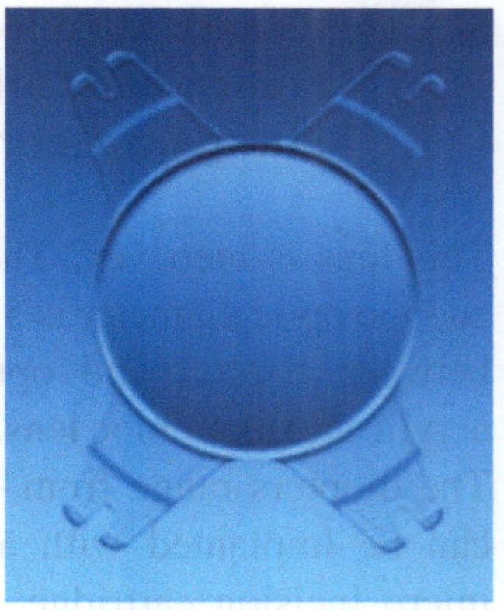

Fig. 8.3 Akreos MI60 AO Micro Incision IOL

Amzallag presented results of 20 patients who received Akreos AO MI60 Micro Incision lenses. The mean size of the microincision group was 1.86 mm. The excellent stability of the lens was confirmed by minimal decentration (0.11 mm) and small PCO rate. In his published data the stretch of the incision was about 0.09 mm. This indicates that this lens can be easily and safely inserted through incisions less than 2.0 mm [17, 18].

Luciano et al. presented 20 cases of patients with Akreos AO MI60 Micro Incision lens implantation through 1.8 mm incision on 87 Congresso Nazionale SOI 2007. The results of this work are very promising. The mean UCVA was 0.89 and BCVA was 1.0. The lens had very good stability in the capsular sac.

We reported during the World Ophthalmology Congress in Hong Kong (2008), results of the optical quality and visual outcomes of MI60 lens in MICS surgery up to 12 months. Preoperative spherical equivalent was −0.53 ± 2.93 D (−9.0 to +8.4 D). The postoperative spherical equivalent was −0.50 ± 0.60 D (−1.75 to +1.0). The mean LogMAR BCVA improved from 0.54 ± 0.23 to 0.11 ± 0.21. At 12 months, LogMAR UCVA was 0.32 ± 0.23. The mean Strehl ratio for the IOL once implanted inside the eye was: 0.26 ± 0.03. Final corneal incision size was sub-1.9 mm in all cases. This demonstrates that this new IOL showed excellent intraocular optical performance with excellent visual and refractive outcomes.

8.1.2.4 IOLtech MICS lens (IOLtech, La Rochelle, France; and Carl Zeiss Meditec, Stuttgard, Germany)

This lens is biconvex. The total diameter is 12.0 mm and the optic diameter is 5.5 mm. The angulation is 13^0 between haptics and optics. This is a hydrophilic acrylic and monobloc lens. This lens has a square edge. The diopters range from +10.5 to +25.5 D. The lens can be implanted with a disposable injector and a micro incision cartridge. This lens shows pseudoaccommodative effect (Fig. 8.4).

Verges et al. (ESCRS congress, Portugal 2005, London 2006) showed data of 48 patients who underwent MICS and implantation of IOLtech MICS lens through 1.8 mm incision. After 1 year follow up, 92% of the patients reported UCDVA 20/25 and 96% BCDVA more than 20/25. Sixty-five percent of the patients achieved near visual acuity J3 with distant correction and 98% of the patients, J5. Only 2 patients needed Nd:YAG capsulotomy.

8.1.2.5 TetraFlex KH-3500 and ZR-1000 (Lenstec, St. Petersburg, FL)

TetraFlex KH-3500 is the accommodating MICS IOL-lens. It is made from hydroxyethylmethacrylate (HEMA) and consists of 26% water and the material is highly flexible. The lens is 11.5 mm in total length and 5.75-mm in optic length with square edges. It is a

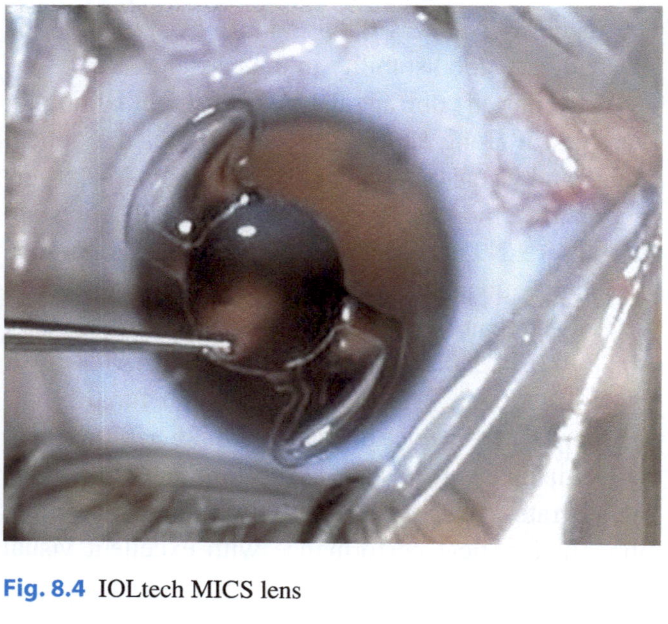

Fig. 8.4 IOLtech MICS lens

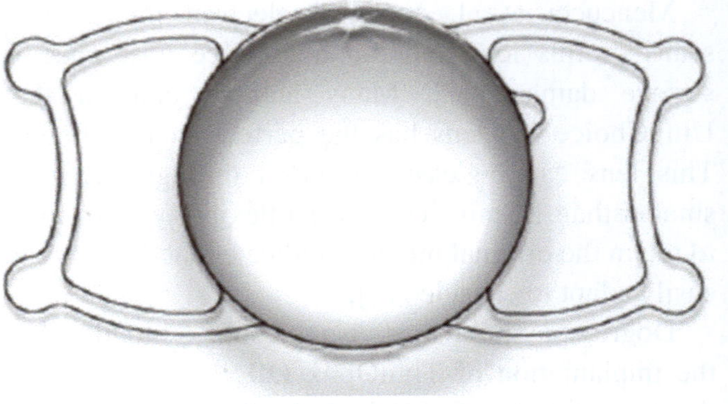

Fig. 8.5 TetraFlex KH-3500

one-piece lens. The lens is available in powers from +5 to +36 D. The TetraFlex KH-3500 uses injector with 1.8-mm cartridge [19] (Fig. 8.5).

Wolffsohn et al. evaluated the accommodative ability of this lens. After surgery, distance BCVA was 0.06 (±0.13) logMAR and 0.58 (±0.2) logMAR at near. The objective accommodation was 0.39 (0.53)D and subjective accommodation was 3.1 (1.6) D. Six months following surgery, posterior subcapsular scatter had increased ($p < 0.01$) in the KH-3500 implanted subjects and near acuity had decreased ($p < 0.05$). In conclusion, authors suggest that the accommodative ability of the lens appears to have decreased by 6 months postsurgery [20].

Chitkara at the ESCRS Winter Refractive Surgery Meeting 2004 reported that the mean accommodation achieved binocularly was 3.42 D. Moreover, 89% of the patients achieved J3 or better unaided binocular near vision at 6 months, and 100% achieved J5 or better [21].

ZR-1000 is the new one-piece lens from Lenstec. The length of this lens is 11.0 mm. The diameter of the optic is 5.5 mm and is made in square edge technology. The optic type is equiconvex and the haptic is plate. The angulation is 0^0. This lens is made of 26% water content acrylic. The diopters of the lens range from +10.0 to +30.0 D. No clinical data are available for this lens (Fig. 8.6, Table 8.3).

8.1.2.6 MicroSlim and SlimFlex MICS IOLs (PhysIOL, Liège, Belgium)

MicroSlim IOL is a hydrophilic acrylic lens with biconvex optics. Optic diameter is 6.15 mm, and overall

Table 8.3 TetraFlex KH-3500 and ZR-1000 lens

Lens	Optic (mm)	Angulation	Range of diopters (D)	Material	Optic characteristic
TetraFlex KH-3500	5.75	5	+5.0 to +36.0	Hydroxyethylmethacrylate (HEMA)	Accommodating lens
ZR-1000	5.5	0	+10.0 to +30.0	26% Water content acrylic	Equiconvex

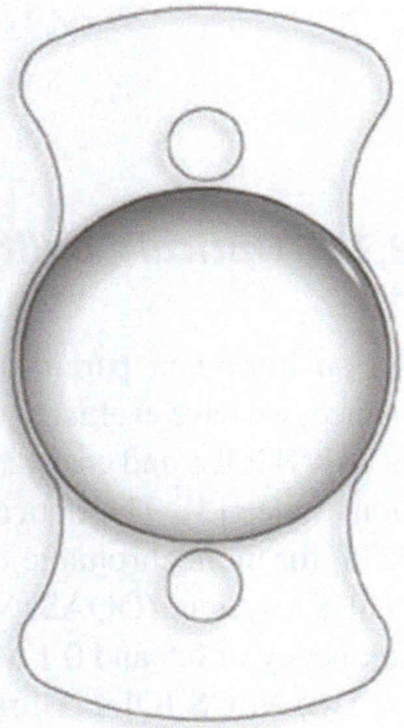

Fig. 8.6 ZR-1000 IOL

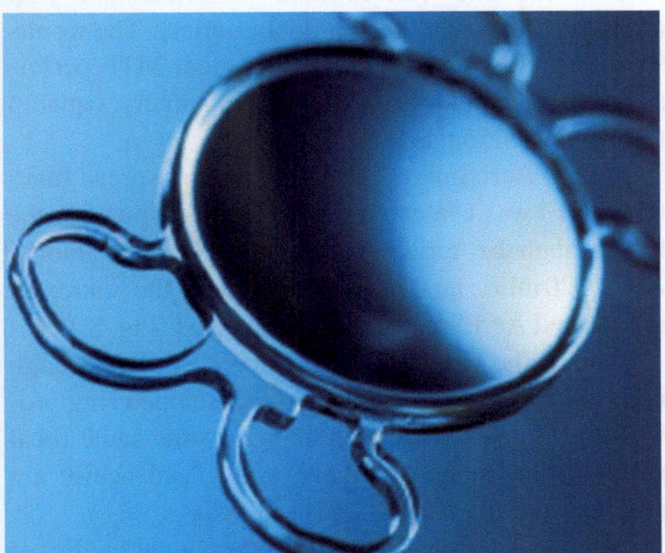

Fig. 8.7 MicroSlim IOL

diameter is 10.75 mm. The angulation is 5^0. The power of the lens range is from +10.0 to +30.0 D. This lens can be injected using Viscoject™ Injector and 1.8 Viscoglide cartridge (Medicel, Widnau, Switzerland). No clinical data are available for this lens (Fig. 8.7).

In the Congress of ESCRS 2006, Vryghem et al. presented their experience in SlimFlex IOL implantation through 1.5 mm incision. A group of 50 patients underwent bilateral MICS with lens implantation. After 6 weeks, mean BCVA was 1.04. Less than 1% of the patients complained about halos or glare, and 3% of lenses resulted in a small damage of the optic or haptics. No clinical data are available for this lens.

8.1.2.7 CareFlex IOL (W20 Medizintechnik AG, Bruchal, Germany)

This is a 26% hydrophilic acrylate, one-piece lens. Optic size is 5.8 mm, overall length is 10.5 mm and the haptic angulation is 0°. The optic design is biconvex. The recommended anterior chamber depth is 5.1 mm. The lens is available from +10.0 to +30.0 D. No clinical data are available for this lens.

8.1.2.8 AcriFlex MICS 46CSE IOL (Acrimed GmbH, Berlin, Germany)

This lens is made of 25% acrylic hydrophilic. The superficial is hydrophobic. The lens diameter is 11.0 mm and optic diameter is 6.0 mm. This is a monobloque type lens with perforated haptics. The angulation is 0°. The optic is biconvex with sharp edges. The lens is available from +15 to +27 D. Clinical data are not available for this lens (Fig. 8.8).

8.1.2.9 Hoya Y-60H (Hoya Corporation, Tokyo, Yapan)

Hoya Y-60H is quite a new lens for micro surgery. This is a hydrophobic foldable lens. No clinical data are available, but Tsuneoka described possibility of implantation of this lens through 1.7 mm incision. He used Hoya F-1 cartridge to inject the lens [22] (Fig. 8.9).

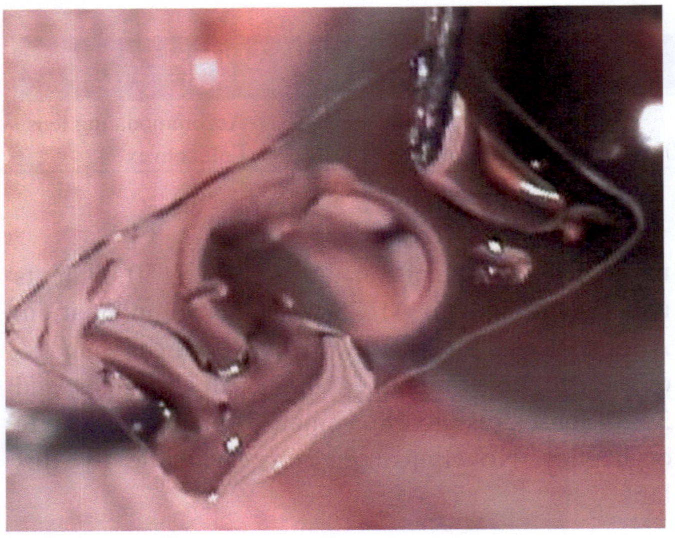

Fig. 8.8 AcriFlex MICS 46CSE IOL

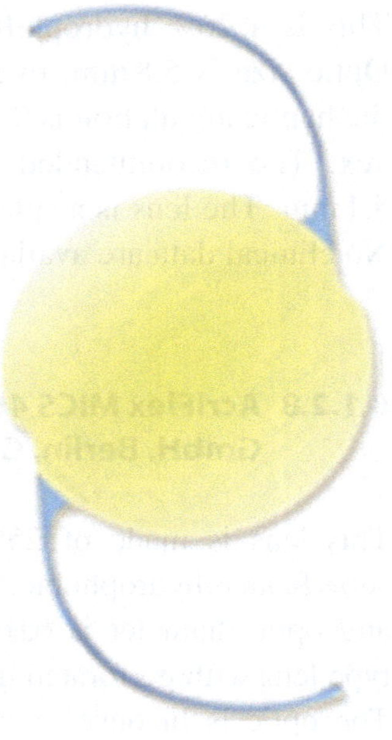

Fig. 8.9 Hoya Y-60H MICS IOL

8.1.2.10 Miniflex IOL (Mediphacos Ltda., Minas Gerais, Brasil)

This is also a new MICS lens and can be implanted through 1.8 mm incision. The material is Flexacryl® Hybrid Acrylic which brings together hydrophobic and hydrophilic monomers. The optics is aberration neutral. The lens can be implanted through 1.8 mm incision using a docking technique. The lens was presented on ESCRS 2008 in Berlin by Carlos Verges (Fig. 8.10).

Fig. 8.10 Miniflex IOL

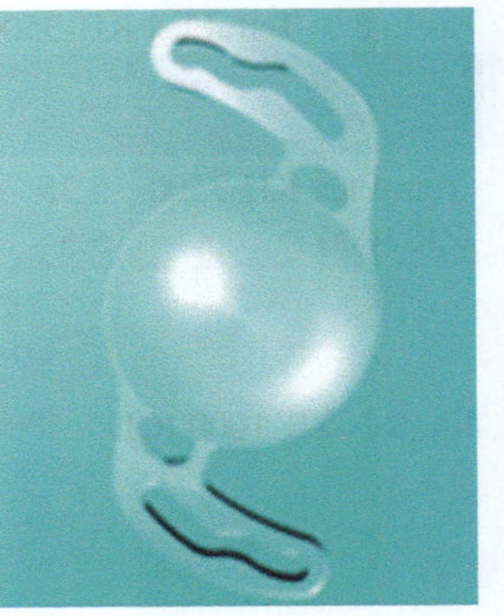

8.1.3 Optical Quality of MICS IOLs

As an important parameter for adequate IOL performance, we have evaluated objectively the optical quality of MICS IOLs and compared it with that of the conventional ones [3]. The optical quality was studied by the MTF for monochromatic light using the optical quality analysis system (OQAS, Visiometrics S.L.) at a spatial frequency of 0.5 and 0.1 MTF of the different IOLs.

Two MICS IOLs (UltraChoice 1.0, ThinOptX, and Acri.Smart 48S, Acri.Tec) were evaluated and compared with one conventional small-incision IOL (AcrySof MA60BM, Alcon Laboratories). The results showed that MICS IOLs have excellent MTF performance when implanted after cataract surgery, equal to that of conventional IOLs (Fig. 8.11).

For the Acri.Smart 48S IOL, the point-spread function (PSF) was evaluated before and after pushing the lens through the Acri.Glide cartridge (Acri.Tec GmbH). After 120 min., no difference between the untreated and treated Acri.Smart could be detected (Fig. 8.12).

Also, in the ThinOptX UltraChoice 1.0 IOL through its tandem fashion of working, each stepped ring provides the same optical information to the same focal point on the retina and MTF and visual acuity are therefore excellent (Fig. 8.13) [23].

We also evaluated the intraocular optical quality of a new MICS IOL Akreos MI60 (Bausch & Lomb) by using our model of intraocular optical quality analysis [24]. With regard to the Strehl ratio, it was 0.26 ± 0.03. The mean value of 0.5 MTF was 3.0 ± 0.5 cycles per degree (cpd) and the mean of MTF cut-off value was 22.3 ± 7.9 cpd (Fig. 8.14).

In order to show the intraocular optical performance of the IOL, intraocular aberrations for a typical eye implanted with Akreos MI60 are shown in (Fig. 8.15) for a 6 mm pupil.

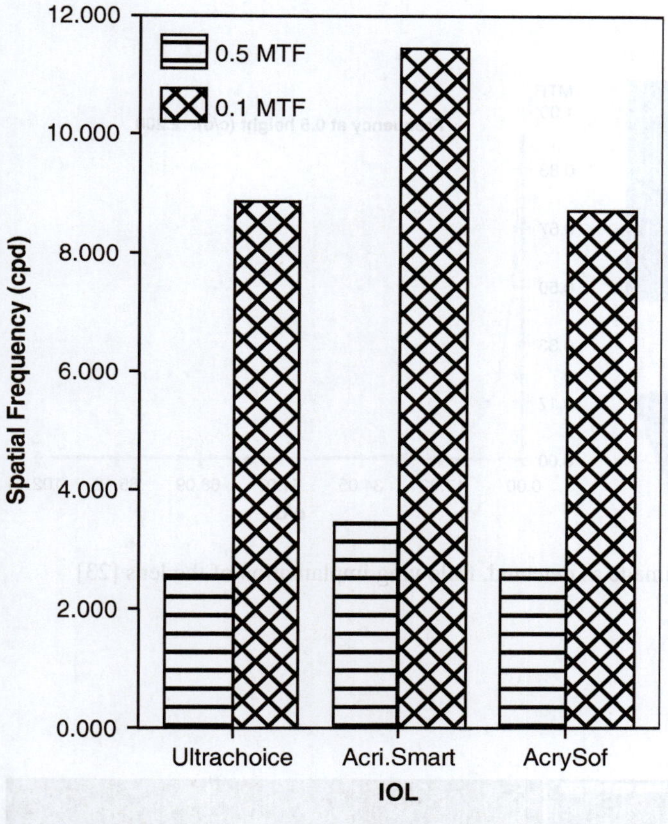

Fig. 8.11 Spatial frequency (cpd) for 0.5 and 0.1 MTF values of Acri.Smart, ThinOptX and AcrySof IOLs [3]

These results showed that MI60 IOL fulfills all the requirements for the modern trend in cataract surgery and MICS, with excellent intraocular optical performance once implanted inside the eye [26].

8.1.4 Conclusion

The number of lenses available for MICS is increasing. Now we have some microincisional lenses which can be injected through sub-2 mm incisions, with clinical data which confirm their perfect characteristics. The decrease of the incision and excellent quality of vision following the surgery, jointly with multifocal capacity to correct refractive errors with precision, makes cataract surgery a part of the refractive surgery. Now we know that MICS lenses have an optical quality equal to or superior to conventional lenses for standard cataract surgery. MICS lenses have excellent capsular bag stability and PCO rate. With the result of postoperative vision after MICS technique and MICS IOLs, we can expect an improvement in the refractive result and optical quality of the eye. In the future an

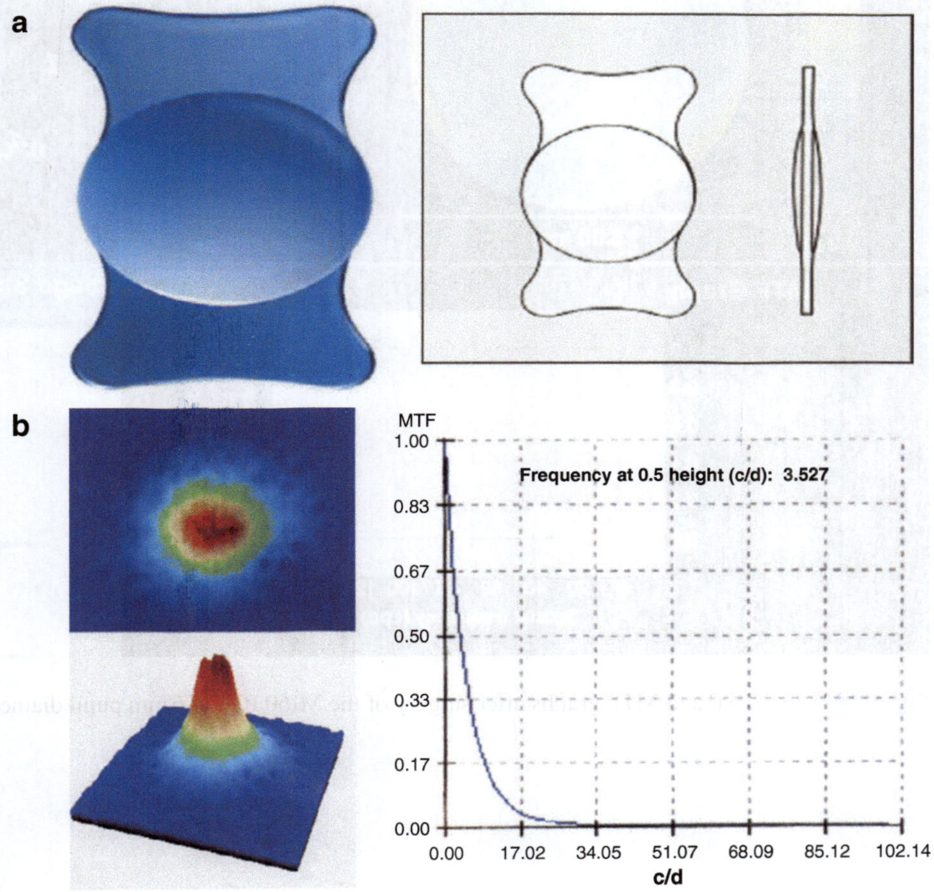

Fig. 8.12 Acri.Smart lens (**a**) Acri. Smart lens. (**b**) Optical quality analysis system (OQAS) image as detected following implantation of the lens [23]

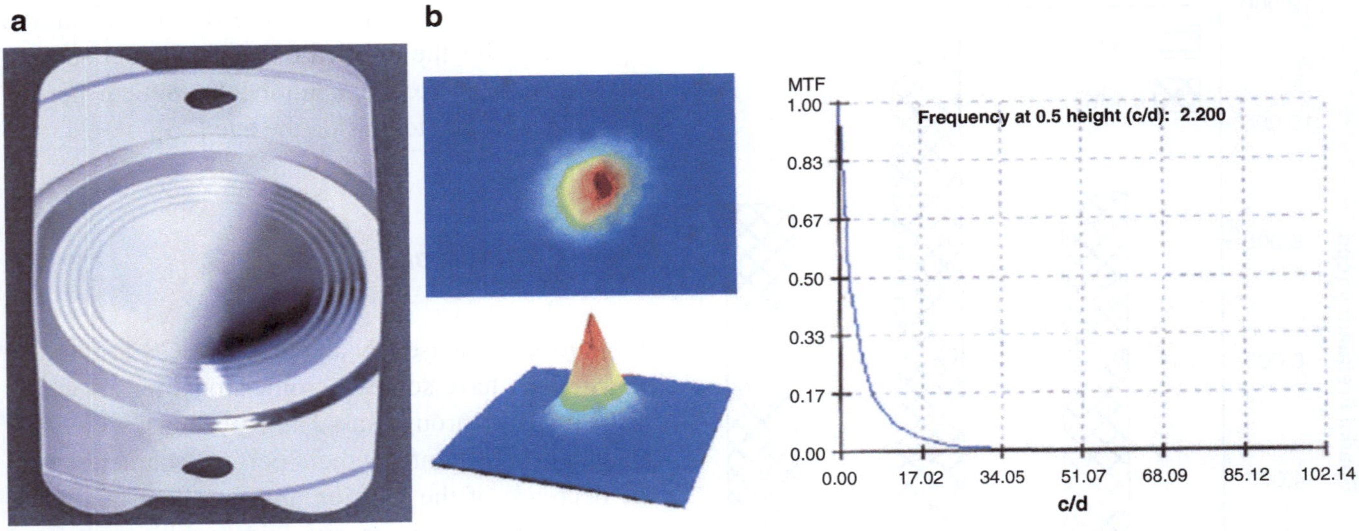

Fig. 8.13 The ThinOptX IOL (**a**) The ThinOptX IOL. (**b**) OQAS image as detected, following implantation of the lens [23]

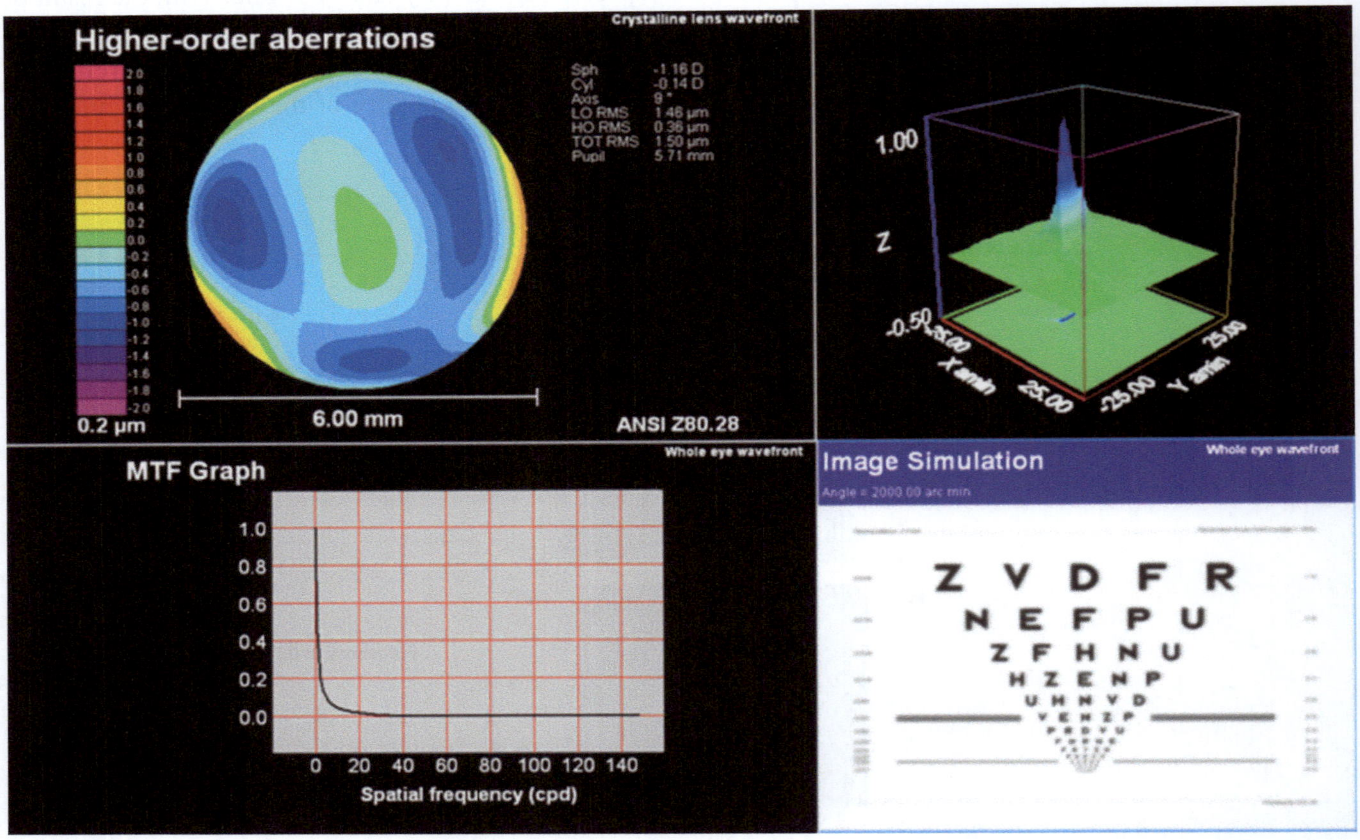

Fig. 8.14 HOA, PSF and MTF graphs after surgery of the MI60 IOL at 6 mm pupil diameter, with E-Snellen simulation

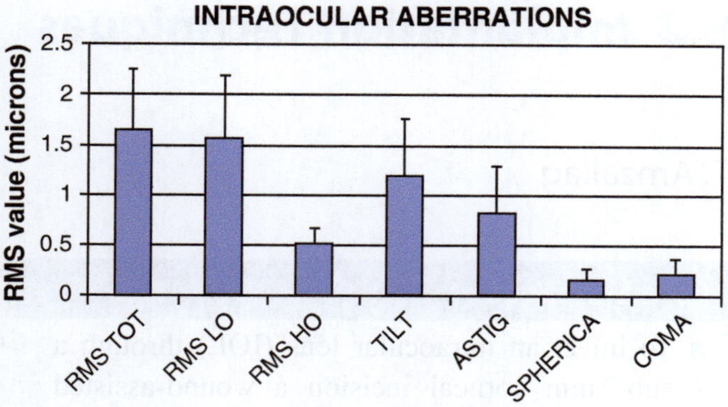

Fig. 8.15 Wavefront intraocular aberrations after surgery of the MI60 IOL

explosive development of MICS IOLs is expected to follow the demand of progress in cataract surgery.

> **Take Home Pearls**
>
> - Ten types of lenses are available today to be used in MICS sub-2 mm
> - MICS lenses fulfill all the demands of modern cataract lenses
> - Modern IOL design, higher index of refraction and improved Abbey factor are the ways to improve MICS IOLs

References

1. Bellucci R, Morselli S. Optimizing higher-order aberrations with intraocular lens technology. Curr Opin Ophthalmol 2007; 18:67–73
2. Alio J, Elkady B, Ortiz D, Bernabeu G. Microincision multifocal intraocular lens with and without a capsular tension ring Optical quality and clinical outcomes. J Cataract Refract Surg 2008; 34(9):1468–1475
3. Alió JL, Schimchak P, Montés-Micó R, Galal A. Retinal image quality after microincision intraocular lens implantation. J Cataract Refract Surg 2005; 31:1557–1560
4. Elkady B, Alió JL, Ortiz D, Montalbán R. Corneal aberrations after microincision cataract surgery. J Cataract Refract Surg. 2008; 34:40–45
5. Wehner W. Microincision intraocular lens with plate haptic design. Evaluation of rotational stability and centering of a microincision intraocular lens with plate haptic design in 12–19 months of follow-up Ophthalmologe 2007; 104: 393–394
6. Lubiñski W, Podboraczyñiska-Jodko K, Barnyk K, Karczewicz D. Microincision cataract surgery with implantation of an Acri.Smart 48S lens Klin Oczna 2007; 109: 267–271
7. Mencucci R, Ponchietti C, Nocentini L, Danielli D, Menchini U. Scanning electron microscopic analysis of acrylic intraocular lenses for microincision cataract surgery. J Cataract Refract Surg 2006; 32:318–323
8. Synder A, Omulecki W, Wilczyñski M, Wilczyñska O. Results of bimanual phacoemulsification with intraocular lens implantation through the micro incision Klin Oczna 2006; 108:20–23
9. Alió JL, Rodriguez-Prats JL, Vianello A, Galal A. Visual outcome of microincision cataract surgery with implantation of an Acri.Smart lens. J Cataract Refract Surg 2005; 31:1549–1556
10. Cavallini GM, Pupino A, Masini C, Campi L, Pelloni S. Bimanual microphacoemulsification and Acri.Smart intraocular lens implantation combined with vitreoretinal surgery. J Cataract Refract Surg 2007; 33:1253–1258
11. Kurz S, Krummenauer F, Thieme H, Dick HB. Contrast sensitivity after implantation of a spherical versus an aspherical intraocular lens in biaxial microincision cataract surgery. J Cataract Refract Surg 2007; 33:393–400
12. Dogru M, Honda R, Omoto M, Fujishima H, Yagi Y, Tsubota K, Kojima T, Matsuyama M, Nishijima S, Yagi Y. Early visual results with the rollable ThinOptX intraocular lens. J Cataract Refract Surg 2004; 30:558–565 (Erratum in: J Cataract Refract Surg 2004; 30:1154)
13. Pandey SK, Werner L, Agarwal A, Agarwal A, Lal V, Patel N, Hoyos JE, Callahan JS, Callahan JD. Phakonit cataract removal through a sub-1.0 mm incision and implantation of the ThinOptX rollable intraocular lens. J Cataract Refract Surg 2002; 28:1710–1713
14. Kaya V, Oztürker ZK, Oztürker C, Yasar O, Sivrikaya H, Ağca A, Yilmaz OF. ThinOptX vs AcrySof: comparison of visual and refractive results, contrast sensitivity, and the incidence of posterior capsule opacification. Eur J Ophthalmol 2007; 17:307–314
15. Cinhüseyinoglu N, Celik L, Yaman A, Arikan G, Kaynak T, Kaynak S. Microincisional cataract surgery and Thinoptx rollable intraocular lens implantation. Graefes Arch Clin Exp Ophthalmol 2006; 244:802–807
16. Prakash P, Kasaby HE, Aggarwal RK, Humfrey S. Microincision bimanual phacoemulsification and Thinoptx implantation through a 1.70 mm incision. Eye 2007; 21:177–182
17. Amzallag T. The Akreos micro-incision lens A clinical evaluation of an IOL for microincisional cataract surgery. J Cataract Refract Surg Today 2006; 4:32–34
18. Nichamin L, Amzallag T. Akreos scores highly for stability and centration Eurotimes 2007; 4:23
19. Doane JF, Jackson RT. Accommodative intraocular lenses: considerations on use, function and design. Curr Opin Ophthalmol 2007; 18:318–324; Review
20. Wolffsohn JS, Naroo SA, Motwani NK, Shah S, Hunt OA, Mantry S, Sira M, Cunliffe IA, Benson MT. Subjective and objective performance of the Lenstec KH-3500 “accommodative” intraocular lens. Br J Ophthalmol 2006; 90:693–669
21. Kellan R. An accommodative IOL with a new approach. Cataract Refract Surg Today 2004; 4:35–36
22. Tsuneoka H. Implantation of a new Hoya-IOL, Y-60H, through a 1.7mm corneal incision. In: Packer M (eds)

Mastering the Techniques of Advanced Phaco Surgery. Jaypee, New Deli, 2008, pp 209–213
23. Alio J, Rodriguez-Prats JL, Galal A. Advances in microincision cataract surgery intraocular lenses. Curr Opin Ophthalmol 2006; 17:80–93
24. Ortiz D, Alió JL, Bernabeu G, Pongo V. Optical quality performance inside the human eye of monofocal and multifocal intraocular lenses. J Cataract Refract Surg 2008; 34:755–762
25. Alio JL, Rodriguez Prats JL, Galal A. MICS Micro-Incision Cataract Surgery. Highlights of Ophthalmology International, Miami, 2004
26. Alio J, Elkady B, Ortiz D, Bernabeu G. Clinical outcomes and intraocular optical quality of a diffractive multifocal intraocular lens with asymmetrical light distribution. J Cataract Refract Surg 2008; 34(6):942–948

8.2 Implantation Techniques

T. Amzallag

Core Messages

- To inject an intraocular lens (IOL) through a sub-2mm corneal incision a wound-assisted visco-injection technique is generally required.
- It is mandatory to understand the IOL characteristics (material, design) and to know how to handle the dedicated injectors.
- The wound-assisted injection technique is the most used as it enables the smallest incision size, to date.
- At every step, the surgeon should keep in mind the exact incision plane in order to follow it closely when injecting.
- The precise loading of the IOL in the cartridge, the loading of the cartridge in the injector and the injection itself should fulfill very precise rules in order to lead to reliable and reproducible results.

Implantation of an intraocular lens through a microincision requires a new technological as well as technical approach, especially as the incision size is decreasing.

A new technological approach is necessary as both the implants and the injectors need to have the expected efficiency.

In spite of the reduction in the volume of the implant, it should have mechanical strength and, after being injected, should maintain the standards of optical quality and postoperative intra-saccular behavior, similar to the best products available.

The injectors and cartridges should be microincision-compatible. Today, it is indeed the internal diameter of the cartridge that determines the incision size. In practice, the internal diameter of the cartridge should be less than 1.4mm while using the wound-assisted technique

T. Amzallag
Ophthalmic Institute of Somain,
28 rue Anatole France, 59490, Somain, France
e-mail: thierry.amzallag@institut-ophtalmique.fr

of injection via an incision of less than 2 mm. Moreover, the integrity of the implant and the intraocular structures should be maintained during the injection.

A new technical approach is necessary as the wound-assisted technique, which does not require introducing the cartridge bevel in the anterior chamber, is currently the only technique of injection that allows making the smallest possible incision. However, for it to be reliable and reproducible the technique should be understood and followed rigorously.

While the sub-2 mm incision, which is the new standard in cataract surgery, is difficult to attain, a sub-1 mm incision goal seems all the more difficult.

This race to achieve the smallest incision size shall continue, since it proves to be beneficial to the patient.

8.2.1 Definition

If we talk specifically about microincisions, the definition of microincisions keeps changing according to the changes in technology, which, as we know, are rapid.

In 1985, Sharing suggested separating ultrasound and irrigation, a little before Agarwal described the Biaxial Phaconit technique using an incision size of less than 1.5 mm.

Jorge Alio [1] suggested the term Micro Incision Cataract Surgery (MICS) for incisions smaller than 2 mm.

Currently, the phacoemulsification by biaxial microincision (Bi-MICS) is used for 1.5 mm to less than 1 mm incisions.

On the other hand, the coaxial microincision (Co-MICS), which is similar to the usual technique, is used for incisions of 1.8 mm and soon, less.

However, because of the constraints of injection (implants, cartridges, injectors), the surgeons supporting the Bi-MICS technique are forced to increase their incision sizes to between 1.5 and 2 mm before implanting.

For this chapter on implantation techniques through microincision, we shall consider an incision size less than 2 mm.

8.2.2 Prerequisites to a Sub-2 Injection

It is necessary to follow certain rules in order to insert an intraocular lens (IOL) through an incision of less than 2.0 mm. There are four prerequisites:

1. The implant material should not be damaged and should be able to bear the high stress of injection. Currently, all the products used for microincision are made of acrylic hydrophilic material. This hydrophilia is one of the factors that help its flexibility.
2. The diameter of the optical zone should be about 6.00 mm at + 20 dpt. Reducing the size of the optical zone excessively has the risk of optical aberrations that could create problems for the patient even in case of a slight decentration.
3. The implant haptics should support 1–2.00 mm compression in the capsular sac without causing optical decentration. The use of large ansae, multiple to divide the efforts or even angular ones to increase the pressure on the posterior capsule and strengthen the effect of the 360° barrier, is recommended. The anterior and the posterior capsule should be able to adhere to each other immediately.
4. The cartridge determines the incision size after injection, mainly the internal diameter of its tip in case of an injection using the wound-assisted technique (without inserting the bevel in the anterior chamber). An empirical rule that allows deciding the post implantation incision measurement according to the internal or external diameter of the cartridge and the injection technique used is as follows:
5. Incision size in mm = [(cartridge diameter at the tip in mm × π)/2] × 0.9.
6. The value of the internal diameter is used for the injections in the wound-assisted technique, whereas the value of the external diameter is used when the bevel is inserted in the anterior chamber. In our experience, this empirical rule correlated very well with our clinical observations.

8.2.3 IOLs Used for Injection Through Microincision

The design of intraocular lenses (IOLs) used in incisions close to 2.2 mm is similar or identical to that usually used in standard incisions of about 3 mm, whereas the IOLs used in microincisions of less than 2 mm require an original and specific design.

In fact, these implants should be resistant enough in order to inject them through the incisions of 1.5–2 mm and they should also have a postoperative intra-saccular behavior comparable with the existing reliable implants.

Only a few materials and designs used today can claim to attain this objective.

The flexibility of the material as well as the design and the volume of the IOL are the characteristics that define the mechanical aptitude of the lens to be injected through a microincision.

8.2.3.1 Material

It is very important to note that the IOLs made of hydrophobic acrylic material whose optical quality and postoperative behavior is well known and proven cannot yet compete with those made of hydrophilic acrylic material, which are more deformable in terms of incision size.

Therefore, two parallel developments could be considered.

Those who support the performance of hydrophobic acrylic material defend the technologies, techniques and IOLs using 2.2 mm incisions [2]. They prefer the known intraocular behavior and the long follow-up of these IOLs.

Whereas those supporting the use of hydrophilic acrylic material are confident about the deformability of this material and the new IOLs having competitive optical capacities, and prefer an incision size of 1.5–1.8 mm [1, 3].

In the case of hydrophilic material, resistance to mechanical stress is a preliminary condition for designing an IOL meant for microincision. In fact, it should allow the insertion of the implant through the injection tunnel of a cartridge with an internal diameter of less than 1.40 mm for incisions less than 2 mm, and 1.10 mm for incisions less than 1.50 mm.

However, this material should not get damaged while trying to conform to the main constraints of microinjection. Properties like deformability and resistance to tear prove to be more important than the refraction index that allows reducing the thickness of optics.

The first hydrophilic acrylic IOLs were poly-HEMA lenses (38% water content) which were found to be extremely deformable in the recovery period. Many companies then decided to work on more rigid hydrophilic material by copolymerizing HEMA with PMMA, and a good result was obtained with a water content rate of approximately 26% (Fig. 8.16), which is now the base of most of the acrylic hydrophilic materials used worldwide.

Currently, the products meant for microincision are made of acrylic hydrophilic material [4] for which the clinical follow-up is more than 10 years.

In future, some new materials will probably allow reducing the incision size further and improve the optical quality and behavior of IOLs.

8.2.3.2 Design

For the first implants meant for microincision, more importance was given to the incision size and the ease of injection than to the postoperative behavior. They were

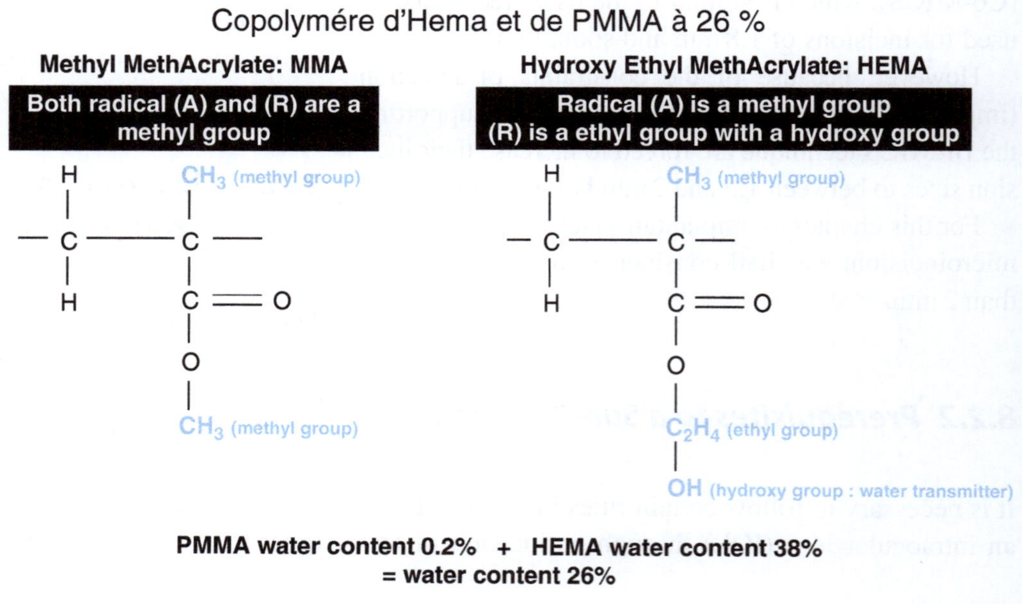

Fig. 8.16 Acrylic hydrophilic material at 26%, copolymer of HEMA and PMMA

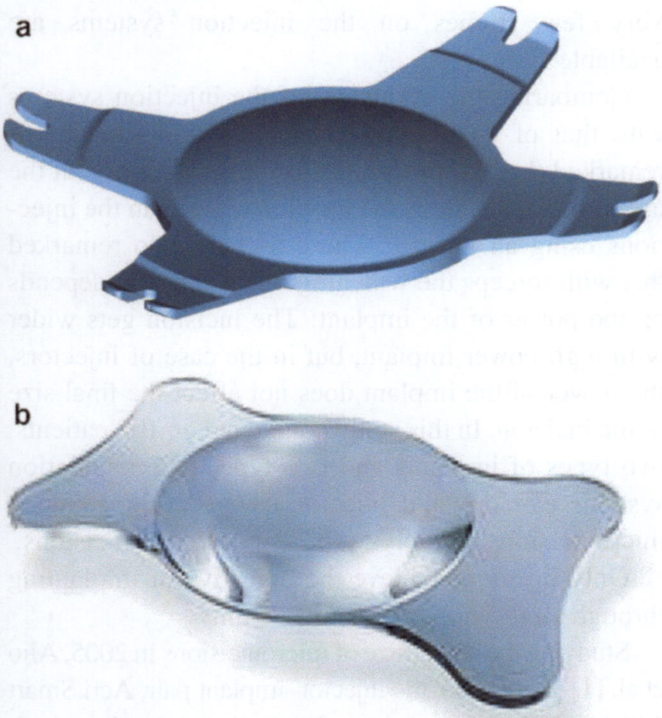

Fig. 8.17 Implants meant for microincision: (**a**) 4 rest areas: Akreos MI 60 (Bausch and Lomb), (**b**) 2 rest areas: Acri.Smart 48 S (ZEISS)

made up of hydrophilic acrylic material and were very thin. They did not have continuous 360° posterior barrier and included two equatorial zones (Fig. 8.17b) that made them likely to favor early postoperative capsular opacifications, excessive saccular contractions that could lead to capsulo-phimosis, or even lens subluxations. The following models have considered these weaknesses to show better medium- and long-term behavior.

8.2.3.3 Optic Design

The optic volume should be reduced in order to follow the microincision. This reduction in thickness can be obtained by various procedures like the use of a confocal optical system (ThinOptix) or by reducing the optical zone diameter. However, the diameter of the optical zone should be about 6.00 mm at +20 dpt. There is a strong desire to reduce this diameter to 5.00 mm or less in order to reduce the central thickness of the implants, and hence their volume during injection. But then there is a high risk of creating optical aberrations that annoy the patient even in case of a slight decentration. Moreover, in case of implants with concentric confocal optics that limit their thickness, there is a possibility of patients frequently complaining about halos or glares.

8.2.3.4 Haptic Design

Haptics are used for stabilizing the optics of the IOL and avoiding any movement during the postoperative saccular contraction. However, if they are numerous and fragile, they can theoretically affect the implantation technique. Their posterior angulation can equally help in limiting the PCO by prematurely increasing the posterior capsular angulation after intervention [5]. These haptics should support 1–2.00 mm compression in the capsular sac without causing optical decentration. This is very important, as reducing the thickness of an implant – an indispensable factor for being able to insert it through a small incision – significantly modifies the stability of the implant and makes it necessary to entirely reconsider the ansae to adapt them according to this new situation. The use of large ansae, multiple to divide the efforts or even angular ones to increase the pressure on the posterior capsule and strengthen the effect of the 360° barrier, is recommended. Thus, the anterior and posterior capsules can adhere to each other earlier on all four locations (Fig. 8.16a).

Though these haptics, which are useful for the right postoperative behavior of the IOL, theoretically make the injection trickier, their specific global design and quality of injection systems do not make it so in practice.

8.2.3.5 Posterior Barrier (360°)

This barrier is mandatory even if it increases the optic thickness and therefore makes the injection more difficult.

8.2.4 Injectors Meant for Microincision

The injectors meant for microincision should have an original design in order to fulfill the requirements. Equipped with high-performance cartridges, they should be efficient, reliable and ergonomic. At the same time, they should protect the IOL and the incision structure.

8.2.4.1 Objectives of Injectors Meant for Microincision

- Efficiency: These injectors should allow an easy, accurate and reproducible implantation through an incision of less than 2 mm, since phacoemulsification through incisions of less than 1 mm is now possible.
- Reliability: These injectors should assure the safety of implantation operations for the eyeball as well as the cartridge and the implant. The cartridge quality and the adequacy of the IOL-cartridge and the plunger-cartridge have a primordial importance. The reliability includes various aspects:

Protecting the integrity of ocular structures, not only at the corneal incision but also at the iris and the posterior capsule: An excessive stretch can lead to a postoperative defect in sealing, increasing the risk of infection. Any damage to the cartridge or implant can cause ocular structure damages of varied severity.

Protecting the integrity of the cartridge: The cartridge can have various damages. It could be a major damage due to bursting of the tip, medium damage due to bleaching and micro fracture of the tip, or minimum damage that can be translated as the "fish mouth" phenomenon or expansion of the cartridge tip. A damaged cartridge can prove to be particularly deleterious for the implant and can cause various damages, from a micro linear laceration in the paracentral optical region to a haptic rupture sometimes with a large optical laceration.

Protecting the integrity of the implant morphologically (optic and haptics should not be affected) as well as optically (bending and other operations necessary for implantation during the injection phase should not alter the optical quality of the implant): The implant surface should not get affected by the injection procedure. The occurrence of lubricant product transfer from the cartridge to the implant during the injection should be kept to a minimum. The microalterations of the implant may lead to adhesion of the inflammatory cells on the optic and could alter its optical quality. They could also induce fibrosis or opacification of the posterior capsule.

- Ergonomics: It can be interpreted as a greater ease in the use of injectors and a short learning curve. The maneuvres should be minimal, simple, fast, reproducible and accurate.

Very few studies on the injection systems are available.

Comparing the efficiency of the injection systems with that of the use of forceps, Mamalis et al. [6] remarked that the procedures of implantation with the use of forceps widens the incision more than the injections using an injector. These authors also remarked that with forceps the widening of the incision depends on the power of the implant: The incision gets wider with high-power implant, but in the case of injectors, the power of the implant does not affect the final size of the incision. In this study conducted on 100 patients, two types of implants and two types of implantation systems (forceps and injectors) were not specific to microincisions but only to the standard size incisions.

Only injectors achieve the objective of implanting through an incision of less than 2 mm.

Studying the actual size of microincisions in 2005, Alio et al. [1] proved that the injector–implant pair, Acri.Smart 48S (Acri.tech), allowed a safe injection through an incision of less than 1.9 mm. This prospective study included 45 patients. The average size of the incision before implantation was 1.46 mm (1.4–1.9 mm). After implantation, the incision size was 1.5 mm or less in 32 out of 45 cases, 1.7 mm in 10 cases and 1.9 mm in three cases.

Three years ago, we completed a pilot study of Akréos MI 60 (Bausch & Lomb) implant meant for microincision, whose structure was designed to optimize the postoperative intra-saccular behavior in terms of stability and posterior capsular opacification. The results at the end of the first year were published [7].

For this study, we used a resterilizable injector and a Medicel 1.8 Viscoglide cartridge (internal diameter 1.23 mm, external diameter 1.65 mm) with a smooth silicone plunger tip. The currently recommended injector (Viscoject, Medicel) is a single use type.

Twenty patients were divided into two groups based on the injection technique used. For 10 patients the injector bevel was inserted in the anterior chamber (IN group). For the remaining 10, the wound-assisted technique of injection was used (OUT group) (Fig. 8.20).

The minimum incision size after injection, measured with the help of calibrators inserted in the incision, was 2.2 mm for the IN group and 1.8 mm for the OUT group.

The incision sizes in the IN group were:

- 2.11 mm before injection (minimum 2, maximum 2.3)

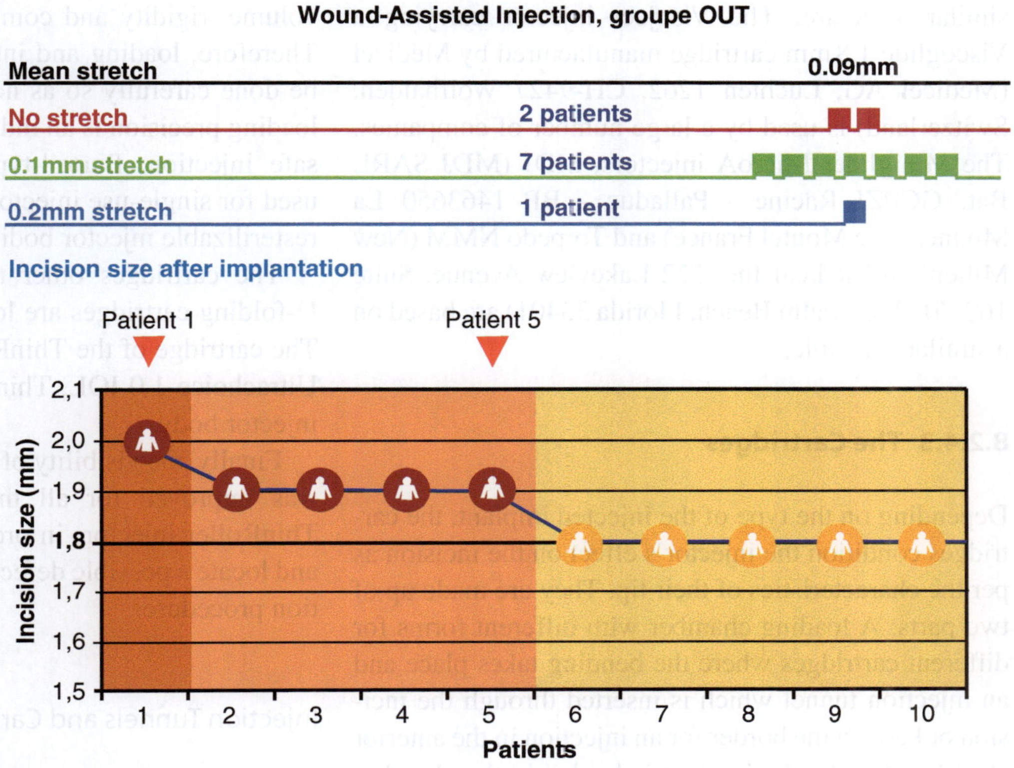

Fig. 8.18 Result of the Akreos MI 60 (Bausch and Lomb) pilot study. Stretch and size of incision after injection

- 2.22 mm after injection, with an average stretch of 0.11 mm and a minimum size of 2.2 mm

The incision sizes in the OUT group were:

- 1.77 mm before injection (minimum 1.7, maximum 1.9)
- 1.86 mm after injection, with an average stretch of 0.09 mm and a minimum size of 1.8 mm

In case of the OUT group, we have also observed a significant reduction in the incision sizes with the expertise acquired (from 2–1.8 mm). We shall probably be able to reduce the incision sizes further by developing the technique (Fig. 8.18). We did not notice any complication.

- For the same Akréos MI 60 (Bausch an Lomb) implant, J. Alió et al. [3] proved that implantation using a Viscoject injector carrying a Viscoglide 1.8 mm cartridge, manufactured by Médicel (Medicel AG, Luchten 1262, CH-9427 Wolfhalden, Switzerland) and having a cartridge with an internal diameter of 1.23 mm, resulted in a slight enlargement of corneal incision when implanted through an incision of 1.68 ± 0.24 mm: the incision size in post-injection became 1.82 ± 0.16 mm, i.e. a variation of 0.14 ± 0.22 mm.
- Belluci et al. did not observe any significant modification in the incision size with the same implant and same injection system while using incisions of 2 mm.
- While studying the reliability of the injection systems meant for microincision, Mencucci et al.[8] used electron microscopy and studied the surface of two implants of microincision after an injection procedure using a special injector: the ThinRoller Injector meant for Ultrachoice 1.0 Rollable Thin Lens IOL and the Acri.shooter Injector meant for the Acrismart implant. Four implants of each type were studied and no significant modification in the morphology of implants was noticed after injection. A small-sized superficial scratch on the haptic was found on the ThinOptx implant of strong magnification. Therefore, it can be stated that inserting an implant through an incision of less than 2 mm does not modify the quality of its optic.

8.2.4.2 Characteristics of Sub-2 Injectors

Other than the ThinRoller injector meant for Ultrachoice 1.0 IOL, ThinOptx, most of the sub-2 injectors have a similar structure. The Visoject injector carrying a Viscoglide 1.8 mm cartridge manufactured by Médicel (Medicel AG, Luchten 1262, CH-9427 Wolfhalden, Switzerland) is used by a large number of companies. The Miniglider MicroA injectors, MDJ (MDJ SARL Bat. GCPZI Racine - Palladuc - BP 1463650 La Monnerie Le Montel France) and Torpedo NMM (New Millenium Medical Inc. 222 Lakeview Avenue, Suite 160-703 West palm Beach, Florida 33401) are based on a similar principle.

8.2.4.3 The Cartridges

Depending on the type of the injected implant, the cartridges condition the injector's effect on the incision as per the characteristics of their tip. They are made up of two parts: A loading chamber with different forms for different cartridges where the bending takes place and an injection tunnel which is inserted through the incision or kept on the border for an injection in the anterior chamber. Firstly, the implant is loaded in the chamber before pushing it towards the injection tunnel. All the cartridges are for single use unlike the injector body.

The cartridges are made of polypropylene and are sterilized using ethylene oxide. Usually they have a shelf life of 2 years. They are equipped with lubricants for an easier insertion of the implant in the loading chamber as well as in the injection tunnel. Blooming and coating are the two principal methods of lubrication. Blooming consists of adding the lubricant in the material of the cartridge. During sterilization, when heated, it oozes out and covers the walls of the cartridge. On the other hand, coating includes lubrication on the cartridge surface. The lubrication of the cartridge should be sufficient, but any transfer of the lubricant onto the optic should be avoided. This could happen if the lubrication technique is used on the one hand and there is lack of adequacy between the injection tunnel's internal diameter and the volume and material of the IOL on the other hand.

Loading Chambers

The referred cartridge is a hinged Bartell-type folding cartridge, the one most commonly used in injection through microincision. It uses a U-folding. It can be easily loaded, although loading depends on the implant. The level of difficulty in loading it depends on the volume, rigidity and complex design of the implant. Therefore, loading and insertion in the tunnel should be done carefully so as not to affect the haptics. The loading precision is an indispensable prerequisite for a safe injection. Bartell-type cartridges are generally used for single-use injectors but can also be used with resterilizable injector bodies.

The cartridges other than these top-loading and U-folding cartridges are loaded in a different manner. The cartridge of the ThinRoller injector meant for the Ultrachoice 1.0 IOL, ThinOptx, is integrated into the injector body.

Finally, the visibility of the implant during injection was improved for all these cartridges (except the ThinRoller injector) in order to verify its progression and locate a possible defect that could revoke the injection procedure.

Injection Tunnels and Cartridge Tips

The thickness of the injection tunnel's wall should be sufficient to resist the mechanical stress of the injection and avoid bursting. The finishing quality has a special importance in cartridges meant for microincision as it avoids any damage to the implant during insertion.

All cartridge tips are bevelled at Howard Fine's instigation. Generally, they are round or oval, along a major horizontal axis, for a flat injection of monobloc implants. These are meant to limit the risk of any gap in the incision (fish mouthing) in case of an incision size that is inadequate for the injector. They also help in achieving good stability of monobloc implants in the injection plane, avoiding any untimely rotation in the tunnel axis or in the perpendicular axis.

Any inadequacy of cartridge (or piston) with the injected implant can be the cause of implant damages regardless of their material. It can be marks, scratches, cracks or deposits on the surfaces. Sometimes these lesions are more severe in cases of bursting of cartridges, separation of a fragment of haptics or optic or the atypical injections dangerous to the integrity of the tissues of the anterior segment. However, in practice such incidents are rare if the manufacturer's instructions are rigorously followed.

The cartridge determines the incision size after injection. As already seen, an empirical rule allows deciding the post implantation incision measurement according to the internal or external diameter of the cartridge and the injection technique used.

Incision size in mm = [(cartridge diameter at the tip in mm × π)/2] × 0.9.

For the wound-assisted technique of injection, we use the value of the internal diameter. Therefore, the internal diameter of the cartridge should be less than 1.4 mm to attain the objective of an incision size of less than 2 mm.

Internal cartridge diameter (mm)	Incision size (mm)
0.7	1
0.85	1.2
1	1.4
1.1	1.5
1.25	1.8
1.6	2.2
2	2.4

8.2.4.4 The Plunger Tips (or plunger)

The plunger tips are very specific and determine the mechanical efficiency of the injector and ensure the preservation of the cartridge and the implant during insertion in the tunnel by their adaptability to the form of implant in the cartridge. The injectors meant for microincision inject only the monobloc implants and not the 3-piece implants that are not appropriate for this incision size. These tips are meant to obtain maximum efficiency while pushing the implant, preserving the haptics and the optic regardless of their form and material. Their form has been designed to avoid the tip getting stuck in the folded implant during insertion, a risk which could affect the efficiency of insertion and increase the possibility of lesion of the implant and the cartridge. These plunger tips can be rigid or soft. Generally, soft plunger tips are made of silicone. The purpose of these soft tips is to limit traumas by their flexibility and to reduce the diameter of the injection tunnel mainly for highly fragile implants. In practice, deformable plunger tips are most commonly used. They allow using a Visco-injection that makes the injection easier and more secure. The principle of "Visco-injection" or "hydraulic injection" using a soft plunger tip usually made of silicone and a viscoelastic substance (VES) is followed by most of the companies claiming an incision of less than 2 mm. In practice, it is of great relevance. In fact, this instrument allows maintaining the VES and the IOL in front of the plunger tip. This serves two purposes: protecting the haptics during injection (they cannot get stuck by the tip) and easing the pressure on the plunger while inserting through smaller diameters. Thus, the injections become easier and more secure. Moreover, the deformability of this plunger tip avoids bursting of tunnel or bevel caused by the required size of a rigid tip.

8.2.4.5 Pushing Systems

The plunger tips can usually be operated by a screw or a piston.

The systems using a screw have the advantage of being more precise and easy to control as they require less force, help making a soft release of the implant and facilitate rotation operations if required. However, they require bimanual usage.

Generally a syringe-type plunger is used for injection through microincision, which allows an injection on planes by simple, mono manual pressure, useful especially if a counter pressure using a second instrument is required. This plunger has a return spring which increases the precision and facilitates its return at the end of injection. The regularity of pressure and control on the implant release can sometimes be tricky during the first injection.

8.2.4.6 Injector Bodies

Injector bodies can be resterilized or be of single-use type.

The resterilizable injectors are the oldest injectors, but as single-use instruments are now the global trend, these injectors are commonly used in injections through microincision. They are mainly meant for monobloc implants.

Currently, preloaded injectors for incision sizes of less than 2 mm do not exist. Their conception proves to be very difficult. In the case of hydrophobic materials, the difficulty in folding a less deformable material creates a problem. In the case of hydrophilic materials, the conservation of lubrication capacity in humid environments becomes problematic.

The ergonomic design of the injector bodies, mostly for single-use, allows an optimal prehension that increases the efficiency and security during the injection procedure.

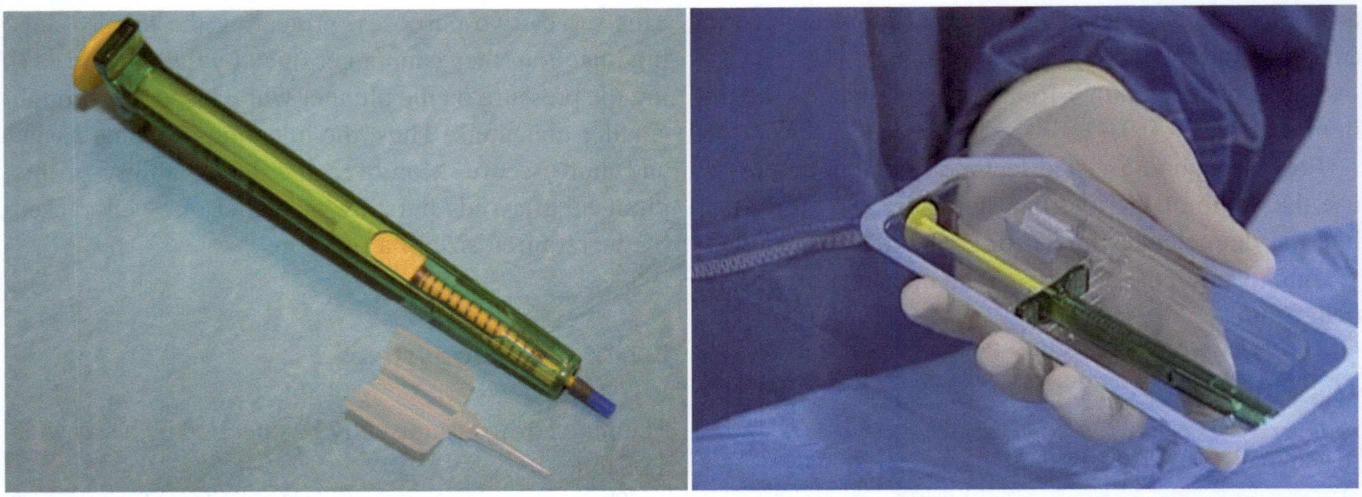

Fig. 8.19 Viscoject injector, Viscoglide 1.8 mm cartridge manufactured by Médicel

8.2.4.7 Principal Sub-2 Injectors

- Viscoject (Medicel) (Fig. 8.19)

The Viscoject injector is manufactured by Médicel (Switzerland) who supplies a large number of laboratories around the world. Through the laboratories that use this injector, Medicel has popularized the use of the Visco-injection. Their Viscoglide 1.8 cartridge makes incision size of 1.8 mm feasible. It injects, among others, the MI 60, Bausch & Lomb and microSlim, Physiol IOLs.

- Thinroller (Thinoptx) (Fig. 8.20)

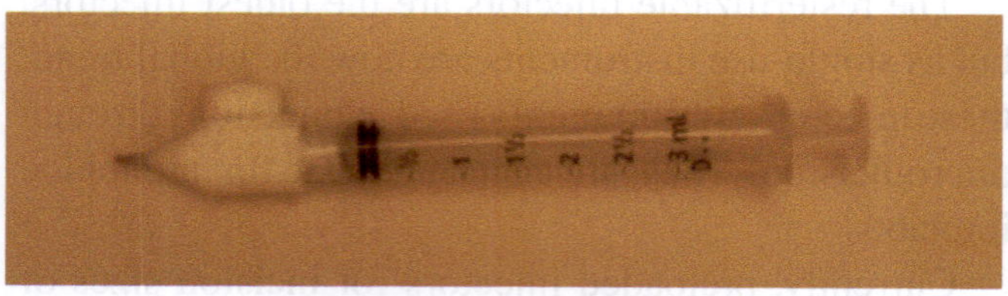

Fig. 8.20 ThinRoller injector meant for the Ultrachoice 1.0 (ThinOptx) IOL

This historical sub-2 injector is meant for the Ultra choice 1.0, ThinOptx confocal hydrophilic acrylic monobloc implant. Its main characteristic, other than the incision size between 1.5 and 2 mm, is that the IOL is rolled in the injector unlike in most of the cases where it is folded in a U-shape. It has a rigid plunger tip, which is not common in sub-2 injectors.

- Acrishooter (Zeiss) (Fig. 8.21)

Meant for Acri.Smart 36 A, Acri.Confort 646 TLC bitorique and Acri.LISA 366 D bifocale difractive IOLs, the Acrishooter is a resterilizable injector having a Laser 2 cartridge (same as for INJ 01) that allows a sub-2 injection.

- INJ 01 (Adriamed) (Fig. 8.22)

Meant for Acri.Smart 36 A, Acri.Confort 646 TLC bitorique and Acri.LISA 366 D bifocale difractive IOLs and having the same Laser 2 cartridge as in Acrishooter, it has a single-usage design made of polycarbonate. The plunger tip is deformable and separated, and a stop collar secures the insertion and prevents excessive pressure on the plunger.

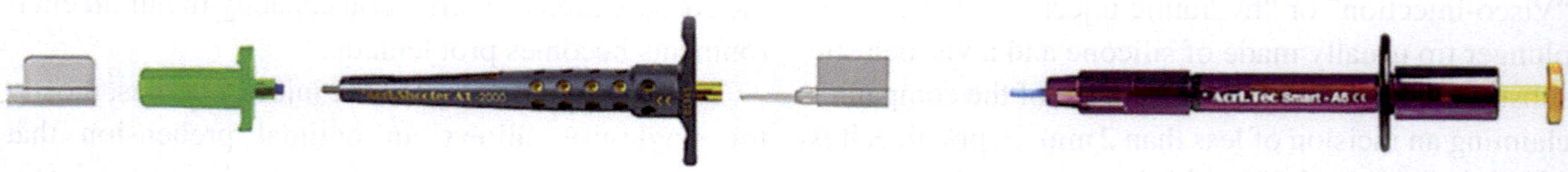

Fig. 8.21 Acrishooter (ZEISS) injector

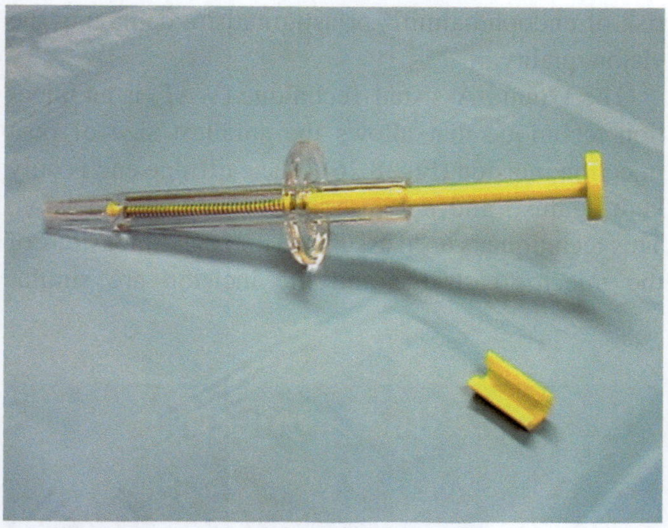

Fig. 8.22 INJ 01 (ADRIAMED) injector

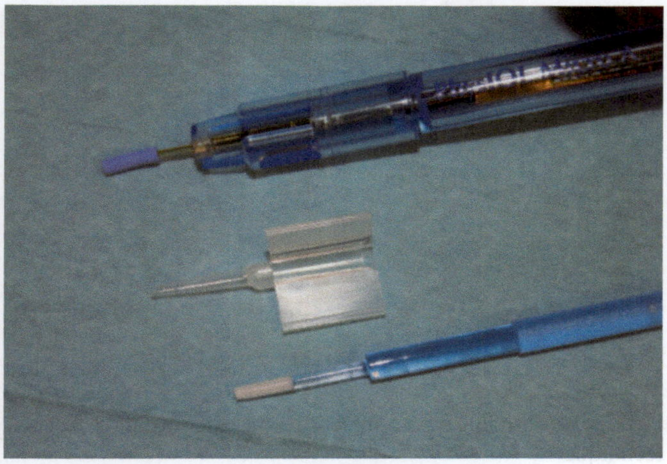

Fig. 8.23 MiniGlider Micro A (MDJ) injector

- Micro A (MDJ) (Fig. 8.23)

Meant for Acryflex 46 CSE and MicroSlim IOLs, whose material was modified according to SlimFlex and YellowFlex, its hydrophilia is different but it has a similar design. For the sub-2 incisions, the Micro A injector is used with a 027 MDJ cartridge, which has an internal diameter of 1.07 mm and external diameter of 1.45 mm.

- Torpedo (NMM) (Fig. 8.24)

Meant for Quadrant NMM IOL made of acrylic hydrophilic material, it has a monobloc design with four rest areas and can be used with various types of cartridges. The RD 100 cartridge having an internal diameter of 1 mm (external diameter 1.3 mm) is

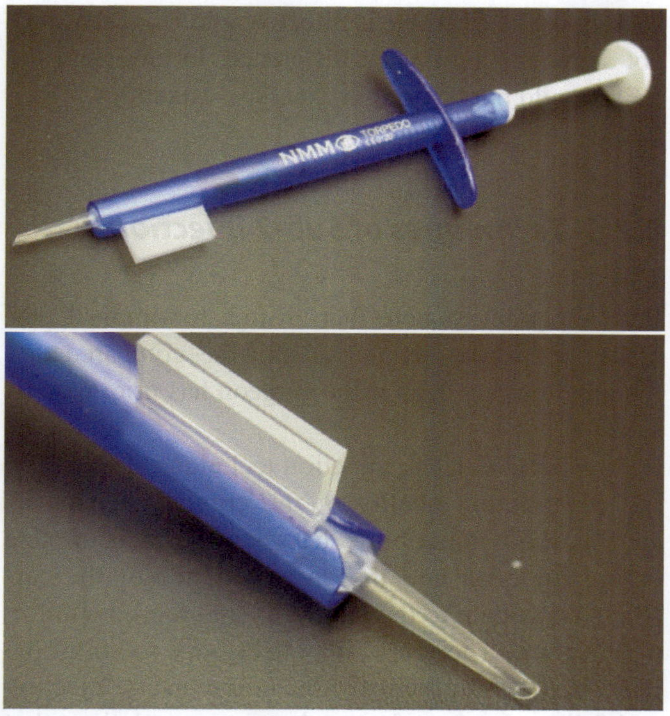

Fig. 8.24 Torpedo (NMM) injector

theoretically compatible with an incision of 1.5 mm, whereas the RD 145 cartridge having an internal diameter of 1.15 mm (external diameter 1.45 mm) is compatible with an incision size of 1.8 mm.

8.2.5 Visco Elastic Substances and Injection Through Microincision

The use of injectors theoretically requires visco elastic substances (VES) with a high coating ability, especially when mechanical constraints are important as for the injections through microincision. The coating ability that measures the adhesion capacity of VES is calculated by the angle formed by the VES with a solid support. The smaller the contact angle, the higher is the coating ability of the VES. This capacity reflects the lubrication capacity of these products. The HPMC (hydroxylpropylmethylcellulose) seems theoretically better adapted. For the same set of reasons, the dispersive VES (low molecular weight, high concentration) seems better adapted than the cohesive VES (high molecular weight, low concentration). In practice, most of the injectors meant for microincision can be used, irrespective of the VES type as long as the coating of the cartridge is effective and clinically does not show any significant difference. In any case, the VES should not be used in excessive quantities.

8.2.6 Techniques of Sub-2 Injection

It is important to note that an injector–implant pair makes a specific set that cannot be compared and requires training even if the surgeon has prior experience [9].

Irrespective of the injection technique (Fig. 8.25), the construction quality of the corneal incision as well as the compatibility between the incision size before injection and the characteristics of the cartridge contribute to the reliability and reproducibility of injection. Therefore, it is necessary to study the characteristics of the cartridge before every injection and follow the manufacturer's recommendations that consider various parameters and a number of in vitro and in vivo tests. It is always interesting and useful to watch a video demonstration and perform the first injection in the presence of a competent delegate after having handled the injector. For most of the injectors, the loading and preparation can be carried out by a trained assistant.

Reduction in incision size can possibly put mechanical stress on the corneal incision during injection. This stress could have immediate postoperative consequences like fault in sealing, hypotonia, an increased risk of endophthalmitis or astigmatism, damaging the vision quality.

The Wound-Assisted Technique (WAT) is an injection technique that allows the smallest size of post injection incision (Fig. 8.26). The cartridge end is only kept against, and not inserted through, the incision. This technique is used assuming that the dimensions of the injector cartridge and the incision are similar

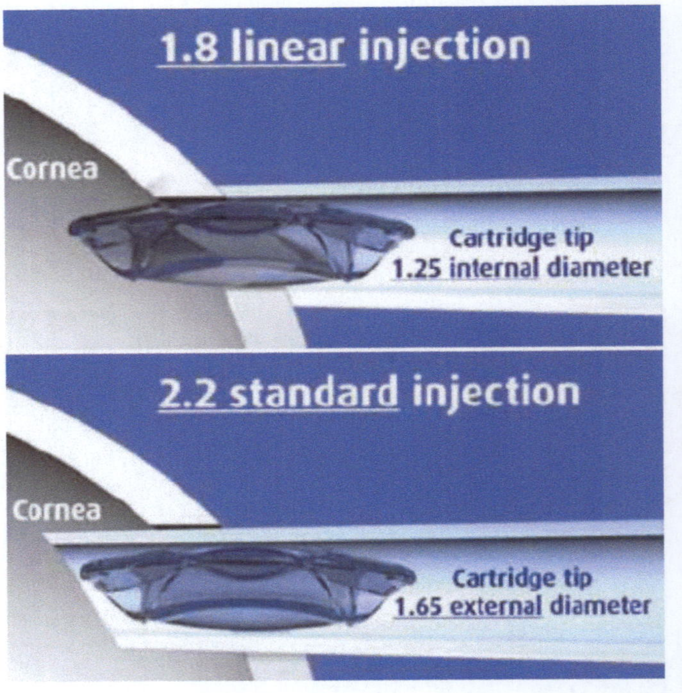

Fig. 8.26 Principles of injection on the wound assisted technique

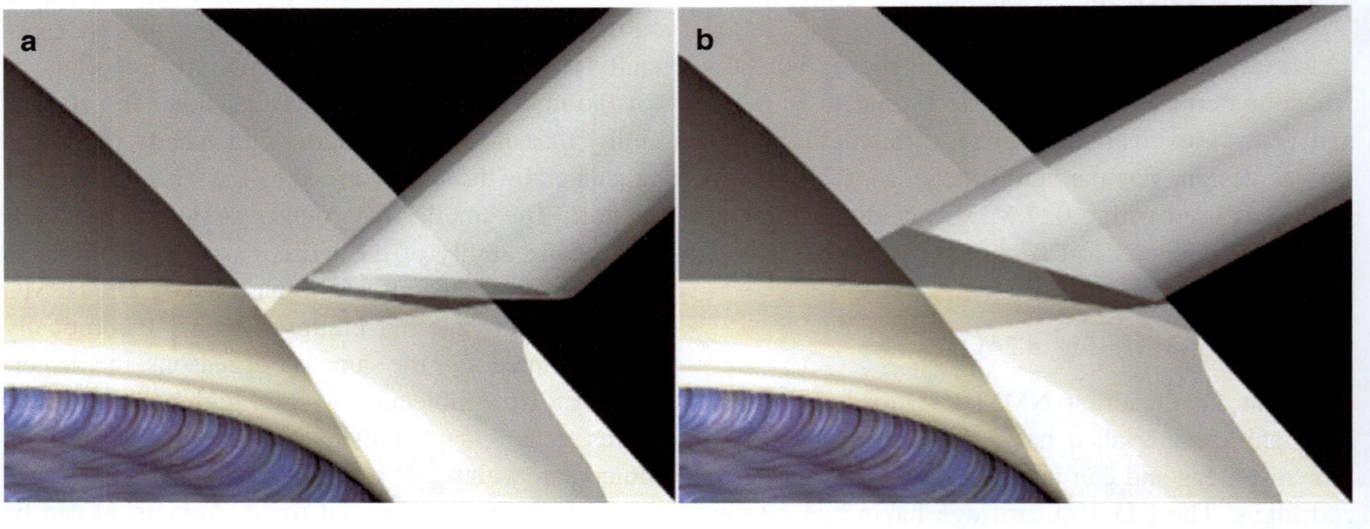

Fig. 8.25 Two principal types of injection: (**a**) wound-assisted technique (**b**) through the incision

enough to create a continuous tunnel of implantation through which the implant will pass. Practically, the internal diameter of the cartridge should be less than, or equal to, the incision size. The injection procedure should not widen the incision excessively (measuring the dimensions of incision pre and post injection using the calibrators allows evaluating clinically the widening of incision caused by the implantation). However, the injection should not cause "fish mouth" (apertognathia of incision) in order to assure perfect sealing in the postoperative phase. The study results confirm that the currently available injectors meant for microincision do not significantly modify the size and architecture of the corneal incision if appropriate dimensions are maintained.

8.2.6.1 Visco-Injection Using Wound-Assisted Technique

Today, the use of the wound-assisted technique to insert an IOL through an incision size between 1.5 and 2 mm is indispensable.

8.2.6.2 Incision Construction

- The construction of the incision should be precise and its size should be as per the injection system in order to avoid any incision leakage after the injection.
- A wrong initial architecture of the incision can cause a gap that could lead to a post operative ocular hypotony. In addition, it could possibly induce a retrograde flow of extraocular fluids through the incision towards the anterior chamber, a potential cause of endophthalmitis. A square-shaped incision seems more resistant and stable than a rectangular incision. A minimum of 2 mm length of incision could help in achieving self-sealing and stability.
- Theoretically, the best-suited incision could be a square-shaped three-plane incision. The first plane or preincision is perpendicular to the corneal plane and its borders can possibly join in case of ocular hypotony. The second plane is a minimum of 2 mm deep in the stromal plane capable of resisting ocular hypertension. Finally, the third plane is induced by using the knife vertically in order to minimize the descemetic traumatism by a penetration in the anterior chamber perpendicular to the corneal plane.
- This well-structured incision has better resistance not only to thermal or mechanical stress of phacoemulsification by microincision irrespective of the technique used, but also to injection stress.

8.2.6.3 Pressurization of the Anterior Chamber

- The anterior chamber is pressurized by injecting a viscoelastic substance which should preferably be cohesive. In fact, the main objective during injection is creating spaces and protecting the cornea and tissues, mainly by maintaining spaces during the maneuvers. A good zero-shear viscosity to create a deep anterior chamber and a high elasticity to amortize the traumatisms are the physical properties required. Cohesive VES attain these objectives better.

8.2.6.4 Loading the Cartridge

In the case of hinged cartridges, a moderate quantity of VES is injected into the grooves of the loading chamber and at the beginning of the injection tunnel. Theoretically, methylcellulose (HPMC) is best suited for this purpose. In practice, any VES can be used for visco-injection. The monobloc hydrophilic acrylic implant is taken out of humid conditioning at the last minute and placed under the locks in the middle of the loading chamber (Fig. 8.27a). Generally, these implants should not remain in nonhydrated conditions for a long time. The IOLs should always be placed in the right direction as most of the implants are angular and aspherical. The posterior angle will be directed towards the rear. It is necessary to position the haptics in the grooves and under the locks and then close the hinges without blocking or affecting any part of the implant. The two jaws of the forceps press the borders of the optic simultaneously while the hinges are folded (Fig. 8.27b). Before folding the hinges, the IOL should be fully loaded and the haptics should not get stuck in the hinges. In some cartridge models, a click sound can signal the closing of hinges which also means that the IOL is correctly loaded. For those models, the click is indispensable before the injection.

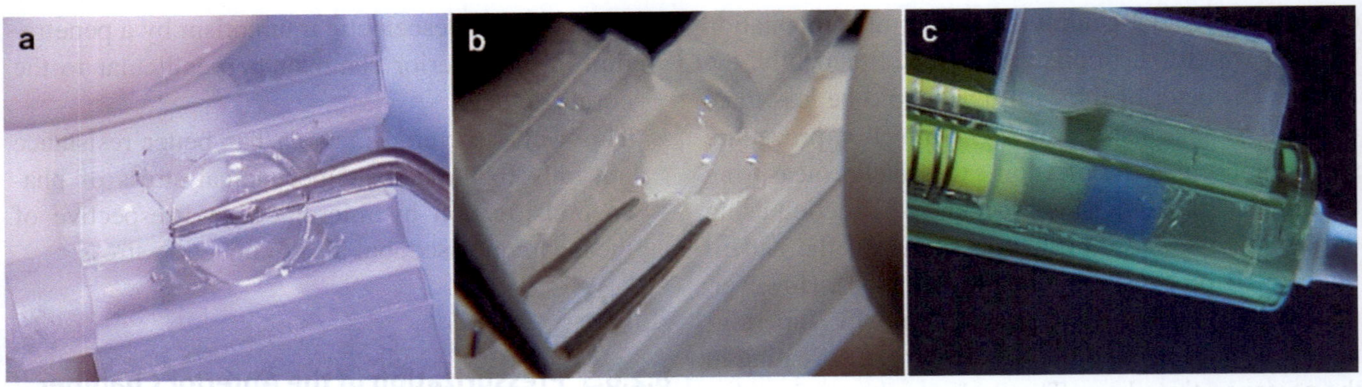

Fig. 8.27 (**a**) Loading the Akreos MI 60 (Bausch and Lomb) IOL in the cartridge, (**b**) closing the cartridge, (**c**) loading the cartridge in the injector body

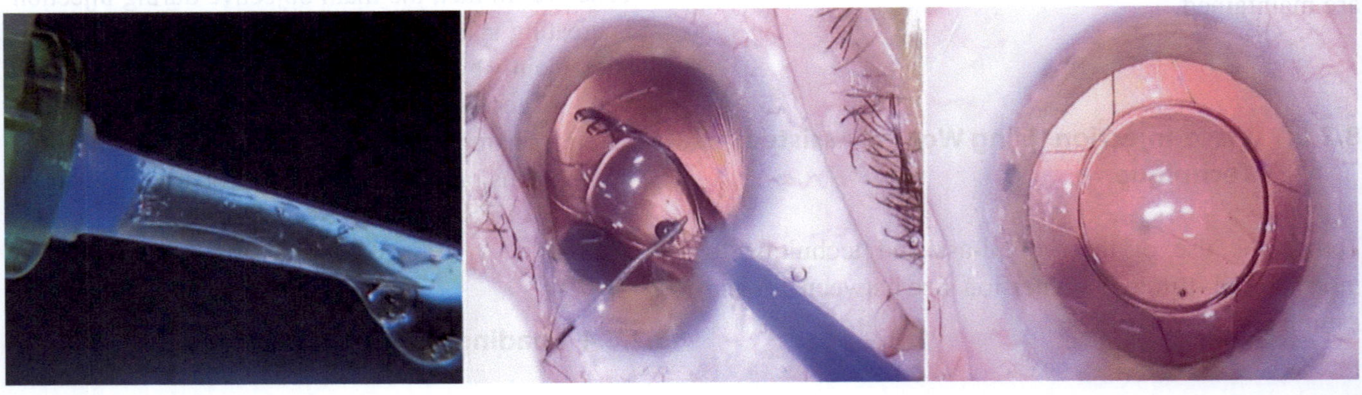

Fig. 8.28 (**a**) Inserting the soft plunger tip in the injection tunnel (**b**) injection on the border with back pressure and simultaneous positioning of the IOL (**c**) verification of the strictly intra saccular position of the Akreos MI 60 (Bausch and Lomb) IOL

8.2.6.5 Loading the Injector

- The cartridge is placed in the injector body (Fig. 8.27c) and should be brought into the chamber by pushing downwards. It should also be pushed backwards to be in contact with the posterior wall of the injector body. This operation is necessary for correct positioning of the soft plunger while inserting it in the loading chamber. As both the injector and the cartridge are transparent, the position of the IOL and the cartridge can be easily verified before the insertion of the plunger tip.

8.2.6.6 Insertion of the Plunger Tip

- The plunger tip is made of silicone and, therefore, is flexible. It should be inserted accurately in the loading chamber. This insertion should be carried out slowly and under observation so as to let the plunger tip deform and acquire a convenient position in the injection's axis (Fig. Fig. 8.28). An incorrect position of the soft tip can cause the bursting of the cartridge. The implant is pushed towards the central one-third of the injection tunnel under observation. The tip starts stretching as the diameter reduces. Since the injection is hydraulic, insertion becomes easy. An excessive resistance could mean anomaly, and hence the injection should be stopped. The injection should be carried out in one go without any latent period.

8.2.6.7 Injection in the Anterior Chamber

The injection can be carried out in favorable conditions after sufficient pressurization of the anterior chamber and proper loading of the IOL and the cartridge in the injector body. The cartridge bevel is then set under the anterior side of the incision. The injector is directed almost horizontally. In fact, the incision plane of the tunnel, parallel to the stroma of the cornea, should be followed, as the incision becomes an extension of the bevel. Any anomaly in the cartridge direction (mainly excessively vertical) can result in the blocking of the IOL in the stroma of the cornea, thus leading to an injection outside the globe or lesions on the incision. If the bevel direction is correct, the counter pressure is not always indispensable although it is useful to stabilize the globe during injection. This counter pressure can be obtained using another instrument or from an irrigation catheter through the second incision. The injection can be carried out when the bevel is correctly placed and directed. The pressure on the plunger should be firm and continuous but not excessive (Fig. 8.28b). Any interruption in the insertion has the risk of blocking the IOL in the incision, which is always difficult to extract (the IOL should be gently pulled out using forceps by letting it deform). The pressure on the plunger is released as soon as the IOL goes into the anterior chamber, as the soft plunger continues to deform and advance even after the insertion. If the soft plunger comes out excessively in the anterior chamber, it can get blocked in the incision. If this happens, it should be taken out slowly to let it stretch. Most of the IOLs available for microincision display good stability during injection, especially as the cartridges are well designed, and get unfolded flat in the anterior chamber.

8.2.6.8 Positioning the IOL in the Capsular Bag

The IOL can be positioned at once in the capsular bag during the injection using a second instrument for counter pressure.

It can also be positioned subsequently in the capsular bag. This easy but indispensable operation should be carried out accurately using a micro-manipulator as the sac is filled with viscoelastic substance. The instrument gently presses the optic's anterior side and, if required, rotates gently in order to place it in the capsular sac. The intra saccular position of all the haptics should be verified before and after removing the viscoelastic substance as these IOLs should necessarily be in an intra saccular position (Fig. 8.28c). Wrong positioning risks subluxation and could require a second intervention to position the IOL correctly.

8.2.6.9 Removing the VES

The VES in the front and the back of the IOL should be removed after implantation in order to restrict the risk of postoperative ocular hypertension and a possible posterior capsular opacification by making a close and premature contact between the posterior side of the IOL and the posterior capsule. The physical characteristics that help attaining these objectives are high pseudoplasticity and cohesion, which help in aspiration. Therefore, cohesive VES are best suited for the purpose. It is possible to use different techniques and care should be taken not to let the IOL move from the capsular sac. We use a direct aspiration of VES in the front and back of the IOL with high values of maximum vacuum and pump output.

8.2.6.10 Thin Roller Injector

The thin roller injector is a specific single-use injector. After assembling the single-use injector, the cartridge end is immersed in the irrigation solution. The hydrated implant is then inserted into the given slit. The implant is rolled in the cartridge's loading chamber by pressing the cap. This compression is maintained for 10 s. No viscoelastic substance is required. Once the implant is rolled, it should be injected quickly through an incision of 1.5–2 mm. After filling and pressurizing the anterior chamber with a viscoelastic substance, the cartridge end is put against the incision border. The implant is injected directly so that it does not unfold in the incision and get blocked. Another instrument is used simultaneously to create a counter pressure (Fig. 8.29a–c). The rolled implant reaches the anterior chamber and unfolds slowly. It should be verified that it unfolds in the correct direction. In fact, this IOL is not symmetrical, and the spurs help in verifying that it is positioned in the correct direction. After verification, the implant is placed in the capsular sac (Fig. 8.30a–c).

8.2.6.11 Conclusion

Injecting through a microincision requires the development of intraocular lenses, injectors and appropriate and innovative injection techniques.

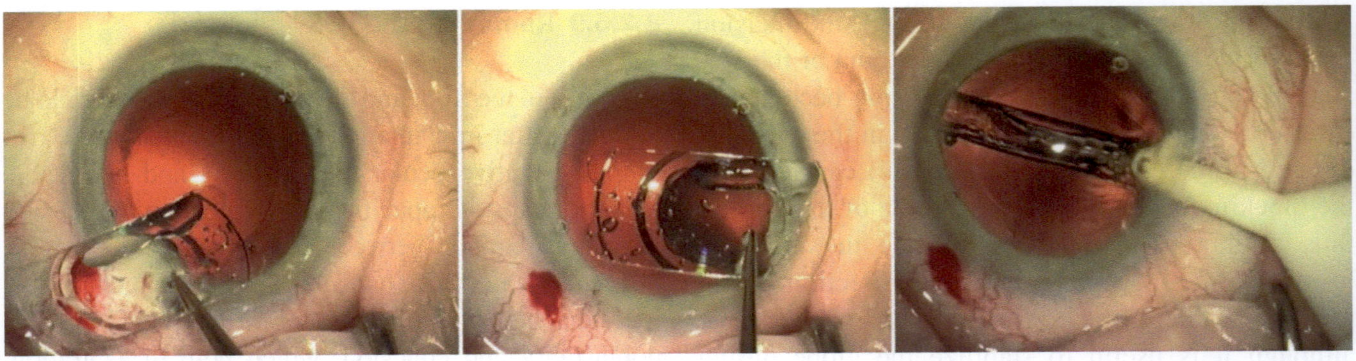

Fig. 8.29 Injection of the Ultrachoice 1.0 (ThinOptx) IOL using the ThinRoller injector

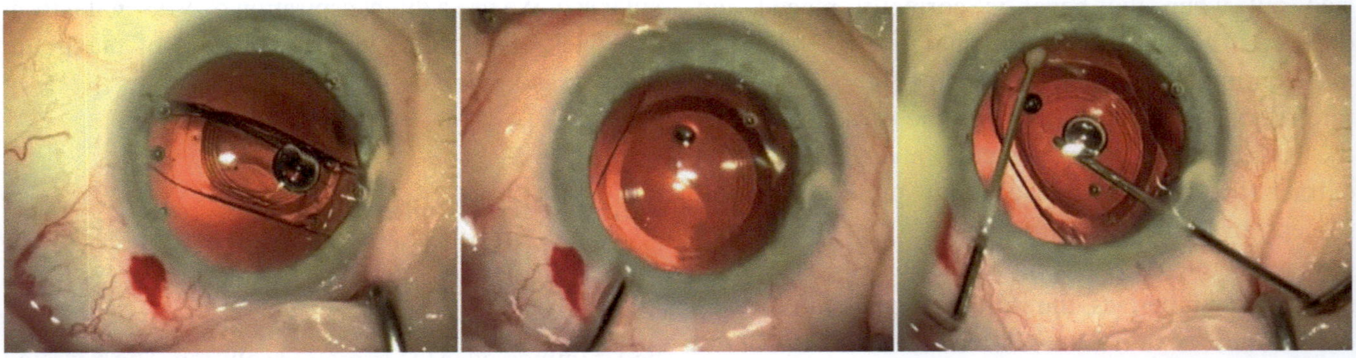

Fig. 8.30 Positioning the Ultrachoice 1.0 (ThinOptx) IOL in the capsular sac

Take Home Pearls

- To achieve a wound-assisted injection of a sub-2 mm IOL, a rigorous technique is mandatory. If the instructions are properly followed, the wound-assisted technique is a reliable and reproducible sub-2 mm injection technique.
- The IOL must be compatible with the sub-2 mm micro incision (material and design) with regard to both the incision size and the post-operative behavior.
- The cartridge and the injector must be reliable, adapted to the IOL and compatible with the micro-incision wound-assisted injection technique (internal diameter less than 1.4 mm).
- During the injection, the injector is angled close to the horizontal plane so that it follows the incision plane.
- The pressure on the plunger must be continuous. Any interruption during the injection has the risk of blocking the IOL in the incision.

The intraocular lenses need to resist the high mechanical stress and preserve their integrity, optic quality and a postoperative behavior similar to the best lenses available.

The injectors should be reliable, competitive and ergonomic. They should protect the IOL and the incision structure.

The implantation techniques adjusted with every injector and implant should be systematic, reliable and reproducible. Today, the Wound Assisted Technique is the most commonly used technique as it allows making the smallest incision.

The last few years has seen significant progress in these three domains that allowed reducing the incision size considerably, towards the patients' quality of vision and a phaco refractive approach of crystalline surgery.

Time will surely confirm this trend to reduce the incision size.

Only the progress made in these three domains shall make it possible.

Acknowledgment We thank Dr Joel Pynson for his precious and continued support.

Reference

1. Alio JL. Visual outcome of microincision cataract surgery with implantation of an Acri.Smart lens. J Cataract Refract Surg 2005; 31(8):1549–5156
2. Osher RH. Microcoaxial phacoemulsification. Part 2: clinical study. J Cataract Refract Surg 2007; 33(3):408–412
3. Alio JL. New MICS IOL:the AKREOS MI60. in European Society of Cataract and Refractive Surgery. 2007. Stockholm
4. Amzallag T, Pynson J. [Lens biomaterials for cataract surgery]. J Fr Ophtalmol 2007; 30(7):757–767
5. Amzallag T. Morphologie des lentilles intra oculaires et cataracte secondaire. In: Milazzo S, Riss I (eds) Cataracte secondaire: physiopathogénie, prévention et traitement. Rapport du BSOF, 2006, pp 155–174
6. Mamalis N. Incision width after phacoemulsification with foldable intraocular lens implantation. J Cataract Refract Surg 2000; 26(2):237–241
7. Amzallag T, Pynson J. Akreos Microincision Lens Pilot Study: 1-Year follow-up. In European Society of Cataract and Refractive Surgery. London, 2006
8. Mencucci R. Scanning electron microscopic analysis of acrylic intraocular lenses for microincision cataract surgery. J Cataract Refract Surg 2006; 32(2):318–323
9. Amzallag T. Implantation intraoculaire. In: Arné J.-L, Turut P, Amzallag T (eds) Chirurgie de la cataracte. Masson, Paris, 2005, pp. 167–198

8.3 Special Lenses

8.3.1 *Toric Posterior Chamber Intraocular Lenses in Cataract Surgery and Refractive Lens Exchange*

Gerd U. Auffarth, Tanja M. Rabsilber, and Miriam Casper

Core Messages

- Toric IOLs have become a new standard in the correction of refractive errors in pseudophakic astigmatism. In future, their use will be widespread due to their advantages in the correction of pseudophakic astigmatism.
- Rotational stability and refractive predictability are the key issues related to the design and the biomaterial of toric IOLs. The clinicians should obtain adequate information in all new toric IOLs regarding these important issues.
- When selecting a toric IOL, corneal astigmatism is the key factor in its calculation.
- Preoperative astigmatism should be left unchanged by cataract surgery. Techniques leading to an increase in the control of postoperative astigmatism are very important in association with the use of toric IOLs.

8.3.1.1 Introduction

For patients with corneal astigmatism (e.g., regular astigmatism or keratoplasty-induced), cataract surgery or refractive lens exchange using standard monofocal posterior chamber intraocular lenses (IOLs) is often unsatisfactory [1, 7, 8, 11, 19, 23].

G. U. Auffarth (✉)
University Eye Hospital Heidelberg, International Vision Correction Research Centre (IVCRC), Ruprechts-Karls-University of Heidelberg, INF 400, 69120 Heidelberg, Germany
e-mail: ga@uni-hd.de

Residual astigmatism requires wearing prescription eyeglasses, which may be acceptable for cataract patients, but is very undesirable for refractive patients [11].

Surgical techniques to correct postoperative astigmatism include "limbal relaxing incisions" (LRI), localization of the incision (temporal/12 o'clock), or "opposite clear corneal incisions" (OCCI). Further treatments with an excimer laser are also possible for astigmatism up to 3 diopters [2, 10].

In addition, there is also the possibility of correction with toric intraocular lenses (T-IOL). A distinction is made between intraocular lenses with a standard torus (usually 2–3 diopters) or individually produced (custom made) toric IOLs with an almost "unlimited" range [3, 6, 8–11, 15, 18, 20, 21].

8.3.1.2 Definitions

The calculation of a T-IOL is usually based on the *K-values* of the cornea [12–14]. These are measured as radii in millimeters. There is a distinction between *flat meridian* with a *large radius* (e.g., 7.90 mm) and *low refractive power* (42 diopters if > 1.0) and the *steep meridian* with a *small radius* (e.g., 7.20 mm) and *high refractive power* (47 diopter if ≤ 1.0) (Fig. 8.31). Conventional keratometer measure only the radii (e.g., IOL Master, topography devices) of the cornea. A direct measurement of the corneal refractive power does not exist. Corneal refractive power in diopters is calculated using the following formula:

$$D = \frac{n-1}{r},$$

Where *n*, the *refractive index* of the model eye is calculated differently with varying devices:

For the Zeiss IOL Master or the Zeiss Ophthalmometer, the value of $n = 1.332$ is used. For Javal-Keratometer or topography devices such as the Orbscan, a value of $n = 1.3375$ is used.

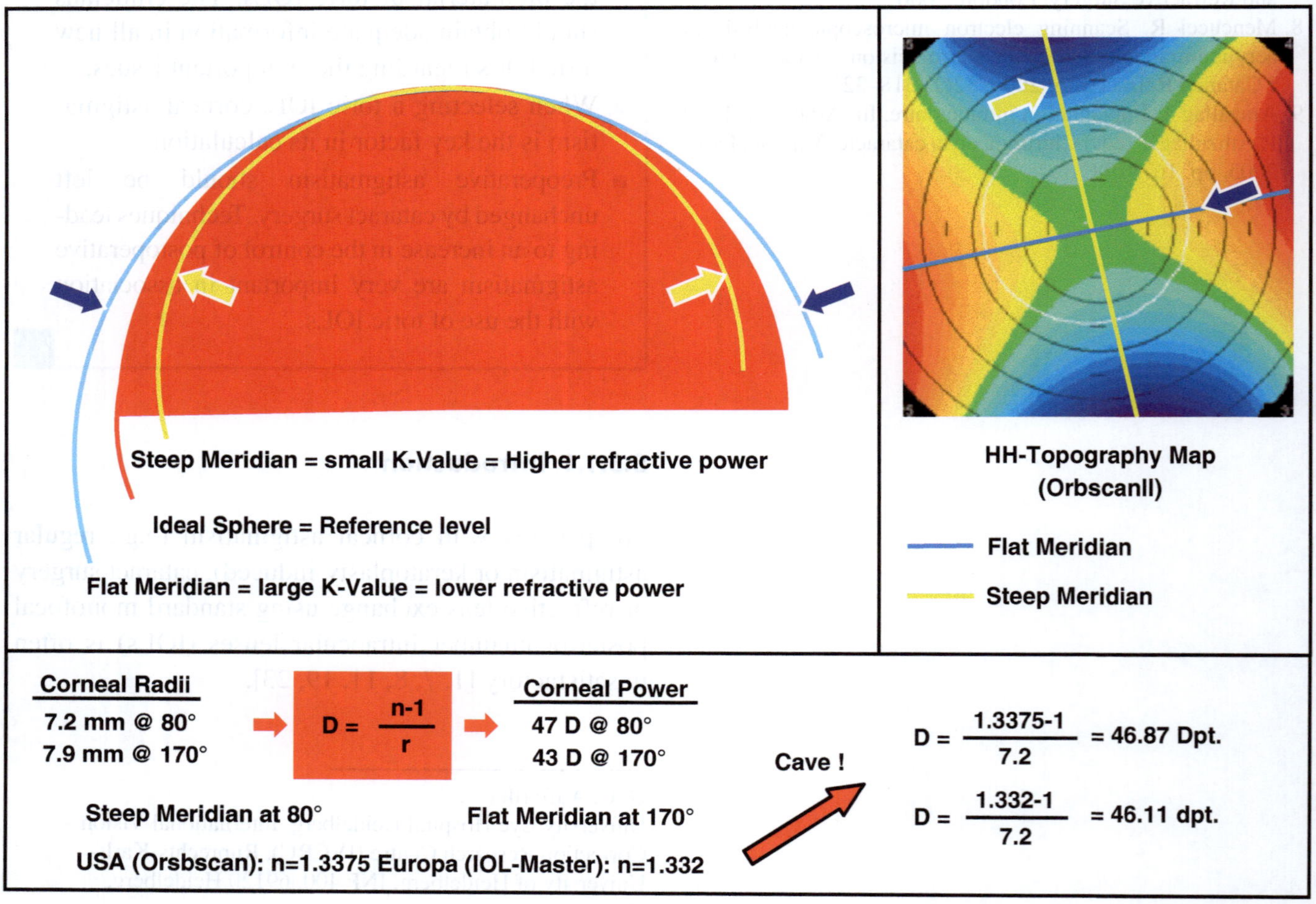

Fig. 8.31 Definitions of astigmatism

This may lead to a difference of 0.75 or 1 diopter:

$$D = \frac{1.3375 - 1}{7.2} = 46.87.\text{diopters}$$

$$D = \frac{1.332 - 1}{7.2} = 46.11.\text{diopters}$$

Therefore, it is important to indicate how the K-values were measured when ordering for a T-IOL (Fig. 8.31).

It is important that the cornea data, whether measured with the IOL Master and/or topography device, is collected at the beginning of the examination. IOP measurement and eye drops administration significantly affect the measurement. Contact lens wearers should be told that they must not wear contact lenses for at least 2 weeks before measurements are taken.

8.3.1.3 T-IOL Calculation

The calculation of a T-IOL is not simple and the task is usually not left to the implanting surgeon. Manufacturing companies usually calculate the intraocular lens power and the torus power using the data received from a mailed or faxed questionnaire. Implantation of the lens is made easier through drawings or available overlays on the operating screen. The company Alcon offers a program that can be accessed over the Internet, which allows users to calculate T-IOLs themselves by entering interactive data. Users may then order the T-IOLs. Figure 8.32 shows how the data should be entered, followed by the calculation of astigmatism on the corneal level. This is done taking into account the incision location and induced astigmatism. The torus is calculated on the plane of the T-IOL placement in the capsular bag, which is usually one or more diopters higher than the spectacle plane.

8.3.1.4 Current T-IOL Models

In Germany, the company Dr. Schmidt/Human Optics has been offering custom-made toric intraocular lenses, model MS 6116 with Z-haptics, for years (Fig. 8.33a). The torus is placed on the posterior surface of the IOL. The MS 6116 TU and the MS 614 T are toric IOLs for the capsular bag, or the sulcus. The model MS 714 TPB is a so-called add-on lens. In cases of pseudophakia, this lens is additionally implanted in the sulcus. The standard range for cylinder correction is up to 12 diopters. In addition, "custom made" IOLs with higher torus should be ordered. The results of cataract surgery with these toric intraocular lenses (e.g., even after keratoplasty) are very good. These toric IOLs are also used in refractive surgery because high ametropia is frequently accompanied by significant astigmatism [3, 7, 11, 18].

Other toric IOL models that are available in Germany are the Rayner 573 and 623 T-IOLs (Fig. 8.3a). The toric IOL model was developed from hydrophilic acrylic material as a "custom made" IOL with maximum torus values of up to 11 diopters [4, 5, 16, 17], on the basis of the one-piece Centerflex 570 H model, which showed good rotational stability. These also showed very good clinical results [17]. A special development by Rayner allowed the world's first toric multifocal, aspheric IOL to be implanted in June 2006 (Fig. 8.34).

The company Acri.Tec (now belonging to Zeiss) brought two different toric IOLs in the market, namely the bitoric IOL Acri.Smart 646 TLC and the Acri.Lyc 543 TLC (Figs. 8.33b and 8.35). The application of torus on both sides of the optics allows for a bit more leeway in the correction of astigmatism. Acri.Tec's bitoric aspherical T-IOLs possess high image quality. The model 646 TLC may be used in the context of micro-incision-cataract-surgery (MICS) techniques.

The company Wavelight (now belonging to Alcon) sells the model LU-804VR. The lens also has a standard torus range of up to 6 diopters and a premium torus range of more than 6 diopters (Fig. 8.33b). Currently, there is no peer-reviewed publication listed in the literature. Rasch (Potsdam) (personal communication) reported good clinical results at various conferences.

The company Staar offers a silicone-plated lens with a fixed torus of 2.0 or 3.5 diopters (Fig. 8.33b). This corresponds to a correction of 1.54 or 2.30, respectively, at the height of the cornea. Besides, the Alcon Acrysof toric IOL, this toric lens is currently, the only approved T-IOL in the United States [6, 10, 19, 20].

The Alcon Acrysof toric IOLs SA60T3/4/5 are also offered with a fixed torus of 1.50, 2.25 or 3.0 diopters (Fig. 8.33b). So far, only the results of the American FDA study of this IOL are known. In the range of 1–2 diopters (on the cornea level), the IOL showed very good results and good rotational stability [12, 21]. Alcon'sprogram for T-IOL calculation is particularly noteworthy (Fig. 8.32).

Pre-Op Refraction: OD: -14.5 -5.0 175 = 20/50

Pre-Op Information

Patient Data	
Flat K	39.67 D
@ Flat Meridian	19°
Steep K	42.19 D
@ Steep Meridian	109°
IOL Spherical Power (P-IOL)	15.5 D
Surgically Induced Cylinder (SIC)	0.50 D
Incision Location (IL)	90°

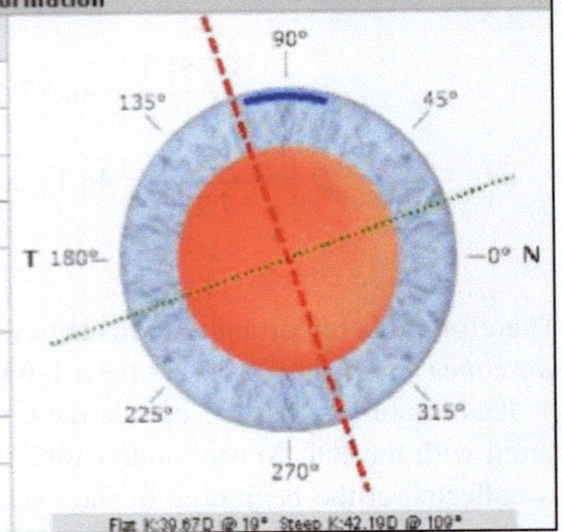

Doctor & Patient Information	
Doctor Name	Prof. Auffarth
Patient Information	[redacted]
Eye Selection	OD (Right)

Lens Details	
AcrySof® Toric IOL	SN60T5
IOL Spherical Equivalent (SE)	15.5 D
Axis of Placement	113°
IOL Cylinder (Cyl)	3.00 D

Calculation Details	
Pre-op Corneal Cylinder:	2.52 X 109°
Surgically Induced Cylinder:	0.50 X 0°
Crossed-Cylinder Result (corneal plane):	2.15 X 113°
Crossed-Cylinder Result (IOL plane):	3.14 X 113°

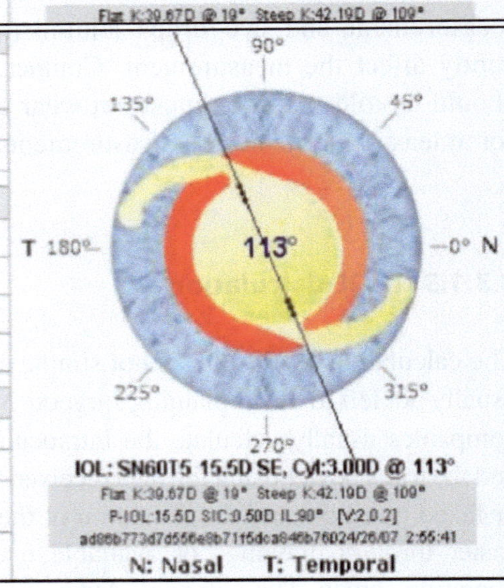

IOL: SN60T5 15.5Dpt 3.0 D Torus

1 d Post-Op OD: ±0 sph = 20/30

Fig. 8.32 Calculation of a toric lens using the Alcon program: Although the patient shows 5 diopters of astigmatism with spectacles, results of the Keratometry shows a corneal astigmatism of 2.52 diopters. Excluding the surgically induced astigmatism, due to incision at 12:00 o'clock, a corneal astigmatism of 2.15 diopters remains. This is 3.14 diopters on the IOL level, therefore an IOL with a torus value 3 diopters is recommended. Postoperative, the patient does not require additional astigmatic correction

8.3.1.5 Preoperative Marking

Before surgery, the patient's eye has to be marked for the axis orientation of the T-IOL. Since general anesthesia, peri, para- or retrobulbar anesthesia or even topical anesthesia can lead to a rotation of the bulbus, it is important to make marks beforehand on the patient when he is awake, seated, looking straight ahead. In general, it is sufficient to mark the horizontal and 90°-meridian, for example, with a surgical pen (Fig. 8.36a). A pendular marker by Geuder (Fig. 8.36b) or other devices can also be used to make marks. It is also often possible to orientate oneself by using certain anatomical characteristics (blood vessels at 12 o'clock, etc.).

8.3.1.6 Clinical Indications

Toric posterior chamber lenses can be implanted during cataract surgery or refractive lens exchange, in patients with existing corneal astigmatism [3, 7, 8, 11, 12, 17]. However, lentogenic and retinal astigmatism cannot be corrected. The production of T-IOLs is always dependent on keratometry. The intraocular fit offers higher correction than spectacle correction, roughly comparable to well-fitted contact lenses. Astigmatism after keratoplasty can be corrected using T-IOLs [1, 8, 15, 17, 22]. For every form of regular, but not irregular astigmatism, T-IOL implantation is promising. Keratokonus should only be corrected using toric posterior chamber lenses under special conditions.

Fig. 8.33 List of toric intraocular lenses: (**a**) Dr. Schmidt/Humanoptics and Fa. Rayner (**b**) Acri.Tec, Wavelight, Staar, and Alcon

a

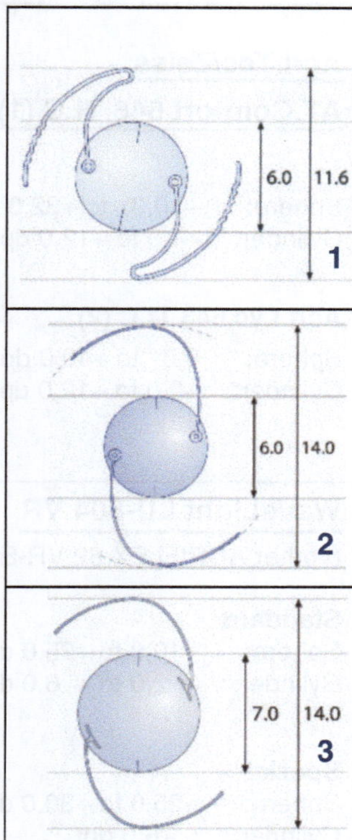

Dr. Schmidt/Humanoptics: MicroSil IOL Line:

MS 6116 TU (1) und MS 614 T (2)

Sphere: +15,0 to +25,0 dpt (in 0,5 dpt steps)
- 3,0 to +14,0 dpt (in 1,0 dpt steps)
+26,0 to +31,0 dpt (in 1,0 dpt steps)
Cyl.: + 2,0 to +12,0 dpt (in 1,0 dpt steps)

MS 714 TPB (3)

Sphere: in relation to cylinder, SE = 0 dpt
Cylinder: +1,0 to +6,0 dpt (in 1,0 dpt steps)

(Customized manufacturing outsinde this range individually possible for all models)

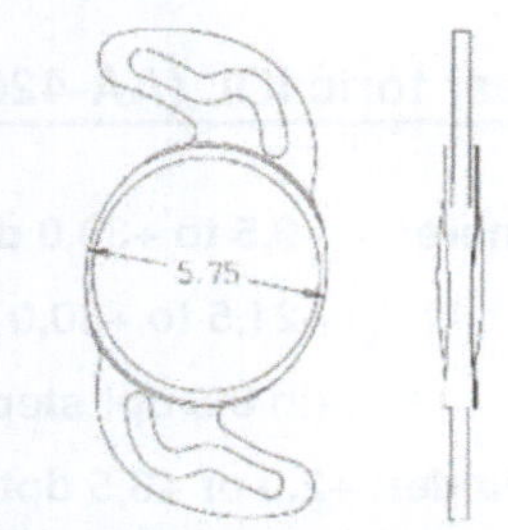

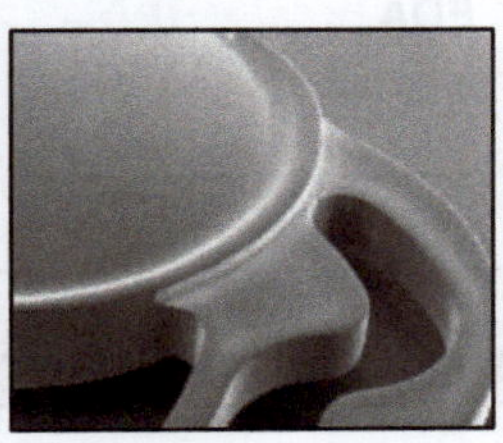

Rayner T-Flex Line

360° sharp edge & Torus on anterior optic
T-flex 573 T based on C-flex 570 C
T-flex 623 T based on Superflex 620 H

Standard
Sphere: +6,0 to +30,0 dpt (in 0,5 dpt steps)
Cylinder: +1,0 to + 6,0 dpt (in 1,0 dpt steps)

Spezial
Sphere: - 5,0 to +32,5 dpt (in 0,5 dpt steps)
Cylinder: +1,0 to +11,0 dpt (in 0,25 dpt steps)

8.3.1.7 Custom-Made Lenses

Besides individually produced T-IOLs, which may have a torus value of up to 30 diopters (Humanoptics), Rayner introduced the M-Flex T- IOL. The M-Flex T- IOL is the world's first customized lens that has an aspheric, toric, and multifocal optics. The first patient to use this lens underwent surgery in June 2006. The patient was a 45-year-old female with a visual acuity of: OD: +8.0/–2.25/170°=0.8 and OS: +10.25/–3.25/5°=0.8. Anterior chamber depth (measured from the endothelium) was 2.45 (OD) and 2.34 mm (OS). The corneal thickness was 528 and 507 µm. Keratometric astigmatism was 3.08 diopter (OD) and 3.68 diopter (OS). After extensive counseling, it was decided that a refractive lens exchange with implantation of a custom made aspherical, toric, multifocal IOL manufactured by the company Rayner, UK, would be carried out. Using

Fig. 8.33 (continued)

b

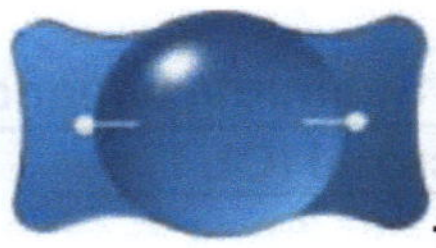

1

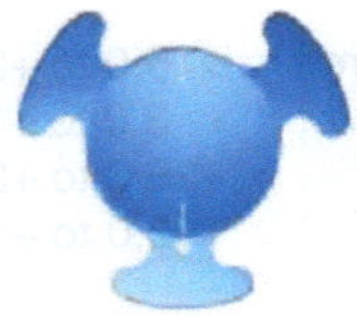

2

Acri.Tec/Zeiss

AT.Comfort 646 TLC (1)

Sphere: −10,0 to +32,0 dpt
Cylinder: +1,0 to +12,0 dpt

Acri.Lyc 643 TLC (2)

Sphere: 0,0 to +40,0 dpt
Cylinder: +2,0 to +12,0 dpt

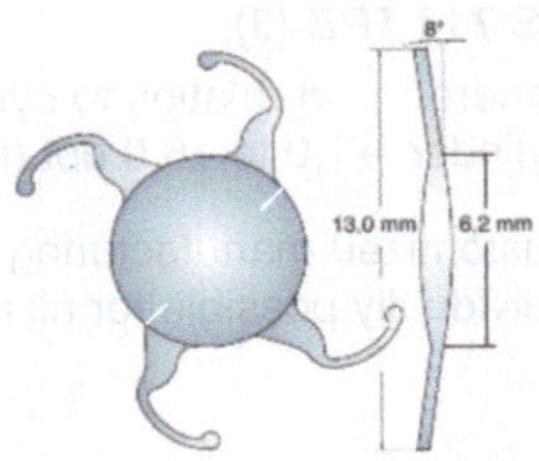

WaveLight LU-804 VR

(vorher ACRIFLEX 62 VR-E)

Standard
Sphere: +10,0 to +25,0 dpt
Cylinder: + 2,0 to + 6,0 dpt

Spezial
Sphere: +25,0 to +30,0 dpt
Cylinder: > +6,0 dpt

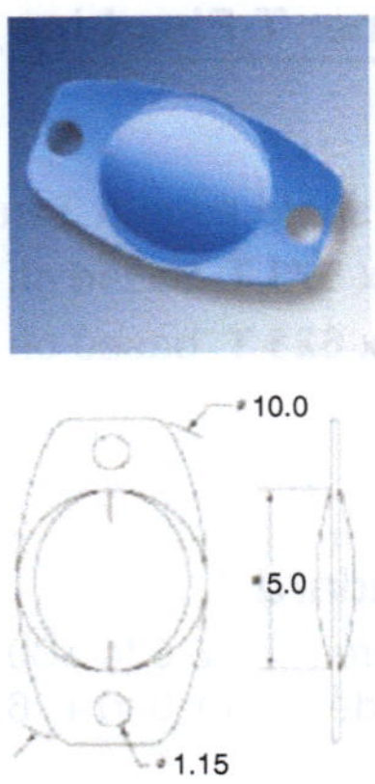

Staar toric IOL (AA-4203 TF or TL)

Sphere: +9,5 to +30,0 dpt /
+21,5 to +30,0 dpt
(in 0,5 dpt steps)

Cylinder: +2,0 or +3,5 dpt

✓ FDA

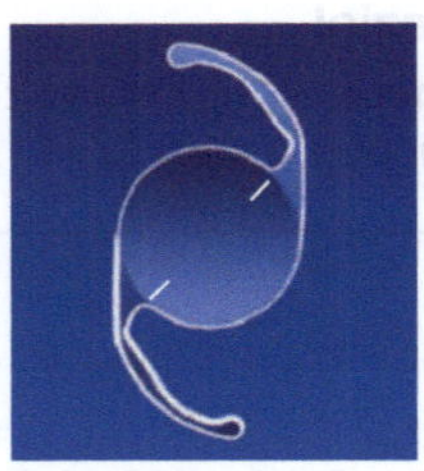

Alcon SN60T3, SN60T4, SN60T5

Torus: 1,50 dpt
2,25 dpt
3,00 dpt

✓ FDA

phakoemulsification, the lens surgery was completed without complications (Fig. 8.34).

On the right eye, the implanted IOL was a Rayner C-flex 588F with +33.5 diopter +3.0 NearAdd, −3.5 torus. On the left eye, the IOL power was +36.5 diopter +3.0 NearAdd, −4.5 diopter torus. The multifocal design corresponded to the Rayner M-Flex, a refractive MIOL with +3 near addition and aspherical intermediate zones. One month post surgery, the uncorrected visual acuity was 0.8 on the right eye and 0.63 on the

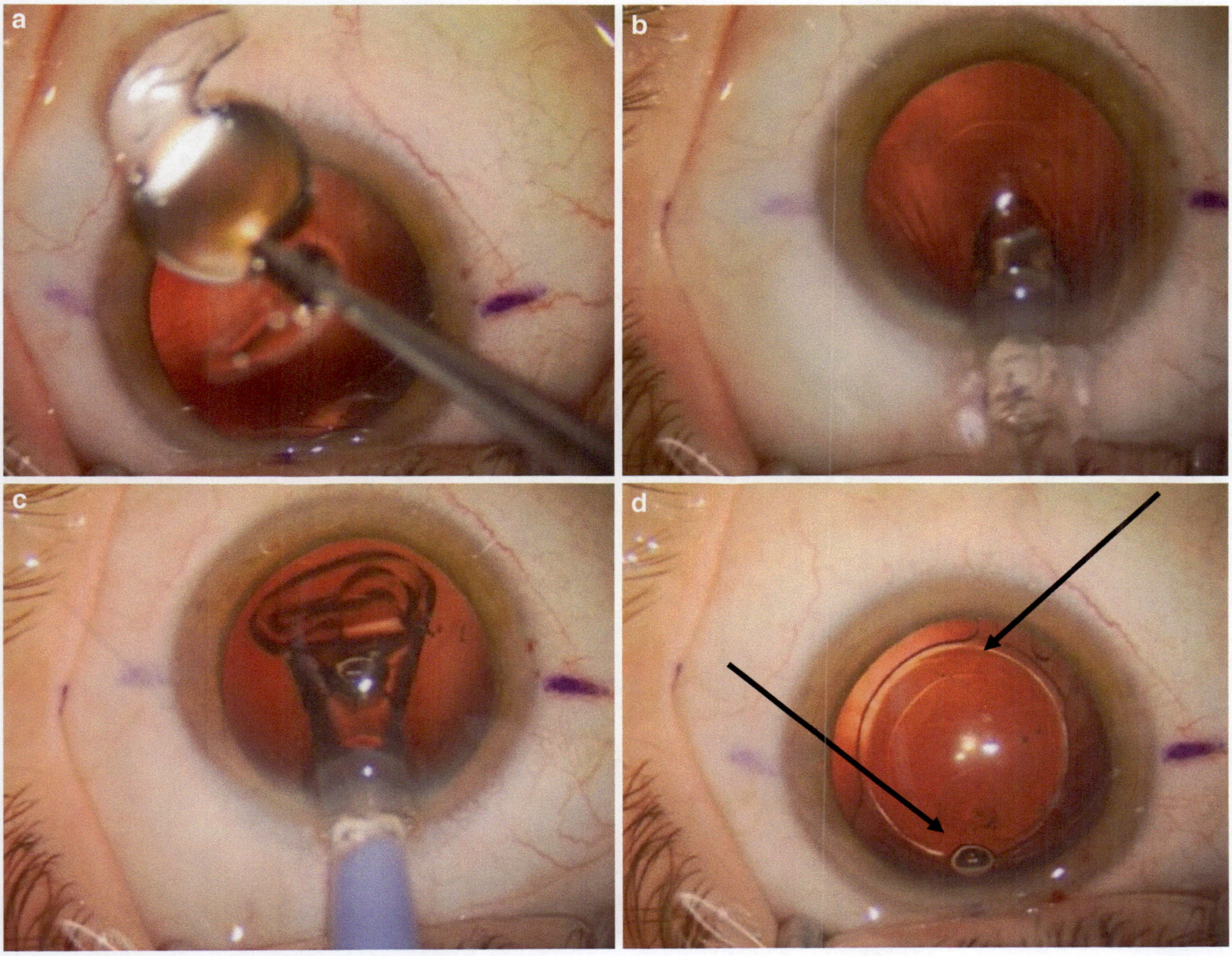

Fig. 8.34 (**a–d**) Implantation sequence of an Acri.Tec 646 TLC 1 Acri.Smart

left eye. Near visual acuity was 0.5 uncorrected. The defocus curve showed an accommodation width of approximately 4–4.5 diopters. A combination of different corrective optical factors of an artificial lens is possible without leading to photic phenomena. This made it possible to create a truly "individually" fitted IOL with good functional results.

In principle, it would be beneficial to develop a multifocal lens, that is, lenses with fixed torus values, for standard surgery (e.g., 2, 4, 6 diopter or 1.5, 2.5, 4.5 diopter), in order to reduce costs and minimize production times.

8.3.1.8 Conclusion for Practice

Toric posterior chamber lenses are becoming increasingly popular. They can be calculated with high accuracy and have shown good functional results. Practitioners should note that since intraocular astigmatism is corrected intraocularly, the Keratometry will continue to show preoperative K-values. Spectacles (if needed) are measured using subjective evaluation rather than being based on Autorefractor results. Clinical results are usually very good and patient satisfaction is high.

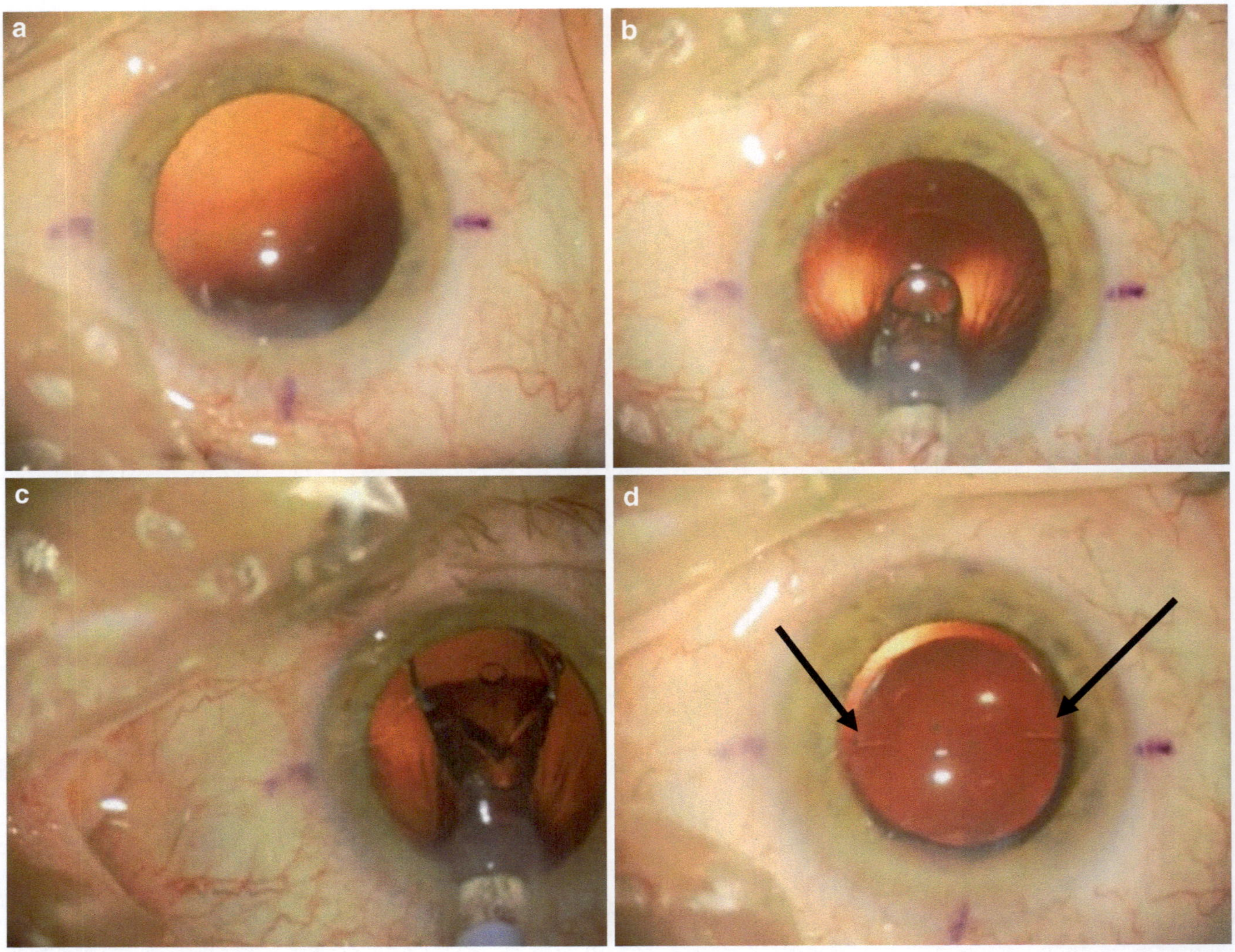

Fig. 8.35 (**a–d**) Marking the axis location on the conjunctiva using a surgical pen (a) or Geuder Pendular Marker (b) on a patient who is upright, seated, and looking straight ahead

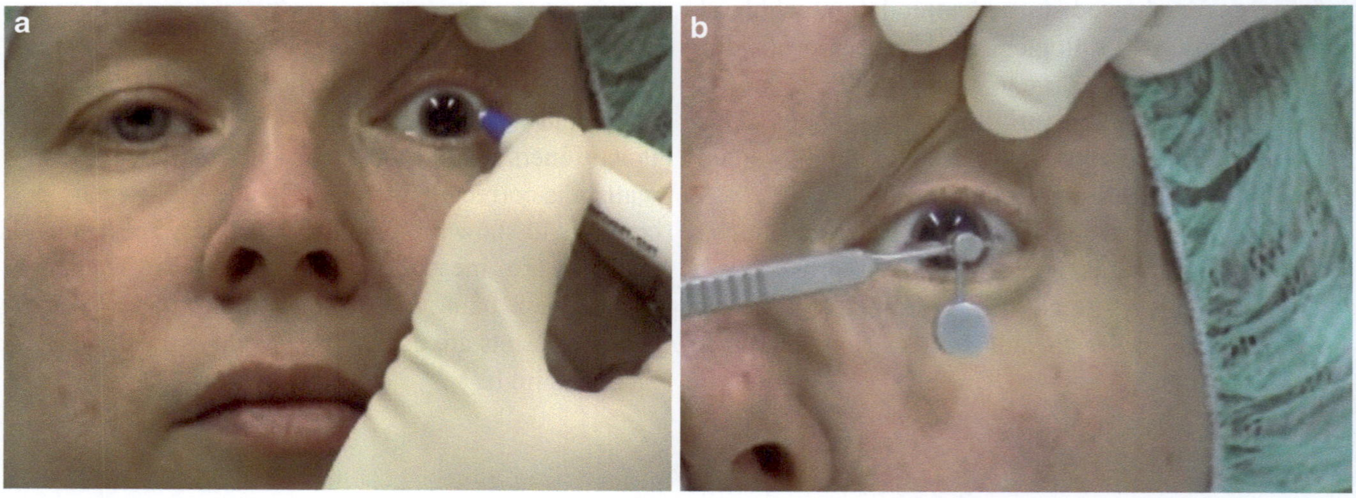

Fig. 8.36 (**a**, **b**) Implantation sequence of a Rayner M-Flex T for the correction of astigmatism and presbyopia

Take Home Pearls

- Toric IOLs provide a much more reliable and a precise way to correct astigmatism in pseudophakia.
- Surgeons should use surgical techniques that control the induction of change in astigmatism in order to make an adequate use of toric IOLs in the surgery.
- In the future, due to their unlimited range, toric IOLs are to be dominant in the correction of astigmatism above 2 diopters. Toric IOL calculation is based on preoperative corneal astigmatism.
- Axis detection, prior to surgery is mandatory before starting the surgery. Preoperative marking of the adequate axis should be performed just before preparing the patient for surgery.

References

1. Amm M, Halberstadt M. [Implantation of toric intraocular lenses for correction of high post-keratoplasty astigmatism]. Ophthalmologe 2002; 99(6):464–469
2. Auffarth GU. (Hrsg.) Aktuelle Laseranwendungen in der refraktiven Chirurgie. Uni-Med Verlag, Bremen, 2004, ISBN 3-89599-806-0
3. Auffarth GU, Holzer MP, Becker KA, Völcker HE. Erste Erfahrungen mit der torischen Silikonintraokularlinse MS6116TU mit Z-Haptik. In: Auffarth GU, Welt R, Demeler U (eds) Kongressband: 17. Kongress der Deutschsprachigen Gesellschaft für Intraokularlinsen Implantation und Refraktive Chirurgie. Biermann, Köln, 2003, pp 171–174
4. Becker KA, Auffarth GU, Volcker HE. Messmethode zur Bestimmung der Rotation und der Dezentrierung von Intraokularlinsen. Ophthalmologe 2004; 101(6):600–603
5. Becker KA, Martin M, Rabsilber TM, Entz BB, Reuland AJ, Auffarth GU. Prospective, non-randomised, long-term clinical evaluation of a foldable hydrophilic single-piece intraocular lens: results of the Centerflex FDA study. Br J Ophthalmol 2006; 90(8):971–974
6. Chang DF. Early rotational stability of the longer Staar toric intraocular lens: fifty consecutive cases. J Cataract Refract Surg 2003; 29(5):935–940
7. De Silva DJ, Ramkissoon YD, Bloom PA. Evaluation of a toric intraocular lens with a Z-haptic. J Cataract Refract Surg 2006; 32(9):1492–1498
8. Dick HB, Krummenauer F, Trober L. [Compensation of corneal astigmatism with toric intraocular lens: results of a multicentre study]. Klin Monatsbl Augenheilkd 2006; 223(7):593–608
9. Gerten G, Michels A, Olmes A. Toric intraocular lenses. Clinical results and rotational stability] Ophthalmologe. 2001; 98(8):715–720
10. Gills J, Van der Karr M, Cherchio M. Combined toric intraocular lens implantation and relaxing incisions to reduce high preexisting astigmatism. J Cataract Refract Surg 2002; 28(9):1585–1588
11. Holzer MP, Auffarth GU, Reuland A.J., Entz BB, Becker KA. Clear Lens Extraction mit Implantation torischer Intraokularlinsen (MS6116 Microsil) als refraktiver Eingriff. In: Pham DT, Auffarth GU, Wirbelauer C, Demeler U (Hrsg.) Kongressband: 18. Kongress der Deutschsprachigen Gesellschaft für Intraokularlinsen Implantation und Refraktive Chirurgie, Biermann, Köln, 2004, pp 377–380
12. Horn JD. Status of toric intraocular lenses. Curr Opin Ophthalmol 2007; 18(1):58–61
13. Langenbucher A, Szentmary N, Seitz B. Calculating the power of toric phakic intraocular lenses. Ophthalmic Physiol Opt 2007; 27(4):373–380
14. Langenbucher A, Viestenz A, Seitz B, Brunner H. Computerized calculation scheme for retinal image size after implantation oftoric intraocular lenses. Acta Ophthalmol Scand 2007; 85(1):92–98
15. Mohammadpour M. Toric IOL and postkeratoplasty astigmatism. Ophthalmology 2007; 114(4):825–826; author reply 826–827
16. Nishi Y, Rabsilber TM, Limberger IJ, Vucic D, Auffarth GU. Influence of 360 degree enhanced optic edge design on secondary cataract development of a hydrophilic acrylic IOL. J Cataract Refract Surg 2007; 33(2):227–231
17. Rabsilber TM, Auffarth GU, Vargas LG, Reuland AJ, Entz BB. Erste Erfahrungen mit der Rayner 570T torischen Intraokularlinse. In: Pham DT, Auffarth GU, Wirbelauer C, Demeler U (Hrsg.) Kongressband: 18. Kongress der Deutschsprachigen Gesellschaft für Intraokularlinsen Implantation und Refraktive Chirurgie, Biermann, Köln, 2004, pp 373–376
18. Ruhswurm I, Scholz U, Zehetmayer M, Hanselmayer G, Vass C, Skorpik C. Astigmatism correction with a foldable toric intraocular lens in cataract patients. J Cataract Refract Surg 2000; 26(7):1022–1027
19. Sun XY, Vicary D, Montgomery P, Griffiths M. Toric intraocular lenses for correcting astigmatism in 130 eyes. Ophthalmology 2000; 107(9):1776–1781
20. Tahzib NG, Eggink FA, Odenthal MT, Nuijts RM. Artisan iris-fixated toric phakic and aphakic intraocular lens implantation for the correction of astigmatic refractive error after radial keratotomy. J Cataract Refract Surg 2007; 33(3):531–535
21. Tehrani M, Dick HB. [Implantation of an ARTISAN toric phakic intraocular lens to correct high astigmatism after penetrating keratoplasty]. Klin Monatsbl Augenheilkd 2002; 219(3):159–163
22. Tehrani M, Schwenn O, Dick HB. [Toric intraocular lens to correct high astigmatism after penetrating keratoplasty in a pseudophakic eye – a case report]. Klin Monatsbl Augenheilkd 2001; 218(12):795–799
23. Till JS, Yoder PR Jr, Wilcox TK, Spielman JL. Toric intraocular lens implantation: 100 consecutive cases. J Cataract Refract Surg 2002; 28(2):295–301

8.3.2 Special Lenses: MF

Hakan Kaymak and Ulrich Mester

Core Messages

- The only multifocal IOL that fits through the 1.5 mm incision size is the *Acri.LISA (*Acri. Tec, Zeiss, Henningsdorf, Germany).
- Acri.LISA is an acronym of the main optical properties of the lens.
- Visual acuity for distance vision is very good with Acri.LISA and is comparable with that of monofocal IOLs, at least under photopic lighting conditions.
- Near vision is also sufficient despite the unequal light distribution of the *Acri.LISA in favor of the far distance.
- Patients with the Acri.LISA have a pseudo-accommodation range of 5.5 diopters.
- Initial results of the toric version of the Acri. LISA are very promising.

The use of multifocal intraocular lenses (MIOL) has been very limited in the past due to several drawbacks and limitations [1]: Surgical techniques were not as refined and predictable as today and accurate biometry to achieve emmetropia was challenging. Moreover, independence from glasses could not be achieved in all patients, particularly for near vision. Many patients complained of photic phenomena [2, 3], and driving was impaired due to reduced contrast sensitivity under mesopic conditions [4, 5].

Meanwhile, a new generation of MIOLs has been developed and investigated in clinical studies. Several new optical concepts were incorporated in these lenses:

The only multifocal IOL that fits through the 1.5 mm incision size is the *Acri.LISA (*Acri.Tec, Zeiss, Henningsdorf, Germany). The characteristics of this MIOL are summarized in Table 8.4. Acri.LISA is the acronym of the main optical properties of the lens (Fig. 8.38).

Table 8.4 Characteristics of Acri.LISA

Optic diameter	6.0 mm	
Total diameter	11.0 mm	*Acri.LISA*
Haptic angulation	0°	
Design	Square edged optic and haptic	
	Single-piece, +3.75 D addition, SMP-technology, refractive / defractive 65:35 aberration-correcting, MICS	
Lens design		
Incision size	1.5 – 1.7 mm	
Material	Foldable acrylate with 25% water content, hydrophobic surface, UV absorber	
Sterilization method	Autoclaving	
Diopter range	±0.0 to +32.0 D, 0.5 D increment	
Package	Sterile, in water for injection	
Recommend A-factor:	Acoustic/optic	
AL < 25.00 mm	117.6/117.9	
AL ≥ 25.00 mm	118.0/118.3	
	A2-2000	
Injector system	Acri.Smart cartridge	

With the application of a diffractive optic, the visual performance became independent of the pupil size, which was a major drawback of the previous MIOL-generation with refractive optics.

The introduction of an aspheric lens design enhanced contrast vision, which could be demonstrated previously in clinical studies with monofocal IOLs [6–8].

Another new concept is that of unequal light distribution for distance and near vision, based on the consideration that most patients prioritize distance vision. This concept may also lead to a reduction of halos.

To reduce the complaints due to straylight, smooth steps within the diffractive pattern were engineered (Fig. 8.38).

Clinical studies were performed with this MIOL.

Thirty patients with bilateral implantation of the *Acri.LISA were examined 1 year after surgery of the second eye.

H. Kaymak (✉)
Department of Ophthalmology, Knappschafts Hospital, Sulzbach, Germany
e-mail: sek-augen@kksulzbach.de

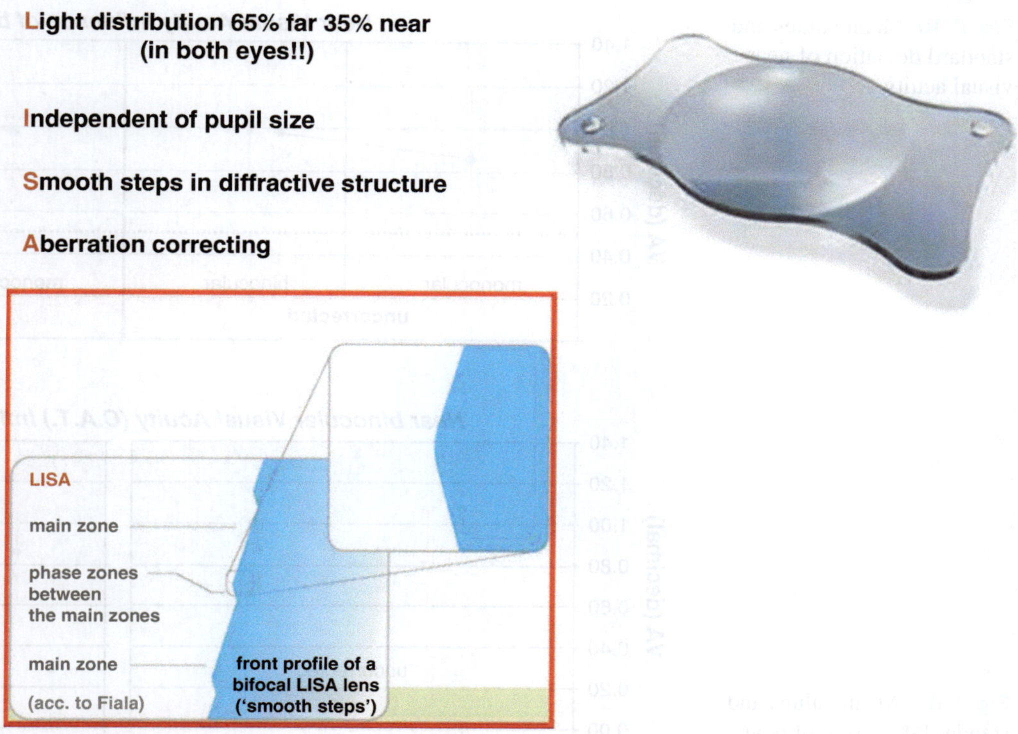

Fig. 8.38 Acri.Lisa

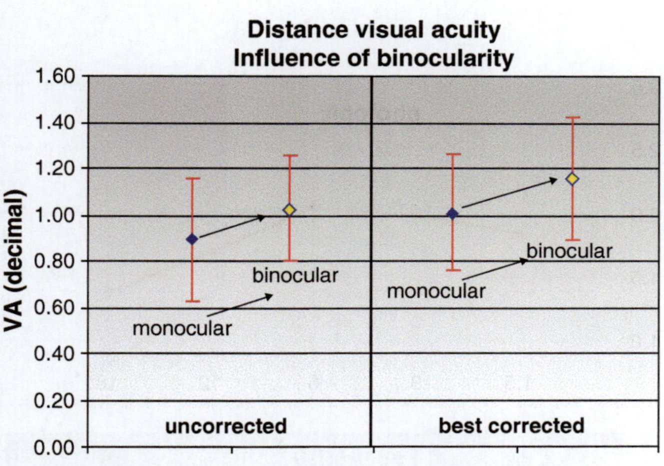

Fig. 8.39 Mean values and standard deviation of distance visual acuity

Monocular and binocular visual acuity (VA) (uncorrected and best corrected) at the 1 year control period are shown in Fig. 8.39. Despite the dominance for far distance of this MIOL, near VA is also very satisfying (uncorrected monocular 0.85, binocular 1.05 under photopic conditions) (Fig. 8.40).

The near uncorrected VA was tested under two lighting conditions demonstrating a luminance depending improvement from 0.8 (80 lux) to 1.0 (350 lux) (Fig. 8.41).

The defocus curve demonstrated the drop of VA at intermediate distance, but not exceeding the critical limit of 0.5 (Fig. 8.42).

The contrast sensitivity was within the normal range under photopic conditions (Fig. 8.43).

With regard to photopic phenomena after 1 year, almost no patient described halos in everyday life.

Overall patients' satisfaction was 8.3 using a scale from 0 to 10 after 1 year (Fig. 8.44).

8.3.2.1 Discussion

The Acri.LISA offered good efficacy, predictability and satisfying functional outcomes. Our results are in accordance with the findings of Alió et al. [1] and Alfonso et al. [2]. Alió et al. [1] demonstrated very good MTF values of the Acri.LISA for 3 and 6 mm pupil sizes which reflected our clinical outcomes.

8.3.2.2 Conclusion

VA for distance vision is very good with Acri.LISA and comparable with monofocal IOLs, at least under photopic lighting conditions.

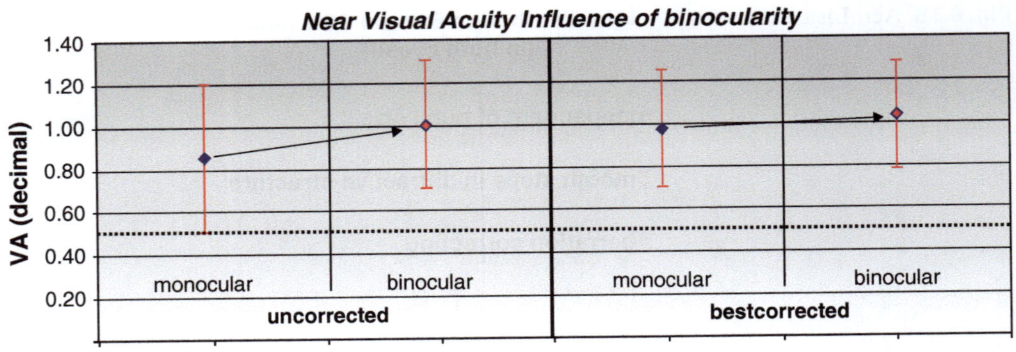

Fig. 8.40 Mean values and standard deviation of near visual acuity

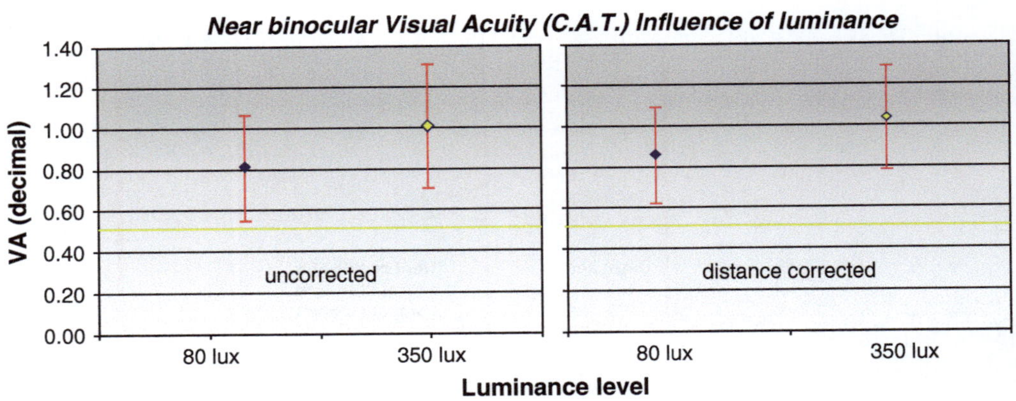

Fig. 8.41 Mean values and standard deviation of near visual acuity under different lighting conditions

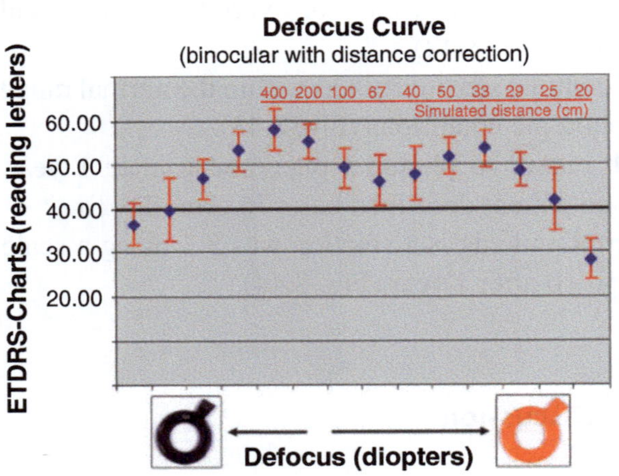

Fig. 8.42 Defocus curve with Acri.LISA

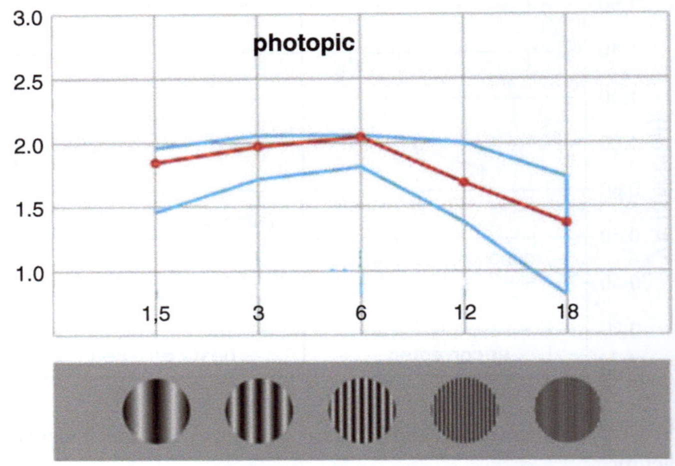

Fig. 8.43 Photopic contrast sensitivity with Acri.LISA (*red*), normal range (*green*)

Near vision is also sufficient despite the unequal light distribution of the *Acri.LISA in favor of the far distance. A better near VA could be achieved with increasing light luminance. Contrast vision is within the normal range.

There is a significant drop of VA at the intermediate distance. This is because of the bifocal optic of the MIOLs. Therefore, it is advisable to speak of bifocal IOLs instead of multifocal lenses to avoid disappointing patients, who might expect to receive IOLs such as progressive glasses. On the other hand, the drop of VA in the intermediate distance did not exceed 0.5, which was sufficient for daily activities for most of the patients.

With the Acri.LISA, more than 80% of the patients gained complete independence from spectacles. This is an enormous improvement compared to just one third of patients getting freedom from glasses with the first generation of MIOLs [13].

Even with these newly developed MIOLs, photic phenomena, particularly halos, have not been totally

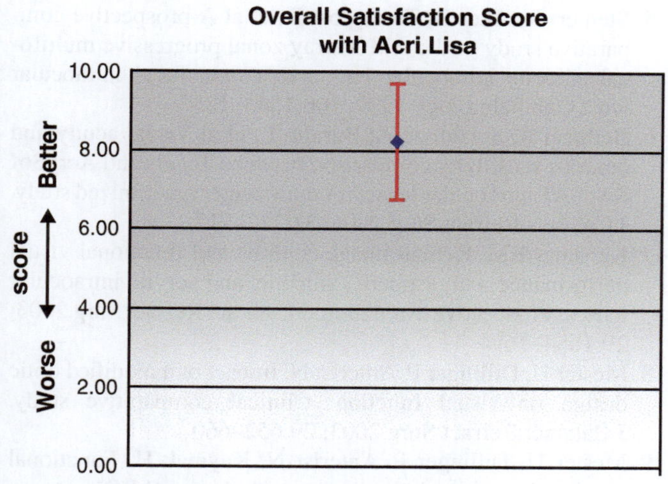

Fig. 8.44 Satisfaction score after 1 year with Acri.LISA

eliminated. These effects seem to be inherent in MIOLs as a result of multiple images, of which only one is in focus. In fact, most patients are usually not disturbed by these optical effects and report that they become less noticeable over time [14, 15].

All the results in our studies were achieved without additional refinement of refraction using photoablative procedures. Using these techniques, further improvement is likely.

One crucial point is exact biometry. We therefore use three different formulas to get as close to emmetropia as possible. Residual refractive errors enhance the side effects of bifocal lenses and should therefore be avoided.

8.3.2.3 Outlook

Until some time, we did not recommend MIOLs for patients with more than 1 diopter of astigmatism and did not accept a second procedure for refinement. Now the toric version of Acri.LISA is available (Table 8.5). First results of this MIOL, which were presented at the ASCRS 2008 in Chicago (Table 8.6), are very promising. A multicenter study comparing the Acri.LISA toric with the Acri.LISA combined with a second refractive procedure, in patients with astigmatism of more than 1.5 D, is under way. The results of the first 6 months are expected in 2009.

Table 8.5 Characteristics of Acri.LISA toric

Optic diameter	6.0 mm	
Total diameter	11.0 mm	*Acri. LISA Toric 466TD*
Haptic angulation	0°	
Lens design	Anterior surface toric, posterior surface bifocal, aberration-free, +3.75 D addition, MICS, SMP-technology	
Incision size	1.5 – 1.7 mm	
Material	Foldable acrylate with 25% water content, hydrophobic surface, UV-absorber	
Sterilization method	Autoclaving	
Diopter range	Spherical: −10.0 D to +32.0 D Cylinder: +1.0 D to +12.0 D Higher diopter on request	
Package	Sterile, in water for injection	
Recommend A-factor	Acoustic/optic	
AL < 25.00 mm	117.6/117.9	
AL ≥ 25.00 mm	118.0/118.3	
Implantation system	Acri.Shooter A2-2000 Acri.Smart cartridge Acri.Smart tip	

Table 8.6 First results with the Acri.LISA toric (with permission of Dr. Breyer, Dusseldorf, Germany)

Patient	Eye	Preop refraction	Target refraction	Postop refraction objective	UCVA near + far	Subjective
1	RA	−8.50 −2.75	+0.21 −0.42	+0.50	1.0 / 0.9	+0.75
	LA	−5.00 −2.50	−0.01 −0.39	−0.25 −0.25	1.0 / 0.9	+0.50 −0.50
2	RA	+8.75 −1.00	+0.50 −0.42	+0.50	0.63 / 0.6	
	LA	+8.75 −0.50	−0.16 −0.60	+0.75 −0.50	0.63 / 0.6	
3	RA	−4.25 −3.00	+0.21 −0.47	−0.50 −0.50	0.6 / 0.8	
	LA	+0.75 −3.25	−0.07 −0.46	−0.75 −0.25	0.6 / 0.8	
4	RA	−7.75 −2.00	+0.05 −0.38	−0.50 −0.50	0.8 / 1.0	
	LA	−9.25 −3.75	−0.23 −0.48	−0.50 −0.75	0.8 / 1.0	
5	RA	+5.75 −2.00	+0.14 −0.28	−0.00 −0.00	1.0 / 0.6	+0.50
	LA	+5.50 −2.25	−0.04 −0.17	−0.00 −0.75	0.8 / 0.6	+0.25

Take Home Pearls

- Several clinical studies and personal experience tell us that visual performance, particularly with MIOLs, will be better after the surgery of the second eye.
- This means that the surgery of the fellow eye should not be postponed, despite the feeling, after the surgery of the first eye, not being as outstanding as expected.
- Dysphotopsia (particularly halos) usually disappears by this time.
- The benefit of the MIOL can easily be demonstrated after the surgery, using a minus 3.0 D glass simulating a monofocal situation. After removing the glass, the patient will appreciate the ability to read without spectacles.
- Slight residual refractive errors (particularly in one eye) must not be corrected in each case: Sometimes this residual error can be used to enhance the vision in intermediate distances.
- There should be no hesitation to perform YAG-capsulotomy even in cases with slight PCO.
- Due to neural adaptation, a time period of up to 6 months is needed for the visual performance to reach its maximum after MIOL implantation. That should be explained to the patient before and be repeated after the surgery.
- Artificial tears are very helpful to improve visual function particularly in the early post-op period.

References

1. Leaming DV. Practice styles and preferences of ASCRS members – 2002 survey. J Cactaract Refract Surg 2003; 29: 1412–1420
2. Dick HB, Tehrani M, Brauweiler P, et al Complications with foldable intraocular lenses with subsequent explantation in 1998 and 1999. Result of a questionaire evaluation. Ophthalmologe 2002; 99:438–444
3. Mamalis N, Davis B, Nilson CD, et al Complications of foldable intraocular lenses requiring explantation or secondary intervention – 2003 survey update. J Cataract Refract Surg 2004; 30:2209–2218
4. Auffarth G, Hunold W, Breitenbach S, et al Contrast and glare sensitivity in patient with multifocal IOLs: Results two years after lens implantation. Klin Monatsbl Augenheilkd 1993; 203:336–340
5. Steinert R, Aker B, Trentacost D, et al A prospective comparative srudy of the AMO array zonal progressive multifocal silicone intraocular lens and a monofocal intraocular lens. Ophthalmology 1999; 106:1243–1255
6. Bellucci R, Scialdone A, Buralto L, et al Visual acuity and contrast sensitivity comparison between Tecnis and AcrySof SA60AT intraocular lenses: A multicenter randomized study. J Cataract Refract Surg 2005; 31:712–717
7. Kershner RM. Retinal image contrast and functional visual performance with aspheric, silicone, and acrylic intraocular lenses: Prospective evaluation. J Cataract Refract Surg 2003; 29:1684–1694
8. Mester U, Dillinger P, Anterist N. Impact of a modified optic design on visual function: Clinical comparative study. J Cataract Refract Surg 2003; 29:652–660
9. Mester U, Dillinger P, Anterist N, Kaymak H. Functional results with two multifocal intraocular lenses (MIOL). Array SA40 versus Acri.Twin. Ophthalmologe 2005; 102:1051–1056
10. Kaymak H, Mester U. Erste Ergebnisse mit einer neuen aberrationskorrigierenden Bifokallinse (*Acri.LISA), Ophthalmologe 2007; 104:1046–1051
11. Alió JL, Elkady B, Ortiz D, Bernabeu G. Clinical outcomes and intraocular optical quality of a diffractive multifocal intraocular lens with asymmetrical light distribution. J Cataract Refract Surg 2008; 34:942–948
12. Alfonso JF, Fernández-Vega L, Señaris A, Montés-Micó R. Prospective study of the Acri.LISA bifocal intraocular lens. J Cataract Refract Surg 2007; 33:1930–1935
13. Mester U, Hunold W, Wesendahl T, Kaymak H. Functional outcomes after implantation of Tecnis ZM900 and Array SA40 multifocal intraocular lenses. J Cataract Refract Surg 2007; 33:1033–1040
14. Dick HB, Krummenauer F, Schwenn O, et al Objective and subjective evaluation of photic phenomena after monofocal and multifocal intraocular lens implantation. Ophthalmology 1999; 106:1878–1886
15. Pieh S, Lackner B, Hanselmayer G, et al Halo size under distance and near conditions in refractive multifocal intraocular lenses. Br J Ophthalmol 2001; 85:816–821

8.3.3 Special Lenses: Aspheric

Mark Packer, I. Howard Fine, and Richard S. Hoffman

Core Messages

- Aspheric intraocular lenses represent an innovative design for enhanced image formation in the eye.
- Aging changes in the crystalline lens cause increasing spherical aberration throughout life.
- Aspheric IOLs offer the cataract surgeons, the opportunity to improve patients' functional vision by minimizing spherical aberration.

In the current era of presbyopia-correcting intraocular lenses (IOLs), toric IOLs and aspheric IOL technology, the practice milieu is changing. Informed consent takes on a new meaning when the surgeon and the patient decide together which IOL technology represents the best fit for a particular lifestyle and its visual demands. Customizing IOL choice is no longer optional; it is essential to the practice of refractive lens surgery.

Because the positive spherical aberration of a spherical pseudophakic IOL tends to increase the total optical aberrations, attention has turned to the development of aspheric IOLs [1]. These designs are intended to reduce or eliminate the spherical aberration of the eye and improve functional vision as compared with that of a spherical pseudophakic implant. Three aspheric IOL designs are currently marketed in the United States: the Tecnis Z9000/2/3 IOLs (AMO, Santa Ana, CA), the AcrySof IQ IOL (Alcon, Ft. Worth, TX) and the SofPort AO IOL (Bausch & Lomb, San Dimas, CA). Other aspheric IOL designs, which are not available in the United States as yet, also promise to reduce spherical aberration [2].

M. Packer (✉)
Oregon Health & Science University, Drs. Fine, Hoffman and Packer, 1550 Oak Street, Suite 5, Eugene, OR 97401, USA
e-mail: mpacker@finemd.com

The Tecnis IOL was designed with a modified prolate anterior surface to compensate for the average corneal spherical aberration found in the adult eye. It introduces –0.27 µm of spherical aberration to the eye measured at the 6 mm optical zone. The clinical investigation of the Tecnis IOL submitted to the US Food and Drug Administration (FDA) demonstrated the elimination of mean spherical aberration as well as significant improvement in functional vision, when compared to a standard spherical IOL [3].

The AcrySof IQ shares the ultraviolet (UV) and blue light-filtering chromophores found in the single-piece acrylic AcrySof Natural IOL. The special feature of the IQ IOL is the posterior aspheric surface, which is designed to reduce spherical aberration by addressing the effects of over-refraction at the periphery. It adds –0.20 µm of spherical aberration to the eye at the 6 mm optical zone. The SofPort Advanced Optics (LI61AO) IOL is an aspheric IOL that has been specifically designed with zero spherical aberration so that it will not contribute to any preexisting higher-order aberrations.

Multiple peer-reviewed, prospective, randomized scientific publications have demonstrated the reduction or elimination of spherical aberrations with the Tecnis modified prolate IOL, when compared to a variety of spherical IOLs [4–13]. Data show that the mean spherical aberration in the eyes implanted with the Tecnis IOL is, in the words approved by the FDA, "not different from zero." Studies have also documented superior functional vision with the Tecnis IOL. Subjects in the FDA monitored randomized double-masked night driving simulation study of the Tecnis IOL, performed functionally better in 20 out of 24 driving conditions (and statistically better in ten conditions), when using best-spectacle correction with the eye implanted with the Tecnis IOL, as compared to best-spectacle correction with the eye implanted with the AcrySof spherical IOL [2]. Data from the night-driving simulation showed a significant correlation between the reduction of spherical aberration and the detection distance for the pedestrian target under rural conditions with glare (the most difficult target to discern).

More recently, peer-reviewed published clinical studies have also supported the reduction of spherical aberration and superior functional vision with the AcrySof IQ when compared with spherical IOLs [14–17]. In fact, the optical advantages of aspheric IOL technology have become fairly well accepted although some controversy remains in the areas of functional benefit as it relates to pupil size, IOL decentration, depth of focus and customization [18]. Some studies have shown little or no benefit of aspheric IOLs with smaller pupils [12, 13], while one laboratory study showed that the SofPort AO provides better optical quality than either a negatively aspheric or a spherical IOL, under conditions of significant decentration [19]. One study has shown diminished distance-corrected near visual acuity, a surrogate measure for the depth of focus, with the AcrySof IQ aspheric IOL as compared to that of the AcrySof SN60AT spherical IOL [17].

Regarding customization of the aspheric correction, it has been suggested that achieving zero total spherical aberration postoperatively provides the best quality of vision. Piers and coauthors utilized an adaptive optics simulator to assess letter acuity and contrast sensitivity for two different values of spherical aberration. The first condition was the average amount of spherical aberration measured in pseudophakic patients with spherical IOLs. The second condition represented the complete correction of the individual's spherical aberration (Z [4,0] = 0). The researchers found an average improvement in visual acuity associated with the correction of spherical aberration of 10 and 38% measured in white and green light, respectively. Similarly, average contrast sensitivity measurements improved to 32 and 57% in white and green light, respectively. When spherical aberration was corrected, visual performance was as good as or better than the normal spherical aberration case for defocus as large as ±1 D. Therefore, these researchers concluded that completely correcting ocular spherical aberration improves spatial vision in the best-focus position, without compromising the subjective tolerance to defocus [20].

On the other hand, it has alternatively been suggested that providing Z [4,0] = +0.1 micron of postoperative spherical aberration represents a better choice [21]. This line of reasoning originated from a study demonstrating that 35 young subjects with uncorrected visual acuity of 20/15 or better had a mean total spherical aberration of Z [4,0] = +0.110 ± 0.077 μm [22]. However, there is no logical basis to infer that the spherical aberration is responsible for the supernormal visual acuity. In fact, the authors of this study concluded that "The amount of ocular HOAs in eyes with natural supernormal vision is not negligible, and is comparable to the reported amount of HOAs in myopic eyes" [22]. This conclusion is brought out by a study performed by Wang and Koch demonstrating a mean total spherical aberration of Z [4,0] = +0.128 ± 0.074 μm in a series of 532 eyes of 306 subjects, presenting for refractive surgery [23]. Nevertheless, Beiko [21] used the Easygraph corneal topographer (Oculus, Lynnwood, WA) to select patients with corneal spherical aberration of +0.37 μm, thus targeting a postoperative total ocular spherical aberration of +0.10 μm following implantation of the Tecnis IOL with −0.27 μm (the Easygraph includes an optional software package that provides Zernike analysis). The selected patient group demonstrated a significantly better contrast sensitivity than an unselected group of control patients, under both mesopic and photopic conditions.

Recently, Beiko, Haigis and Steinmueller presented data from a series of 696 eyes confirming the mean corneal spherical aberration of +0.27 μm used in the design of the Tecnis IOL [24]. They found a wide standard deviation of 0.089 μm, with a range from +0.041 to +0.632 μm, and significantly different corneal spherical aberration means in men and women. In some cases the corneal spherical aberration differed significantly between fellow eyes. The authors concluded that "individuals' eyes should be measured to determine their unique value when considering correction of this aberration" [24]. In addition, they noted that keratometry and the corneal Q value do not correlate well with spherical aberration, and therefore, corneal spherical aberration must be measured directly with a topographer.

One method of proceeding with customized selection of aspheric IOLs involves the following protocol:

1. Preoperative testing to include corneal topography as well as axial length determination, anterior chamber depth, phakic lens thickness and corneal white-to-white diameter
2. Application of a software package such as VOL-CT (Sarver and Associates, Carbondale, IL) or the use of corneal topographer such as the i-Trace (Tracey Technologies, Houston, TX) to transform the topography elevation data into preoperative corneal Zernike coefficients, with special attention to Z [4,0], fourth order spherical aberration at the 6 mm optical zone
3. Application of an IOL calculation formula, such as the Holladay 2 (available as part of the Holladay IOL Consultant & Surgical Outcomes Assessment Program, Jack T. Holladay, Houston, TX) to determine

the correct IOL power for desired postoperative spherical equivalent
4. Determination of desired postoperative total ocular spherical aberration and selection of the IOL type

For example, if the desired postoperative total ocular spherical aberration is zero, and the preoperative corneal spherical aberration measures about + 0.27 μm, the Tecnis with –0.27 μm would be selected. In general, the aspheric IOL that comes closest to providing the desired correction should be selected.

Initial results for customizing the selection of aspheric IOLs have shown promise.

A prospective study was undertaken to determine the feasibility of selectively targeting zero total postoperative spherical aberration, by selecting the best fit aspheric IOL, based on preoperative topographically derived corneal spherical aberration (Fig. 8.45). Candidates for unilateral or bilateral cataract surgery who did not desire presbyopia-correcting IOLs were offered customized selection of aspheric lenses. Subjects with a history of previous keratorefractive surgery, ocular pathology, judged to limit potential visual acuity to 20/30 or less, or sufficient corneal astigmatism to indicate peripheral corneal relaxing incisions, were excluded. Informed consent for cataract surgery was obtained from all subjects. Preoperative evaluation included a complete ophthalmologic examination, including manifest refraction, best-corrected visual acuity and brightness acuity testing, if indicated.

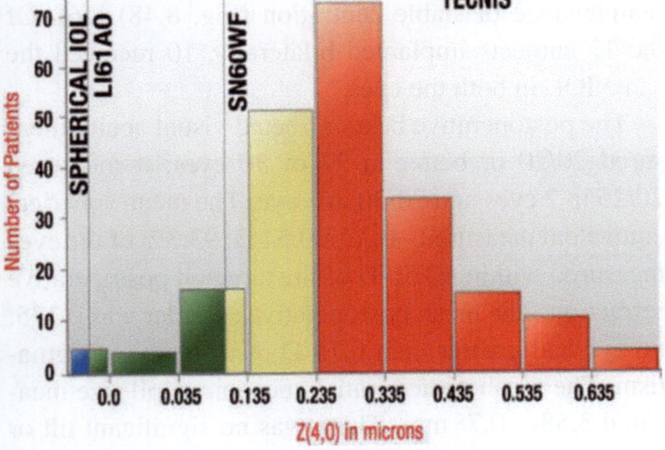

Fig. 8.45 Aspheric IOL selection chart based on the frequency distribution of corneal spherical aberration in the population (for background information, see [1, 24]

In some cases, a visual function questionnaire was administered to help ascertain whether cataract surgery was indicated. Axial length measurement, keratometry, anterior chamber depth and corneal white-to-white measurements were obtained with the IOL Master (Carl Zeiss Meditec, Inc., Dublin, CA). The preoperative corneal topographic spherical aberration (Z [4,0]) was measured at the 6 mm optical zone (iTrace, Tracey Technologies) (Fig. 8.46).

IOL power calculation was performed with the Holladay IOL Consultant using the Holladay II formula (Jack Holladay, Bellaire, TX). An aspheric IOL was selected for implantation in each eye based on the preoperative corneal spherical aberration and the labeled IOL spherical aberration, such that the arithmetic sum of these two values was closest to zero. Thus, for corneal spherical aberration less than + 0.1 μm, the LI61AO was selected; for corneal spherical aberration greater than + 0.1 μm but less than +0.235 μm, the SN60WF was selected; and, for corneal spherical aberration greater than +0.235 μm, the Tecnis Z9000 or Tecnis Z9002 was selected.

At 4–6 weeks postoperatively, the subjects returned for evaluation, including manifest refraction, best-corrected visual acuity, pupillometry and dilated wavefront aberrometry (WASCA, Wavefront Sciences, Inc.). The measured total ocular spherical aberration Z [4,0] for a maximal 6 mm pupil size was compared with the predicted value given mathematically by the sum of the preoperative corneal spherical aberration and the labeled IOL spherical aberration.

Data from 30 eyes of 18 consecutive subjects (9 men and 9 women) were available for analysis. The mean age of the subjects was 72.8 ± 6.2 years (range: 62–86 years). The mean preoperative corneal spherical aberration, measured at the 6 mm zone for the entire population was +0.26 ± 0.089 μm. One eye had Z [4,0] less than + 0.1 μm and therefore was selected to receive the LI61AO IOL. The corneal spherical aberration of this eye measured +0.065 μm. Eleven eyes had Z [4,0] greater than +0.1 μm, but less than +0.235 μm, and therefore were selected to receive the SN60WF. The mean corneal spherical aberration of this group measured +0.18 ± 0.037 μm. Eighteen eyes had corneal spherical aberration greater than +0.235 μm, and therefore received the Tecnis IOL. The mean corneal spherical aberration of this group measured +0.31 ± 0.063 μm. The frequency distribution of the preoperative corneal spherical aberration is shown in Fig. 8.47.

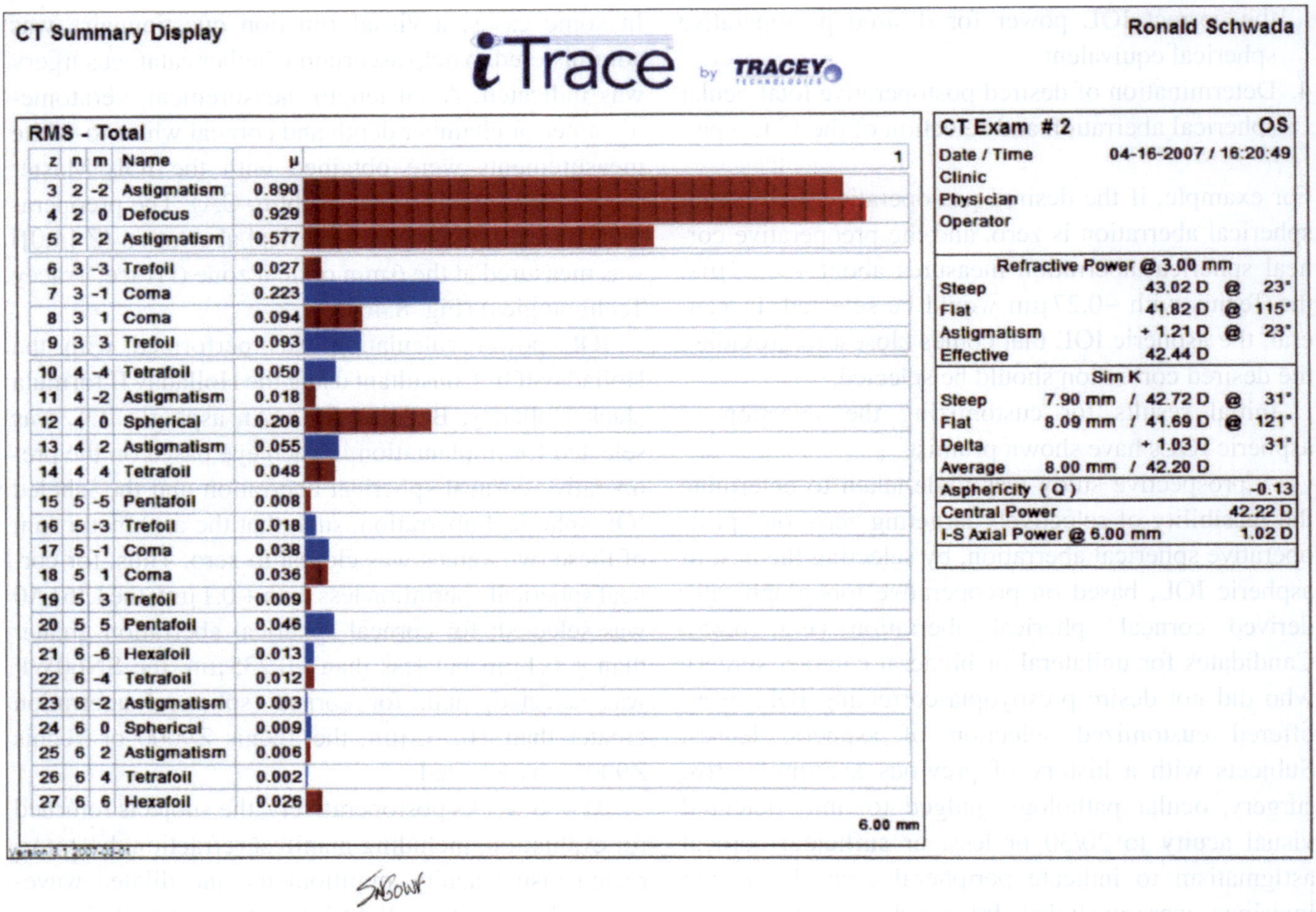

Fig. 8.46 Data from iTrace (Tracey Technologies) showing Zernike coefficients derived from corneal topography at the 6 mm optical zone

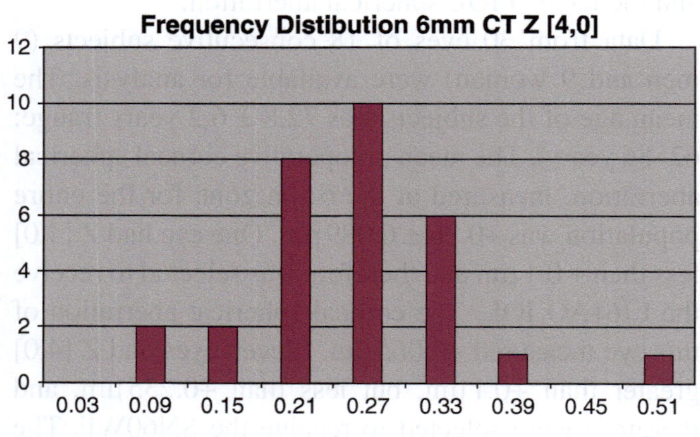

Fig. 8.47 Frequency distribution of corneal topographic wavefront spherical aberration Z [4,0] in the study population (mean +0.26 ± 0.089 μm)

All patients underwent uneventful phacoemulsification and IOL implantation by one surgeon (MP) utilizing a biaxial micro incision technique [25]. The capsulorhexis diameter was intentionally sized at approximately 4.5–5.0 mm in all cases in order to facilitate the "shrink wrap effect" of the IOL for a long-term prevention of posterior capsular opacification and maintenance of stable centration (Fig. 8.48) [26]. Of the 12 subjects implanted bilaterally, 10 received the same IOL in both the eyes.

The postoperative best-corrected visual acuity measured 20/20 or better in 27 of 30 eyes; it measured 20/25 in 2 eyes and 20/30 in 1 eye. The mean spherical equivalent measured –0.32 ± 0.54 D; 93.3% of the eyes measured within ±0.50 D of the targeted postoperative refraction. The mean postoperative cylinder was 0.375; no eye had greater than 0.75 D of refractive astigmatism. The mean postoperative mesopic pupil size measured 3.58 ± 0.78 mm. There was no significant tilt or decentration greater than 0.25 mm of any IOL, as measured by Guyton's method [27, 28].

The total postoperative ocular spherical aberration for the entire population measured –0.013 ± 0.072 μm. The total ocular spherical aberration for the eye implanted with the LI61AO IOL measured +0.025 µm. This single eye was excluded from further comparative statistical analysis, but included in the descriptive

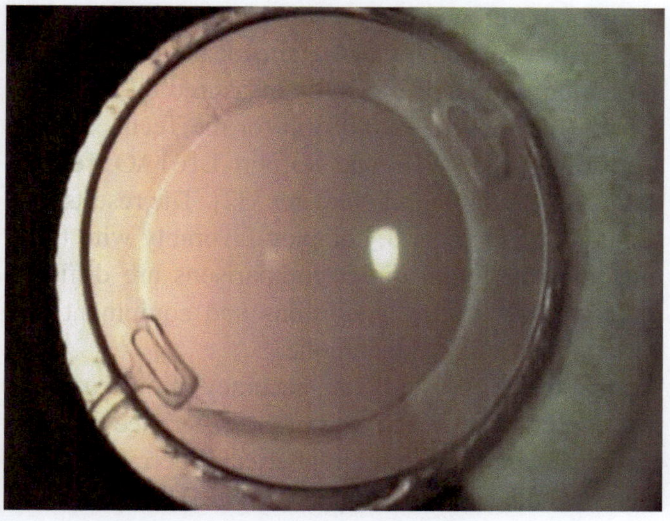

Fig. 8.48 The anterior capsule margin overlies the edge of the Tecnis Z9000 IOL, effectively reducing the aperture (despite wide pupil dilation) to 4.5 mm

statistics for the entire population. For the eyes implanted with the SN60WF, the mean total postoperative ocular spherical aberration measured + 0.010 ± 0.053 µm. For the eyes implanted with the Tecnis, the mean total postoperative ocular spherical aberration measured −0.015 ± 0.052 µm. There was no statistically significant difference between the postoperative ocular spherical aberration of the SN60WF group vs. the Tecnis group (two sample *t*-test assuming equal variances, $p = 0.22$).

Examination of the difference between the predicted and measured postoperative spherical aberration for the entire group shows that the mean absolute error measured 0.058 ± 0.056 µm. For the eyes implanted with the SN60WF, the mean absolute error measured 0.052 ± 0.040 µm. For the eyes implanted with the Tecnis, the mean absolute error measured 0.063 ± 0.066 µm. A two sample *t*-test assuming equal variances did not reveal any statistically significant difference between the mean absolute errors for the SN60WF and Tecnis eyes ($p = 0.63$). Figure 8.49 shows a scatter plot of predicted vs. measured Z [4,0] for all the eyes. As expected from the values and standard deviations

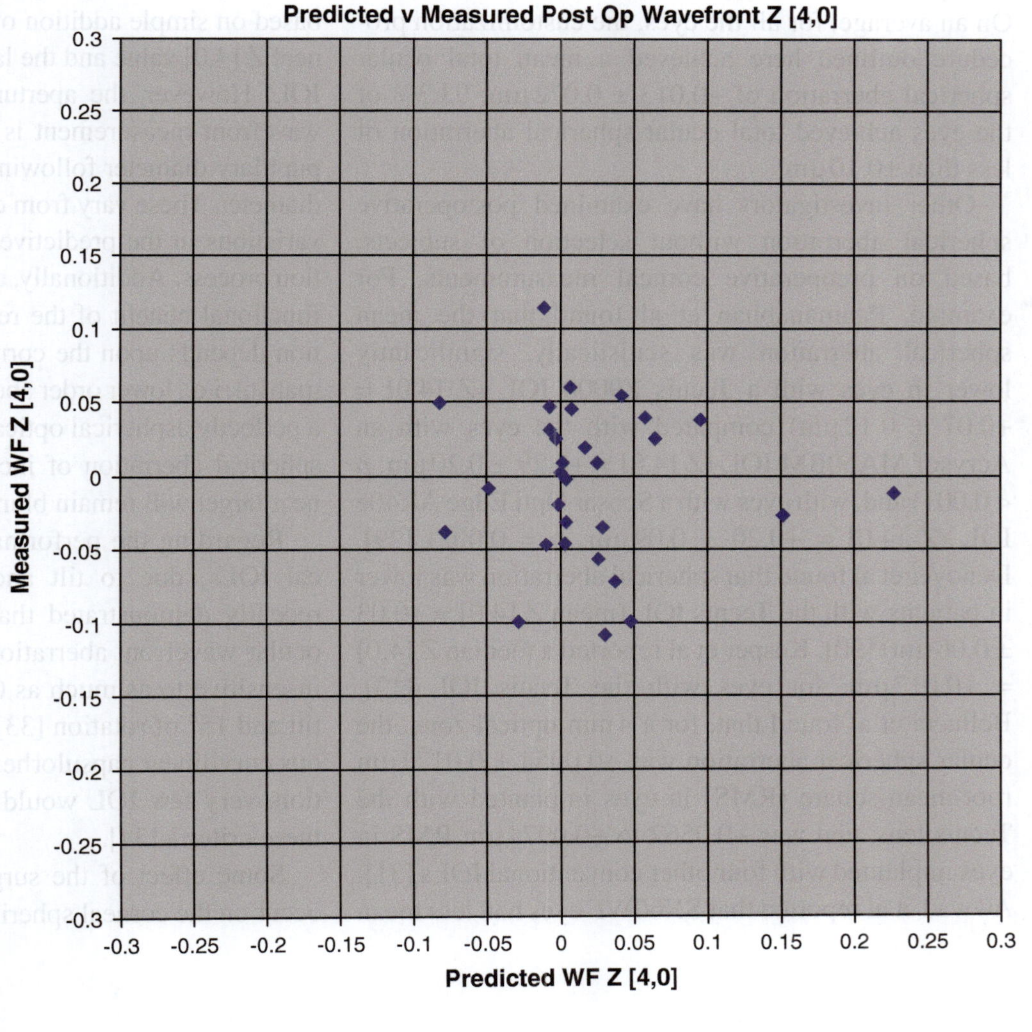

Fig. 8.49 Predicted vs. measured post operative wavefront spherical aberration Z [4,0] for the entire study population. 86.7% of the paired data points lie within ±0.1 µm of zero, and 53.3% lie within ±0.05 µm of zero

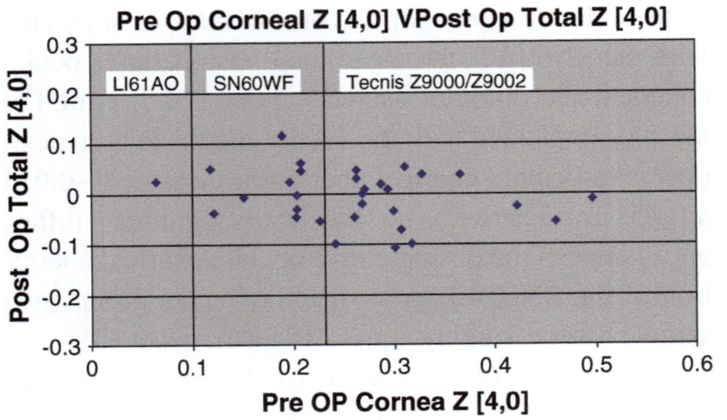

Fig. 8.50 The plot of preoperative corneal spherical aberration (*x*-axis) and postoperative total wavefront spherical aberration (*y*-axis) shows the distribution of IOLs among the subjects

for mean absolute error, almost all the points lie within 0.10 μm of zero, and approximately half the points lie within 0.050 μm of zero. Figure 8.50 demonstrates the relationship between the preoperative corneal spherical aberration and the postoperative total spherical aberration, with reference to the selected aspheric IOLs.

The value of customizing any refractive or wavefront parameter can only reside in enhanced outcomes. On an average, for all the eyes, the customization procedure outlined here achieved a mean total ocular spherical aberration of –0.013 ± 0.072 μm; 93.3% of the eyes achieved total ocular spherical aberration of less than ±0.10 μm.

Other investigators have examined postoperative spherical aberration without selection of subjects, based on preoperative corneal measurements. For example, Padmanabhan et al found that the mean spherical aberration was statistically, significantly lower in eyes with a Tecnis Z9000 IOL (Z [4,0] = +0.07 ± 0.12 μm) compared with the eyes with an Acrysof MA60BM IOL (Z [4,0] = +0.29 ± 0.20 μm, $p < 0.001$) and, with eyes with a Sensar Opti Edge AR40e IOL (Z [4,0] = +0.20 ± 0.09 μm, $p = 0.002$) [29]. Denoyer et al found that spherical aberration was lower in patients with the Tecnis IOL (mean Z [4,0] = +0.03 ± 0.06 μm) [30]. Kasper et al reported a median Z [4,0] = +0.017 μm, for eyes with the Tecnis IOL [13]. Bellucci et al found that, for a 4 mm optical zone, the ocular spherical aberration was +0.0054 ± 0.0172 μm root-mean-square (RMS) in eyes implanted with the Tecnis lens, and was +0.0562 to +0.0974 μm RMS in eyes implanted with four other conventional IOLs [31]. Awwad et al reported that SN60WF eyes had less mean absolute spherical aberration than SN60AT eyes, both at 4 mm (+0.04 ± 0.03 vs. +0.11 ± 0.03 RMS, $p < 0.0001$) and 6 mm pupils (+0.09 ± 0.04 vs. +0.43 ± 0.12 RMS, $p < 0.0001$) [14]. Rocha et al found a mean spherical aberration of +0.03 ± 0.05 μm in their AcrySof IQ groups in two separate publications [16, 17]. Caporossi et al found that the mean total spherical aberration with aspheric IOLs measured 0.05 ± 0.06, 0.11 ± 0.1, and 0.19 ± 0.08 μm for the Tecnis Z9000, Acrysof IQ SN60WF, and Sofport L161AO, respectively, for a 5 mm pupil diameter [32]. The results presented here, in general, compare favorably with these outcomes, although direct comparisons are difficult, given various testing conditions and equipment and variations in surgical technique.

As a feasibility study, the accuracy of our customization procedure is reflected in the difference between predicted and measured spherical aberration. The mean absolute error measured 0.058 ± 0.056 μm for all the eyes. Several factors such as, effective postoperative pupil size, tilt or decentration of the IOL and surgically induced spherical aberration may influence these results, and should be considered in our evaluation.

The predicted postoperative spherical aberration is based on simple addition of the 6 mm preoperative corneal Z [4,0] value and the labeled 6 mm Z [4,0] for each IOL. However, the aperture size of the postoperative wavefront measurement is limited by the reduction of pupillary diameter following dilation and capsulorhexis diameter. These vary from case to case and will produce variations in the predictive accuracy of the customization process. Additionally, an important limitation of the functional benefit of the reduction of spherical aberration depends upon the correction of defocus and astigmatism, i.e., lower order aberrations. Furthermore, while a perfectly aspherical optical system may correct for the spherical aberration of incoming parallel light rays, a near target will remain blurred, because of defocus.

Regarding the performance limitations of aspherical IOLs, due to tilt and decentration, Piers et al recently demonstrated that customized correction of ocular wavefront aberrations with an IOL is relatively insensitive to as much as 0.8 mm decentration, 10° of tilt and 15° of rotation [33]. Fortunately, with continuous curvilinear capsulorhexis and in-the-bag IOL fixation, very few IOL would be expected to fall outside these criteria [34].

Some effect of the surgery should be expected to occur on the corneal spherical aberration and therefore, another variable should be added to the system. In fact, Guirao et al determined that the mean surgically induced spherical aberration, following cataract extraction through a 3.5 mm clear corneal incision, with implantation of a monofocal IOL for a 6 mm pupil, calculated by ray-tracing from the corneal topography, measures 0.03 ± 0.17 μm (spherical aberration mean: pre, +0.32 ± 0.12 μm, and post, +0.34 ± 0.19 μm) [35]. However, with a mean absolute error of 0.058 ± 0.056 μm for all the eyes in this study, this degree of surgically induced spherical aberration could explain the majority of inaccuracies in the results. Postoperative topography was not included as an outcome measure in the present study and remains a topic for further research.

Another limitation of this feasibility study is the absence of psychometric testing or contrast sensitivity measurements to evaluate the functional results. Analysis of the functional impact of customized selection of aspheric IOLs must eventually rely upon such data, which represent an important area for future study.

Along these lines, research in "just-noticeable differences" of refractive and wavefront errors indicates that 0.04 μm of RMS aberration should be considered as the threshold [36]. While on a population average, the benefit of aspheric IOL selection based on corneal wavefront measurements may reside below this threshold, for a specific individual, the difference may in fact be quite noticeable. Customization is particularly important for patients who have had prior keratorefractive surgery, such as LASIK. Selection of aspheric IOLs in this population remains a topic for future research.

Take Home Pearls

- Aspheric intraocular lenses offer superior mean functional vision and contrast sensitivity for most patients.
- Selecting the best fit aspheric IOL on the basis of corneal topography may enhance the results.

References

1. Holladay JT, Piers PA, Koranyi G, van der Mooren M, Norrby S. A new intraocular lens design to reduce spherical aberration of pseudophakic eyes. J Refract Surg 2002; 18:683–691
2. Kurz S, Krummenauer F, Thieme H, Dick HB. Contrast sensitivity after implantation of a spherical versus an aspherical intraocular lens in biaxial microincision cataract surgery. J Cataract Refract Surg 2007; 33(3):393–400
3. Tecnis Foldable Ultraviolet Light-Absorbing Posterior Chamber IOL [package insert]. Advanced Medical Optics, Santa Ana, CA, 2005
4. Packer M, Fine IH, Hoffman RS, Piers PA. Initial clinical experience with an anterior surface modified prolate intraocular lens. J Refract Surg 2002; 18:692–696
5. Mester U, Dillinger P, Anterist N. Impact of a modified optic design on visual function: Clinical comparative study. J Cataract Refract Surg 2003; 29(4):652–660
6. Packer M, Fine IH, Hoffman RS, Piers PA. Improved functional vision with a modified prolate intraocular lens. J Cataract Refract Surg 2004; 30:986–992
7. Bellucci R, Scialdone A, Buratto L, Morselli S, Chierego C, Criscuoli A, Moretti G, Piers P. Visual acuity and contrast sensitivity comparison between Tecnis and AcrySof SA60AT intraocular lenses: A multicenter randomized study. J Cataract Refract Surg 2005; 31(4):712–717
8. Kennis H, Huygens M, Callebaut F. Comparing the contrast sensitivity of a modified prolate anterior surface IOL and of two spherical IOLs. Bull Soc Belge Ophtalmol 2004; 294:49–58
9. Kershner RM. Retinal image contrast and functional visual performance with aspheric, silicone, and acrylic intraocular lenses: prospective evaluation. J Cataract Refract Surg 2003; 29:1684–1694
10. Ricci F, Scuderi G, Missiroli F, Regine F, Cerulli A. Low contrast visual acuity in pseudophakic patients implanted with an anterior surface modified prolate intraocular lens. Acta Ophthalmol Scand 2004; 82(6):718–722
11. Martinez Palmer A, Palacin Miranda B, Castilla Cespedes M, Comas Serrano M, Punti Badosa A. Spherical aberration influence in visual function after cataract surgery: Prospective randomized trial [in Spanish]. Arch Soc Esp Oftalmol 2005; 80(2):71–77
12. Munoz G, Albarran-Diego C, Montes-Mico R, Rodriguez-Galietero A, Alio JL. Spherical aberration and contrast sensitivity after cataract surgery with the Tecnis Z9000 intraocular lens. J Cataract Refract Surg 2006; 32(8):1320–1327
13. Kasper T, Buhren J, Kohnen T. Visual performance of aspherical and spherical intraocular lenses: intraindividual comparison of visual acuity, contrast sensitivity, and higher-order aberrations. J Cataract Refract Surg 2006; 32(12): 2022–2029
14. Awwad ST, Lehmann JD, McCulley JP, Bowman RW. A comparison of higher order aberrations in eyes implanted with AcrySof IQ SN60WF and AcrySof SN60AT intraocular lenses. Eur J Ophthalmol 2007; 17(3):320–326
15. Sandoval HP, Fernández de Castro LE, Vroman DT, Solomon KD. Comparison of visual outcomes, photopic contrast sensitivity, wavefront analysis, and patient satisfaction following cataract extraction and IOL implantation: aspheric vs spherical acrylic lenses. Eye 2008; 22(12):1469–1475
16. Rocha KM, Soriano ES, Chalita MR, Yamada AC, Bottos K, Bottos J, Morimoto L, Nose W. Wavefront analysis and contrast sensitivity of aspheric and spherical intraocular lenses: a randomized prospective study. Am J Ophthalmol 2006; 142(5):750–756

17. Rocha KM, Soriano ES, Chamon W, Chalita MR, Nosé W. Spherical aberration and depth of focus in eyes implanted with aspheric and spherical intraocular lenses: a prospective randomized study. Ophthalmology 2007; 114(11):2050–2054
18. Werner L, Olson RJ, Mamalis N. New technology IOL optics. Ophthalmol Clin North Am 2006; 19(4):469–483
19. Altmann GE, Nichamin LD, Lane SS, Pepose JS. Optical performance of 3 intraocular lens designs in the presence of decentration. J Cataract Refract Surg 2005; 31(3):574–585
20. Piers PA, Fernandez EJ, Manzanera S, Norrby S, Artal P. Adaptive optics simulation of intraocular lenses with modified spherical aberration. Invest Ophthalmol Vis Sci 2004; 45(12):4601–4610
21. Beiko G. Personalized Correction of Spherical Aberration in Cataract Surgery. In: Annual Meeting of the American Academy of Ophthalmology, Chicago, IL, 18 October 2006
22. Levy Y, Segal O, Avni I, Zadok D. Ocular higher-order aberrations in eyes with supernormal vision. Am J Ophthalmol 2005; 139(2):225–228
23. Wang L, Koch DD. Ocular higher-order aberrations in individuals screened for refractive surgery. J Cataract Refract Surg 2003; 29(10):1896–1903
24. Beiko GH, Haigis W, Steinmueller A. Distribution of corneal spherical aberration in a comprehensive ophthalmology practice and whether keratometry can predict aberration values. J Cataract Refract Surg 2007; 33(5):848–858
25. Packer M, Fine IH, Hoffman RS. Bimanual ultrasound phacoemulsification. In: Fine IH, Packer M, Hoffman RS (eds) Refractive Lens Surgery. Springer, Heidelberg, 2005, pp 193–198
26. Apple DJ, Peng Q, Visessook N, Werner L, Pandey SK, Escobar-Gomez M, Ram J, Whiteside SB, Schoderbeck R, Ready EL, Guindi A. Surgical prevention of posterior capsule opacification. Part 1: Progress in eliminating this complication of cataract surgery. J Cataract Refract Surg 2000; 26(2):180–187
27. Guyton DL, Uozato H, Wisnicki HJ. Rapid determination of intraocular lens tilt and decentration through the undilated pupil. Ophthalmology 1990; 97(10):1259–1264
28. Wu M, Li H, Cheng W. Determination of intraocular lens tilt and decentration using simple and rapid method. Yan Ke Xue Bao 1998; 14(1):13–16; 26
29. Padmanabhan P, Rao SK, Jayasree R, Chowdhry M, Roy J. Monochromatic aberrations in eyes with different intraocular lens optic designs. J Refract Surg 2006; 22(2):172–177
30. Denoyer A, Roger F, Majzoub S, Pisella PJ. [Quality of vision after cataract surgery in patients with prolate aspherical lens]. J Fr Ophtalmol 2006; 29(2):157–163
31. Bellucci R, Morselli S, Piers P. Comparison of wavefront aberrations and optical quality of eyes implanted with five different intraocular lenses. J Refract Surg 2004; 20(4):297–306
32. Caporossi A, Martone G, Casprini F, Rapisarda L. Prospective randomized study of clinical performance of 3 aspheric and 2 spherical intraocular lenses in 250 eyes. J Refract Surg 2007; 23:639–648
33. Piers PA, Weeber HA, Artal P, Norrby S. Theoretical comparison of aberration-correcting customized and aspheric intraocular lenses. J Refract Surg 2007; 23(4):374–384
34. Packer M. Tilt and decentration: Toward a new definition of tolerance. In: Fine IH (ed) Perspectives in Lens and IOL Surgery. EyeWorld 2005; 10(6):65–66
35. Guirao A, Tejedor J, Artal P. Corneal aberrations before and after small-incision cataract surgery. Invest Ophthalmol Vis Sci 2004; 45:4312–4319
36. Legras R, Chateau N, Charman WN. Assessment of just-noticeable differences for refractive errors and spherical aberration using visual simulation. Optom Vis Sci 2004; 81(9):718–728

8.3.4 *Intraocular Lenses to Restore and Preserve Vision Following Cataract Surgery*

Robert J. Cionni and David Hair

Core Messages

- Our ability to restore the vision lost due to cataracts has improved tremendously over the last few decades.
- More focus on maintaining the vision is essential, especially for patients with macular degeneration.
- Blue light has been shown to be potentially damaging to the retina.
- The normal human crystalline lens filters out a significant amount of high frequency blue wavelength light. Removal of this lens and placing a colorless UV blocking IOL leaves the retina exposed to higher levels of blue light.
- IOLs are now available that can filter out blue light similar to the normal human lens.
- Blue light filtering IOLs have been shown to have no negative effect on visual acuity, contrast sensitivity, color perception, or night vision.

8.3.4.1 Introduction

Advancing surgical and intraocular lens technologies now offer our patients the opportunity of excellent vision following surgery. Newer multifocal and accommodating IOLs now offer the possibility of restoring vision to the pre-presbyopia state and thus, reduce spectacle dependency for both distance and near vision [1–4]. Unfortunately, many of our cataract patients also suffer from, or may later develop, age-related macular degeneration. Despite our successes at restoring vision for our cataract patients, we have not gained significant ground in preserving the vision for those patients with macular degenerative disease. Over the last few decades, more literature has surfaced suggesting that blue light may be one of the factors related to the progression of age-related macular degeneration [5]. Additionally, the role of blue light and its association with the increased risk of choroidal melanoma is becoming more apparent [6].

In addition to ultraviolet light, it is well known that the normal human crystalline lens filters much of the high frequency blue wavelength. Thus, when we remove the crystalline lens, clear or cataractous, and replace it with a clear, nonfiltering IOL, we may be decreasing the eye's natural ability to protect against worsening ARMD or malignant melanoma. In this chapter, we will investigate the rationale for implanting blue light filtering IOLs. We will also evaluate the differences in the various blue light filtering IOLs available in the market today.

8.3.4.2 Why Filter Blue Light?

It is well known that pseudophakic eyes are more susceptible to retinal damage from near ultraviolet light sources [7, 8]. Pollack et al., followed 47 patients with bilateral early ARMD after they underwent extracapsular cataract extraction and implantation of an UV-blocking IOL in one eye, with the fellow eye as a phakic control [9]. Neovascular ARMD developed in nine of the pseudophakic eyes vs. two of the control eyes, which the authors suggested, might be due to the loss of the "yellow barrier" provided by the natural crystalline lens.

Data from the Age-Related Eye Disease Study (AREDS) suggest a heightened risk of central geographic retinal atrophy in pseudophakic eyes [10]. The retina appears to be susceptible to chronic repetitive exposure to low-radiance light as well as brief exposure to higher-radiance light [11–14]. Chronic, low-level exposure (Class 1) injury occurs at the level of the photoreceptors and is caused by the absorption of photons by certain visual pigments with subsequent destabilization of the photoreceptor cell membranes. Sparrow and colleagues have demonstrated that a component of lipofuscin, known as A2E, is integral in blue light-induced retinal pigment epithelium (RPE) damage [15–17]. Although the retina has inherent

R. J. Cionni (✉)
The Eye Institute of Utah, Salt Lake City, UT 84107, USA
e-mail: rcionni@theeyeinstitute.com

protective mechanisms from Class 1 photochemical damage, the aging retina is less able to provide sufficient protection from insults like blue light [18, 19].

Several epidemiological studies have concluded that cataract surgery and/or subsequent increased blue wavelength light exposure may be associated with the progression of macular degeneration [20, 21]. Still, other epidemiologic studies have failed to come to this conclusion [22–24]. Such conflicting epidemiological results are not unexpected since age-related macular diseases is felt to be a multifactorial biologic process. Therefore, many of the studies concerning the effect of blue light on the retina have been conducted in animals and in vitro [25–30]. Many of these laboratory studies demonstrate a susceptibility of the RPE to damage, when exposed to blue light [31, 32].

Since blue light can potentially induce retinal injury, the etiology or the mechanism of this damage needs to be studied. It is well known that lipofuscin accumulates in the RPE cells as we age. One component of lipofuscin, known as A2E, is believed to be a key culprit in RPE cell death. A2E has an excitation maximum in the blue wavelength region (441 nm) and when excited by blue light, A2E generates oxygen free radicals. These free radicals are believed to cause RPE damage and ultimately cell death. At Columbia University, Sparrow and colleagues exposed cultured human retinal pigment epithelial cells laden with A2E, to blue light and observed extensive cell death. They then placed different UV blocking IOLs or combined UV blocking/blue light filtering IOL in the path of the blue light and evaluated the effect. The results of this study demonstrated that cell death was extensive with all UV blocking colorless IOLs, but cell death significantly diminished with the combined UV and blue light filtering IOL [33]. These experiments were conducted in vitro and therefore could not take into account any natural protective mechanisms that might be present in vivo. Additionally, the light exposure employed is a mere representative of high-level short term exposure rather than low level chronic exposure, experienced by the natural eye. Still, this work demonstrates clearly that blue light filtering IOLs can help the A2E-ladden RPE cells to survive the phototoxic insult of the blue light.

The link between uveal melanoma and blue light has recently begun to receive increased attention. Burnier and colleagues investigated the effect of blue light on the proliferation rates of four human uveal melanoma cell lines [6]. This study clearly demonstrated the increased proliferation of the melanoma cells after exposure to blue light compared to the cells without exposure. When comparing cells that had UV only and cells with blue filtering lenses present during light exposure, it was evident that the UV only subgroup had a higher proliferation rate. Again, it must be realized that this in an in vitro study and its significance clinically is unknown.

Summary

A growing body of literature suggests that blue light exposure may be one of the factors in the progression of macular degeneration. Also, blue light exposure may be a factor in the development of uveal melanoma. In vitro evidence suggests that blocking blue light may have a protective effect against these two entities.

8.3.4.3 Importance of Blue Light to Cataract and Refractive Lens Exchange Patients

The human crystalline lens normally filters ultraviolet light and much of the light throughout the blue wavelength spectrum [34]. When the natural lens is removed during cataract or RLE surgery, blue-wavelength light then, has the potential to reach the retina at significantly increased levels. If a *colorless* UV blocking IOL is implanted, the RPE cells remain exposed to this increased level of potentially damaging blue light. Until now, three manufacturers have developed IOLs that filter blue light in addition to UV light.

The AcrySof® Natural (Alconlabs, Inc, Fort Worth, TX) is a hydrophobic acrylic foldable IOL, that incorporates a yellow chromophore cross-linked to the acrylic molecules. This yellow chromophore allows the IOL to filter not only UV light, but also specific levels of light in the blue wavelength region. Aging studies with this lens have shown that the chromophore will not leach out or discolor [35]. The AcrySof® Natural IOL was approved for use in Europe in 2002 and in the USA in 2003. Evaluation of its light transmission curve demonstrates that this IOL approximates the transmission spectrum of the normal human crystalline lens in the blue light spectrum (Fig. 8.51). Therefore, in addition to benefiting from less blue light exposure of the retina, color perception should seem more natural to these patients as opposed to the

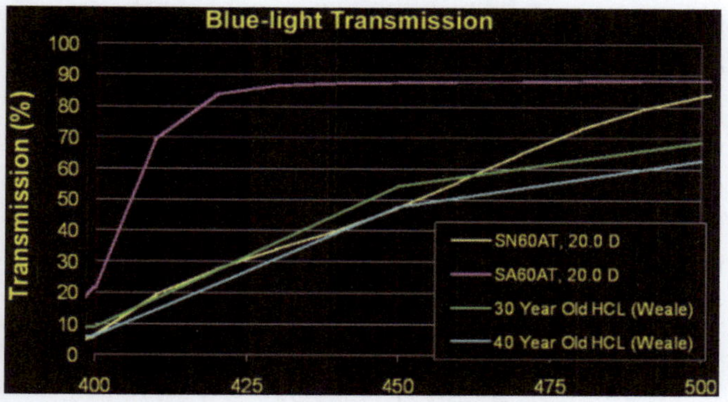

Fig. 8.51 Light transmission spectrum of a 20 diopter AcrySof Natural IOL compared to a 30 year old and 40-year-old human crystalline lens and a 20 diopter colorless UV-blocking IOL [36]

increased blue hues seen by patients who have received colorless UV blocking IOLs [37]. Hoya introduced blue light filtering IOLs in Japan in 1991 (three-piece PMMA Model HOYA UVCY) and in 1994 (single-piece PMMA Model HOYA UVCY-1P). The blue light filtering characteristics of the HOYA and the AcrySof Natural differ only slightly. Clinical studies of these blue light filtering IOLs have been carried out in Japan. One study found that pseudophakic color vision with a yellow-tinted IOL approximated the vision of 20-year-old control subjects in the blue light range [38]. Another study found some improvement in photopic and mesopic contrast sensitivity, as well as a decrease in the effects of central glare on contrast sensitivity, in pseudophakic eyes with a tinted IOL vs. a standard lens with UV-blocker only [39].

Recently, Bausch and Lomb introduced the SoftPort AO lens which is designed to block purple light. UV and purple light are considered more toxic than blue light, and it is felt by some that blocking UV and purple light should be sufficient.

Although blue light is known to be less toxic, it has clearly been shown to have deleterious effects and so blocking only purple wavelengths may put the retina at risk.

Summary

Removing the cataractous or noncataractous human lens, removes the eye's natural blue light filter and exposes the retina to higher levels of blue light, than ever before. IOLs are now available that can filter out much of that blue wavelength light similar to the normal noncataractous human lens. Purple wavelength blocking IOLs may still leave the retina exposed to blue light.

8.3.4.4 Quality of Vision with Blue Light Filtering IOLs

A multi-centered, randomized prospective FDA evaluation of the AcrySof® Natural IOL was carried out before the lens gained approval for use in the USA. Three hundred patients were randomized to bilateral implantation of the AcrySof® Natural IOL or the clear AcrySof Single-Piece IOL. All the patients were screened to ascertain normal preoperative color vision before being deemed eligible for the study. Postoperative parameters measured, included visual acuity, photopic and mesopic contrast sensitivity, and color perception using the Farnsworth D-15 test. Results demonstrated no difference between the AcrySof® Natural IOL and the clear AcrySof® IOL in any of these parameters. More substantial color perception testing, using the Farnsworth-Munsel 100 Hue Test has also demonstrated that there is no difference in color perception between the AcrySof Natural IOL and the clear AcrySof IOL [40].

Although the contrast sensitivity tests performed under mesopic conditions in the FDA trials demonstrated that the AcrySof® Natural IOL does not negatively affect mesopic vision, some have raised concerns about mesopic and scotopic vision in patients with blue light filtering IOLs, since blue light is imperative for night vision. Mesopic vision begins at approximately 0.001 cd/m^2 and extends up to 5 cd/m^2 for a 3° diameter centrally fixated target [41]. The upper range could extend up to 15 cd/m^2 for a 25° diameter target; however, 3 cd/m^2 is the most often cited upper limit for mesopic vision. One can liken this to the low-light conditions on a cloudless night with a full moon. Scotopic refers to light levels below the mesopic range, which can be likened to a moonless, starry night.

Certainly, if all the blue light were blocked, one might expect some decrease in scotopic vision. However, neither the HOYA nor the AcrySof® Natural IOL blocks all blue light. It is well recognized that the most important wavelengths for scotopic vision are at and around 507 nm [42]. The AcrySof® Natural IOL allows transmission of approximately 85% of light at

507 nm. In comparison, a UV blocking colorless IOL transmits only 4% more light at this wavelength. It is also important to note that the normal human crystalline lens at any age transmits significantly *less* light at and near 507 nm than does the AcrySof® Natural IOL and therefore, patients implanted with the AcrySof® Natural IOL should have enhanced scoptopic vision. It would be counterintuitive to believe that scotopic vision would be diminished instead of being enhanced.

A study presented at the ASCRS Annual Meeting in 2005 evaluated the detection thresholds for a Goldmann size V target at wavelengths of 410, 450, 500 nm using a modified Humphrey Field Analyzer in patients, with and without yellow clips that approximated the filtering ability of the AcrySof® Natural IOL [43]. Each test was carried out with a single wavelength of light. The results showed decreased ability to perceive objects when only 410 or 450 nm light was present, but no significant decrease in perception ability at 500 nm. This decrease was more significant in patients with ARMD. The results are exactly what would be expected, based on the light transmission spectrum of these IOLs. However, the study fails to provide insight into mesopic or scotopic vision as it does not represent mesopic or scotopic conditions. In the real life environment, there is always a spectrum of light present, not just one wavelength. This is also true of mesopic and scotopic conditions, where there is more 500 nm and longer wavelength light than 410 or 450 nm. (Fig. 8.52)

In 2008, Drs Turner and Mainster questioned the effect of blue light filtering IOLs on the circadian

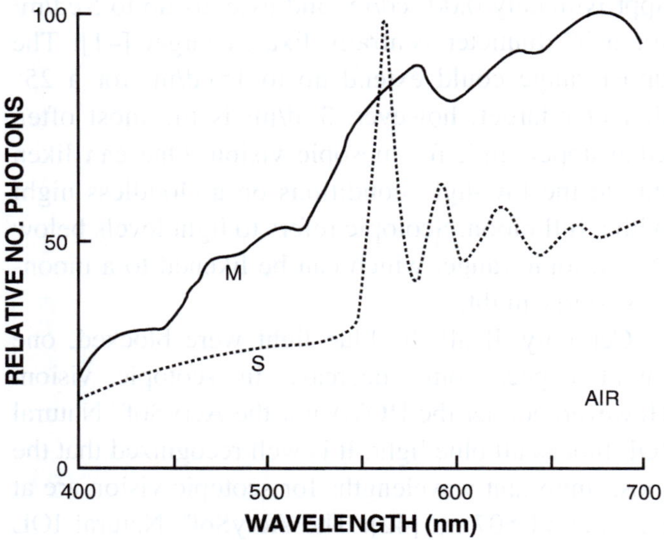

Fig. 8.52 Spectral light distribution in air under mesopic (M) and scotopic (S) conditions [44]

rhythm and perhaps, as a result, on the sleep patterns of the patients receiving these IOLs [45]. However, no peer reviewed literature could be found to corroborate their concerns. Indeed, until today, only one study seems to disprove these claims. Patel and Dacey examined the relative effectiveness of photoentrainment of the circadian rhythm by a blue light-filtering tinted intraocular lens (AcrySof Natural SN60), an UV-only filtering IOL (AcrySof SA60), compared to human lenses in four age groups. They found that with the most recently published action spectra for circadian photoentrainment, blue light filtering IOLs were significantly more effective for photoentrainment of the circadian action rhythm than with previously cited action spectra. These results suggest that the effectiveness of the blue light filtering SN60 IOLs placed in 60- to 85-year-old patients would be within +6 to −13% of that in 30- to 39-year-olds, and that both SN60 and SA60 IOLs should be effective for melatonin suppression under average household illumination [46]. Separately, in a recent clinical study, Landers et al. evaluated sleep patterns in 31 patients implanted with UV-only blocking IOLs and compared them to the sleep patterns of 18 patients receiving UV and blue light filtering IOLs [47]. They found no significant difference in sleep patterns between these two groups and concluded that the blue light filtering IOLs had no deleterious effect on circadian rhythm or sleep patterns.

Summary

Clinical studies demonstrate no clinically significant difference between colorless, UV-blocking IOLs and blue light filtering IOLs in terms of visual acuity, contrast sensitivity, color vision, night vision, circadian rhythm or sleep patterns.

8.3.4.5 Clinical Experience

Having implanted many thousand AcrySof® Natural IOLs, I have had the opportunity to gain insight to the quality of vision provided by this unique IOL. The visual results in my patients have been excellent without any complaints of color perception or night vision problems. I have implanted blue light filtering IOL in the fellow eye of many patients previously implanted with colorless UV-filtering IOLs. When asked to compare the color of a white tissue paper, 70% do not see a difference between the two eyes. Of the 30% that could tell a difference, none perceived the difference before I checked and none felt the difference was bothersome. With more than 40,000,000 AcrySof® Natural IOLs implanted worldwide at the time of this writing, the authors are not aware of any confirmed reports of color perception night vision or circadian rhythm problems.

Summary

Clinical experience with blue light filtering IOLs showed no difficulty with color perception or night vision.

8.3.4.6 Unresolved Issues and Future Considerations

Laboratory studies have demonstrated the protective benefit provided by filtering blue light for cultured RPE cells. However, the benefits of blue-light filtering IOLs in preventing the development, or worsening of macular degeneration or uveal melanoma have not been proven clinically. A large multicentered prospective clinical study will be necessary to determine if these IOLs truly provide a protective effect. Additionally, there may be a role for different levels of blue light filtering capabilities in these lenses in an effort to maximize retinal protection while minimizing any possible compromise to the quality of vision.

Take Home Pearls

- Newer technologies provide us the opportunity to improve vision following cataract or RLE surgery more substantially and predictably than ever before.
- We now need to make efforts to maintain that vision long-term.
- Given the growing body of evidence, implicating blue light as a potential factor in the worsening of ARMD and the positive collective clinical experience with blue light filtering IOLs, it makes sense to implant these protective IOLs, when possible.
- Blue light filtering IOLs will eventually become the standard of care in cataract and RLE surgery.

References

1. Alio J, Tavolato M, De la Hoz F, Claramonte P, Rodriguez-Prats J, Galal A. Near vision restoration with refractive lens exchange and pseudoaccommodating and multifocal refractive and diffractive intraocular lenses: comparative clinical study. J Cataract Refract Surg 2004; 30:2494–2503
2. Stachs O, Schneider H, Stave J, Guthoff R. Potentially accommodating intraocular lenses – an in vitro and in vivo study using three-dimensional high-frequency ultrasound. J Refract Surg 2005; 21:37–45
3. Nuijts R, et al Clinical outcomes and patient satisfaction after cataract surgery with the array and AcrySof ReSTOR multifocal IOLs. In: The ASCRS Annual Meeting, 2005
4. Chang D. Prospective functional and clinical comparison of bilateral ReZoom and ReSTOR intraocular lenses I patients 70 years or younger. J Cataract Refract Surg 2008; 34:934–941
5. Ham W, Mueller A, Sliney DH. Retinal sensitivity to short wavelength light. Nature 1976; 260:153–155
6. Marshall JC, Gordon KD, McCauley CS, de Souza Filho JP, Burnier MN. The effect of blue light exposure and use of intraocular lenses on human uveal melanoma cell lines. Melanoma Res 2006; 16(6):537–541
7. Lerman S. Biologic and chemical effects of ultraviolet radiation. Radiant Energy and the Eye. Macmillan, New York, 1980, pp 132–133
8. Mainster MA. Spectral transmittance of intraocular lenses and retinal damage from intense light sources. Am J Ophthalmol 1978; 85:167–170
9. Pollack A, et al Age-related macular degeneration after extracapsular cataract extraction with intraocular lens implantation. Ophthalmology 1996; 103:1546–1554
10. Age-Related Eye Disease Study Group. Risk factors associated with age-related macular degeneration. A case-control study in the Age-Related Eye Disease Study: Age-Related Eye Disease Study report number 3. Ophthalmology 2000; 107(12):2224–2232
11. Marshall J. The effects of ultraviolet radiation and blue light on the eye. In Cronly-Dillon J (ed) Susceptible Visual Apparatus (Vision and Visual Dysfunction; vol. 16). Macmillan, London, 1991
12. Marshall J, Mellerio J, Palmer DA. Damage to pigeon retinae by commercial light sources operating at moderate levels. Vision Res 1971; 11(10):1198–1199
13. Sperling HG, Johnson C, Harwerth RS. Differential spectral photic damage to primate cones. Vision Res 1980; 20(12): 1117–1125
14. Sykes SM, Robison WG Jr, Waxler M, Kuwabara T. Damage to the monkey retina by broad-spectrum fluorescent light. Invest Ophthalmol Vis Sci 1981; 20(4):425–434
15. Sparrow JR, Cai B. Blue light-induced apoptosis of A2E-containing RPE: involvement of caspase-3 and protection by Bcl-2. Invest Ophthalmol Vis Sci 2001; 42(6):1356–1362
16. Ben-Shabat S, Parish CA, Vollmer HR, Itagaki Y, Fishkin N, Nakanishi K, Sparrow JR. Biosynthetic studies of A2E, a major fluorophore of retinal pigment epithelial lipofuscin. J Biol Chem 2002; 277(9):7183–7190
17. Liu J, Itagaki Y, Ben-Shabat S, Nakanishi K, Sparrow JR. The biosynthesis of A2E, a fluorophore of aging retina, involves the formation of the precursor, A2-PE, in the photoreceptor outer segment membrane. J Biol Chem 2000; 275(38):29354–29360

18. Winkler BS, Boulton ME, Gottsch JD, Sternberg P. Oxidative damage and age-related macular degeneration. Mol Vis 1999; 5:32
19. Roberts JE. Ocular phototoxicity. J Photochem Photobiol 2001; 64(2–3):136–143
20. Taylor HR, West S, Munoz B, et al The long-term effects of visible light on the eye. Arch Ophthalmol 1992; 110:99–104
21. Cruickshanks KJ, Klein R, Klein BE, Nondahl DM. Sunlight and the 5-year incidence of early age-related maculopathy: the beaver dam eye study. Arch Ophthalmol 2001; 119:246–250
22. Darzins P, Mitchell P, Heller RF. Sun exposure and age-related macular degeneration. An Australian case-control study. Ophthalmology 1997; 104:770–776
23. Delcourt C, Carriere I, Ponton-Sanchez A, et al Light exposure and the risk of age related macular degeneration: the Pathologies Oculaires Liees a l'Age (POLA) study. Arch Ophthalmol 2001; 119:1463–1468
24. McCarty CA, Mukesh BN, Fu CL, et al Risk factors for age-related maculopathy: The Visual Impairment Project. Arch Ophthalmol 2001; 119:1455–1462
25. Mainster MA. Light and macular degeneration: a biophysical and clinical perspective. Eye 1987; 1:304–310
26. Nilsson SE, Textorius O, Andersson BE, Swenson B. Clear PMMA versus yellow intraocular lens material. An electrophysiologic study on pigmented rabbits regarding "the blue light hazard". Prog Clin Biol Res 1989; 314:539–553
27. Li ZL, Tso MO, Jampol LM, Miller SA, Waxler M. Retinal injury induced by near-ultraviolet radiation in aphakic and pseudophakic monkey eyes. A preliminary report. Retina 1990; 10:301–314
28. Marshall J. The effects of ultraviolet radiation and blue light on the eye. In: Cronly-Dillon J (ed) Susceptible Visual Apparatus (Vision and Visual Dysfunction; vol. 16). London: Macmillan, 1991
29. Rapp LM, Smith SC. Morphologic comparisons between rhodopsin-mediated and short-wavelength classes of retinal light damage. Invest Ophthalmol Vis Sci 1992; 33:3367–3377
30. Pang J, Seko Y, Tokoro T, Ichinose S, Yamamoto H. Observation of ultrastructural changes in cultured retinal pigment epithelium following exposure to blue light. Graefe's Arch Clin Exp Ophthalmol 1998; 236:696–701
31. Sparrow JR, Cai B. Blue light-induced apoptosis of A2E-containing RPE: involvement of caspase-3 and protection by Bcl-2. Invest Ophthalmol Vis Sci 2001; 42:1356–1362
32. Schutt F, Davies S, Kopitz J, Holz FG, Boulton ME. Photodamage to human RPE cells by A2-E, a retinoid component of lipofuscin. Invest Ophthalmol Vis Sci 2000; 41:2303–2308
33. Sparrow J, Miller A, Zhou J. Blue light-absorbing intraocular lens and retinal pigment epithelium protection in vitro. J Cataract Refract Surg 2004; 30:873–878
34. Lerman S, Borkman R. Spectroscopic evaluation of classification of the normal, aging and cataractous lens. Opthalmol Res 1976; 8:335–353
35. Data on file, Alcon Laboratories, Fort Worth, TX, USA
36. Lerman S, Borkman R. Spectroscopic evaluation of classification of the normal, aging and cataractous lens. Opthalmol Res 1976; 8:335–353
37. Yuan Z, Reinach P, Yuan J. Contrast sensitivity and color vision with a yellow intraocular lens. Am J Ophthalmol 2004; 138:138–140
38. Ishida M, Yanashima K, Miwa W, et al [Influence of the yellow-tinted intraocular lens on spectral sensitivity] (Article in Japanese). Nippon Ganka Gakkai Zasshi 1994; 98(2):192–196
39. Niwa K, Yoshino Y, Okuyama F, Tokoro T. Effects of tinted intraocular lens on contrast sensitivity. Ophthalmic Physiol Opt 1996; 16(4):297–302
40. Cionni R, Tsai J. Color perception evaluation of the AcrySof natural IOL and the AcrySof single piece IOL in photopic and mesopic conditions. J Cataract Refract Surg
41. Wyszecki G, Stiles WS. Color Science Concepts and Methods, Quantitative Data and Formulae. 2nd edn. Wiley, New York, 1982
42. Swanson WH, Cohen JM. Color vision. Ophthalmol Clin N Am 2003; 16:179–203
43. Jackson G. Pilot study of the effect of a blue-light-blocking IOL on Rod-Mediated (Scotopic) vision. In: ASCRS Annual Meeting, 2005
44. Munz F, McFarland W. Evolutionary adaptations of fishes to the photic environment. In: Crescitelli F (ed) The Visual System of Vertebrates. Springer, New York, 1977, pp 194–274
45. Turner P, Mainster M. Circadian photoreception: ageing and the eye's important role in systemic health. Br J Ophthalmol 2008; 92:1439–1444; Review
46. Patel AS, Dacey DM. Relative effectiveness of a blue light-filtering intraocular lens for photoentrainment of the circadian rhythm. J Cataract Refract Surg 2009; 35:529–539
47. Landers J, Tamblyn D, Perriam D. Effect of a blue-light-blocking intraocular lens on the quality of sleep. J Cataract Refract Surg 2009; 35:83–88

8.3.5 Microincision Intraocular Lenses: Others

Richard S. Hoffman, I. Howard Fine, and Mark Packer

Core Messages

- Current limitations in the available IOL technology have impeded full utilization of a biaxial microincisional approach to cataract surgery by many surgeons.
- There are numerous IOLs available internationally that can be injected through 1.5–2.2 mm incisions.
- IOLs that are multifocal and toric are being manufactured and implanted through sub-2.0 mm incisions.
- Injectable polymer lenses hold the promise of making full utilization of a biaxial microincisional technique without the need for incision enlargement, although further research and development needs to transpire.

Continuing advances in phacoemulsification technology have allowed for safer lens extraction through smaller and smaller incisions. Removal of the crystalline lens utilizing microincisions has improved our technique not so much because of the use of smaller incisions, but through the virtues of performing the lens extraction by means of a biaxial approach. In reality, reducing incision sizes below 2.5 mm has diminishing returns with regard to astigmatism reduction, since the induced astigmatism for these incision sizes is practically neutral. Although there may be some added safety inherent in smaller incisions with regard to incision trauma, incision leakage, and endophthalmitis, the true power in removing cataracts through 1.0–1.2 mm incisions lies in the added options inherent in a biaxial approach with separated infusion and aspiration.

A biaxial approach through microincisions allows the lens to be approached from two different directions by easily switching aspiration and irrigation handpieces between two microincisions. This has added safety for difficult and challenging cases such as eyes with weakened zonules resulting from trauma, pseudoexfoliation, or genetic diseases such as the Marfan syndrome. The biaxial approach has also been found to be helpful in reducing vitreous loss in the presence of ruptured posterior capsules and reducing the incidence of posterior capsule rupture in eyes with weakened or defective posterior capsules, such as posterior polar cataracts. Bimanual irrigation and aspiration of cortical material has also allowed for the safer removal of subincisional cortex, especially in the presence of a small capsulorhexis.

The advantages of a biaxial approach are numerous. Despite this, there has been a slow incorporation of this method, especially within the United States, because of perceived difficulties in achieving proficiency with this technique and perceived limited advantages without the access to microincision intraocular lenses (IOLs) that can be inserted through these microincisions. Currently available IOLs within the US require 2.0–3.0 mm incisions for implantation. Thus, in order to complete a biaxial microincision procedure, a third incision of the appropriate size would need to be created between the biaxial microincisions, or one of the microincisions would need to be enlarged to accommodate IOL insertion. Despite this current drawback, the benefits of a biaxial approach far outweigh the need for a larger incision for IOL insertion. This advantage is somewhat analogous to the advantages that were presented years ago with the introduction of 3.2 mm phacoemulsification that still required wound enlargement for 6 mm PMMA IOLs. It was not until the introduction of foldable IOLs that could fit through 3 mm incisions that the full benefits of 3 mm phacoemulsification could be realized.

IOL technology has tended to lag behind phacoemulsification technology, and the same is true for current microincision phacoemulsification. The microincision IOLs that are currently being produced and developed are such that they can be inserted into smaller and smaller incisions, taking us one step closer to the ideal IOL that can deliver the full benefit of a microincision technique, and especially a biaxial

R S. Hoffman (✉)
Drs. Fine, Hoffman & Packer, LLC, 1550 Oak Street, Suite 5, Eugene, OR 97403, USA
e-mail: rshoffman@finemd.com

microincision technique. Some of the lenses and lens technologies that may be instrumental in furthering the utility of microincision lens extraction are reviewed below.

8.3.5.1 ThinOptX®

The ThinOptX IOL is a hydrophilic acrylic IOL with a special annular ring design that allows the 5.5 mm optic of the lens to be no thicker than 300–400 µm [9]. The posterior surface of the lens has a 3 mm central optic surrounded by a series of concentric annular rings of increasing diameters (Fig. 8.53). The rings form optically cooperative image-forming sections that create a single well-focused image without significant optical aberrations. Each ring contains the desired refractive power and contains a step that leads into the next ring segment, minimizing the thickness of the refractive ring. Each step is perpendicular to the curve of the ring at that point allowing each ring to focus incoming images at the desired focal point, while maintaining the thickness of each ring to approximately 50 µm [24].

The rings of the ThinOptX IOL appear similar in design to that of a Fresnel lens. However, the lines on a Fresnel lens function as a series of prisms with a diffractive design that has multiple focal points. The ThinOptX IOL is refractive with the posterior surface designed to assist the front surface in focusing light at a single point. Thus, it is not a true Fresnel lens but does share the quality of an ultrathin structure by virtue of a concentric ring construction. This ultrathin design of the ThinOptX lens has been reported to yield modulation transfer function (MTF) that exceeds 100% when conventional testing methods are utilized. This is believed to be due to the limitations of current MTF devices that assume the presence of some optical aberrations that may not be present on the ThinOptx IOLs [24]. Other studies have confirmed excellent MTF in the ThinOptX IOL but found the results to be no different than conventional foldable acrylic IOLs [2].

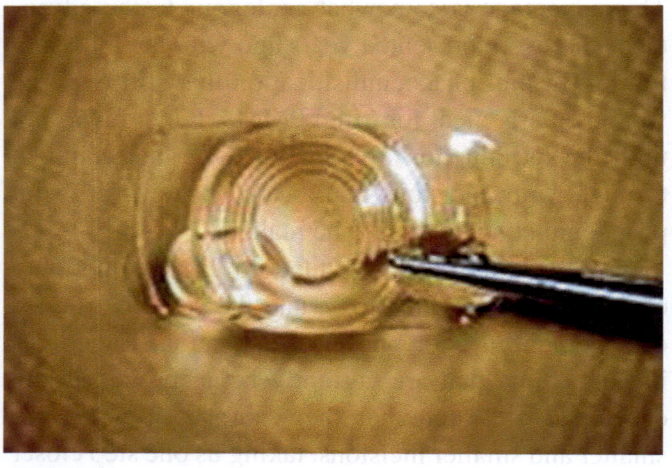

Fig. 8.53 The ThinOptX IOL demonstrating concentric annular rings of increasing diameters

The unique thin design of the ThinOptX lens has produced some interesting advantages and some potential drawbacks. A recent study by Ouchi demonstrated better contrast sensitivity and lower spherical aberration with the ThinOptX IOL compared to the Alcon AcrySof lens [20]. Dogru also demonstrated higher contrast sensitivities in the ThinOptX compared to the three-piece AcrySof IOL [7]. Pseudo-accommodation has also been demonstrated with the ThinOptX IOL. Vejarano measured over 2 D of accommodation with the push-up method and similar amplitudes with trial lenses [31]. In a pilot study of the IOL performed by Alio, ultrasound biomicroscopy revealed forward movement of the IOL during accommodation that may be contributing to improved near vision results [24].

Although none of the 10 patients in Alio's study reported glare or halos, a larger recent study of 50 eyes by Prakash revealed a 61% incidence of colored halos around artificial lights and a 64% posterior capsule opacification (PCO) rate at 15 months postoperatively [21]. A greater tendency for PCO was also discovered when the ThinOptX was compared to the three-piece AcrySof IOL [11].

The greatest advantage of the ThinOptX IOL with regard to microincision surgery is the ability to implant the lens through incision sizes of 1.4–1.7 mm [9, 21, 24]. Secondary to the ultrathin construction of the IOL, it can be rolled and injected into the eye with gentle atraumatic unfolding within the capsular bag. An injector system is available that does not require a cartridge to be placed within the incision and scanning electron studies have demonstrated no signs of surface damage or alterations, after the IOL has passed through the dedicated injector [15]. Although the IOL has been shown to move forward during accommodation, none of the eyes in Alio's pilot study were reported to demonstrate any permanent change in IOL position, significant decentration, or lens tilt, 1 year following surgery.

8.3.5.2 Smart IOL

One of the more interesting prospects for microincision IOLs involves a technology being developed by Medennium. The Smart IOL is a lens constructed of a thermodynamic hydrophobic acrylic material. Wax is chemically bonded to the acrylic in order to create a material that remains solid at room temperature [6]. At room temperature, the lens is packaged as a 2 mm wide × 30 mm long solid rod. When inserted into the eye and warmed to body temperature, the rod transforms into a soft elastic disc that has dimensions that closely mimic those of the natural crystalline lens (9.5 × 3.5 mm) (Fig. 8.54). Before the IOL is packaged as a rod, it is imprinted with a precise dioptric power and after 30 s at body temperature, it expands into an elastic lens with the desired lens power [34].

There are many potential advantages of the IOL design. In addition to allowing for implantation through a microincision, the lens completely fills the average capsular bag (Fig. 8.55). There should be no open space for cell growth, no edge glare, no spherical aberration, and no decentration in the presence of an intact capsular bag. The hydrophobic acrylic material should promote adherence to the capsular bag, reducing the incidence of PCO. The acrylic is highly flexible (Fig. 8.56) and has a high refractive index of 1.47, thus, there is an anticipation that minute changes in lens shape through accommodative effort may result in significant changes in lens power shift-yielding high amplitudes of accommodation [34].

There is also the possibility of changing the current rod dimensions in order to facilitate IOL insertion through smaller microincisions. The Smart IOL is currently in the preliminary stages of development although cadaver studies and optical bench studies have been performed.

8.3.5.3 Afinity™

The Staar Afinity IOL (Fig. 8.57) is a single piece plate haptic IOL designed to be injected through a 2.2 mm incision utilizing the Staar nanoPOINT™ injector

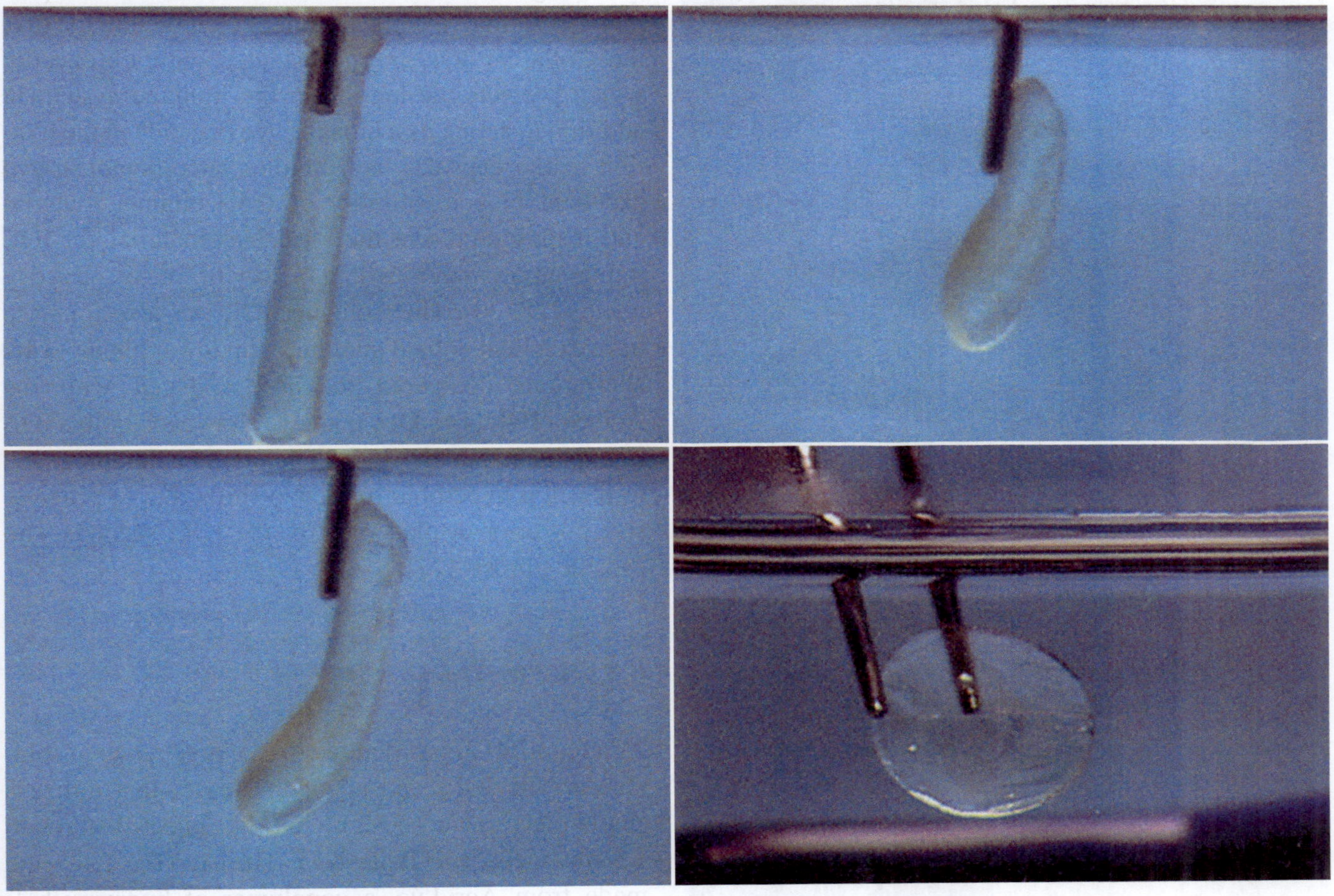

Fig. 8.54 The Medennium Smart IOL demonstrating transformation from a rod to a 9.5 × 3.5 mm disc after 30 s in a warm saline bath

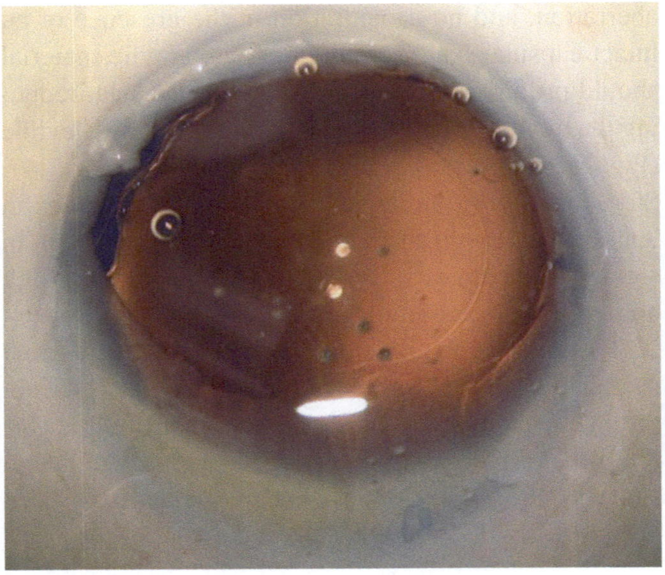

Fig. 8.55 The Smart IOL in situ (cadaver eye) fills the capsular bag completely (Courtesy of Nick Mamalis)

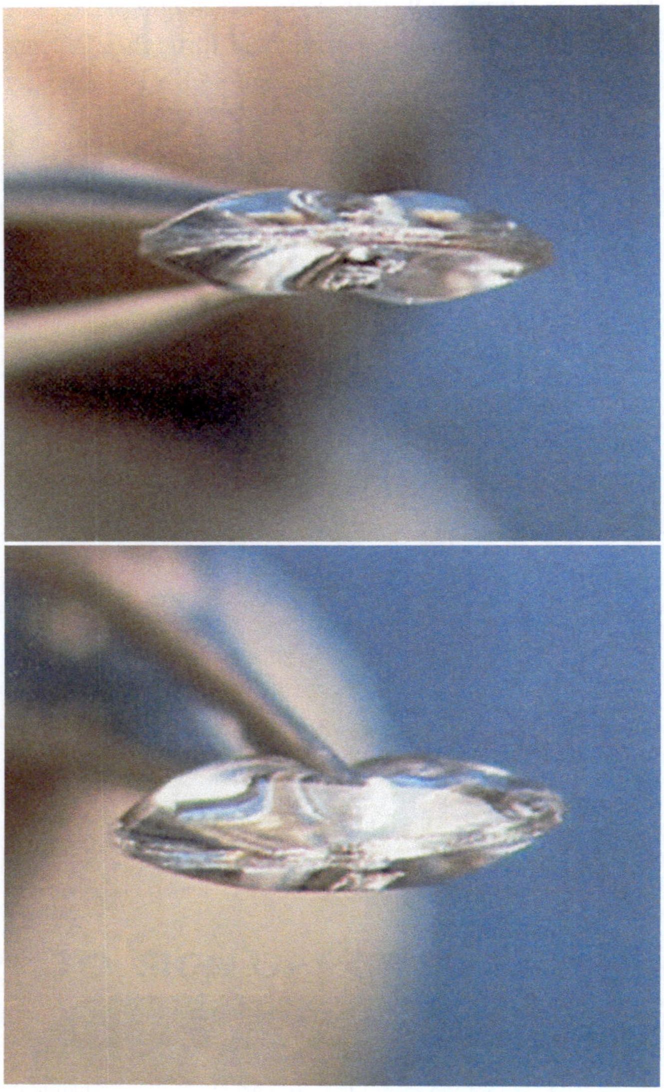

Fig. 8.56 Elastic quality of the Smart IOL

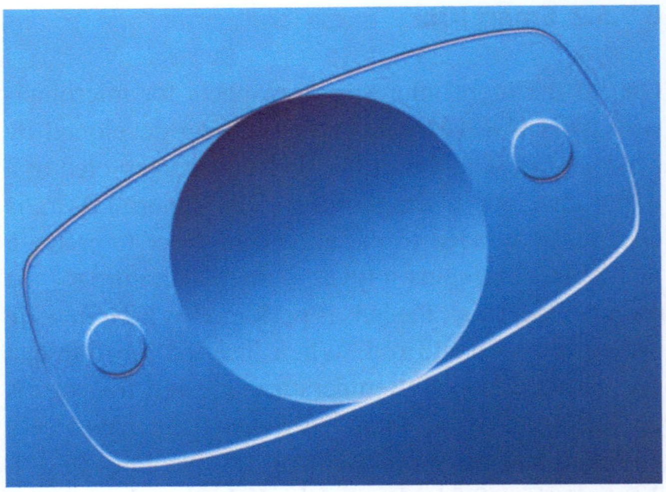

Fig. 8.57 Staar Afinity single piece plate haptic IOL (Courtesy of Staar Surgical)

system (Fig. 8.58). Collamer is a proprietary hydrophilic material made from a combination of collagen and Poly-HEMA hydrogel. A benzophenone chromophore is covalently bonded to the poly-HEMA copolymer to create the final UV filtering Collamer material.

Collagen within the Collamer material inhibits protein deposition. Shortly after implantation into the eye, the Collamer IOL is encapsulated with fibronectin, which protects the lens from the immune system in addition to acting as a bioadhesive that aids in the fixation to the capsular bag. Studies have demonstrated excellent biocompatibility of the Collamer material and it may represent the ideal lens material for IOL implantation in eyes with a history of uveitis or active uveitis [28, 30]. The Collamer IOL was also found to have excellent optical qualities with lower higher order aberrations compared to those induced with the AcrySof IOL [14]. One potential drawback of this IOL is its plate haptic design which has been demonstrated to develop hyperopic refractive shifts due to progressive posterior displacement of the IOL, secondary to capsule fibrosis [27].

8.3.5.4 AcriTec

AcriTec (Carl Zeiss Meditec) has a large range of foldable acrylic IOLs and all of the lenses that utilize a single-piece plate design can be injected through 1.5 mm incisions (Table 8.7). The AcriTec IOLs are made from Acri.Lyc, a copolymer of hydroxyethylmethacrylate and ethoxymethacrylate with a UV absorber. The Acri.Lyc material is 25% hydrophilic but

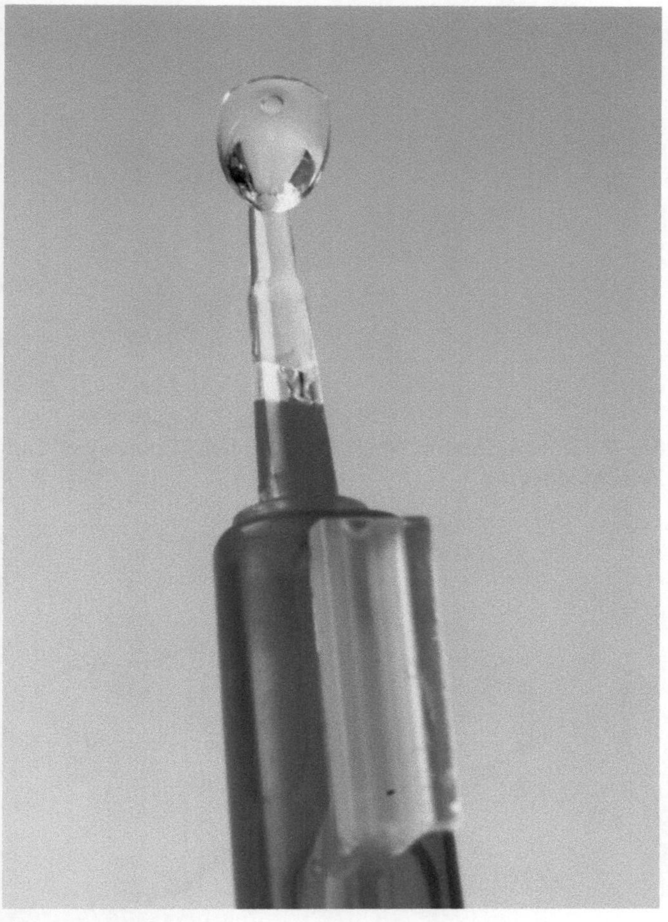

Fig. 8.58 Staar Afinity being ejected from the Staar nanoPO-INT™ injector system (Courtesy of Staar Surgical)

maintains a hydrophobic surface. The material has a strong memory that does not change its curvature or power after rolling and unfolding and no surface damage develops after microincision injection [15]. The IOLs can be injected through a 1.5 mm microincision utilizing the Acri.Smart Glide System (Acri.Shooter A2-2000 and Acri.Smart Glide cartridge). Extensive tests measuring point spread functions before and 120 min after injection through the cartridge system confirmed that optical performance of the IOLs was not altered. Initial studies of the Acri.Smart IOLs demonstrated good centration, absence of tilt, very low induced astigmatism, and low Nd:YAG capsulotomy rates [24].

The Acri.Smart series of Acri.Tec lenses were some of the earliest microincision IOLs developed in the world. The initial design utilized a 5.5 mm optic but this has now been replaced with three newer versions of the Acri.Smart IOLs that incorporate a 6 mm diameter optic – Acri.Smart 46S, Acri.Smart 36A, and Acri.Smart 46LC (Fig. 8.59). These three microincision IOLs basically have the same plate IOL design and are made from the same Acri.Lyc material. They differ only in the aspect that the Acri.Smart 46S lens is spherical while the Acri.Smart 46LC is aspherical, and the Acri.Smart 36A is "aberration-correcting," in that it is designed to neutralize corneal spherical aberration.

Table 8.7 Acri.Tec microincision IOLS

	Acri.Smart 36A	Acri.Smart 46S	Acri.Smart 46LC	Acri.Comfort 646TLC	Acri.LISA 366D	Acri.LISAtoric 466TD
Lens design	Single-piece monofocal aspheric	Single-piece monofocal	Single-piece monofocal aspheric	Single-piece bitoric	Single-piece bifocal +3.75	Single-piece toric/bifocal
Material	Foldable acrylate	Foldable acrylate	Foldable acrylate	Foldable acrylate	Foldable acrylate	Foldable acrylate
Optic diameter (mm)	6.0	6.0	6.0	6.0	6.0	6.0
Length (mm)	11.0	11.0	11.0	11.0	11.0	11.0
Incision size (mm)	1.5–1.7	1.5–1.7	1.5–1.7	1.5–1.7	1.5–1.7	1.5–1.7
Recommend A-factor acoustic/optic						
AL < 25 mm	117.6/117.9	117.6/117.9	117.6/117.9	117.6/117.9	117.6/117.9	117.6/117.9
AL ≥ 25 mm	118.0/118.3	118.0/118.3	118.0/118.3	118.0/118.3	118.0/118.3	118.0/118.3
Diopter range	0–10 D 1 D increment 10–32 D 0.5 D increment	16–27 D 0.5 D Increment	0–10 D 1 D increment 10–32 D 0.5 D increment	Sphere −10 to +32 D Cylinder +1 to +12 D	0–32 D 0.5 D Increment	Sphere −10 to +32 D Cylinder +1 to +12 D
Implantation injector cartridge	A2–2000 Acri.Smart	A2–2000 Acri.Smart	A2–2000 Acri.Smart	A2–2000 Acri.Smart	A2–2000 Acri.Smart	A2–2000 Acri.Smart

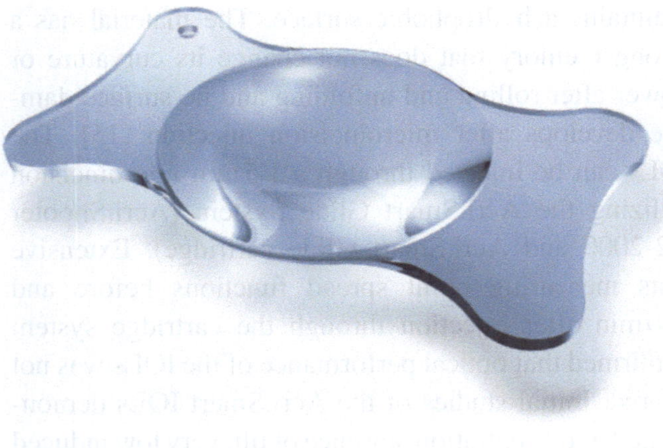

Fig. 8.59 Acri.Smart plate IOL design (Courtesy of Carl Zeiss Meditec)

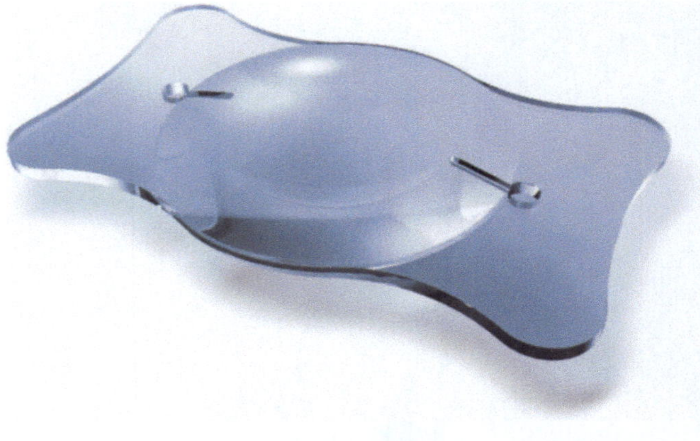

Fig. 8.60 Acri.Comfort 646TLC bitoric IOL (Courtesy of Carl Zeiss Meditec)

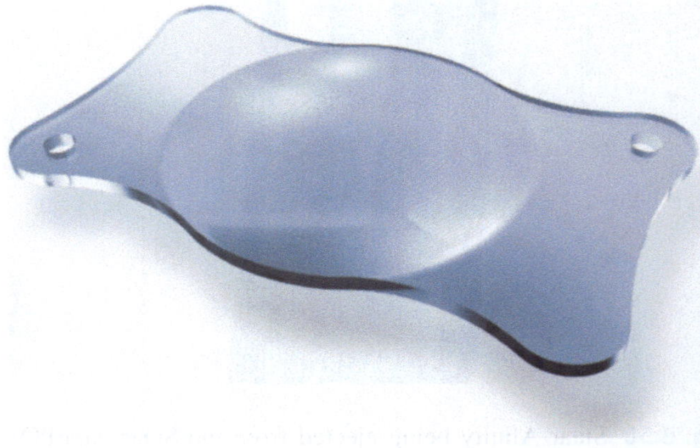

Fig. 8.61 Acri.LISA 366D biconvex diffractive-refractive single-piece IOL with a 6.0 mm aspheric optic (Courtesy of Carl Zeiss Meditec)

Acri.Tec produces two bitoric IOLs designed to treat astigmatism. The Acri.Comfort 643TLC is a bitoric foldable IOL with a tripod design that can be injected through a 2.2 mm incision. The Acri.Comfort 646TLC (Fig. 8.60) is also bitoric and can be injected through a 1.5 mm incision utilizing the Acri.Smart Glide System injector. The cylinder correction is symmetrically distributed over the front and back surface of the IOLs. Due to the reduction of the difference in the radii of curvature, image quality is claimed to be superior to traditional monotoric IOLs. The truly remarkable feature of these toric IOLs is the range of cylinder correction. Spherical power ranges from −10.0 to +32.0 D and cylindrical power ranges from +1.0 to +12.0 D. Higher powers can also be manufactured with special request.

Acri.Tec has also released a new generation bifocal IOL – the Acri.LISA (Fig. 8.61). The Acri.LISA 366D is a biconvex diffractive-refractive single-piece IOL with a 6.0 mm aspheric optic. The aspheric profile is designed to neutralize positive corneal spherical aberration. The lens has an overall diameter of 11.0 mm with 0° angulation. The diffractive-refractive optic of the Acri.LISA is based on patented SMP technology (smooth micro phase). The SMP technology produces a lens surface that does not exhibit any square edges or right angles. This technology is claimed to produce ideal image quality with a marked reduction of scattered light unlike common diffractive IOLs that incorporate a saw-tooth design on the surface of the lens. Incident light is distributed 65% for distance and 35% for near focus and the bifocal optic functions independent of the pupil size. The IOL power ranges from 0 to +32 D and incorporates a +3.75 D near add that corresponds to a +3.00 D add at the spectacle plane. Note: LISA is an acronym for (L) light distribution for 65% distance and 35% near, (I) independent of pupil size, (S) smooth micro phase refractive/diffractive optic, and (A) aberration correcting-optimized aspheric optic.

Recent studies of the Acri.LISA bifocal IOL have demonstrated good performance with a satisfactory full range of vision. Alfonso reported on 81 patients implanted bilaterally with the Acri.LISA and found mean binocular distance-corrected near vision of approximately 20/20. The mean binocular distance-corrected intermediate acuity ranged from 20/20 at 33 cm. to 20/40 at 70 cm. Contrast sensitivity was within normal limits under photopic and mesopic conditions and improved at all spatial frequencies with binocular testing [1].

Alio reported on 69 eyes of 52 patients implanted with the Acri.LISA 366D and found good efficacy and safety, good predictability, and excellent distance and near visual acuity . Distance-corrected near acuity averaged 0.90 ± 0.14 (between 20/20 and 20/25). This study also evaluated the intraocular performance and demonstrated good intraocular aberration, Strehl ratio, and MTF values [3].

The latest addition to the Acri.Tec inventory of microincision IOLs is the Acri.LISAtoric 466TD. This lens has a diffractive bifocal aspheric front surface and a toric aspheric back surface. Similar to the Acri.LISA bifocal IOL, the Acri.LISAtoric distributes 65% of incident light for distance focus and 35% for near focus, functions independent of pupil size, and incorporates a 3.75 D add that corresponds to a +3.00 D add at the spectacle plane. The advantage of this IOL is the ability to correct large amounts of cylinder at the time of implantation of the bifocal optic, which would improve final visual acuities relative to procedures that require large limbal relaxing incisions for astigmatic reduction. The rotational stability of the Acri.Tec single-piece plate lenses has been demonstrated to be excellent with Reiter [23] reporting less than 4° of rotation in 98% of eyes at 6 months follow-up and Wehner [32] reporting no rotation or decentration of the Acri.Smart IOL, 12–19 months postoperatively. Thus, the capacity to stably correct up to +12 D of cylinder while simultaneously implanting a high quality bifocal IOL would make this lens a popular option for presbyopia correction in the future.

Breyer recently reported early results of ten bilateral implantations in 5 patients which included eyes with high astigmatism and myopia. At the 5 month follow-up, mean spherical equivalent improved from −5.25 to 0.4 D and the mean cylinder improved from 2.25 to 0.44 D. Uncorrected mean postoperative acuity was 0.69 (approximately 20/30) for distance and 0.78 (approximately 20/25) for near [19].

8.3.5.5 Akreos

The Bausch & Lomb Akreos AO MI60 (Fig. 8.62) is one of the several IOLs in the Akreos inventory that can be injected through a 1.8 mm incision. The Akreos IOLs are one-piece equiconvex hydrophilic acrylic lenses made from a poly-HEMA/MMA copolymer. The Akreos AO MI60 has a thin, aspherical, aberration-free optic with a 360° posterior square edge to reduce PCO. The lens has four haptics that provide for four-point fixation while stabilizing the optic in three dimensions. This transpires by virtue of conforming tips at the end of each haptic that are able to bend as the capsular bag contracts and avoid transferring these contraction forces to the optic (Fig. 8.63). A 10° angulation of the haptics enhances the contact of the optic

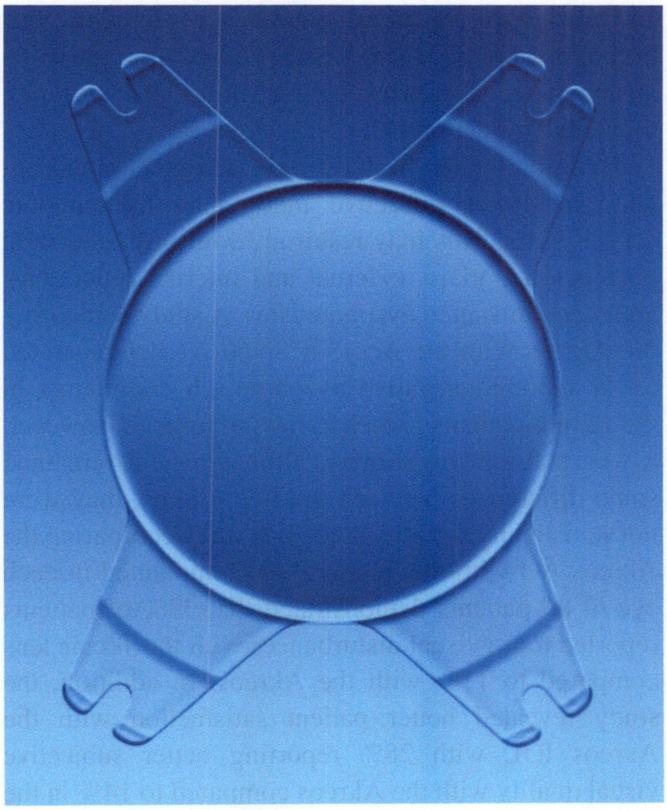

Fig. 8.62 Bausch & Lomb Akreos AO MI60 (Courtesy of Bausch & Lomb)

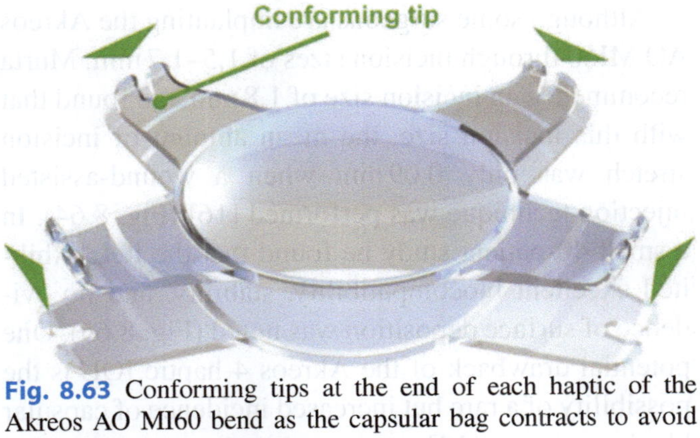

Fig. 8.63 Conforming tips at the end of each haptic of the Akreos AO MI60 bend as the capsular bag contracts to avoid transferring contraction forces to the optic

with the posterior capsule to further reduce the development of PCO [4].

The Akreos AO MI60 is available in powers ranging from +10.0 to +30.0 D. In order to maximize stability of the IOL and posterior edge contact, regardless of the capsular bag size, the IOL is manufactured in three different diameters with three optic sizes depending on the lens power. For IOL powers between 10 and 15 D, the overall diameter is 11.0 mm with an optic diameter of 6.2 mm. For powers between 15.5 and 22.0 D, the overall diameter is 10.7 mm with an optic diameter of 6.0 mm. For higher powered IOLs of 22.5 D and greater, the overall diameter decreases to 10.5 mm with an optic diameter of 5.6 mm [4].

Hydrophilic acrylic IOLs have a higher water content and lower refractive index than hydrophobic acrylic IOLs. This may result in fewer problems with postoperative glare, external and internal reflections, and other unwanted dysphotopsias. A study comparing the Akreos with the AcrySof SN60-AT demonstrated fewer reported negative dysphotopsia complaints in the Akreos patients 1 week following surgery. However, 8 weeks following surgery, although there remained some differences between the two groups, they were not statistically significant [22]. A study comparing the Akreos AO with the Tecnis Z9000 implanted in each eye of 80 patients demonstrated that 33% of patients reported more visual disturbances with the Tecnis lens compared to 11% with the Akreos. In addition, the study revealed better patient satisfaction with the Akreos IOL with 28% reporting better subjective visual quality with the Akreos compared to 14% in the Tecnis eye. The Akreos IOL was found to provide a larger depth of field than the Tecnis lens which may have been partially responsible for the perceived higher quality of vision [10].

Although some surgeons are implanting the Akreos AO MI60 through incision sizes of 1.5–1.7 mm, Murta recommends an incision size of 1.8 mm and found that with this incision size, the mean amount of incision stretch was only 0.09 mm when a wound-assisted injection technique was performed [16] (Fig. 8.64). In a small 40-patient study he found that the IOL exhibited excellent biocompatibility, stability, and no evidence of surface deposition was noted (Fig. 8.65). One potential drawback of the Akreos 4 haptic IOL is the possibility of a rare but increased incidence of capsular block syndrome [13].

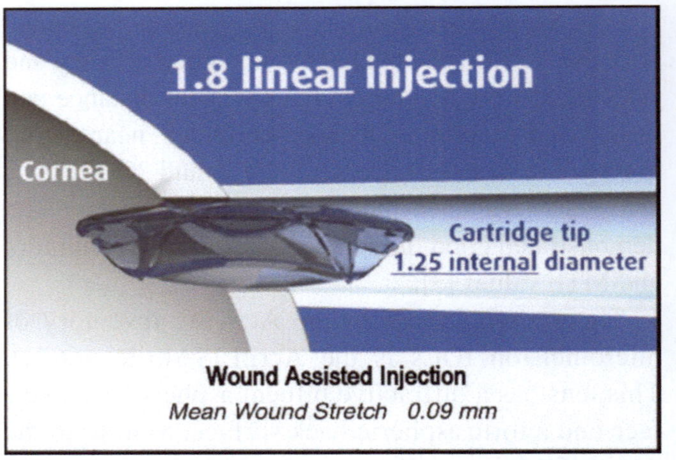

Fig. 8.64 Wound-assisted injection of Akreos AO MI60 through an incision size of 1.8 mm. The mean amount of incision stretch was 0.09 mm. (Courtesy of Joaquin Murta)

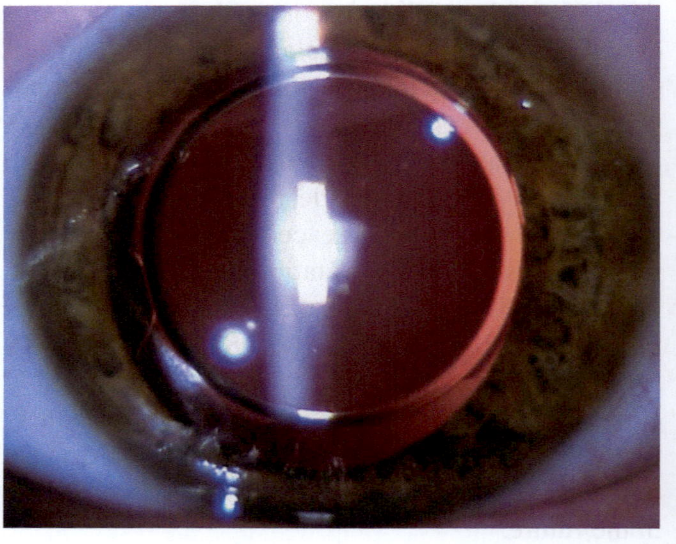

Fig. 8.65 Akreos AO MI60 in situ (Courtesy of Joaquin Murta)

8.3.5.6 Tetraflex

The Lenstec Kellan Tetraflex (model KH-3500) is a poly-HEMA accommodating IOL that can be injected through a 2 mm incision using a 1.8 mm cartridge system. The IOL has a square-edge design with a 5.75 mm optic (Fig. 8.66). The lens is designed to angulate forward, away from the posterior capsule in the resting state. In contrast to hinged-accommodating IOLs, the Tetraflex has no hinges and has a unique mechanism of accommodation that does not depend on vitreous pressure during accommodative effort. The haptic design of the IOL are proposed to allow the lens to move forward with the capsular bag during accommodation [12].

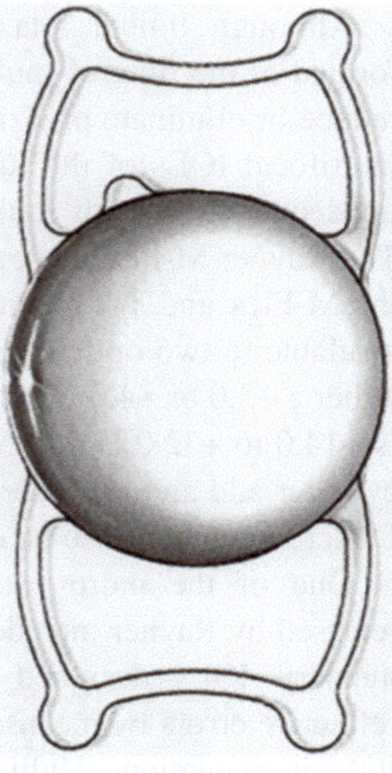

Fig. 8.66 The Lenstec Kellan Tetraflex (model KH-3500)

Sanders reported on 95 eyes of 59 patients implanted with the tetraflex. Six months following surgery, 63% of the eyes had a distance-corrected near acuity of 20/40, or better. Of the patients who were implanted bilaterally, all the patients were reported to have achieved 1 D of accommodative ability and 96% had at least 2 D [25]. In a separate paper, Sanders found that 88% of the Tetraflex eyes obtained distance corrected near acuities that were sufficient to read a newspaper and telephone directory print and 63% could read classified ads, stock quotes, and pocket bibles. When tested binocularly, these percentages increased to 96 and 89% [26]. The prospects of an accommodating IOL that yields good functional near vision in a large majority of patients, while being implantable through an incision of 2 mm holds great promise. Further studies and research will be needed to confirm the viability and efficacy of this IOL.

8.3.5.7 Rayner

Rayner Intraocular Lenses (East Sussex, England) has a vast inventory of lenses that can be injected through their single use soft-tipped IOL injector (R-INJ-04). The injector has an outer nozzle tip diameter of 2.0 mm and the company claims that their lenses can be injected through a sub 2.0 mm incision utilizing a wound-assisted injection technique. Regardless of the minimal incision size that these IOLs can be inserted through, they do have special qualities that deserve mention.

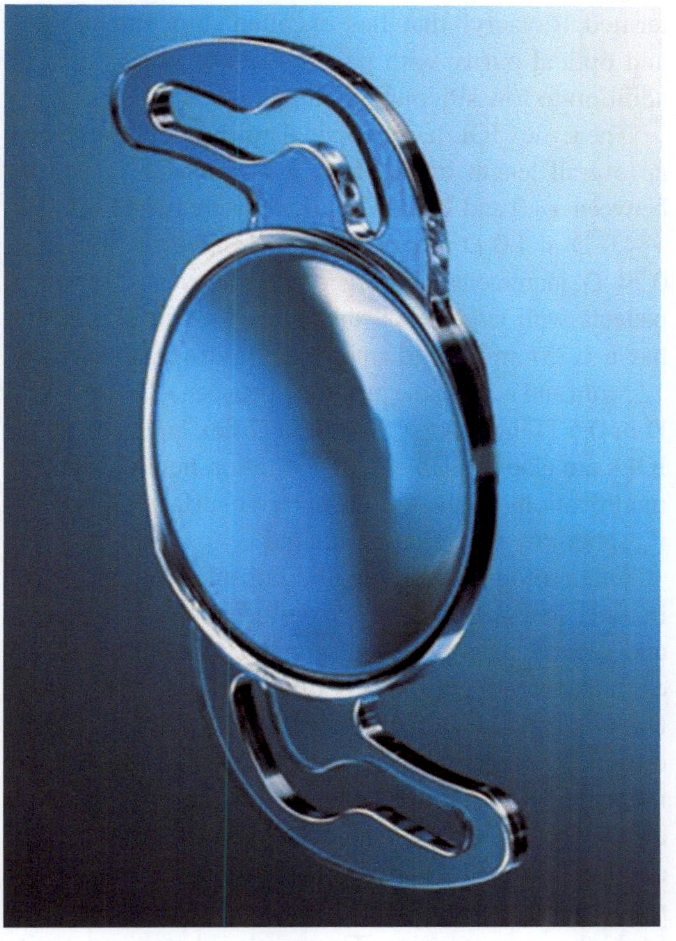

Fig. 8.67 Angled view of the Raynor C-flex (570C) IOL demonstrating the unique AVH technology (Photo courtesy of Rayner)

The two major classes of foldable IOLs that Rayner produces are designed for in-the-bag and sulcus implantation. The in-the-bag IOLs include the C-flex, Superflex®, T-flex®, M-flex®, and M-flex® T lenses. The lenses designed for sulcus implantation include the Sulcoflex® Aspheric, Sulcoflex® Toric, and Sulcoflex® Multifocal IOLs.

All of the capsular bag lenses are produced on a similar lens platform that incorporates a single-piece hydrophilic acrylic design with unique anti-vaulting haptic (AVH) technology (Fig. 8.67). The AVH technology allows for capsular bag contraction to develop without affecting IOL centration, rotation, or stability within the capsular bag. The lens platform also contains the Amon-Apple Enhanced Square Edge design that features a 360° posterior square edge to the optic that includes the vulnerable optic-haptic junctions in order to reduce the incidence of PCO [5, 17, 33]. The hydrophilic acrylic material is a propriety copolymer termed Rayacryl that has excellent biocompatibility and optical purity with no vacuoles or glistenings, in addition to low silicone oil adherence.

The C-flex IOL has an optic diameter of 5.75 mm and an overall length of 12.0 mm. It is available in powers between +8.0 and +30.0 D in 0.5 D increments, +30.0 to +34.0 D in 1.0 D increments, and +18.0 to +23.75 D in 0.24 D increments. In larger myopic eyes or younger patients with larger pupil diameters, the Superflex® lens has a 6.25 mm optic diameter and an overall length of 12.5 mm and is available in powers between −10.0 to +25.5 D in 0.5 D increments. Both the C-flex and Superflex® IOLs are also available with aberration-neutral aspheric modifications applied to the anterior surface of the IOL if asphericity of the lens is desired.

Other modifications to the capsular bag platform include a toric IOL (T-flex®), multifocal IOL (M-flex®), and combined multifocal toric IOL (M-flex® T). The excellent rotational stability offered by the AVH haptic technology makes the Rayner platform ideal for a toric design. The T-flex® has the toric component implemented on the anterior surface of the optic and is available in two models. Model 623T has a 6.25 mm optic and is designed for low and medium power lenses and model 573T contains a 5.75 mm optic and is designed for higher power lenses. The standard lenses are available with powers ranging from +6.0 to +26.0 D in 0.5 D incremental steps with +1.0 to +6.0 D of cylindrical correction in 1.0 D increments. Alternative powers are also available with −10.0 to +35.0 D with up to +11.0 D of cylindrical correction in 0.25 D increments.

The Rayner M-flex® is a multi-zoned refractive aspheric IOL with either four or five annular zones (depending on IOL base power) that are available with either +3.0 or +4.0 D of additional near power (equivalent to +2.25 or +3.0 D respectively at the spectacle plane). These alternate near powers give the option of the same power bilateral implantation or "mix and match" implantation, utilizing the same IOL multifocal design platform with two different adds. The M-flex® optic incorporates multi-aspheric aberration-neutral surfaces with the interface between each annular zone designed to reduce halo and glare. At each zonal interface, the aspheric correction is adjusted and the aspheric coefficients are recalculated to create a precise zonal blend. This lens contains a 6.25 mm optic with an overall length of 12.5 mm. The powers range from +14.0 to +25.0 D in 1.0 D increments and +18.5 to +23.5 D in 0.5 D increments, for both add powers.

Although limbal relaxing incisions can be performed at the time of multifocal IOL implantation to reduce or eliminate preexisting astigmatism, the ideal multifocal IOLs of the future will have toric corrections combined with multifocality on one platform. The Rayner M-flex® T combines all of the features of the M-Flex and T-flex lenses in one IOL model. It is available in two optic sizes of 5.75 and 6.25 mm with either a +3.0 or +4.0 D add. The standard power range is +14.0 to +32.0 D in 0.5 D increments with a 2.0 D cylinder add and toric corrections of 1.0–6.0 D in 0.5 D increments can also be ordered.

One of the more exciting technologies recently released by Rayner include their pseudophakic supplementary IOLs designed to eliminate postoperative refractive errors by means of ciliary sulcus piggy-back IOL implantation. Unlike conventional piggy-back IOLs, the Rayner Sulcoflex® lenses have a unique concave posterior surface that avoids physical contact between the two IOLs. This would reduce the likelihood of optic surface distortion, unwanted photopic effects, and hyperopic defocus. The wide 6.5 mm round-edged optic and undulating round-edged haptics with 10° angulation (Fig. 8.68) would reduce the risk of dysphotopsias, optic-iris capture, and uveal contact with pigment dispersion, while providing excellent centration and rotational stability.

The Sulcoflex platform comes in an aspheric model, toric model, and multifocal model. These models allow the surgeon to adjust postoperative spherical errors with the Sulcoflex® Aspheric (653L) and postoperative residual cylinder with the Sulcoflex® Toric (653T) (Fig. 8.69), and also allows currently, monofocal pseudophakic patients, the opportunity to attempt to correct their pseudophakic presbyopia with a Sulcoflex® Multifocal IOL (653F) (Fig. 8.70). If a patient is dissatisfied with the quality of the toric or multifocal optics, the sulcus lens can be easily explanted.

The Sulcoflex® Aspheric IOL comes available in powers −10.0 to +10.0 D in 0.5 D increments. The Sulcoflex Multifocal comes available in powers from −5.0 to +5.0 D in 0.5 D increments and a +3.50 D add. The Sulcoflex® Toric is available in spherical powers between −9.0 and +3.0 D and with cylindrical powers from 1.0 to 6.0 D in 0.5 D increments.

Over all, the Rayner inventory of foldable hydrophilic acrylic capsular bag and sulcus lenses encompasses an exciting array of choices, for enhancing patient outcomes immediately, and several years

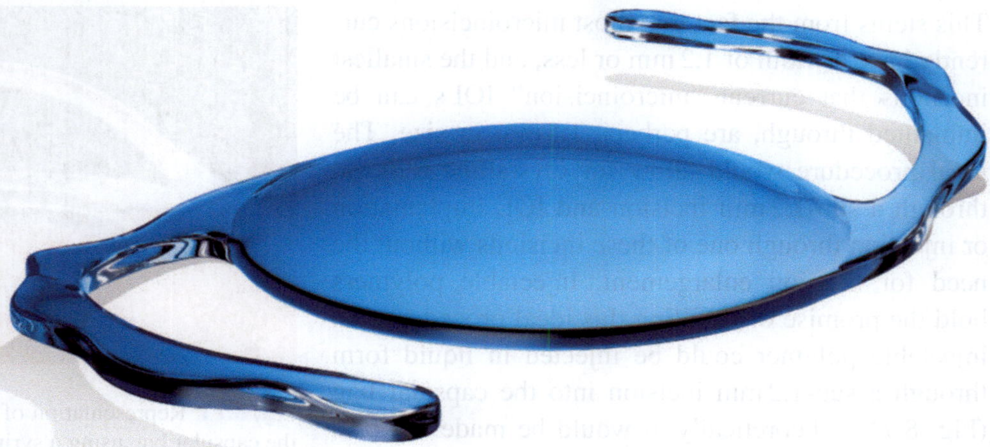

Fig. 8.68 Angled view of the Rayner Sulcoflex Aspheric IOL demonstrating 10° angled undulating haptics (Courtesy of Rayner)

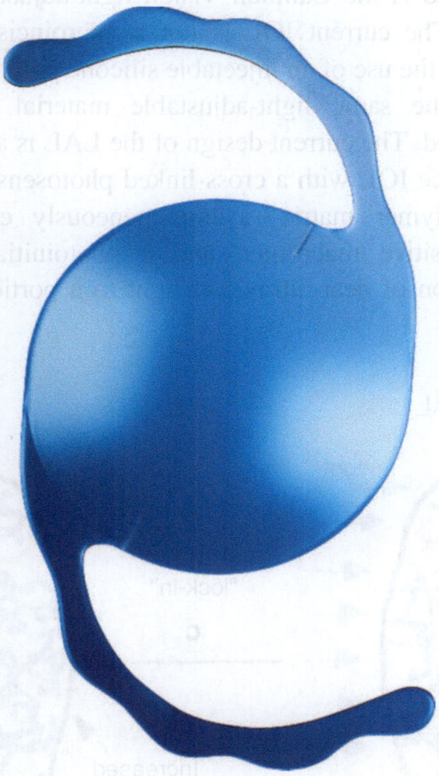

Fig. 8.69 Rayner Sulcoflex Toric IOL (Courtesy of Rayner)

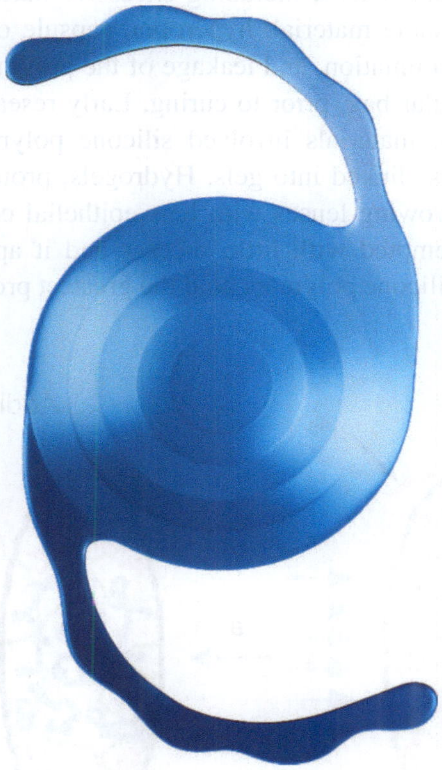

Fig. 8.70 Rayner Sulcoflex Multifocal IOL (Courtesy of Rayner)

following lens extraction and IOL implantation. Further utilization and additional future publications regarding these lenses will ultimately determine the incision size limitations with the current IOL injector model.

8.3.5.8 Injectable Polymers

Common to all of the IOL technologies discussed so far, is the need to create a new incision or widen a microincision in order to accommodate the IOL insertion.

This stems from the fact that most microincisions currently have a width of 1.2 mm or less, and the smallest incisions that current "microincision" IOLs can be implanted through, are perhaps 1.5 mm in size. The ideal procedure would allow for crystalline removal through a sub-1.2 mm incision and IOL implantation or injection through one of these incisions without the need for incision enlargement. Injectable polymers hold the promise of fulfilling this ideal procedure. An injectable polymer could be injected in liquid form through a sub-1.2 mm incision into the capsular bag (Fig. 8.71). Theoretically, it would be made out of a material whose final congealed state would be elastic enough to restore some accommodative ability.

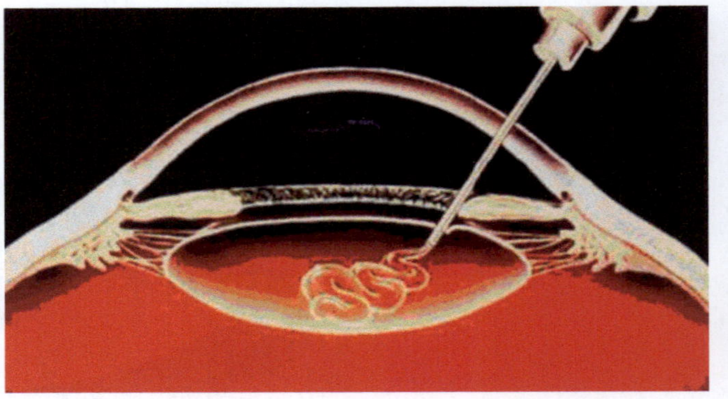

Fig. 8.71 Representation of liquid polymer being injected into the capsular bag using a syringe through a 1.0 mm paracentesis

One of the first pioneers to attempt refilling the capsular bag with Silastic was Kessler in the 1960s. Others continued the work on injectable polymers but ran into various drawbacks, including excessive hardening of the injectable material, hyperopia, capsule opacification, inflammation, and leakage of the polymer out of the capsular bag, prior to curing. Early research with injectable materials involved silicone polymers that were cross-linked into gels. Hydrogels, proteins, and even regrowing lenses with lens epithelial cells have been attempted with little success and it appears as though silicone polymers hold the greatest promise for a functioning injectable polymer with the best chances for restoring accommodation [18].

One of the most intriguing IOL technologies being researched is the Calhoun Vision light-adjustable lens (LAL). The current IOL is not a microincision lens, however, the use of an injectable silicone polymer made out of the same light-adjustable material is being researched. The current design of the LAL is a foldable three-piece IOL with a cross-linked photosensitive silicone polymer matrix, a homogeneously embedded photosensitive macromer, and a photoinitiator. The application of near-ultraviolet light to a portion of the

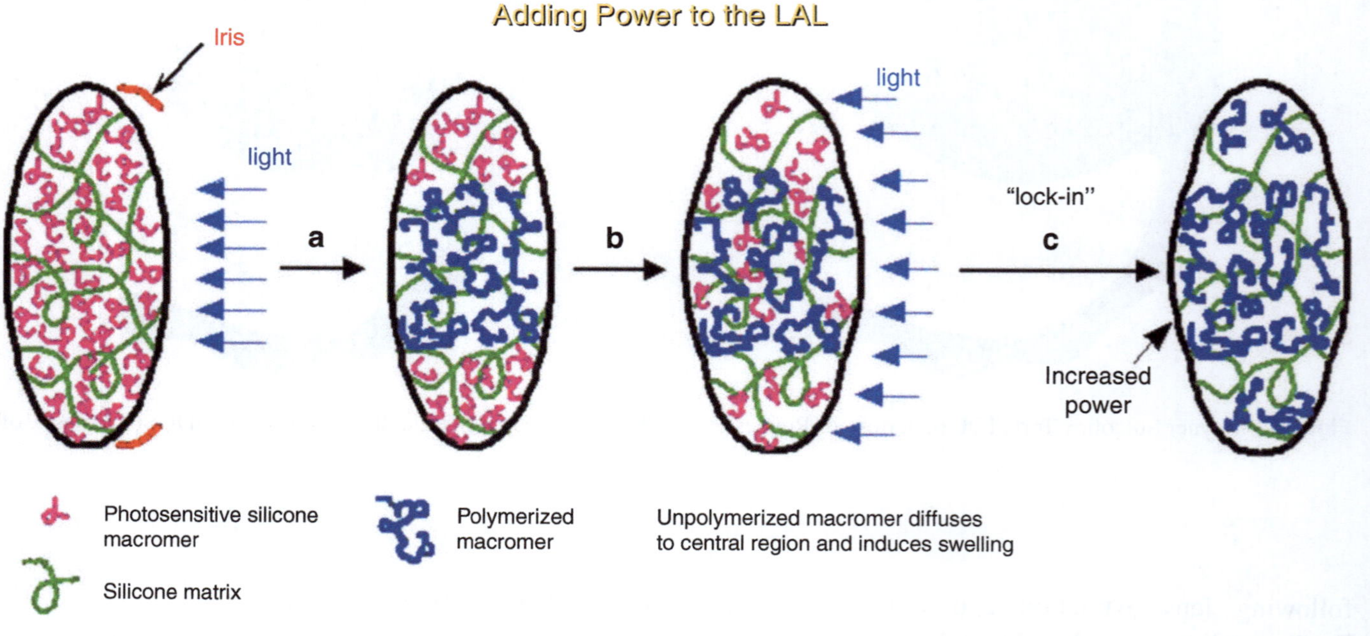

Fig. 8.72 Cross sectional schematic illustration of the mechanism for treating hyperopic correction. (**a**) Selective irradiation of the central portion of the lens polymerizes macromer, creating a chemical gradient between irradiated and nonirradiated regions; (**b**) in order to reestablish equilibrium, macromer from the peripheral lens diffuses into the central irradiated region leading to the swelling of the central zone; (**c**) irradiation of the entire lens polymerizes the remaining macromer and "locks-in" the new lens shape (Courtesy of Calhoun Vision, Inc.)

lens optic results in disassociation of the photoinitiator to form reactive radicals that initiate polymerization of the photosensitive macromers within the irradiated region of the silicone matrix. Polymerization itself does not result in changes in lens power, however, it does create a concentration gradient within the lens, resulting in the migration of nonirradiated macromers into the region, that is now devoid of macromer as a result of polymerization. Equilibration from migration of the macromers into the irradiated area causes swelling within that region of the lens with an associated change in the radius of curvature and power. Once the desired power change is achieved, irradiation of the entire lens to polymerize all remaining macromer "locks-in" the adjustment so that no further power changes can occur [29].

This IOL was designed to offer the possibility of fine-tuning the refractive result following implantation. If following implantation, an eye was hyperopic, treatment to the central portion of the optic would increase the power and resolve the hyperopia (Fig 8.72). Similarly, treatment to the peripheral portion of the optic in an annular pattern would decrease the power of the IOL and resolve residual myopia. Treatment along a toric meridian could treat cylinder and using a patented digital light delivery device, higher order corrections could also be applied [8].

This technology holds the promise of correcting all residual refractive errors including lower and higher order aberrations. As an injectable polymer, it also addresses one of the major issues of past polymer studies, which was hyperopic refractive errors and an inability to accurately determine the amount of polymer to inject in order to achieve emmetropia. With an injectable polymer made out of a light adjustable material, an IOL could be injected through a 1 mm incision and then adjusted postoperatively in order to eliminate or reduce any lower and higher order refractive errors. Although the three-piece version of the LAL has been implanted in human eyes, the injectable polymer version is still in the early stages of research and development.

8.3.5.9 Final Comments

Cataract surgery and crystalline lens based refractive surgery continue to improve in small incremental steps. The transition from a coaxial approach to lens surgery to a biaxial technique through microincisions offers numerous advantages. One of the main limitations for acceptance of this newer technique has been the inability to fully utilize these microincisions for IOL implantation. However, just as the transition from large extracapsular incisions to 3 mm phacoemulsification incisions offered added benefits, despite the need to enlarge the incisions to 6 mm for implantation of nonfoldable PMMA IOLs, the benefits of a biaxial approach through microincisions also outweighs the need for incision enlargement for IOL implantation. IOL technology has always lagged behind surgical technique technology but eventually IOLs are created that can fully realize the newer techniques without incisional adjustments.

IOLs are now being produced that can fit through 2.0 mm and smaller incisions. Outside the US, these lenses are being utilized with increasing frequency and will eventually be available to all the surgeons. With continued research and development, IOLs that can be injected through 1.2–1.4 mm microincisions or smaller will eventually be designed. If injectable polymer research can be fully perfected, we may, one day, be performing lens-based surgery through sub-1.0 mm incisions with adjustable injectable polymers. The future of IOL technology is still unfolding.

Take Home Pearls

- A biaxial technique for cataract surgery has the advantage of approaching the lens nucleus from two different directions. This can help reduce zonular stress in patients who have a compromised zonular apparatus, in addition to facilitating cortex removal
- IOLs that can be injected through sub-2.0 mm incisions are increasing in numbers. Many of these IOLs can be inserted through 1.5 mm incisions using injector cartridge systems and wound-assisted injection techniques
- Multifocal and toric technologies are available on some of these microincision implants which would help increase their utilization and the use of a biaxial microincision technique
- Lens technology will continue to improve in the future allowing for injection of IOLs through smaller and smaller incisions. This will eventually create the impetus for a fully biaxial microincision approach for cataract and lens-based surgery that will eliminate the need for the creation of a third incision or incision enlargement for IOL implantation

References

1. Alfonso JF, Fernandez-Vega L, Senaris A, Montes-Mico R. Prospective study of the Acri.LISA bifocal intraocular lens. J Cataract Refractive Surgery 2007; 33:1930–1935
2. Alio JL, Schimchak P, Montes-Mico R, Galal A. Retinal image quality after microincision intraocular lens implantation. J Cataract Refract Surg 2005; 31:1557–1560
3. Alio JL, Elkady B, Ortiz D, Bernabeu G. Clinical outcomes and intraocular optical quality of a diffractive multifocal intraocular lens with asymmetrical light distribution. J Cataract Refract Surg 2008; 34:942–948
4. Assouline M, Weber K, Welt R, Barrett GD. Akreos Acrylic IOLs: Clinical Evidence Continues to Support Biocompatibility and Design Features. Bausch & Lomb Incorporated internal memo, 2004
5. Becker KA, Martin M, Rabsilber TM, et al Prospective, non-randomised, long term clinical evaluation of a foldable hydrophilic single piece intraocular lens: results of the Centerflex FDA study. Br J Ophthalmolo 2006; 90:971–974
6. Chang DF. Next-generation IOLs. Cataract Refract Surg Today 2005; 71–76
7. Dogru M, Honda R, Omoto M, et al Early visual results with the rollable ThinOptX intraocular lens. J Cataract Refract Surg 2004; 30:558–565
8. Hoffman RS, Fine IH, Packer M. The light-adjustable lens. In: Fine IH, Packer M, Hoffman RS (eds) Refractive Lens Surgery. Springer, Berlin, 2005, pp 162–171
9. Hunkeler JD Update on the Thinoptx IOL. Cataract Refract Surg Today, 2004; 83–85
10. Johansson B, Sundelin S, Wikberg-Matsson A, et al Visual and optical performance of the Akreos Adapt Advanced Optics and Tecnis Z9000 intraocular lenses: Swedish multicenter study. J Cataract Refract Surg 2007; 33:1565–1572
11. Kaya V, Ozturker ZK, Ozturker C, et al ThinOptX vs AcrySof: Comparison of visual and refractive results, contrast sensitivity, and the incidence of posterior capsule opacification. Eur J Ophthalmol 2007; 17:307–314
12. Kellan RE Next-generation IOLs: Lenstecs's Kellan tetraflex IOL. Cataract Refract Surg Today 2005; 71–76
13. Kim HK, Shin JP. Capsular block syndrome after cataract surgery: Clinical analysis and classificiation. J Cataract Refract Surg 2008; 34:357–363
14. Martin RG, Sanders DR. A comparison of higher order aberrations following implantation of four foldable intraocular lens designs. J Refract Surg 2005; 21:716–721
15. Mencucci R, Ponchietti C, Nocentini, et al Scanning electron microscopic analysis of acrylic intraocular lenses for microincision cataract surgery. J Cataract Refract Surg 2006; 32:318–323
16. Murta J. Bimanual microphacoemulsification and the new Akreos MI60 through 1.8 mm incision. In: The 25th Congress of the European Society of Cataract and Refractive Surgery, Stockholm, Sweden, 2007
17. Nishi Y, Rabsilber TM, Limberger IJ, et al Influence of 360-degree enhanced optic edge design of a hydrophilic acrylic intraocular lens on posterior capsule opacification. J Cataract Refract Surg 2007; 33:227–231
18. Norrby S. Injectable polymer. In: Fine IH, Packer M, Hoffman RS (eds) Refractive Lens Surgery. Springer, Berlin, 2005, pp 174–186
19. O'hEineachain R. New microincision IOL provides multifocality and corrects astigmatism. EuroTimes 2008; 13(5):31
20. Ouchi M, Kinoshita S. Aberration-correcting effect of ThinOptX IOL. Eye 2007 (Online publication)
21. Prakash P, Kasaby HE, Aggarwal RK, Humfrey S. Microincision bimanual phacoemulsification and Thinoptx implantation through a 1.70 mm incision. Eye 2007; 21:177–182
22. Radford SW, Carlsson AM, Barrett GD. Comparison of pseudophakic dysphotopsia with Akreos Adapt and SN60-AT intraocular lenses. J Cataract Refract Surg 2007; 33:88–93
23. Reiter J. Rotational stability of two posterior chamber intraocular lens designs: a comparative study. In: The 26th Congress of European Society of Cataract and Refractive Surgeons Annual Meeting; London, 12 September 2006
24. Rodriguez Prats JL, Alio JL, Galal A. MICS and new intraocular lens technologies. In: Alio JL, Rodriguez Prats JL, Galal A (eds) Micro-Incision Cataract Surgery. Highlights of Ophthalmology International, El Dorado, Panama, 2005, pp 67–91
25. Sanders DR, Sanders ML. Visual performance results after Tetraflex accommodating intraocular lens implantation. Ophthalmology 2007; 114:1679–1684
26. Sanders DR, Sanders ML. Near visual acuity for everyday activities with accommodative and monofocal intraocular lenses. J Refract Surg 2007; 23:747–751
27. Sanders DR, Higginbotham RW, Opatowsky IE, Confino J. Hyperopic shift in refraction associated with implantation of the single-piece Collamer intraocular lens. J Cataract Refract Surg 2006; 32:2110–2112
28. Schild G, Amon M, Abela-Formanek C, et al Uveal and capsular biocompatibility of a single-piece, sharp-edged hydrophilic acrylic intraocular lens with collagen (Collamer): 1-year results. J Cataract Refract Surg 2004; 30:1254–1258
29. Schwiegerling JT, Schwartz DM, Sandstedt CA, Jethmalani J. Light-adjustable intraocular lenses. Review of Refractive Surgery. Jobson, Newtown Square, 2002
30. Till JS. Collamer intraocular lens implantation with active uveitis. J Cataract Refract Surg 2003; 29:2439–2443
31. Vejarano LF, Vejarano A, Vejarano M, et al The safest and most effective technique in microincision cataract surgery. Highlights Ophthalmol 2004; 32:13–19
32. Wehner W. Microincision intraocular lens with plate haptic design. Evaluation of rotational stability and centering of a microincision intraocular lens with plate haptic design in 12–19 months of follow-up. Ophthalmologe 2007; 104:393–398
33. Werner L, Mamalis N, Pandey SK, et al Posterior capsule opacification in rabbit eyes implanted with hydrophilic acrylic intraocular lenses with enhanced square edge. J Cataract Refract Surg 2004; 30:2403–2409
34. Werner L, Olson RJ, Mamalis N. New technology IOL optics. Ophthalmol Clin Am 2006; 19:469–483

Outcomes

9.1 Safety: MICS versus Coaxial Phaco

George H. H. Beiko

> **Core Messages**
>
> - Microincisional cataract surgery (MICS) is a recent innovation upon standard coaxial cataract phacoemulsification.
> - MICS meets the safety benchmark of coaxial phacoemulsification, and surpasses it in some aspects.
> - Visual rehabilitation and outcomes with MICS meet or surpass that of coaxial phacoemulsification.

9.1.1 Introduction

The separation of irrigation and aspiration in cataract surgery, termed "biaxial technique," was first described in the early 1970s [1, 2]. In 1985, Shearing advocated the use of the biaxial technique for cataract extraction; however, his technique required the enlargement of the incision to 7 mm in order to insert the intraocular lens [3]. It was not until the advent of the ability to modulate power in phacoemulsification that sleeveless phaco tips could be inserted safely through small incisions, and microincision surgery was born.

Microincision cataract surgery (MICS) was first coined by Professor Alio in 2001 to describe cataract surgery through sub-2.0 mm incisions [4]. The term "MICS" was patented by Alio in 2003 (Alio, personal communication).

The benefits of the biaxial approach in MICS are described in other chapters in this book, but briefly can be listed as the following [5]:

- Better control of rhexis
- Improved surgical efficiency by decreased effective phaco time (EPT)
- Better fluidic control
- Enhanced chamber stability
- Better followability through fluid dynamics by separation of irrigation and aspiration so as to minimize opposition between the two
- Access to entire anterior chamber with either irrigation or aspiration by inserting the instruments through either incision
- Ease of removal of subincisional cortex; lower posterior capsular opacification rates
- Increased ability to handle complications, including the ability to avoid areas of zonular weakness
- Ability to use the irrigating fluid as a tool to manipulate material within the capsular bag or anterior chamber
- Reduction of vitreous prolapse in cases of posterior capsular tear or rupture
- Increased suitability for complicated cases

The purpose of this chapter is to investigate the safety of MICS, by looking at visual outcome, incision damage, corneal changes and complications.

G. H. H. Beiko
Assistant Professor in Ophthalmology, McMaster University, Lecturer in Ophthalmology, University of Toronto, Hamilton, ON, Canada
e-mail: george.beiko@sympatico.ca

J. L. Alió, I. H. Fine (eds.), *Minimizing Incisions and Maximizing Outcomes in Cataract Surgery*,
DOI: 10.1007/978-3-642-02862-5_9, © Springer-Verlag Berlin Heidelberg 2010

9.1.2 Visual Outcomes

The true test of a new technique or instrument in cataract surgery is visual outcome. Whenever a new lens is introduced, the point of comparison is the visual outcome compared to the current standard lens. Similarly, at the very least, MICS should be able to attain vision comparable to standard coaxial phacoemulsification; otherwise, any perceived benefit would be compromised.

Howard Fine and colleagues compared visual outcomes with bimanual phaco with those of standard phaco in a number of phaco systems and found that vision was improved similarly, irrespective of the technique [6] (see Fig. 9.1.1).

In studying the visual rehabilitation following cataract surgery, it has been reported that MICS patients gain vision faster than coaxial patients. Kurz et al. [7] studied 70 patients prospectively, equally divided between MICS and coaxial; their findings are reproduced in Fig 9.1.2 and demonstrate a smaller interquartile range in MICS.

MICS has been reported to have a significantly decreased mean total phaco time and mean EPT [7, 8] (see Fig. 9.1.3). As phaco time is believed to be directly related to corneal damage, less phaco time should translate into less corneal trauma and quicker visual recovery.

In point of fact, it has been reported that MICS brings about more rapid visual rehabilitation due to reduced postoperative inflammation as a result of decreased chamber turbulence [9–11]. Similarly, it has been reported that postoperative inflammation using flare readings, were decreased significantly in MICS eyes compared to coaxial phaco eyes at 1 week [12]. Thus, decreased inflammation should also mean faster visual recovery.

In terms of visual rehabilitation, MICS has certainly been demonstrated to be similar to coaxial phaco, and in some authors' hands, to be superior since visual recovery occurs sooner.

Machine	Coaxial Results	Bimanual Results
Series 20000 Legacy with Neosonix	96%	93%
Millennium with Phaco Burst	100%	95%
Staar Sonic Wave*	74%	100%
Sovereign phaco system with Whitestar Technology	94%	95%

*P<.01

Fig. 9.1.1 Percentage of eyes with UCVA of 20/40 or better, 2–24 h postoperatively, comparison of coaxial and bimanual phaco (from Fine et al. [6])

Post operative BVCA in Biaxial MICS compared With Coaxial Small Incision Clear Cornea Cataract Surgery[15]

	Biaxial MICS	Coaxial SICS	P value
Pre-op	20/40	20/40	0.970
3 hour post op	20/40 (20/400-20/25)	20/63 (20/400-20/15)	/
1 day post op	20/25 (20/50-20/15)	20/30 (20/400-20/15)	0.018
3 days post op	20/25 (20/30-20/15)	20/30 (20/400-20/15)	0.002
7 days post op	20/25 (20/40-20/15)	20/25 (20/200-20/15)	0.605
8 weeks post op	20/20	20/25	0.015

Note. MICS: 35 eyes, final incision size 1.5 - 1.7mm; SICS: 35 eyes, final incision size 2.75mm

Fig. 9.1.2 Visual rehabilitation following cataract surgery; comparison of MICS and coaxial techniques (from Kurz et al. [7])

EPT for Biaxial MICS versus Coaxial Phaco[11]

	MICS	Coaxial phaco	P value
Mean phacoemulsification time (s)	0.38±0.41	0.41±0.44	0.259
Mean total phacoemulsification (%)	5.28±3.91	19.2±10.98	0.001
Mean effective phacoemulsification	2.19±2.77	9.2±12.38	0.001

Fig. 9.1.3 Comparison of effective phaco time [EPT]; MICS vs. coaxial (Alio et al. [8]) ("mean effective phacoemulsification" was defined as the mean EPT in seconds in this study as it "represented the estimated phacoemulsification time if 100% phacoemulsification power in continuous mode had been used" [8])

9.1.3 Incision Damage

Examination of the incision should reveal the extent of trauma or injury at the incision sites. Ideally, the incision should allow access to the eye without compromising the ability of the incision to seal post-op and to minimize the amount of permanent change such as induced astigmatism.

In a scanning electron microscope comparison study of incision damage in cadaver eyes [13] (see Fig. 9.1.4), it has been suggested that incision leakage occurred in all MICS eyes under test conditions when the IOP was raised to 125 mmHg for 30 s and in none of microincisional coaxial eyes under similar conditions. It was also

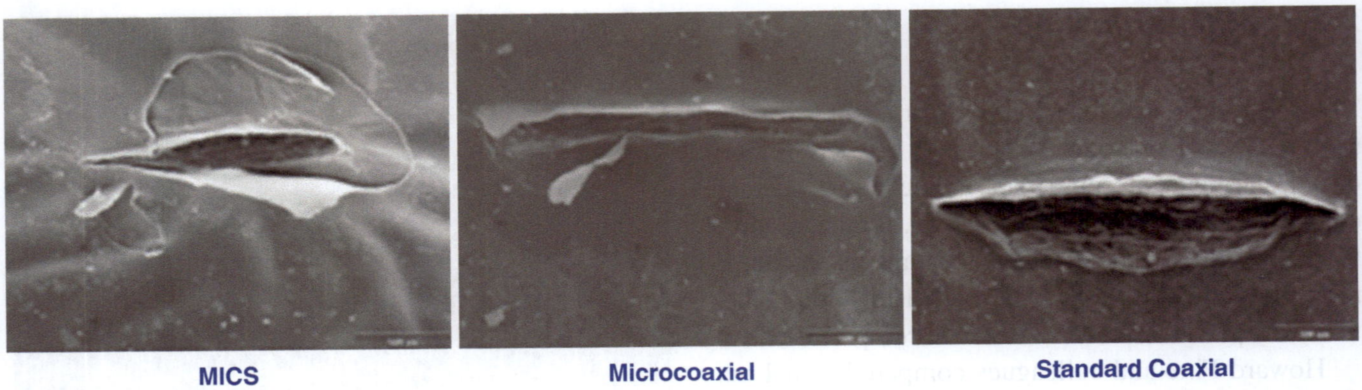

Fig 9.1.4 Scanning EM images of endothelial surface of clear corneal incisions after phacoemulsification in cadaver eyes (from Berdahl et al. [13])

reported that whitening of the incision occurred in 4 or 5 MICS eyes, suggesting that incision burn would occur. However, the criticism of this study has been made that the investigators were inexperienced with MICS and that incision construction was inaccurate (Alio, personal communication).

In a similar cadaver study, the changes in incision architecture were also studied by the authors who compared MICS with microincisional coaxial incisions [14]. It was found that both types of incisions were slightly larger post-op compared to the incision made. However, Descemet's tear extensions were greater at the MICS phaco site than the microincisional coaxial phaco site while tears were similar at the irrigation sites in both. Also, endothelial cell loss [ECL] was similar in both, although there was a greater loss near the phaco site of microincisional coaxial than MICS and no difference at the irrigation site in both. This study would suggest that although minimal differences exist between MICS and microcoaxial incisions, there is likely no significant impact on corneal endothelial function, incision leak or induced astigmatism when the two are compared.

9.1.4 Corneal Incision Burn

Corneal incision burns (see Fig. 9.1.5) can result in significant distortion of the incision, resulting in the necessity of incision closure with sutures and significant induced astigmatism. Incision burns occur as a result of thermal damage to corneal collagen, and this occurs when tissue temperatures exceed 60°C [15, 16]. It is for this reason, that irrigating sleeves on the phaco tip were introduced in traditional coaxial phaco. When considering conversion to sleeveless phaco for MICS, this is of paramount concern as there is a perception that the loss of the irrigating sleeve will allow friction of the phaco tip with the cornea tissue, causing incision temperatures to rise and incision burns to occur.

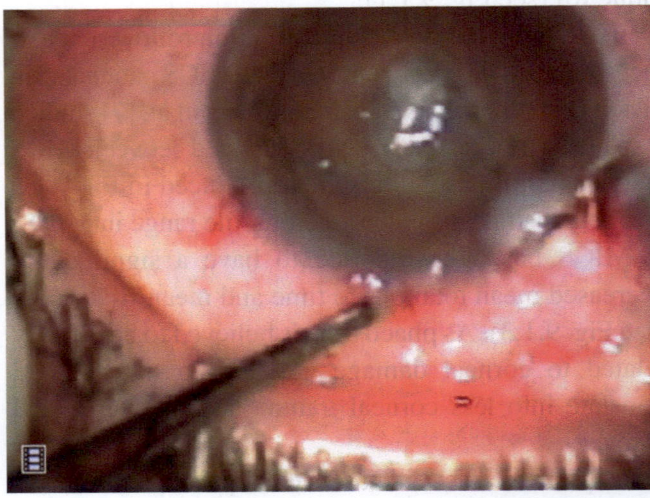

Fig. 9.1.5 Corneal incision burn

In MICS, it is almost a necessity for the phaco tip to make contact with the corneal tissue when micro incisions are employed. Power modulations of phaco energies through variation of burst and pulse modes have allowed the safe use of sleeveless phaco tips in direct contact with corneal tissue without the creation of corneal incision burns. The proof of this is as follows.

Steinert and Schafer [17] used a thermal camera in a laboratory setup to investigate the rise in temperature, comparing continuous ultrasound with Whitestar micropulse technology (AMO, Santa Ana, USA). Their findings were that, continuous ultrasound resulted in a phaco tip temperature of 61°C, while the Whitestar micropulse phaco tip temperature never rose above 35°C. Thus, clinically, continuous ultrasound would induce incision burn while the Whitestar settings would prevent this due to the decrease of at least 20°C in incision temperature, and well below 60°C which would cause incision burn.

In a cadaver eye study, using sleeveless phaco, it was found that the incision temperature never rose above 41.8°C and that the incision remained clear [10].

Clinically, using a thermocouple attachment in cataract patients, it has been shown that a sleeveless phaco tip with Whitestar modulations results in temperature rises in the 24–34°C range; far short of the temperature for incision burn [18].

Similarly, other clinical studies have also determined that the wound temperature with MICS does not rise above 40°C under normal clinical conditions [19, 20]. In a series of 637 patients who underwent MICS, there was no report of corneal incision burn [21].

As corneal incision burn is dependent on the temperature, the impact of ultrasonic phaco handpieces, tip geometries and operating modes is significant. In a laboratory setting, it has been shown that there are differences between the various phaco systems currently available. Using high speed thermal imaging of phaco tips, it was found that the greatest temperature rise was with the Alcon Inifinity system with Torsional handpieces; B & L Stellaris and AMO Signature with Ellips had the least temperature rise, as demonstrated in Fig. 9.1.6 [22].

Thus, not only is there considerable laboratory and clinical evidence to support the use of sleeveless phaco tips in MICS, but also some indication that the AMO Signature Ellips system may be least likely to cause incision burn.

9.1.5 Corneal Changes

a. Clarity

Clarity of the cornea following cataract surgery is an indication of the trauma incurred during surgery. In a study comparing MICS and standard coaxial phaco, no difference was found between the techniques [3], as Fig. 9.1.7 illustrates.

Thus, MICS and standard coaxial phaco, at the very least, induce comparable minimal trauma to the eye.

b. Induced corneal aberrations

As cataract surgery has evolved over the past two decades, so have corneal incisions decreased from greater than 10 mm with ICCE, 8–10 mm with ECCE, 6.0–7.0 mm with phaco and PMMA lenses, and less than 3.5 mm with phaco and foldable IOLs. With each incremental decrease in incision size, there has been a decrease in induced corneal astigmatism. Scleral

Machine	Coaxial Results	Bimanual Results
Series 20000 Legacy with Neosonix (Alcon Laboratories, Inc. Fort Worth, TX)	98%	100%
Millennium with Phaco Brust (Baush & Lomb, Rochester, NY)	100%	100%
Staar Sonic Wave (Staar Surgical Company, Monrovic, CA)	95%	100%
Sovereign Phaco system with Whitestar Technology (Advanced Medical Optics, INC, Santa Ana, CA)	100%	97%

*P<.05 for all comparisons

Fig. 9.1.7 Percentage of eyes with clear corneas, 2–24 h postoperatively (from Fine et al. [6])

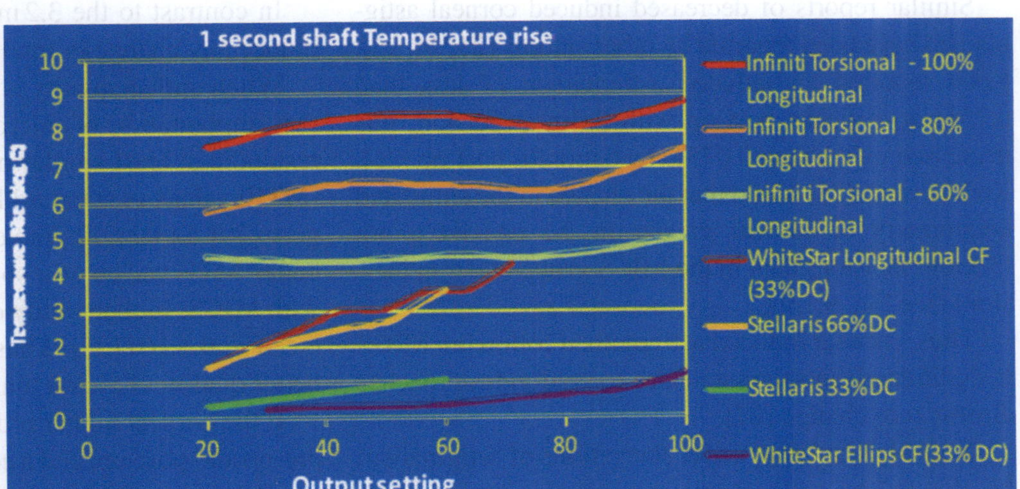

Fig. 9.1.6 Temperature rise in shaft of phaco tip after 1 s (from Schafer [22])

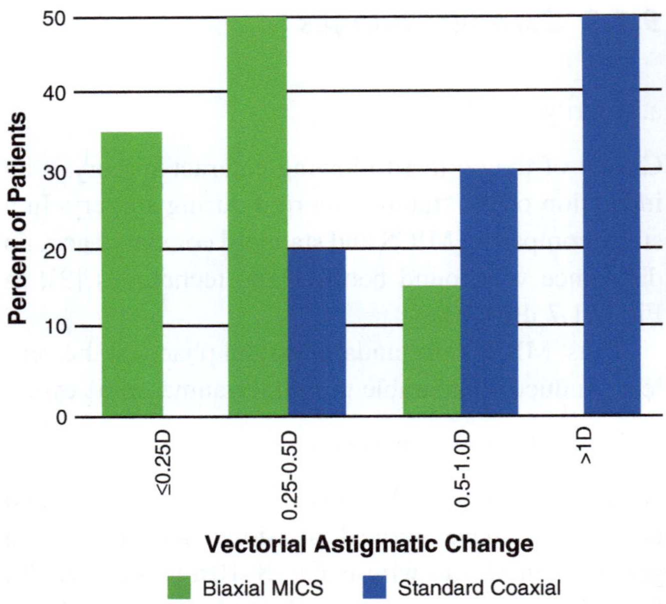

Fig. 9.1.8 Vectoral astigmatic analysis of surgically induced astigmatism in biaxial MICS compared with coaxial cataract surgery (from Alio et al. [8])

incisions have been associated with less induced astigmatism than corneal incisions [23].

In a prospective, randomized study of 100 patients, comparing MICS and standard coaxial phaco, Alio et al. [8] analyzed the surgically induced astigmatism using vectoral analysis. The MICS group had a mean incision size of 1.71 ± 0.21 mm compared to the coaxial group of 3.1 ± 0.25 mm. They reported a mean change of 0.36 ± 0.232 D in the MICS group compared to a significantly greater increase of 1.2 ± 0.74 D in the standard coaxial phaco group. An interesting finding was that more than 50% of the coaxial group had more than 1 D of induced astigmatism while none of the MICS group had this (see Fig. 9.1.8).

Similar reports of decreased induced corneal astigmatism have been reported by other authors [21, 24, 25]. Koch reported an induced astigmatism of less than 0.25 D at 4 weeks post-op with 2.0 mm incision; this decreased to less than 0.075 D by 6 months post-op [26]. Ke Yao et al. [25] found that the change in the simulated keratometry value was greater in the coaxial group (3.2 mm incision) than in the MICS group (1.7 mm incision) (see Fig. 9.1.9).

Thus, corneal induced astigmatism following MICS is significantly less than standard coaxial and approaches almost zero change [27].

Not only can lower order aberrations of astigmatism be affected by cataract surgery, but also higher-order

Comparative results on corneal astigmatism for Microincision Incision Cataract Surgery versus Small Incision Cataract Surgery[10]

	MICS	SICS	P value
Preoperative ΔSim k (D)	0.7 ± 0.34	0.66 ± 0.38	0.669
Postoperative ΔSim k (D)	0.78 ± 0.68	1.29 ± 0.68	0.001

Note. ΔSim k represent the difference in power between the steep and flat meridians. MICS: 30 eyes, 1.7 ± 0.1mm; SICS: 30 eyes, 3.2mm

Fig. 9.1.9 Changes in the simulated keratometry values; comparison of MICS and coaxial cataract surgery (from Ke Yao et al. [25])

Comparative results on corneal astigmatism for Microincision Incision Cataract Surgery versus Small Incision Cataract Surgery[10]

Spatial Frequency (cpd)	MICS	SICS	P value
0.5 MTF	3.13±0.30	2.75±0.63	0.004
0.1 MTF	9.37±3.72	7.24±3.43	0.134

Note. MICS: 30 eyes, 1.7 ± 0.1mm; SICS: 30 eyes, 3.2mm
MTF (modulation transfer function) are the metrics to indicate retinal image quality from an incoming object

Fig. 9.1.10 Comparison of MTF with MICS and coaxial phaco (from Ke Yao et al. [25])

aberrations. A 3.2 mm superior clear corneal incision "induced consistent and significant changes in several corneal Zernicke terms (vertical astigmatism, trefoil and tetrafoil) resulting in a significantly increased overall corneal RMS wavefront error" [28]. However, the 3.2 mm incision did not induce significant changes in spherical aberration or coma terms. The amount and orientation of the aberrations induced depended on the surgical meridian and incision location.

In contrast to the 3.2 mm incision, MICS does not induce any change in total RMS value [27].

When optical quality is evaluated, it has been found that implantation of micro incision IOLs with MICS results in at least similar modulation transfer function (MTF) values as standard IOLs in coaxial cataract surgery [29]. In fact, Ke Yao et al. reported a significantly better MTF values at a spatial frequency of 0.5 MTF with MICS, in their study of MICS vs. coaxial surgery (see Fig 9.1.10) [25]. Thus, MICS provides similar or better quality of vision than coaxial.

If the corneal higher order aberrations are measured pre-op and post-op, and a comparison is made of MICS vs. 3.2 mm coaxial cataract surgery, an increase in

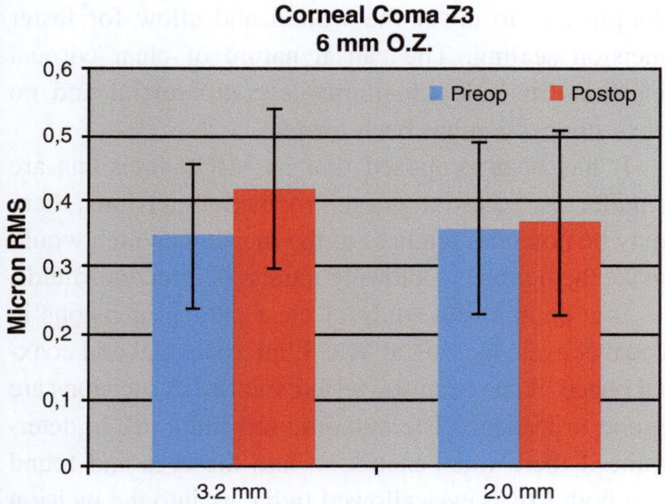

Fig. 9.1.11 Comparison of total corneal coma; MICS vs. coaxial cataract surgery (from Bellucci and Morselli [30])

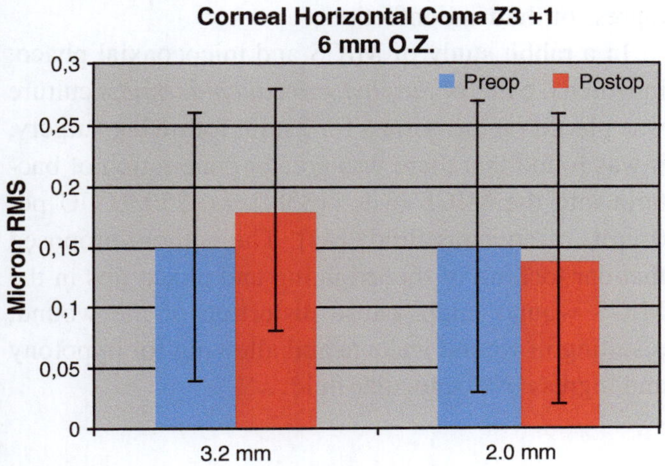

Fig. 9.1.12 Comparison of horizontal corneal coma; MICS vs. coaxial cataract surgery (from Bellucci and Morselli [30]

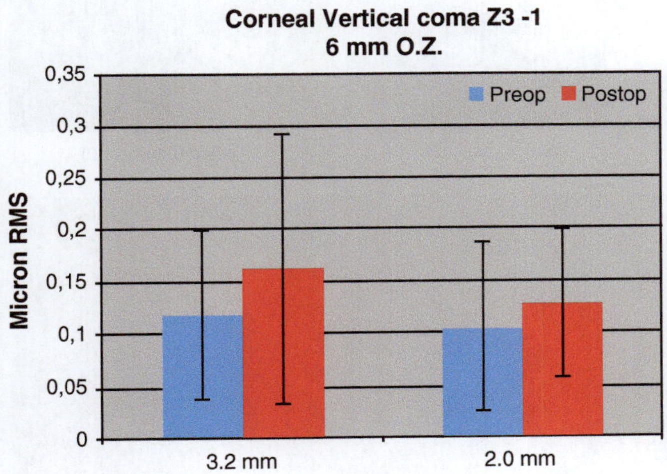

Fig. 9.1.13 Comparison of vertical corneal coma; MICS vs. coaxial cataract surgery (from Bellucci and Morselli [30])

induced coma has been reported in the latter group [30]. This increased coma would result in degradation of the quality of vision (See Figs 9.1.11–9.1.13).

All studies support the conclusion that smaller incision with MICS result in less induced corneal aberrations, whether of lower order (astigmatism) or higher order (coma). Lower aberrations result in better vision.

c. Endothelial cell loss

In this chapter, it has been shown that MICS is associated with decreased phaco time, decreased inflammation and less ocular trauma; in theory, this should result in lower ECL.

Before looking in depth into this aspect of MICS, it is important to understand the measurement of ECL. Measurements of endothelial cell counts are highly reproducible by a model of specular microscope but the results are *not interchangeable* between different models of specular microscopes [31]; thus in comparing ECL, it is essential that the same type of specular microscope is used. Cell loss of 10% is within confidence interval of measurement error with a specular microscope [32]. In multicentre studies, precision of only 8–10% can be expected; improved precision of 2% can be anticipated only if one centre and experienced staff are employed for the interpretation of the data [33].

In standard coaxial phaco, ECL of 6.4–8.8% at 90 days post cataract surgery has been reported. To be determined that MICS is safe, it must be shown that at least comparable ECL occurs. A number of studies prospectively comparing coaxial phaco to MICS have confirmed this [7, 8, 34–39]) (see Fig. 9.1.14 for summary of the data)

	No. Eyes	Endothelial Cell Loss (%) 3 mos	
		Coaxial	MICS
Crema 2007	60	4.7±6.1	4.5±5.1
Cavallini 2007	100	10.1±11.7	11.9±15.2
Mencucci 2006	80	6.5	6.3
Kurz 2006	70	4.7±6.1	4.5±5.1
Kahraman 2006	66	3.1±6.5	6.2±5.1
Alio 2005	100	11.7±16.0	7.4±9.2

Fig. 9.1.14 Comparison of ECL between MICS and coaxial phaco

Fig. 9.1.15 ECL related to cataract density in MICS (from Tsuneoka et al. [21])

Cataract Grade	Endo Cell Loss %
1	4.6 +/- 12.8
2	6.9 +/- 16.5
3	10.8 +/- 12.4
4-5	15.6 +/- 13.7

The amount of ECL is proportional to the density of cataract being emulsified, and this is also true for MICS, as has been reported by Tsuneoka et al. [21] (see Fig. 9.1.15).

Corneal damage as assessed by ECL is similar whether coaxial phaco or MICS is employed to remove cataracts.

9.1.6 Infection

Endophthalmitis in cataract surgery has been proposed to be associated with many factors including incision construction and location; preoperative, intraoperative, and postoperative use of antibiotics; surgical trauma; and patient health. Some authors have claimed that clear corneal incisions compared to scleral incisions are at increased risk of endophthalmitis due to decreased integrity of the incision and delayed incision healing [40–43]. Scleral and near limbal incisions are thought to have decreased infection due to the ability of the conjunctiva to cover the wound and allow for faster incision sealing. The causal nature of clear corneal incisions in endophthalmitis is controversial and no clear connection has been made.

It has been proposed that as MICS incisions are smaller than coaxial and microcoaxial incisions, there may be potential features of the incisions which would make them prone to allowing ingress of infectious fluids.

In a comparison study of clear corneal incisions in cadaver eyes, looking at MICS, microcoaxial and coaxial phaco, it has been suggested that MICS incisions are prone to leakage. The authors used India ink to determine if there was penetration into the eyes and found that both MICS eyes allowed India ink into the incision compared to one standard coaxial and none of the microcoaxial eyes [13] (see Fig. 9.1.16a, b). They hypothesized that MICS incisions would be prone to allowing ingress of fluid and infection.

In a rabbit study of MICS and micocoaxial phaco, in which 0.5 mL of *Staphylococcal epidermidis* culture was placed on the cornea for 2 min, following surgery, it was found that there was greater penetration of bacteria into the MICS eyes (1358.1 vs. 250.9 CFU per 0.1 mL of aqueous fluid) [44]. The authors proposed that oar locking of the irrigating and phaco tips in the MICS wound might cause distortion of the wound, resulting in wound leakage and allowing for hypotony and ingress of extraocular fluid.

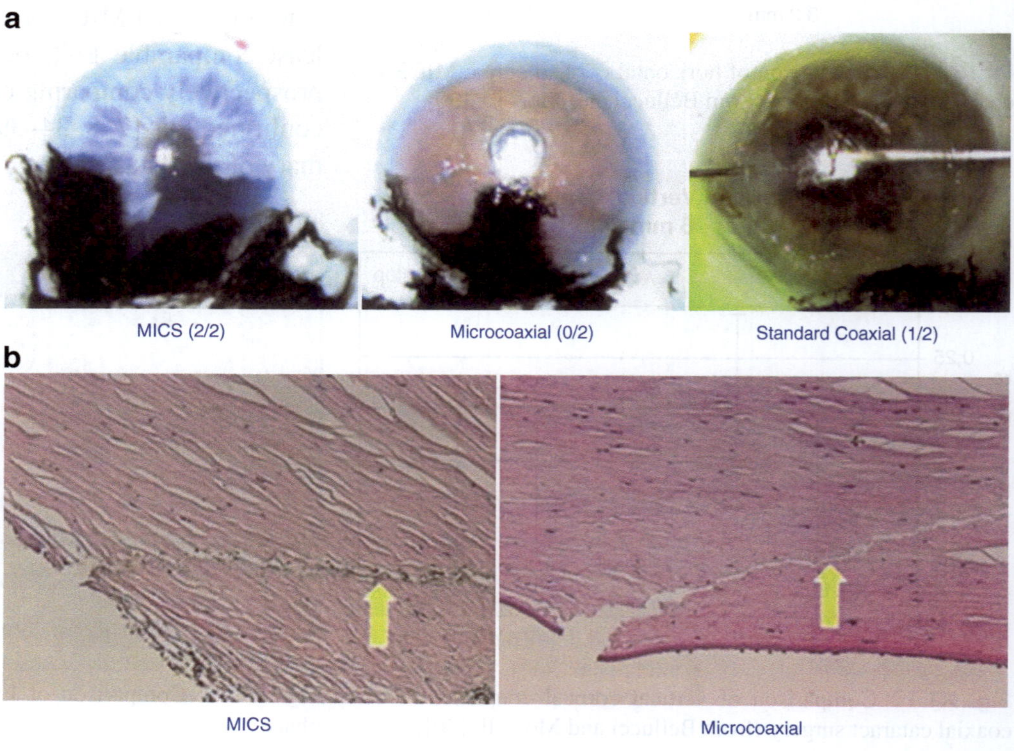

Fig. 9.1.16 (**a**) India ink penetration: clear corneal incisions after phacoemulsification in cadaver eyes (from Berdahl et al. [13]) (**b**) India ink penetration: clear corneal incisions after phacoemulsification in cadaver eyes (from Berdahl et al. [13])

In these studies, incisions with parallel sides were constructed which facilitates greater damage from oar locking than if trapezoidal incisions had been made. With trapezoidal incisions, the oar locking only occurs at the internal lip of the incision and thus trauma is minimized (Fine, personal communication).

Despite these laboratory studies suggesting greater risk of endophthalmitis with MICS, there have been no reports of any epidemics of infection with MICS. In fact, a literature search found a mention of one case report, in which endophthalmitis developed on day 4 post-op. Clinically, there was fibrin present at the incision at 7 o'clock incision, which was in contact with the inferior fornix. This infection grew alpha-hemolytic *Streptococcus* [45].

It is this author's opinion that the lack of clinical correlation to the laboratory findings is that the smaller MICS incisions, if properly hydrated at the end of the case, are closed tighter than larger coaxial incisions. This would explain the lack of increased endophthalmitis.

9.1.7 Summary

This author has been performing exclusively MICS for the past 6 years. All the reasons stated at the beginning of the chapter were the appeal in transitioning to MICS. There have been no safety concerns related to MICS. The control during surgery and the visual outcomes are the main reasons for my continued implementation of this technique.

Take Home Pearls

- Visual outcomes and rehabilitation with MICS superior than coaxial surgery
- Incision damage minimal and comparable to coaxial phaco
- No increase in corneal incision burn despite use of sleeveless phaco tip
- Superior vision with MICS than coaxial due to less induced astigmatism and higher-order aberrations
- Endothelial cell loss comparable to coaxial phaco
- No increase in infection with MICS compared to coaxial phaco

References

1. Shock JP (1972) Removal of cataracts with ultrasonic fragmentation and continuous irrigation. Trans Pac Coast Otoophthalmol Soc Annu Meet 53:139–144
2. Girard LJ (1978) Ultrasonic fragmentation for cataract extraction and cataract complications. Adv Ophthalmol 37: 127–135
3. Shearing SP, Relyca RL, Louiza A et al (1985) Routine phacoemulsification through a one millimeter non-sutured incision. Cataract 2:6–11
4. Alio JL (2004) What does MICS require? In: Alio JL, Rodriquez-Prats JL, Gala A (eds) MICS micro-incision cataract surgery. Highlights of Ophthalmlogy International, Miami
5. Brooks L, Cipres MC 1.8 mm Biaxial White Paper. A review of the literature; B & L internal document
6. Fine IH, Hoffman RS, Packer M (2004) Why we prefer bimanual microincisional phacoemulsification. Cataract Ref Surg Today 9:43–46
7. Kurz S, Krummenauer F Gabriel P, Pfeiffer N, Dick HB (2006) Biaxial microincision versus coaxial small incision clear corneal cataract surgery. Ophthalmology 113(10):1818–1826
8. Alio J, Rodriguez-Prats JL, Galal A, Ramzy M (2005) Outcomes of microincision cataract surgery versus coaxial phacoemulsification. Ophthalmology 112(11):1997–2003
9. Fine IH, Hoffman RS, Packer M (2004) Optimizing refractive lens exchange with bimanual microincision phacoemulsification. J Cataract Refract Surg. 30:550–554
10. Braga-Mele R, Lui E (2003) Feasibility of sleeveless bimanual phacoemulsification with the millenium microsurgical system. J Cataract Refract Surg 29:2199–2203
11. Agarwal A, Agarwal A Agarwal S et al (2001) Phaconit: phacoemulsification through a 0.9 mm corneal incision. J Cataract Refract Surg. 27(10):1548–1552
12. Krootila K, Matilla J (2006) Effect of fluidics on postoperative outcomes in bimanual phaco using the Whitestar micropulse technology. In: ESCRS Annual Meeting, London
13. Berdahl JP et al (2007) Corneal wound architecture and integrity after phacoemulsification. Evaluation of coaxial, micorincisional coaxial and microincisional bimanual techniques. J Cataract Refract Surg 33(3):510–515
14. Weikert M, Koch D (2006) Corneal wound architecture in bimanual and coaxial microincisional cataract surgery. In: ESCRS Annual Meeting, London
15. Sporl E, Genth U, Schmalfuss K, Seiler T (1997) Thermomechanical behaviour of the cornea. Ger J Ophthalmol 6:322–327
16. Goldblatt WS, Finger PT, Perry HD et al (1989) Hyperthermic treatment of rabbit corneas. Invest Ophthalmol Vis Sci 30: 1778–1783
17. Steinert RF, Schafer ME (2003) Thermal energy and turbulence with WhiteStar and conventional phacoemulsification. In: Annual Meeting of ASCRS
18. Donnenfeld E et al (2003) Efficacy and wound-temperature gradient of WhiteStar phacoemulsification through a 1.2 m incision. J Cataract Refract Surg 29(6):1097–1100
19. Soscia W et al (2002) Microphacoemulsification with WhiteStar: a wound-temperature study. J Cataract Refract Surg 28: 1044–1046
20. Fabian E (2002) Bimanual phaco and temperature using new phaco-software (WhiteStar). In: ESCRS, Nice, France

21. Tsuneoka H, Shiba T, Takahashi Y (2002) Ultrasonic phacoemulsification using 1.4 mm incision: clinical results. J Cataract Refract Surg 28:81–86
22. Schafer ME (2008) Thermal characterization of phacoemulsification tips. In: ESCRS Annual Meeting, Berlin
23. Pesudovs K, Dietze H, Stewart OG et al (2005) Effect of cataract surgery incision location and intraocular lens type on ocular aberrations. J Cataract Refract Surg 31:725–734
24. Tsuneoka H, Shiba T, Takahashi Y (2001) Feasibility of ultrasound cataract surgery with a 1.4 mm incision. J Cataract Refract Surg 27:934–940
25. Ke Yao, Xiajing Tang, Panpan Ye (2006) Corneal astigmatism, higher order aberrations, and optical quality after cataract surgery: microincision versus small incision. J Refract Surg 22:S1079–S1082
26. Koch D (2003) Cataract surgery through a 2.0 mm incision: results of bimanual phaco-chop technique and acrylic IOL implantation. In: ASCRS Meeting, San Francisco
27. Elkady B, Ortiz D, Montalbán R (2008) Corneal aberrations after microincision cataract surgery. J Cataract Refract Surg 34(1):40–45
28. Marcos S et al (2007) Change in corneal aberrations after cataract surgery with two types of aspherical intraocular lenses. JCRS 33(2):217–226
29. Alió JL, Schimchak P, Montés-Micó R, Galal A (2005) Retinal image quality after microincision intraocular lens implantation. J Cataract Refract Surg 31(8):1557–1560
30. Bellucci R, Morselli S (2008) Aberration control in cataract surgery with the Akreos MI60 microincision IOL. In: ASCRS Presentation, Chicago
31. Landesz M, Siertsema JV, Van Rij G (1995) Comparative study of three semiautomated specular microscopes. J Cataract Refract Surg 21(4):409–416
32. Probst LE, Hakim OJ, Nichols BD (1994) Phacoemulsification with aspirated or retained Viscoat. J Cataract Refract Surg 20(2):145–149
33. Edelhauser HF, Sanders DR, Azar R, Lamielle H; ICL in Treatment of Myopia Study Group (2004) Corneal endothelial assessment after ICL implantation. J Cataract Refract Surg 30(3):576–583
34. Crema AS et al (2007) Comparative study of coaxial phacoemulsificaiton and microincisonal cataract surgery. J Cataract Refract Surg 33:1014–1018
35. Mencucci R et al (2006) Corneal endothelial damage after cataract surgery: MICS vs standard technique. J Cataract Refract Surg 32:1351–1354
36. Mathys K et al (2007) Determining factors for corneal endothelial cell loss by using bimanual microincisional phacoemulsification and power modulation. Cornea 26(9): 1049–1055
37. Cavallini GM, Campi L, Masini C, Pelloni S, Pupino A (2007) Bimanual microphacoemulsification versus coaxial miniphacoemulsification: prospective study. J Cataract Refract Surg 33(3):387–392
38. Kahraman G, Franz C, Prinz A, Abela-Formanek C (2007) Intraindividual comparison of surgical trauma after bimanual microincision and conventional small-incision coaxial phacoemulsification. J Cataract Refract Surg 33(4):618–622
39. Beiko GHH (2005) Endothelial cell loss with micro-incisional cataract surgery. In: Presented ASCRS Annual Meeting, Washington
40. McDonnell PJ et al (2003) Dynamic morphology of clear corneal cataract incisions. Ophthal 110:2342–2348
41. Taban M et al (2004) Dynamic morphology of sutureless cataract wounds-effect of incision angle and location. Surv Ophthal 49(Suppl 2):S62–S72
42. Taban M et al (2005) Ingress of India ink into the anterior chamber through sutureless clear corneal cataract wounds. Arch Ophthal 123:643–648
43. John ME, Noblitt R (2001) Endophthalmitis: scleral tunnel versus clear corneal incision. In: Buzzard K, Friedlander MH Febbraro JL (eds) The blue line incision and refractive phacoemulisification. Slack, NJ
44. Gajjar D et al (2007) Ingress of bacterial inoculum into the anterior chamber after bimanual and microcoaxial phacoemulsification in rabbits. J Cataract Refract Surg 33(12): 2129–2134
45. Chee SP (2005) Bascal K-endophthalmitis after microincisional cataract surgery. J Cataract Refract Surg 31: 1834–1835

9.2 Control of Corneal Astigmatism and Aberrations

Jorge L. Alió and Bassam El Kady

Core Messages

- Sub-2 mm incision of MICS manipulates the tissues gently with minimal surgical trauma and distortion of the surrounding tissues.
- Among the major advantages of MICS is the reduction of surgical trauma resulting in a reduction of surgically induced astigmatism (SIA).
- MICS is superior to standard coaxial phaco with regard to corneal aberration induction.
- Excellent incision quality in MICS demonstrated immediate postoperative visual recovery, equivalent to that of microcoaxial 2.2 incision.
- Corneal OCT is an excellent way to study the postoperative evolution of cataract surgery incision.

9.2.1 Introduction: Impacts of MICS Incision on the Outcomes of Cataract Surgery

An important aspect in the modern techniques of cataract surgery is to provide the patient with an immediate postoperative visual recovery with good quality of vision. To a great extent the optical quality of the cornea is an essential factor for such rapid and excellent visual and refractive outcomes, as it plays an important role in the recovery of visual function after cataract surgery. This idea is one of the basic concepts and principals in MICS through providing a recent and innovative surgical technique of cataract extraction with a refractive touch, thanks to a reduction of incision size down to the minimum possible size [1].

J. L. Alió (✉)
Department of Ophthalmology, Miguel Hernández University, Alicante, Spain
e-mail: jlalio@vissum.com

The reason behind this is that the micro sub-2 mm incision of MICS manipulates the tissues gently with minimal surgical trauma and distortion of the surrounding tissues, leading to reduction of surgically induced astigmatism (SIA) and aberrations, with subsequent improvement of the corneal optical quality ending in excellent visual outcome and high patient satisfaction [1–5].

So, it is important to study the corneal incision as in MICS there is a bare phaco tip hitting the cornea with potential damage for the corneal lamellae. This might have an influence in the immediate outcome of cataract surgery, especially in filtration [1, 2].

9.2.2 Objective Evaluation of Corneal Incision

Visual function after cataract surgery is determined by a combination of corneal and internal aberrations generated by the IOL and those induced by the surgery. These corneal refractive changes are attributed to the location and size of the corneal incision applying the fact that the smaller the incision, the lower the aberrations, the better the optical quality [1, 6–8].

Degraded optical quality of the cornea after incisional cataract surgery would limit the performance of the pseudophakic eye. So, it is important not to increase or to induce astigmatism and/or corneal aberrations after cataract surgery [9]. MICS could achieve reduction of the astigmatism and higher-order corneal aberrations [8].The need to study this with new technology evolved as clinical evaluation is insufficient to evaluate minimal changes in the incision configuration. Corneal topography, aberrometry and corneal optical coherence tomography (OCT) were the main tools for adequate and objective analysis of corneal incision and the best means to know whether this corneal trauma is affecting the quality of corneal optics [10, 11].

9.2.3 Control of Corneal Aberration and Astigmatism with MICS

We have described the improved control on corneal SIA with MICS when compared to conventional 3 mm phacoemulsification. A great advantage of MICS is the reduction of SIA and that the microincision does not produce an increase in astigmatism [1].The shorter the incision, the less the corneal astigmatism, as it was estimated that the magnitude of the SIA studied by vector analysis is around 0.44 and 0.88 D, rising as the size of the incision increases [12, 13].

Also, sutureless small-incision 3.5-mm surgery does not systematically degrade the optical quality of the anterior corneal surface. However, it introduces changes in some aberrations, especially in nonrotationally symmetric terms such as astigmatism, coma, and trefoil [14]; therefore, one has to expect better results and lesser changes with sub-2 mm incision (MICS).This is further supported by the finding that the corneal incision of sub-2 mm had no impact on corneal curvature [8, 15, 16].

All of these factors were the driving forces for us to carry out an objective study to investigate if MICS sub 2 mm incision effectively decreases the induction or changes in corneal higher-order aberrations (HOA) during cataract surgery, evaluating its effect on the corneal optical quality [10]. We studied 25 eyes of 25 patients with nuclear or corticonuclear cataracts graded from +2 to +4 (lens opacities classification system III) [17]. All of them underwent MICS through a 1.6–1.8 mm clear corneal incision, placed on the axis of the positive corneal meridian, and using low ultrasound power. An Acri.Smart 48S lens (Acri.Tec, Germany) was implanted in all eyes. Seidel aberration root mean square (RMS) values were obtained for a 6-mm pupil using the CSO topographer (CSO, Firenze, Italy) preoperatively, 1 and 3 months after surgery [10].

9.2.4 Role of Corneal Aberrometry in Evaluating MICS Incision

Owing to its role in providing the most important metrics for evaluating the visual function, we used the corneal aberrometry to evaluate corneal optical quality, as about 80% of all aberrations of the human eye occur in the corneal surface [18]. The topography system we used (CSO topographer) analyzes up to 6,144 corneal points within the corneal zone between 0.33 and 10 mm with respect to corneal vertex, with more expressive analysis and assessment for up to the seventh order aberration by using the Zernike polynomials. In addition, it avoids superimposing of the light spots associated to different parts of the wavefront produced by highly aberrated eye. Finally, with some kind of global aberrometry, it is assumed that the slope of the wavefront in each analyzed portion is locally flat; this could induce significant errors in the calculated final results [18].

Corneal aberrations were derived from the data of the anterior surface of the cornea obtained from this topography system, the software of this topography system, the EyeTop2005 (CSO), makes the conversion of the corneal elevation profile into corneal wavefront data using the Zernike polynomials with an expansion up to the seventh order. The RMS of the wave aberration (Seidel aberrations) was studied at 6-mm pupil diameter for: total, coma (Z3 ± 1), spherical (Z40), reported with its sign, astigmatism (Z2 ± 2) and HOA. Measurements were performed preoperatively, as well as 1 and 3 months postoperatively [10].

9.2.5 Role of OCT in Evaluating MICS Incision

The OCT system Visante proved its usefulness as a very helpful tool in assessing corneal incision quality for different types of cataract surgery. It allows dynamic evaluation of incision behaviour and its effect on the corneal tissue as a sensitive indicator of corneal function and incision quality. Additionally, it provides a new non-contact device which is able to accurately evaluate incision quality and to detect even mild signs undetectable by slit-lamp [11]

OCT, being a non-contact method, is able to study and evaluate all the parameters of the incision and so any degree of incision deformability is attributable to ocular dynamics without external forces being applied to the wound. This confirms the role of OCT as an accurate quantitative tool assessing the incision effect and quality [11].

9.2.6 Our Experience in Corneal Aberrations and Astigmatism After MICS

The comparison between corneal topography and aberrometry maps preoperative vs. 1 and 3 months after

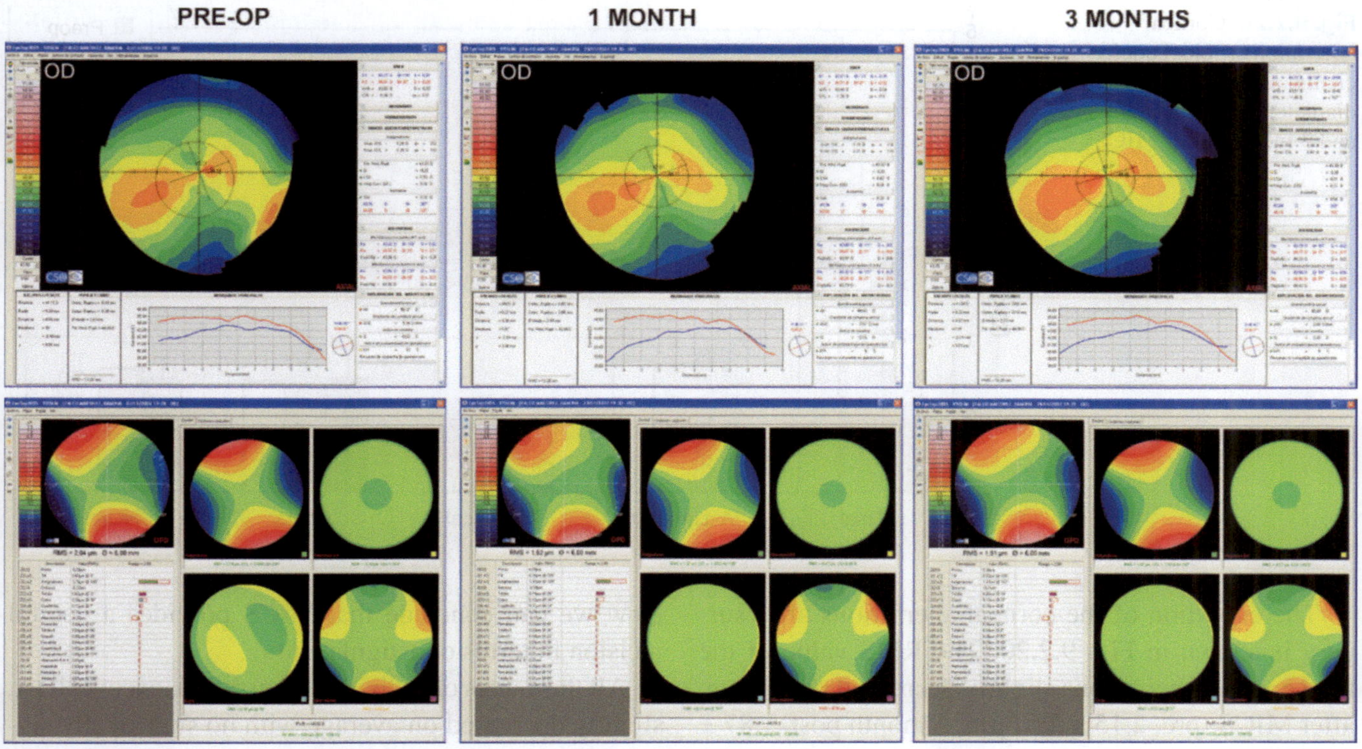

Fig 9.2.17 *Top*: Corneal topography map (axial map) preoperative (*left*) vs. 1 month (*center*) and 3 months (*right*) after MICS surgery for one of the 25 eyes of the study. *Bottom*: Corneal aberrometry map (*Seidel panel*) preoperative (*left*) vs. 1 month (*center*) and 3 months (*right*) after MICS surgery for one of the 25 eyes of the study

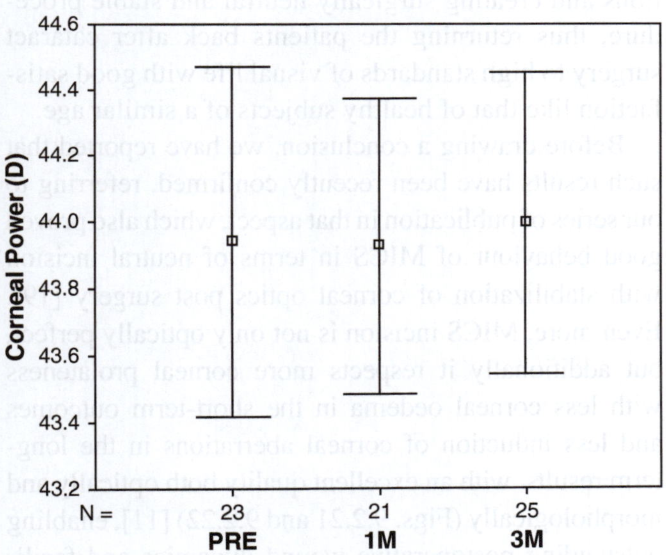

Fig. 9.2.18 Corneal power in diopters (D). Preoperative vs. 1, 3 months after surgery

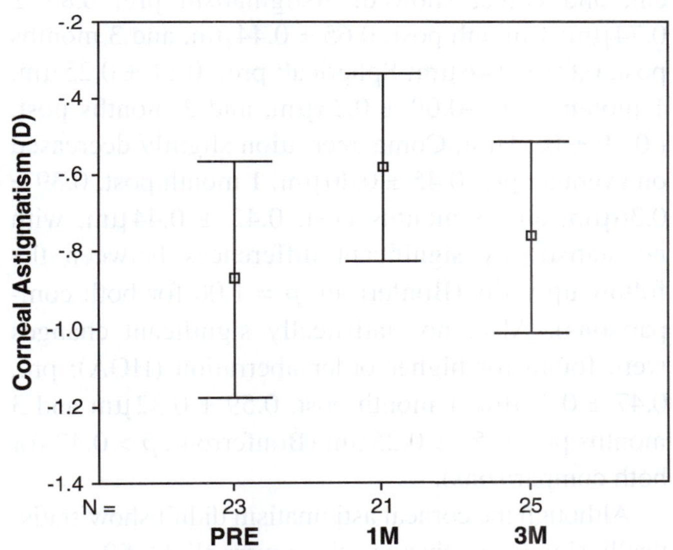

Fig. 9.2.19 Corneal astigmatism in diopters (D). Preoperative vs. 1, 3 months after surgery

MICS surgery is shown in Fig. 9.2.17, in order to illustrate the slight change induced by the surgery. The corneal power slightly changed after surgery (Fig. 9.2.18): preoperative, 44.08 ± 1.21 D; 1 month, 43.97 ± 1.05 D, and 3 months, 44.17 ± 1.18 D. There were no statistical differences between the different follow-up visits (Bonferroni, $p > 0.05$), even when comparing the corneal power at 1 and 3 months after surgery ($p = 1.00$). Also, the corneal astigmatism (Fig. 9.2.19) did not show statistically significant changes (pre: −0.80 ± 0.76 D; 1 month post: −0.61 ± 0.57; 3 months post −0.63 ± 0.62) (Bonferroni, $p > 0.05$ for all comparisons). The mean change in corneal astigmatism preoperatively to 3 months was −0.19 ± 0.40 D.

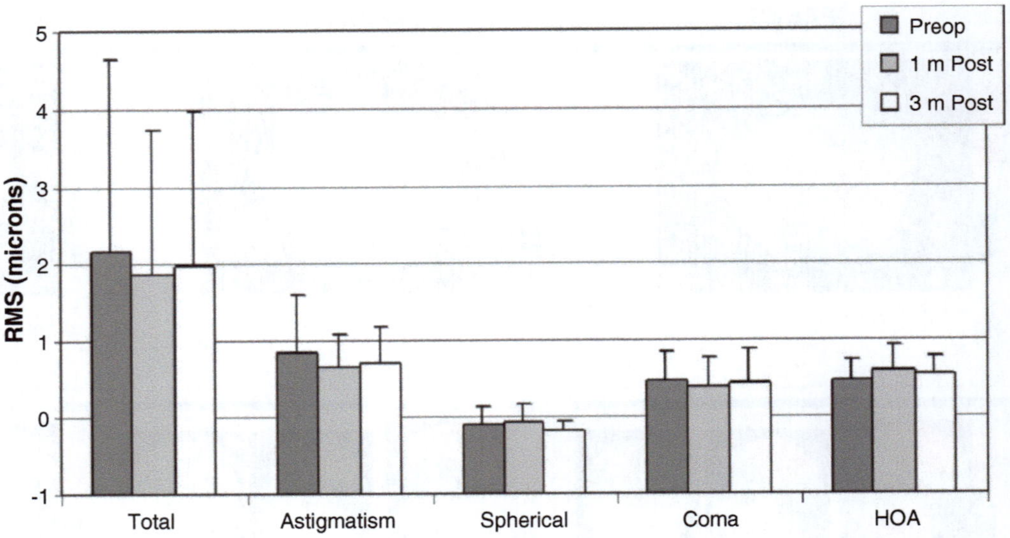

Fig. 9.2.20 Corneal aberrations (Seidel coefficients) at 6-mm pupil diameter before, and 1 and 3 months after MICS

The evolution of the corneal aberrations after surgery is shown in Fig. 9.2.20. The RMS value of the total corneal aberrations slightly decreased on average after MICS (pre, 2.15 ± 2.51 µm; 1 month post, 1.87 ± 1.87 µm; 3 months post, 1.96 ± 2.01 µm), but the difference were no statistically significant (Bonferroni, $p = 1.00$ for both comparisons). The analysis of some individual Zernike terms, such as astigmatism, spherical, and coma, showed: Astigmatism pre, 0.85 ± 0.74 µm; 1 month post, 0.65 ± 0.44 µm, and 3 months post, 0.69 ± 0.46 µm; Spherical: pre,–0.11 ± 0.25 µm, 1 month post, –0.09 ± 0.25 µm, and 3 months post, –0.19 ± 0.13 µm. Coma aberration slightly decreased on average: pre, 0.45 ± 0.40 µm, 1 month post, 0.39 ± 0.36 µm, and 3 months post, 0.42 ± 0.44 µm, with no statistically significant differences between the follow-up visits (Bonferroni, $p = 1.00$ for both comparisons). Also, no statistically significant changes were found for higher order aberration (HOA): pre, 0.47 ± 0.26 µm, 1 month post, 0.59 ± 0.32 µm and 3 months post 0.54 ± 0.25 µm (Bonferroni, $p > 0.47$ for both comparisons).

Although the corneal astigmatism didn't show statistically significant changes, there were slight differences between preoperative, 1 and 3 month postoperative values (Bonferroni, $p > 0.05$ for all comparisons). The mean change in corneal astigmatism preoperatively to 3 months was –0.19 ± 0.40 D, with little difference between 1 and 3 month measures, indicating that MICS provides completely stable incision for up to 3 months postoperatively. This results supports the previously published studies [1, 8, 9, 13], augmenting the advantage of MICS over traditional small incision cataract surgery, which induces low levels of astigmatism [9]. Now we can conclude that MICS provides a neutral incision in terms of astigmatism.

All the values of individual aberration, except HOA, slightly decreased on average with no statistically significant differences between the follow-up visits. The whole measures were stable with no changes for up to 3 months, indicating the successful golden role of MICS in avoiding induction of higher order aberrations and creating surgically neutral and stable procedure, thus returning the patients back after cataract surgery to high standards of visual life with good satisfaction like that of healthy subjects of a similar age.

Before drawing a conclusion, we have reported that such results have been recently confirmed, referring to our series of publication in that aspect, which also proved good behaviour of MICS in terms of neutral incision with stabilization of corneal optics post surgery [19]. Even more, MICS incision is not only optically perfect, but additionally it respects more corneal prolateness with less corneal oedema in the short-term outcomes and less induction of corneal aberrations in the long-term results, with an excellent quality both optically and morphologically (Figs. 9.2.21 and 9.2.22) [11], enabling outstanding postoperative wound dynamics and facilitating faster visual recovery and early postoperative patient ambulation [11].

9.2.7 Conclusion

Finally, we can conclude that MICS sub 2 mm incision surgery is effective in stabilizing the cornea after surgery, effectively decreasing the induction of corneal HOA. It does not degrade the corneal optical quality

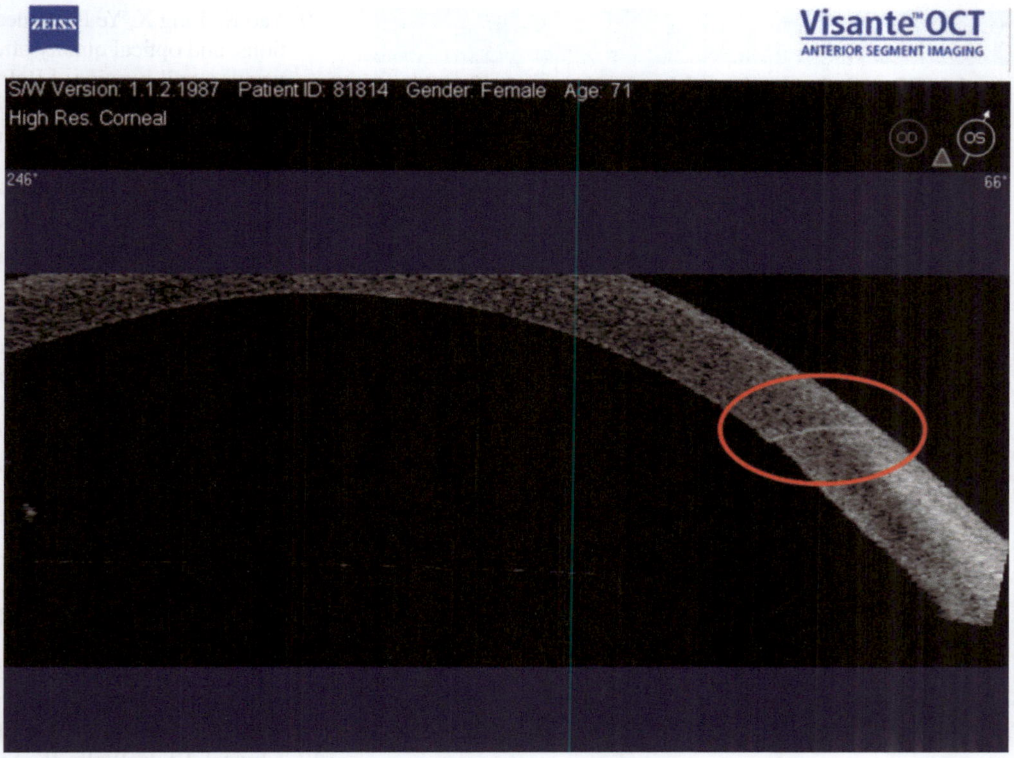

Fig. 9.2.21 OCT image of an MICS incision showing the characteristic appearance of the incision with accurate configuration

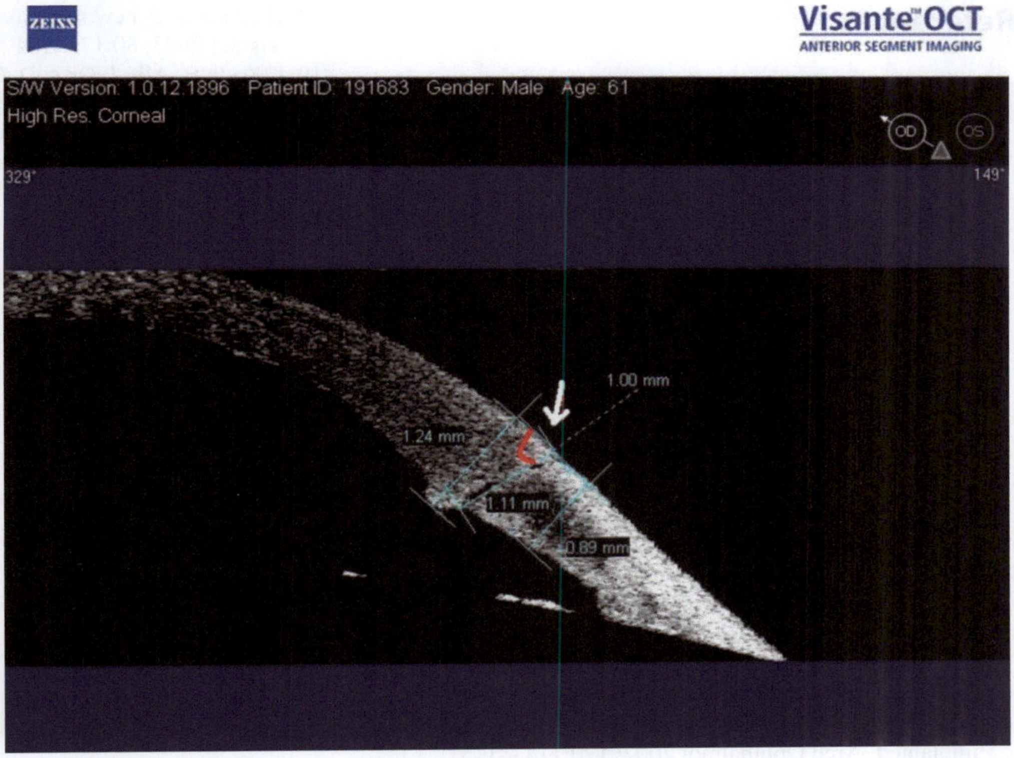

Fig. 9.2.22 OCT image of an MICS incision showing our model for measuring angle of the incision (*white arrows*)

nor induces modification of the corneal astigmatism, even in the axis. This demonstrates that a maximum reduction to sub-2 mm in incision size improves the control of the optical performance of the human eye. Stable corneal optics with MICS frames this technique as a refractive procedure through controlling and even decreasing astigmatism and HOA, so minimized incision maximized the outcomes.

Take Home Pearls

- MICS sub-2 mm incision surgery is effective in stabilizing the corneal optics after surgery.
- MICS surgery technique compared to standard coaxial phacoemulsification diminishes surgically induced astigmatism.
- With MICS, we can achieve a reduction of astigmatism and higher-order corneal aberrations.
- OCT is a very useful tool in assessing corneal incision quality in MICS.
- Corneal OCT provides a standardized model and protocol to objectively evaluate incision quality in MICS.
- Corneal OCT concluded that MICS incision has an excellent morphological and optical behaviour in short- and long-term outcomes.

References

1. Alió J, Rodríguez-Prats JL, Galal A, Ramzy M. Outcomes of microincision cataract surgery versus coaxial phacoemulsification. Ophthalmology 2005; 112:1997–2003
2. Alió JL, Klonowski P, Rodríguez-Prats JL, El Kady B. MICS (microincision cataract surgery). In: Garg A, Fine IH, Alió JL, et al (eds) Mastering the techniques of advanced phaco surgery. Jaypee Brothers, New Delhi, 2008, pp 121–136
3. Alió JL, Klonowski P, Rodríguez-Prats JL, El Kady B. MICS (microincision cataract surgery). In: Garg A, Fine IH, Alió JL, Chang DF, Weinstock RJ, Mehta KR, Bovet JJ, Tsuneoka H, Malyugin B, Pinelli R, Pajic B, Mehta CK. Mastering the techniques of advanced phaco surgery. Jaypee Brothers, New Delhi, 2008, pp 121–136
4. Alio J, Rodriguez-Prats JL, Galal A. Advances in microincision cataract surgery intraocular lenses. Curr Opin Ophthalmol 2006; 17:80–93
5. Naeser K, Knudsen EB, Hansen MK. Bivariate polar value analysis of surgically induced astigmatism. J Refract Surg 2002; 18:72–78
6. Guirao A, Redondo M, Geraghty E, Piers P, Norrby S, Artal P. Corneal optical aberrations and retinal image quality in patients in whom monofocal intraocular lenses were implanted. Arch Ophthalmol 2002; 120:1143–1151
7. Holladay JT. Optical quality and refractive surgery. Int Ophthalmol Clin 2003; 43:119–136
8. Jiang Y, Le Q, Yang J, Lu Y. Changes in corneal astigmatism and high order aberrations after clear corneal tunnel phacoemulsification guided by corneal topography. J Refract Surg 2006; 22:S1083–S1088
9. Yao K, Tang X, Ye P. Corneal astigmatism, high order aberrations, and optical quality after cataract surgery: microincision versus small-incision. J Refract Surg 2006; 22:S1079–S1082
10. El Kady B, Alió J, Ortiz D, Montalbán R. Corneal aberrations after microincision cataract surgery. J Cataract Refract Surg 2008; 34:40–45
11. Elkady B, Piñero D, Alió JL. Corneal incision quality: microincision cataract surgery versus microcoaxial phacoemulsification. J Cataract Refract Surg 2009; 35(3): 466–474
12. Simsek S, Yasar T, Demirok A, Cinal A, Yilmaz OF. Effect of superior and temporal clear corneal incisions on astigmatism after sutureless phacoemulsification. J Cataract Refract Surg 1998; 24:515–518
13. Masket S, Tennen DG. Astigmatic stabilization of 3.0 mm temporal clear corneal cataract incisions. J Cataract Refract Surg 1996; 22:1451–1455
14. Guirao A, Tejedor J, Artal P. Corneal aberrations before and after small-incision cataract surgery. Inves Ophthalmol Vis Sci 2004; 45:4312–4319
15. Olson RJ, Crandall AS. Prospective randomized comparison of phacoemulsification cataract surgery with a 3.2-mm vs. a 5.5-mm sutureless incision. Am J Ophthalmol 1998; 125:612–620
16. Oshika T, Tsuboi S. Astigmatic and refractive stabilization after cataract surgery. Ophthalmic Surg 1995; 26:309–315
17. Chylack LT Jr, Wolfe JK, Singer DM, et al The lens opacities classification system III. The longitudinal study of Cataract Study Group. Arch Ophthalmol 1993; 111:831–836
18. Hamam H. A new measure for optical performance. Optom Vis Sci 2003; 80:175–184
19. E Kady B, Alió J, Ortiz D. Corneal optical quality following microincision cataract surgery (MICS) vs. microcoaxial phacoemulsification (microphaco). 2008; (In process)

9.3 Corneal Endothelium and Other Safety Issues

H. Burkhard Dick[1]

Core Messages

- Many surgeons are still apprehensive to convert their surgical technique for fear of increased complications, including endothelial cell loss, intraocular pressure, and endophthalmitis. The density of the nucleus affects endothelial cell loss because of the number of small, hard fragments in the anterior chamber.
- When MICS is performed correctly, risk of these complications is minimized.
- It is important to learn to avoid complications during MICS, such as endothelial cell loss and elevated intraocular pressure, as well as manage these complications when they arise.
- Endothelial cell loss was only weakly associated with the average of phaco power used in foot position three.
- Using power modulation as well as pulse/hyperpulse and burst/hyperburst should not only reduce the loss of endothelial cells but also provide quicker visual recovery for the patient.
- The longer standard coaxial as well as microcoaxial phacoemulsification lasts and the more power that is used, the greater is the endothelial cell loss.
- The correlation between endothelial cell loss and total phacoemulsification energy and length of the procedure is weak.
- Additional risk factors for an increase in endothelial cell loss include operating on harder cataracts, size of the cataractous nucleus, infusion volume, and total phaco energy.
- Accepting the challenge to convert comes with many rewards, including less wound-related complications and quicker visual recovery.

[1]The author has no financial interest in any materials or products mentioned in the article.

H. B. Dick
Center for Vision Science, Ruhr University Eye Hospital, In der Schornau 23-25, 44892 Bochum, Germany
e-mail: burkhard.dick@kk-bochum.de

The evolution of cataract surgery in the past few years has been bountiful. In addition to innovative technologies, new and enhanced surgical techniques and smaller incision sizes have increased the development of cataract surgery. Patients are enjoying improved results and faster visual recovery. However, the threat of intra- and postoperative complications, including endothelial cell loss, is enough for some surgeons to shy away from tackling a small-incision technique.

Most complications are avoidable, and the advantages of minimizing cataract surgery incisions to sub-2 mm outweigh the potential complications associated with it. Although a learning curve can be expected for those surgeons who have not previously used small-incision cataract surgery, it is relatively short and may easily be overcome by paying close attention to details and quickly learning to manage complications or difficulties that arise.

When discussing incision lengths, I like to use the following terms to distinguish the size of the incision:

- *Long-incision cataract surgery*. This term coincides with extra- or intracapsular cataract extraction via a 10-mm incision.
- *Small-incision cataract surgery*. This term is meant for phacoemulsification with a PMMA IOL with a 6-mm incision.
- *Mini-incision cataract surgery*. When a foldable IOL is inserted through a 3-mm incision, I refer to it as mini-incision cataract surgery.
- *Microincision cataract surgery*. Any procedure employing a 1.5-mm or smaller incision is referred to as microincision cataract surgery (MICS).

For the purpose of this article, we will be discussing mini-incision and microincision surgery. Although the size of the incision is likely to vary depending on the surgeon's preference, such as his choice of instrumentation, and skill level, any decrease in incision size may come with the benefits of: decreased postoperative intraocular inflammation, less wound-related complications and surgically induced astigmatism, and shorter surgical and rehabilitation time [1]. Additionally, biaxial and coaxial MICS allows the surgeon to vary the power during the surgery, thus decreasing the necessary amount of ultrasound energy, creating a stable anterior chamber, and promoting clearer corneas and faster visual rehabilitation [2].

Reducing the incision size during cataract surgery has recently become more common worldwide; however, the techniques of MICS are still evolving. Many surgeons debate the safest and easiest options for MICS or mini-incision cataract surgery. While some surgeons use unsleeved phaco tips through two 1.5-mm incisions and enlarging the incision size to 2.8 mm for IOL insertion (i.e., biaxial MICS), others use sleeved phaco tips through larger, 2-mm incisions (i.e., coaxial phacoemulsification). The controversy regarding which of these two methods is better will continue, just as some surgeons will continue to argue that reducing the incision size is altogether unnecessary.

The advantages of mini-incision cataract surgery and MICS compared with standard phacoemulsification are well documented [1, 3, 4]; however, many surgeons are still apprehensive to convert their surgical technique for fear of increased complications, including endothelial cell loss [3, 5], intraocular pressure [6], and endophthalmitis [7]. The density of the nucleus affects endothelial cell loss because of the number of small, hard fragments in the anterior chamber [2]; however, when MICS is performed correctly, risk of these complications is minimized. Mencucci et al. [3] performed biaxial MICS with a stop-and-chop phacoemulsification technique and compared endothelial cell loss with that during standard cataract surgery. The investigators found that endothelial cell loss and endothelial morphology was not significantly different between the two groups (difference between the standard group and the MICS group: baseline, 25 cells/mm^2; 1 month, 19 cells/mm^2; 3 months, 19 cells/mm^2).

Any time a surgeon changes the surgical technique, there is the risk of increased complications. This is no different when upgrading from standard phacoemulsification to biaxial or coaxial MICS technique; however, learning to (1) avoid complications and (2) manage them if and when they occur will help the surgeon to overcome the learning curve quickly. Bausch & Lomb developed its so-called MICS Platform to address the issue of the learning curve and make the MICS conversion easier and minimize complications.

First, it helps to understand how MICS works. In biaxial MICS, irrigation and aspiration are separate, allowing the surgeon to create and use smaller incisions during phacoemulsification. Using a sub-1.5-mm incision, biaxial MICS employs a sleeveless phaco tip and a separate irrigating chopper (Fig. 9.3.23). In most instances, one incision is enlarged to at least 1.8 mm to allowing insertion of a foldable IOL (Fig. 9.3.24). However, the use of smaller incisions during the phacoemulsification period means decreasing the outflow and vacuum and increasing the inflow, thus creating a stable anterior chamber. Biaxial MICS also gives the surgeon the ability to control power modulation with

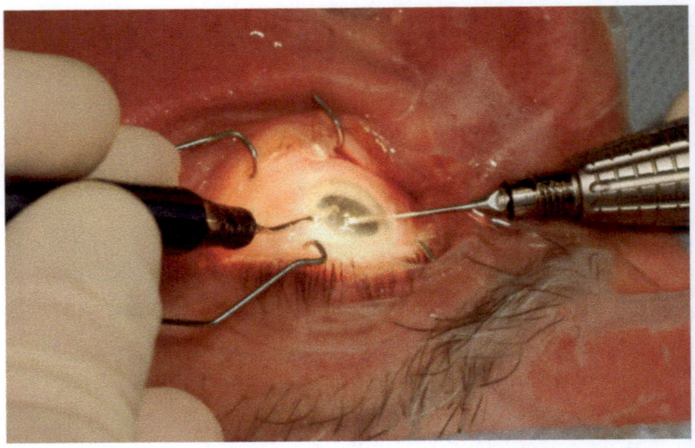

Fig. 9.3.23 Biaxial phacoemulsification: ergonomic balanced light-weight handpiece employing six crystals for increased stroke length with tighter curve for more precise and accurate delivery of US power on demand (optimised 28.5 Hz cavitation)

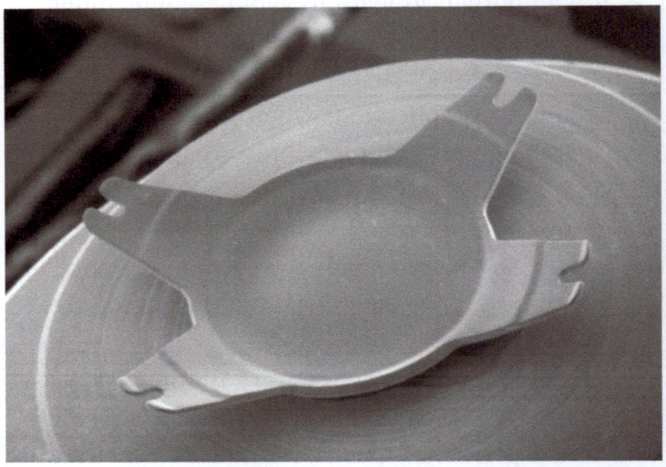

Fig. 9.3.24 Hydrophilic acrylic foldable one-piece aspheric IOL (MI60, B and L) with 360° sharp edge design for MICS (overview, scanning electron microscopy)

fixed or linear control of on- and off-times. One advantage of controlling the power modulation is a reduced risk of wound burn [8]. Coaxial small-incision surgery is also a newer phacoemulsification technique that is gaining popularity. In coaxial, a sleeved phaco tip is used, and the incision size is often enlarged from 1.5 to 1.8-mm (as in my technique). For example, the Stellaris system (Bausch & Lomb) features a 1.8-mm sleeved phaco tip for coaxial MICS in addition to its biaxial MICS phaco tip. The 6-crystal handpiece operates at a lower frequency of 28.5 kHz, using a longer stroke length to optimize cutting and minimize the thermal loading. When using the vacuum mode, additional chamber stability is provided by the StableChamber Tubing System (B&L). The tubing system incorporates restricted tubing and a mesh to capture lens material over 5 mm to protect against post occlusion surge.

Second, the surgeon should know what types of complications are the most common during MICS or mini-incision cataract surgery. During biaxial MICS, complications include occlusion of the phaco tip, which most likely will occur if a high viscosity ophthalmic viscosurgical device (OVD) is used; folds in the cornea, occurring when a small incision is manipulated and the wound stretches; and anterior chamber instability, sometimes caused by a larger incision that creates turbulence in the anterior chamber. Additionally, the surgeon must keep in mind that the use of a small irrigating chopper will limit the amount of irrigation in the eye, which has the tendency to result in an unstable anterior chamber if high vacuum is used [9].

Although some surgeons worry that endothelial cell loss is associated with the use of MICS, Mathys et al. [2] concluded that endothelial cell loss was only weakly associated with the average of phaco power used in foot position three. Although phaco time was slightly longer when using biaxial MICS, endothelial cell loss and proportional loss of cells were not affected by the duration of the procedure. Perhaps the use of OVDs or disorders such as subclinical endothelial or systemic diseases also affect endothelial cell loss. Using power modulation as well as pulse/hyperpulse and burst/hyperburst, such as the custom control software II (CCS II, B and L), should not only reduce the loss of endothelial cells but also provide quicker visual recovery for the patient [10].

Several clinical trials found a greater endothelial cell loss with greater phacoemulsification time and power used [11–14]. Other studies found either no correlation or only a weak association between endothelial cell loss and total phacoemulsification energy and length of procedure [15, 16]. Additional risk factors for an increase in endothelial cell loss include operating on harder cataracts, the size of the cataractous nucleus, infusion volume, and total phaco energy [15, 17]. Mathys et al. [2] found that the nuclear color strongly correlated to the loss of endothelial cells. Furthermore, power modulation during biaxial MICS showed less correlation to central endothelial cell loss, phacoemulsification time, and energy used during surgery.

Recently, my colleagues and I studied the use of biaxial MICS vs. coaxial small-incision in complicated cataract cases, such as exfoliation syndrome, uveitis, anterior or posterior synchia, phacodonesis, or previous intraocular surgery [18]. Of the 94 eyes (94 patients), half underwent biaxial MICS via a 1.5-mm incision and the other half underwent coaxial small-incision phaco with pulsed ultrasound energy and variable duty cycles. The endothelial cell loss in the biaxial vs. coaxial group was similar, 8 weeks after surgery (343 cells/mm^2 vs. 222 cells/mm^2). Complications included early postoperative corneal edema surrounding the tunnel, a fibrin reaction in the anterior chamber, and pupillary distortion; however, the most common complications after cataract surgery often include transient corneal edema, wound leakage, elevated intraocular pressure, and fibrin reaction [19–25], and, therefore, our rate of complications was not uncommon. Additionally, we did not have any incidence of elevated intraocular pressure or wound leakage. When biaxial MICS was used, effective phaco time was statistically significantly lower than when coaxial small-incision phaco was performed (median, 1.34 vs. 5.4 s, respectively). Mean phaco power was also lower (3.3 vs. 12.9%, respectively).

Many other surgeons have had success with biaxial MICS as well. Dada et al. [26] performed biaxial MICS in a vitrectomized eye. In combination with silicone oil removal, Data and colleagues concluded that biaxial MICS was a safe alternative to standard phacoemulsification in vitrectomized eyes. Kurz et al. [27] found that patients who underwent biaxial MICS experienced an earlier visual rehabilitation time than standard phacoemulsification. Furthermore, according to Alió et al. [28] biaxial MICS in healthy eyes had a significantly lower mean phaoemulsification time, mean total phacoemulsification percent, mean efficient phacoemulsification time, and surgically induced astigmatism compared with conventional phacoemulsification.

As of recently, many studies have compared the advantages and disadvantages of MICS with standard cataract surgery techniques. Other studies have compared biaxial and coaxial MICS [29–31]; both techniques have been found to be safe and effective alternatives for phacoemulsification. Only time will tell which method will be the most advantageous. In the time being, I suggest researching several MICS techniques and crafting your own.

I am well versed in both coaxial and biaxial MICS. For biaxial MICS, I create a 1.2-mm corneal incision at the 11-o'clock position, parallel to the limbus (in the plane of the cornea). I choose to use the front of a trapezoidal microkeratome. I begin the second incision at the 2-o'clock position (Fig. 9.3.25) and insert the irrigating sleeve through this 1-mm incision. After filling the anterior chamber with Healon (Advanced Medical

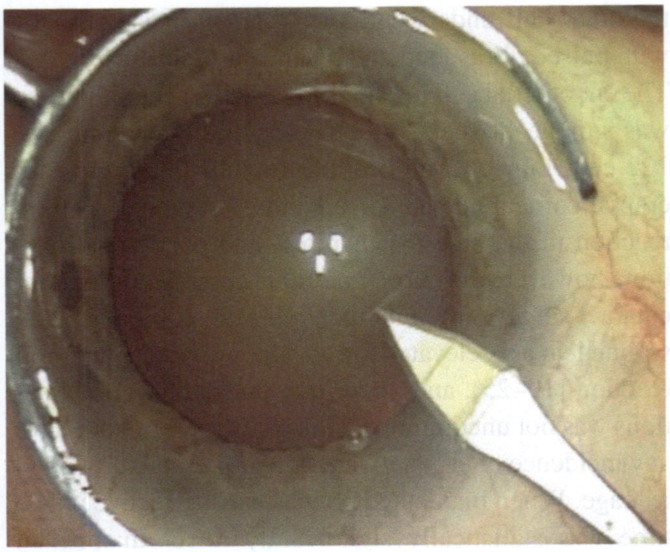

Fig. 9.3.25 Trapezoidal two-step self-sealing tunnel incision to maintain chamber stability allows more lateral maneuverability and limit collateral fluid loss

Optics, Inc., Santa Ana, California), I create a continuous curvilinear capsulorhexis with a 24-gauge bent needle. Alternatively, you can use a capsulorhexis forceps designed for MICS. Then, I perform hydrodissection and hydrodelineation. The phaco tip is inserted through the 11-o'clock incision, using my right hand, and the 19-gauge irrigating chopper is inserted through the 2-o'clock incision with my left hand. The irrigating handpiece should go in first to expand the anterior chamber before the phaco tip. If you put the phaco tip in first, you may shallow the anterior chamber and not be able to get the irrigating handpiece in.

Rose [32] suggested that biaxial MICS is the appropriate option for patients with small pupils, endothelial disease, pseudoexfoliation, traumatic cataracts, zonular loss, and high myopia. Rose's study also suggested, much like Dada et al. [26], that biaxial MICS is safe to use in vitrectomized eyes.

My technique is different for coaxial small-incision surgery. I use a metal microkeratome and make a 2.75-mm clear corneal tunnel incision, in two steps, at the 12-o'clock or temporal position. The second step is to use another steel microkeratome to create two 1-mm incisions at the 10- and 2-o'clock positions. I again fill the anterior chamber with Healon and perform the capsulorhexis, hydrodissection, and hydrodelineation just as I would for biaxial MICS. I use a 19-gauge, sleeved phaco tip, and two irrigating choppers are inserted into the sideport incisions. A manual chopper is inserted at the 2-o'clock position.

Choosing to learn a MICS technique is, of course, a surgeon's individual choice; however, accepting the challenge to convert comes with many rewards, including less wound-related complications and quicker visual recovery. Additionally, handling difficult situations and complicated cases is sometimes easier with MICS than with standard phacoemulsification. For these reasons, I suggest investing time and energy in developing a MICS technique. Once the short learning curve is overcome, MICS enhances the surgeon's ability to offer patients the best surgical option, care, and outcomes possible.

Take Home Pearls

- Using power modulation as well as pulse/hyperpulse and burst/hyperburst should not only reduce the loss of endothelial cells but also provide quicker visual recovery for the patient.
- Additional risk factors for an increase in endothelial cell loss include operating on harder cataracts, the size of the cataractous nucleus, infusion volume, and total phaco energy.
- Biaxial MICS has a shorter effective phaco time and a lower mean phaco power as compared with coaxial small-incision cataract surgery. Biaxial MICS also provides patients with an earlier visual rehabilitation time.
- MICS is a safe alternative to standard cataract surgery, with a low rate of complications.

References

1. Alió JA, Rodríguez-Prats JL, Galal A, et al Outcomes of microincision cataract surgery versus coaxial phacoemulsification. Ophthalmology. 2005;112(11):1997–2003
2. Mathys KC, Cohen KL, Armstrong BD. Determining factors for corneal endothelial cell loss by using bimanual microincision phacoemulsification and power modulation. Cornea. 2007;26(9):1049–1055
3. Mencucci R, Ponchietti C, Virgili G, Giansanti F, Menchini U. Corneal endothelial damage after cataract surgery: microincision versus standard technique. J Cataract Refract Surg. 2006;32:1351–1354
4. Fine IH, Packer M, Hoffman RS. Power modulations in new phacoemulsification technology: improved outcomes. J Cataract Refract Surg. 2004;30:1014–1019
5. Wilczynski M, Drobniewski I, Snyder A, Omulecki W. Evaluation of early endothelial cell loss in bimanual microincision

cataract surgery (MICS) in comparison with standard phacoemulsification. Eur J Ophthalmol. 2006;16:798–803
6. Khng C, Packer M, Fine IH, Hoffman RS, Moreira FB. Intraocular pressure during phacoemulsification. J Cataract Refract Surg. 2006;32:301–308
7. Chee SP, Bacsal K. Endophthalmitis after microincision cataract surgery. J Cataract Refract Surg. 2005;31:1834–1835
8. Braga-Mele R, Liu E. Feasibility of sleeveless bimanual phacoemulsification with the Milennium microsurgical system. J Cataract Refract Surg. 2003;29:2199–2203
9. Fine IH, Hoffman RS, Packer M. Power modulations in new phacoemulsification technology: improved outcomes. J Cataract Refract Surg. 2004;30:1014–1019
10. Devgan U. Phaco fluidics and phaco ultrasound power modulations. Ophthalmol Clin North Am. 2006;19:457–468
11. Dick HB, Kohnen T, Jacobi FK, et al Long-term endothelial cell loss following phacoemulsification through a temporal clear corneal incision. J Cataract Refract Surg. 1996;22:63–71
12. Beltrame G, Salvetat ML, Driussi G, et al Effect of incision size and site on corneal endothelial changes in cataract surgery. J Cataract Refract Surg. 2002;28:118–125
13. Hayashi K, Nakao F, Hayashi F. Corneal endothelial cell loss following phacoemulsification using the small-port phaco. Ophthalmic Surg. 1994;25:510–513
14. Walkow T, Anders N, Klebe S. Endothelial cell loss after phacoemulsification: relation to preoperative and intraoperative parameters. J Cataract Refract Surg. 2000;26:727–732
15. Lundberg B, Jonsson M, Behndig A. Postoperative corneal swelling correlates strongly to corneal endothelial loss after phacoemulsification cataract surgery. Am J Ophthalmol. 2005;139:1035–1041
16. Zetterstrom C, Laurell C. Comparison of endothelial cell loss and phacoemulsification energy during endocapsular phacoemulsification surgery. J Cataract Refract Surg. 1995; 21:55–58
17. Hayashi K, Hayasky H, Nakao F, et al Risk factors for corneal endothelial injury during phacoemulsification. J Cataract Refract Surg. 1996;22:1079–1084
18. Kurz S, Jrummenauer F, Morgenstern J, Dick B. Biaxial microincision versus coaxial small incision in complicated cataract surgery. [submitted for publication, under review]
19. Desai P. The national cataract surgery survey, II: clinical outcomes. Eye. 1993;7:489–494
20. Norregaard JC, Bernth-Petersen P, Bellan L. Intraoperative clinical practice and risk of early complications after cataract extraction in the United States, Canada, Denmark, and Spain. Ophthalmology. 1999;106:42–48
21. Nishi O. Vitreous loss in posterior chamber lens implantation. J Cataract Refract Surg. 1987;13:424–427
22. Willerscheidt AB, Healey ML, Ireland M. Cataract surgery outcomes: importance of comorbidities in case mix. J Cataract Refract Surg. 1995;21:177–181
23. Holland GN, Earl DT, Wheeler NC, et al Results of inpatient and outpatient cataract surgery: a historical cohort comparison. Ophthalmology. 1992;99:845–852
24. Chambless WS. Incidence of anterior and posterior segment complications over 3,000 cases of extracapsular cataract extractions: intact and open capsules. J Cataract Refract Surg. 1985;11:146–148
25. Chitkara DK, Smerdon DL. Risk factors, complications, and results in extracapsular cataract extraction. J Cataract Refract Surg. 1997;23:570–574
26. Dada T, Subrata M, Anand A, et al Microincision cataract surgery in a vitrectomized eye. J Cataract Refract Surg. 2007;33:618–622
27. Kurz S, Krummenauer F, Gabriel P, et al Biaxial microincision versus coaxial small-incision clear cornea cataract surgery. Ophthalmology. 2006;113(10):1818–1826
28. Alio J, Rodriguez-Prats JL, Galal A, et al Outcomes of microincision cataract surgery versus coaxial phacoemulsification. Ophthalmology. 2005;112(1):1997–2003
29. Osher R. Microcoaxial phacoemulsification. J Cataract Refract Surg. 2007;22:408–412
30. Cavallini GM, Campi L, Masini C, et al Bimanual microphacoemulsification versus coaxial miniphaoemulsification: prospective study. J Cataract Refract Surg. 2007;33:387–392
31. Kahraman G, Amon M, Franz C, et al Intraindividual comparison of surgical trauma after bimanual microincision and conventional small-incision coaxial phacoemulsification. J Cataract Refract Surg. 2007;33:618–622
32. Rose AD. Coaxial and bimanual phacoemulsification; considerations in patient and technique selection. Tech Ophthalmol. 2005;3:63–70

9.4 Incision Quality in MICS

Bassam El Kady and Jorge L. Alió

Core Messages

- Minimization of the incision is a consequence of a natural evolution of the cataract surgery technique.
- Good-quality incision is the cornerstone for the success of any type of cataract surgery.
- Microincision cataract surgery (BMICS) provides not only a small incision size of 1.5 mm, but also an incision of good quality with minimal tissue damage.
- Excellent incision quality in BMICS provides immediate, postoperative, unaided visual rehabilitation and early patient satisfaction.
- One of the major advantages of BMICS is the reduction of surgical trauma resulting in a reduction of surgically induced astigmatism (SIA) and corneal high-order aberrations.
- By using the optical coherence tomography (OCT), Visante Anterior Segment OCT we are able to develop a standardized model and protocol to objectively evaluate incision quality in BMICS.
- This high-quality incision opened the door for BMICS to be the surgery of choice for refractive lens exchange.

9.4.1 Introduction: History of Incision Size Reduction

Being a cornerstone and one of the major limbs for the success of any type of cataract surgery, the incision performed has been subjected to revolutionary transformations over many years aiming towards its reduction in size.

B. El Kady (✉)
Ain Shams University, Cairo, Egypt
bisoelkadi@yahoo.com

Consequently, the incision size has been subjected to many waves of development. The history started years ago with a 10 mm, or even larger, incision size for intracapsular and then extracapsular cataract extraction techniques through a corneoscleral incision. The operating incision was approximately 180° around the limbus and this caused considerable damage to the outside layers of the eye with subsequent large numbers of intraoperative and postoperative complications. Owing to surgical advances, the incision size further reduced down to 7–8 mm for the extracapsular era [1].

Then, the method of lens phacoemulsification with the help of ultrasound discovered by Charles Kelman in the late 1960s was a turning point [2] that allowed further reduction of incision size from 3.4 to 2.8 mm, which was the minimum incision performed before the recent era of microincision cataract surgery (BMICS) [1, 3]. Nowadays, BMICS can provide an incision of 1.5 mm or smaller [3–5].

9.4.2 The Trends Towards Microincision Cataract Surgery (BMICS)

With the advantages and benefits of innovative technologies, BMICS has become an increasingly utilized phaco technique, and this modality has been investigated by many authors such as Shock and Girard in the 1970s [6–7], Shearing in 1985 [8], Hara in 1989 [9], as well as Amar Agarwal in 1998 [10], and more recently by Jorge Alió in 2001 [1]. The goal is to achieve smaller incisions with excellent quality, less invasive surgical techniques, and more rapid visual rehabilitation [3].

These trends towards minimizing the incision size had driven us to the biaxiality technique, which requires separation of function for irrigation and aspiration using a bare phacoemulsification tip [3]. Two separate microincisions provide minimal operative stress to the cornea, better incision stability, less astigmatism, and corneal aberrations [11–16].

9.4.3 Advantages of Minimizing the Incision Size

In addition to aforementioned optical benefits of BMICS incision and its ability in stabilizing the corneal optics, such a type of incision, being of a tiny size, allows minimal tissue manipulation and functional disturbances, and hence is considered anatomically capable of providing many other advantages. The decrease in incision size has proved to be associated with a significant decrease in postoperative intraocular inflammation and endophthalmitis [17, 18], less incision-related complications, less surgical time, and shorter postoperative rehabilitation [1, 3], in addition to lower incidents of vitreous loss, iris extrusion, better management of intraoperative floppy iris syndrome (IFIS) [19, 20], and less CME [1, 4, 11, 13].

9.4.4 Model for the Analysis of Corneal Incision Quality [21]

BMICS, in conjunction with microincision IOLs, new phaco technology and fluidic technology, and microinstruments, represents a major breakthrough in cataract surgery. Using the Visante Anterior Segment OCT, we are able to analyze incision quality [21].

The optical coherence tomography system, the Visante OCT, uses infrared light of a 1,310-nm wavelength [22]. The system is connected to a computer with a software that provides different options for image capture and measurement. We developed the following model for analysis.

The patient is well positioned and the related data is introduced in the software. After this, the option "High Res Corneal" is chosen in order to obtain accurate scans of the corneal structure. The patient is asked to fixate on an object located on the opposite direction of the corneal incision in order to obtain a complete cross-sectional scan. A linear scan is used with the same orientation of the incision. This linear scan is rotated 10° in a clockwise direction and 10° in a counterclockwise direction in order to find the image with the best resolution. After this, the scanning is performed and an image is acquired. All scans have a characteristic appearance with arcuate configuration (Fig. 9.4.26).

After obtaining the image, it is analyzed. The following characteristics are determined:

- Angle of the incision: continuously variable, angle formed between the line joining the epithelial and endothelial edges and the tangent line to the epithelial edge of the incision (Fig. 9.4.27). The distances are measured and the angle is calculated by trigonometry.
- Sealing of the epithelial edge: sealed or not sealed (Fig. 9.4.28).
- Sealing of the endothelial edge: sealed or not sealed (Fig. 9.4.29).

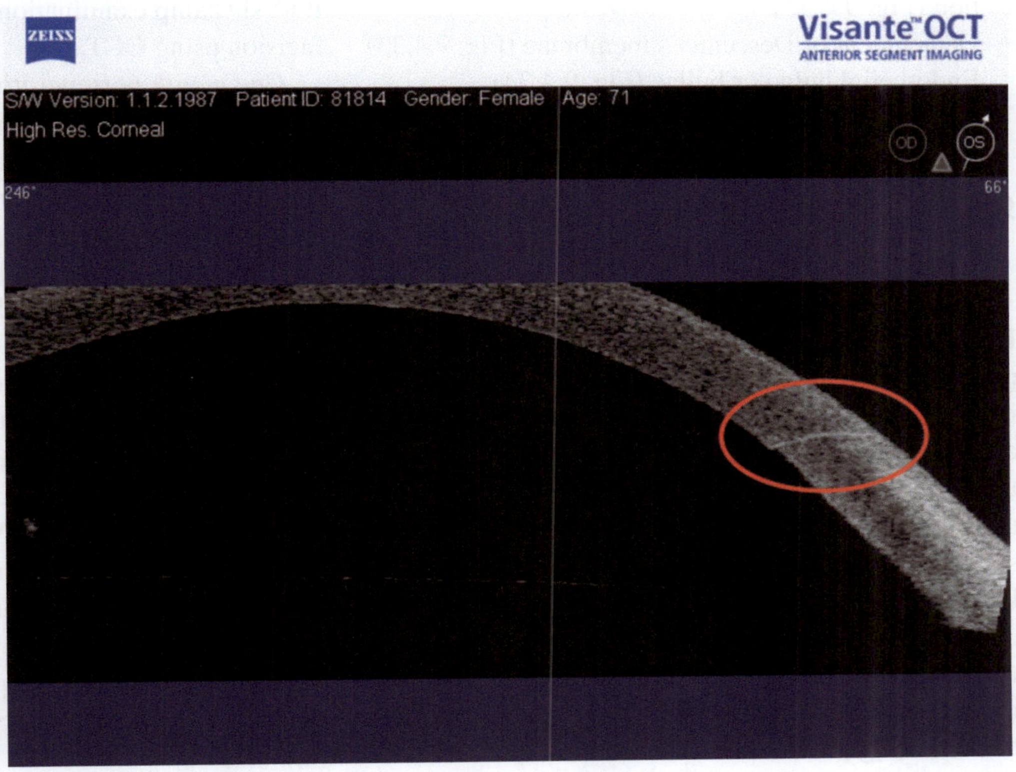

Fig. 9.4.26 OCT image of an MICS incision showing the characteristic appearance of the incision with arcuate configuration

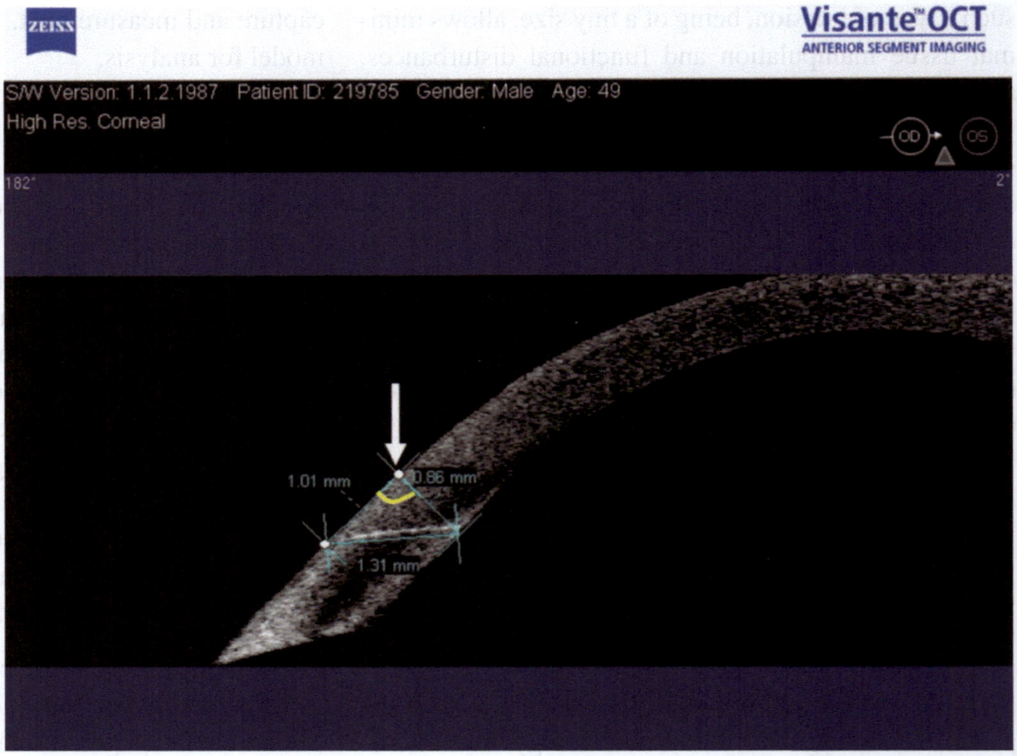

Fig. 9.4.27 OCT image of an MICS incision showing our model for measuring angle of the incision (*white arrow*)

- Thickness of the cornea in the area of the incision and at 1 mm at each side of the incision (Fig. 9.4.30).
- Central corneal thickness and mean thickness in an area of 2–5 and 5–7 mm of the cornea (pachymetric map) (Fig. 9.4.31).
- Percentage of the incision length without coaptation (Fig. 9.4.32).
- Detachment of Descemet's membrane (Fig. 9.4.33).
- Endothelial bulge or bullae (Fig. 9.4.34).

9.4.5 Our Protocol for Evaluation of Incision Quality in BMICS [21]

Based on our experience with BMICS [1, 3, 4], and our published data that documents the ability of BMICS incision to neutralize the corneal optics and to reduce aberrations and astigmatism [11], we created our protocol for adequate objective evaluation of BMICS incisions in both short and long-term outcomes, and subsequently its impact on visual outcomes and optical behavior. Our protocol is as follows:

Patients are scheduled for the postoperative follow-up visits with the clinical examinations and specific measurements are performed at each visit according to the following protocol:

Thirty minutes after surgery: clinical slit-lamp examination with localization of the incision.

One day postoperative: visual acuity, IOP, slit-lamp examination, Seidel's test to check for incision leakage and analysis of the corneal incision using OCT.

One week postoperative: visual acuity, refraction, IOP, slit-lamp examination and analysis of the corneal incision using OCT.

One month postoperative: visual acuity, refraction, IOP, slit-lamp examination, analysis of the corneal incision using OCT, corneal topography, corneal aberrometry and ocular aberrometry.

The stability of corneal incision is analyzed 30 min after surgery with the slit lamp biomicroscopy and its localization is detected. The sealing of the corneal incision is analyzed using fluorescein Seidel's test (Colircusi fluotest® 3 mL (2.5 mg fluorescein sodium + 4 mg Oxibuprocaine chloride) Alcon Cusi, Barcelona-Spain). Any epithelial or stromal alteration is recorded and analyzed. After slit lamp biomicroscopic evaluation, the analysis with the Visante OCT is performed.

We can observe that 1 month postoperatively, corneal topography, corneal and total ocular aberrometry are performed in order to evaluate the incision quality.

Twenty-five eyes of 16 patients with nuclear or corticonuclear cataracts underwent MICS surgery through 1.8 mm incision with IOL implantation. For adequate

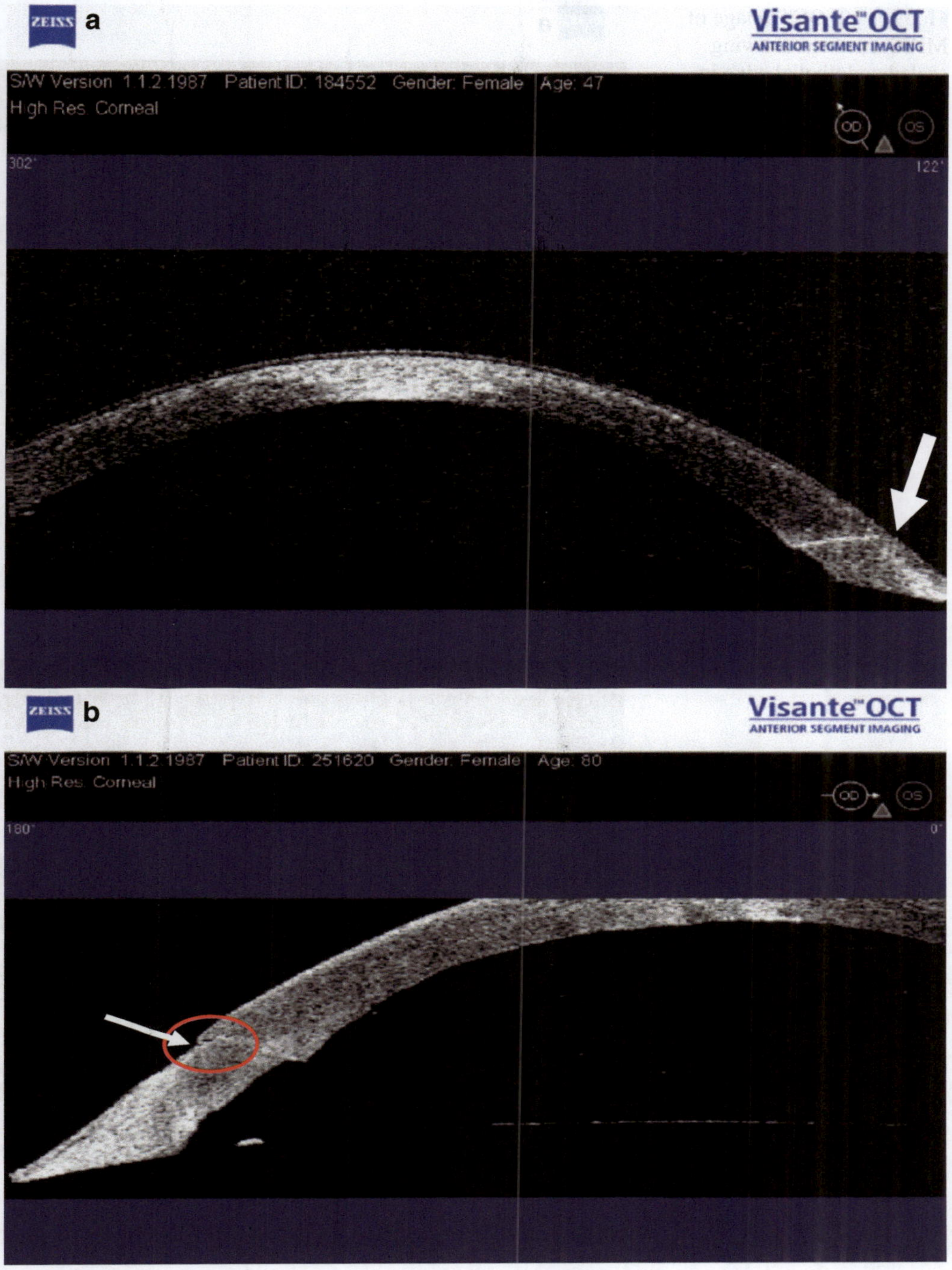

Fig. 9.4.28 OCT image of MICS incisions showing sealed epithelial edge in one case (**a**) and slightly gaped epithelial edge in another one (**b**) (*white arrows*)

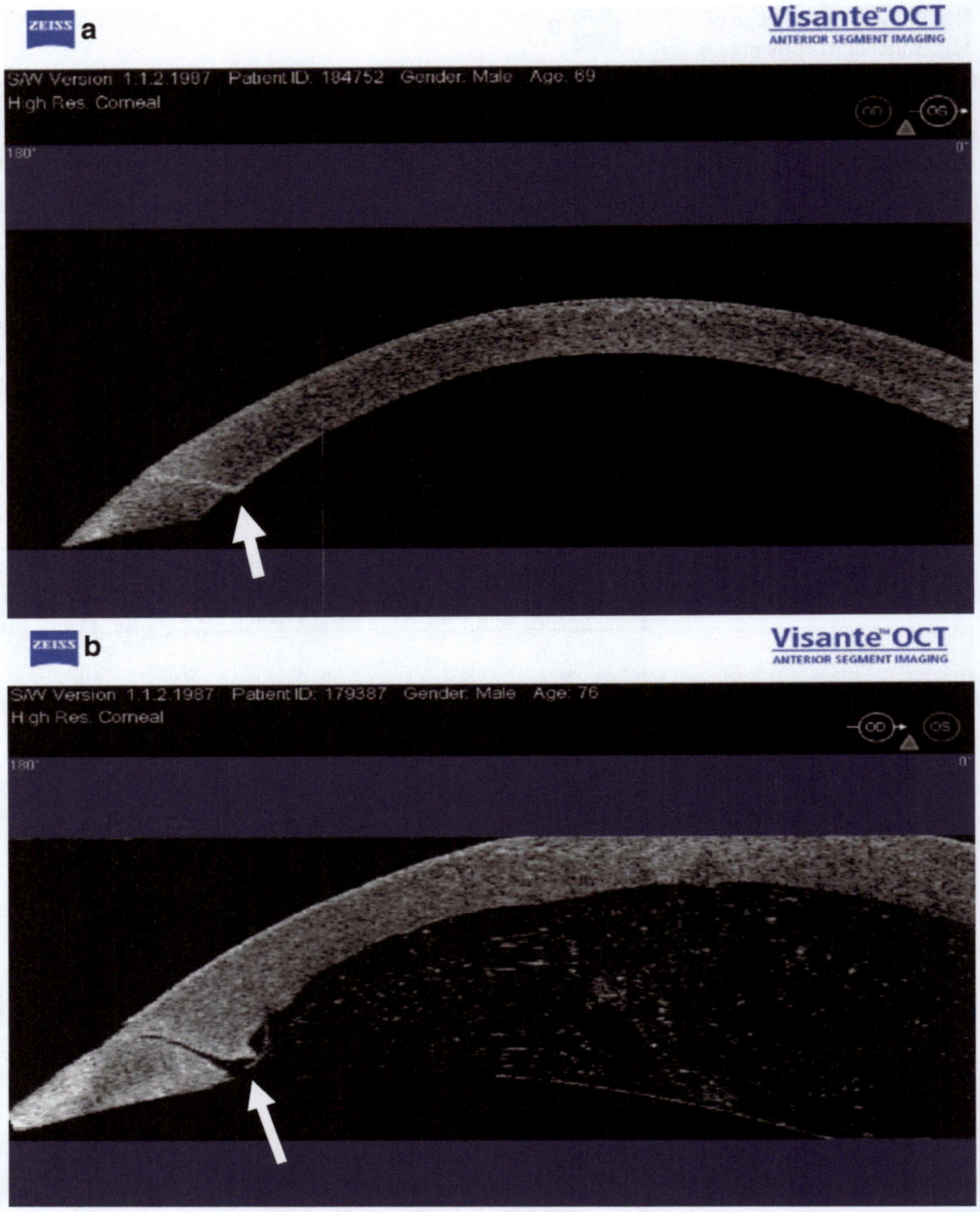

Fig. 9.4.29 OCT image of MICS incisions showing sealed endothelial edge in one case (**a**) and gaped endothelial edge in another one (**b**) (*white arrows*)

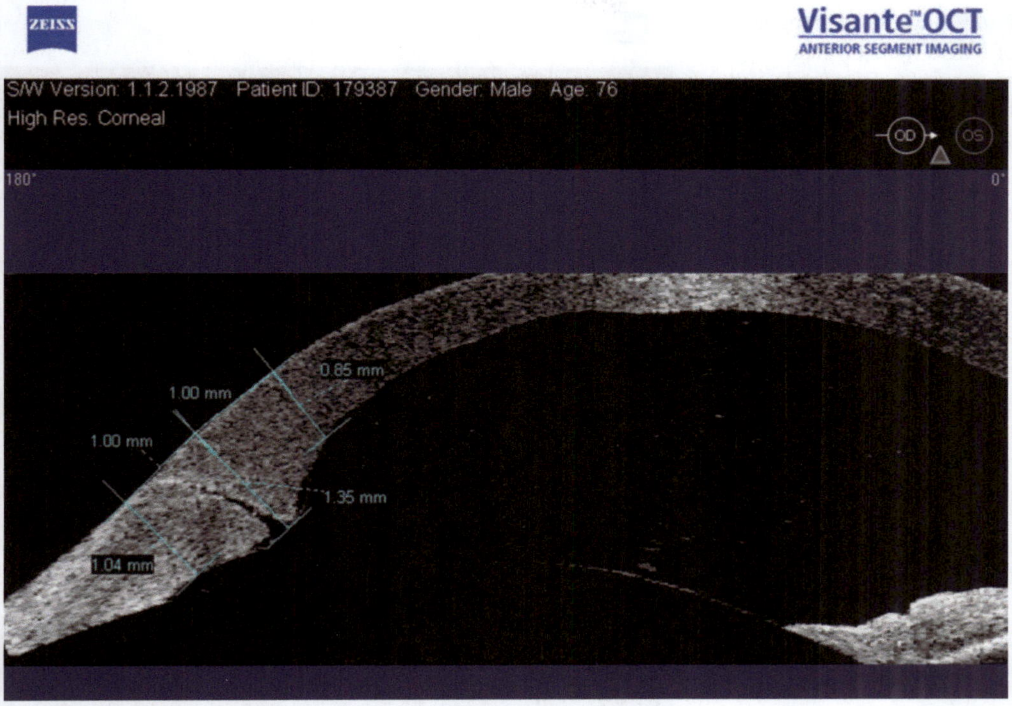

Fig. 9.4.30 OCT image of an MICS incision showing our model for measuring corneal thickness in the area of the incision and at 1 mm at each side of the incision

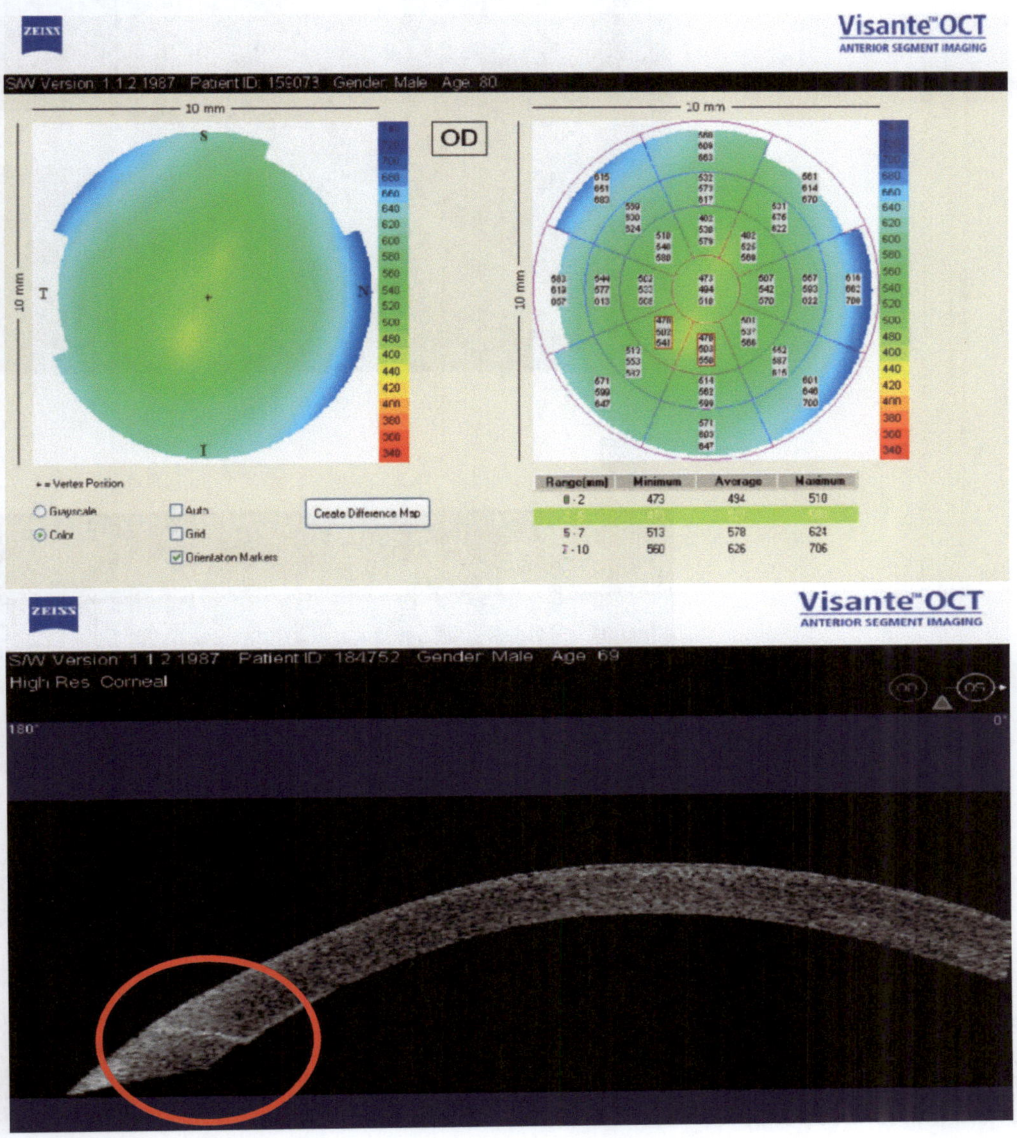

Fig. 9.4.31 Pachymetric map showing central corneal thickness and mean thickness in an area of 2–5 and 5–7 mm of the cornea with the OCT imaging appearance of the same incision (a case of normal corneal thickness)

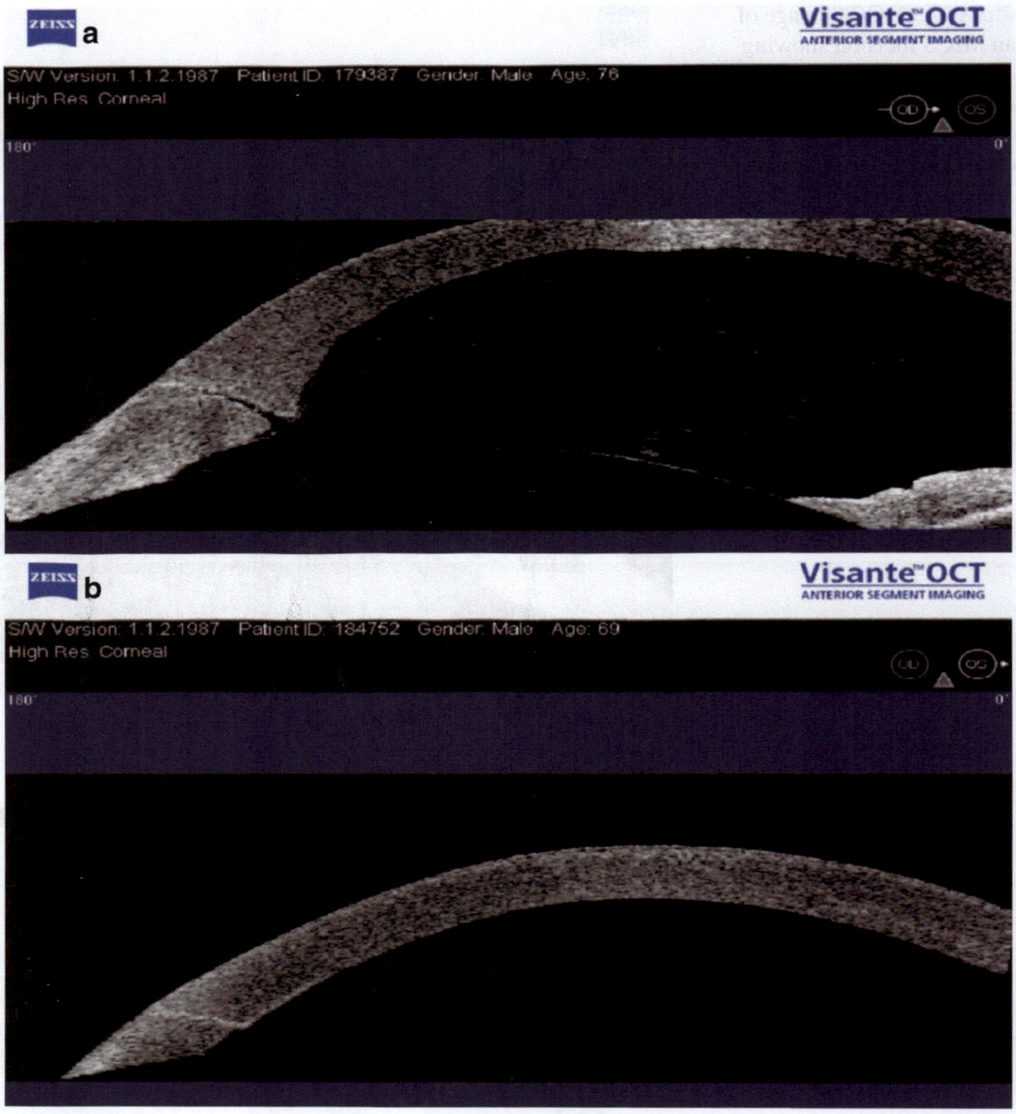

Fig. 9.4.32 OCT images of MICS incisions showing an example of a gaped incision (**a**) and a completely sealed incision (**b**)

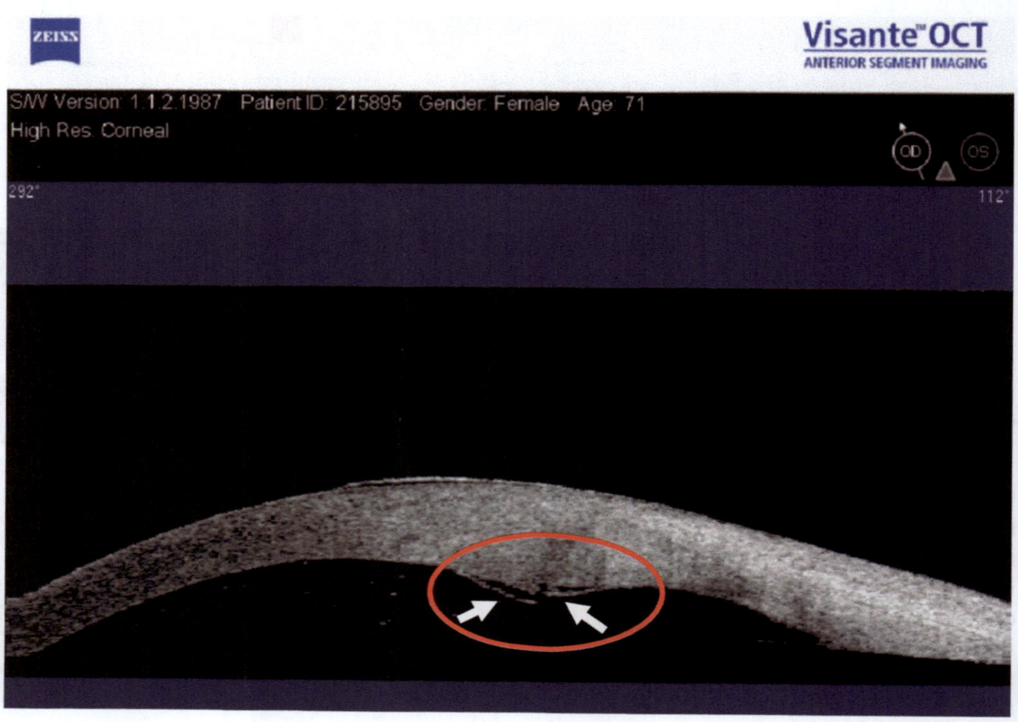

Fig. 9.4.33 OCT image of an MICS incision showing Descemet's membrane detachment (*white arrows*)

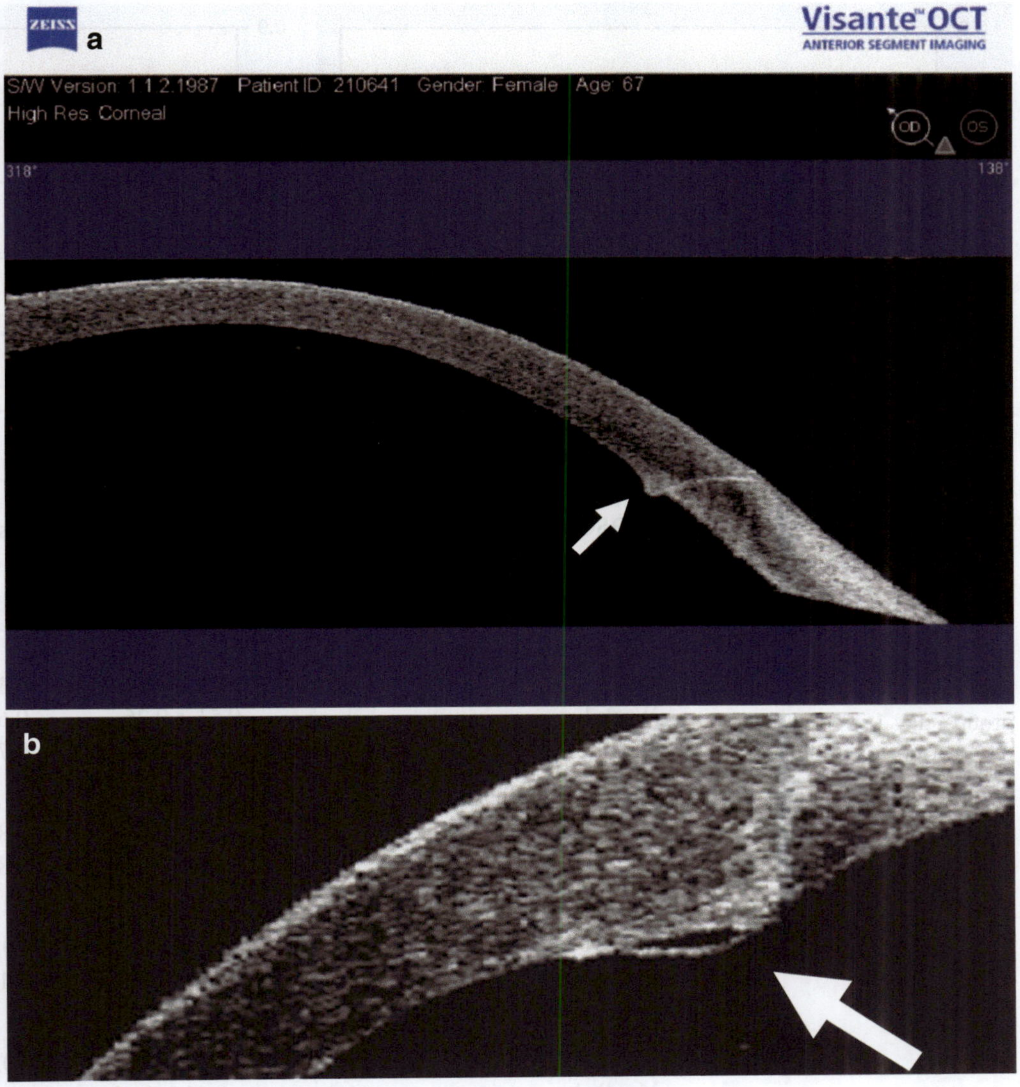

Fig. 9.4.34 OCT images of MICS incisions showing an example of endothelial bulge (**a**) and endothelial bullae (**b**) (*white arrows*)

evaluation of the incision, these group of eyes with BMICS have been compared with an equal number of eyes (25) having the same grade of cataract deepening on the Lens Opacities Classification System III [23]. The second group of patients underwent surgery using the other method currently available for microincision lens surgery using a protected (sleeved) tip, which is the microcoaxial phacoemulsification with an incision of 2.2 mm (microphaco) [24–26].

9.4.6 Results

9.4.6.1 Visual, Refractive and Biomicroscopic Outcomes

Only UCVA (uncorrected visual acuity) at 1 week and 1 month postoperatively were statistically significant. However, BSCVA (best spectacle corrected visual acuity), postoperative sphere and cylinder showed no statistical difference (Fig. 9.4.35, Table 9.4.1).

MICS showed less corneal edema at the first postoperative day by slit-lamp biomicroscopy (Table 9.4.1).

9.4.6.2 Incision Imaging (OCT) Outcomes

Three different OCT incision parameters were evaluated: pachymetric (corneal thickness) values, qualitative (non numerical) incision data and quantitative (numerical) incision data. When comparing both groups, we observed the following results:

Pachemetry measurements (Fig. 9.4.36): BMICS showed less corneal thickness in an area of 5–7 mm of the cornea but only on day-1 (659.92 ± 56.74 vs. 697.00 ± 80.56 $\propto$cm; $p = 0.066$).

Qualitative (descriptive) incision data are summarized in (Table 9.4.2) from which we had the following observations: No misalignment of epithelial edge were

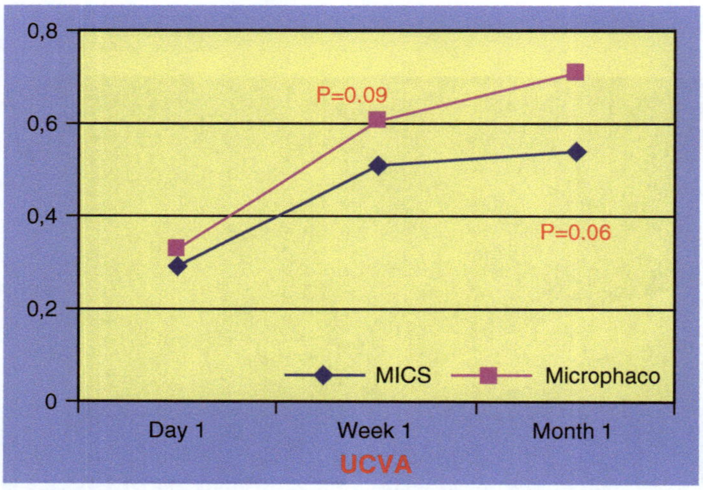

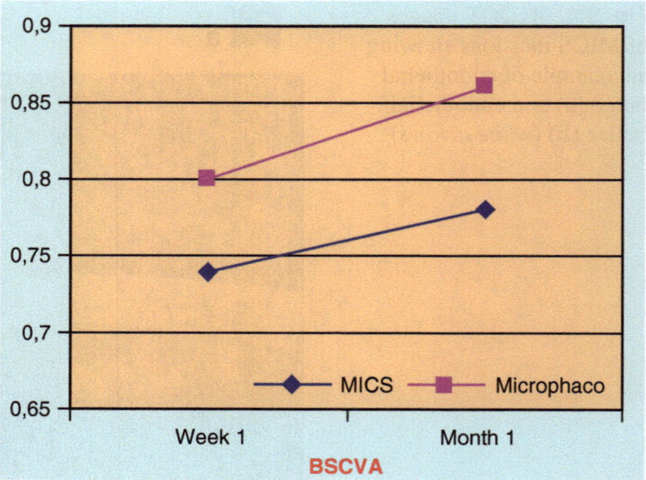

Fig. 9.4.35 Evolution of UCVA and BSCVA, MICS vs. microphaco, throughout the follow-up visits

Table 9.4.1 Comparison of visual acuities, refraction, slit-lamp examination and IOP between both study groups, day 1, week 1 and month 1 postoperatively.

Parameter	MICS	Microphaco	*p* value
UCDVA (mean ± SD)			
Day 1	0.29 ± 0.20	0.33 ± 0.19	0.58
Week 1	0.51 ± 0.26	0.64 ± 0.27	0.09
Month 1	0.54 ± 0.23	0.71 ± 0.27	0.06
BSCDVA (mean ± SD)			
Week 1	0.74 ± 0.26	0.8 ± 0.19	0.42
Month 1	0.78 ± 0.27	0.86 ± 0.20	0.32
Sphere D (mean ± SD)			
Week 1	0.11 ± 0.90	–0.02 ± 0.81	0.60
Month 1	0.16 ± 0.97	0.15 ± 0.96	0.90
Cylinder D (mean ± SD)			
Week 1	–0.75 ± 0.53	–0.96 ± 1.11	0.40
Month 1	–0.61 ± 0.62	–0.65 ± 0.75	0.50
IOP (mmHg) (mean ± SD)			
Day 1	14.32 ± 4.4	16.41 ± 6.19	0.19
Week 1	13.88 ± 2.64	14.09 ± 3.72	0.82
Month 1	13.75 ± 2.77	14.38 ± 3.03	0.43
Flare (%)			
Day 1	56.00	30.4	0.09
Week 1	16.00	4.2	0.35
Month 1	0.00	0.00	–
Edema (%)			
Day 1	44.00	87.00	0.003
Week 1	12.00	4.2	0.61
Month 1	0.00	0.00	–
Seidel (%)			
Day 1	8.00	0.00	0.49
Week 1	0.00	0.00	–
Month 1	0.00	0.00	–
PCO (%)			
Day 1	4.00	8.7	0.60
Week 1	4.00	4.2	1.00
Month 1	4.00	0.00	1.00

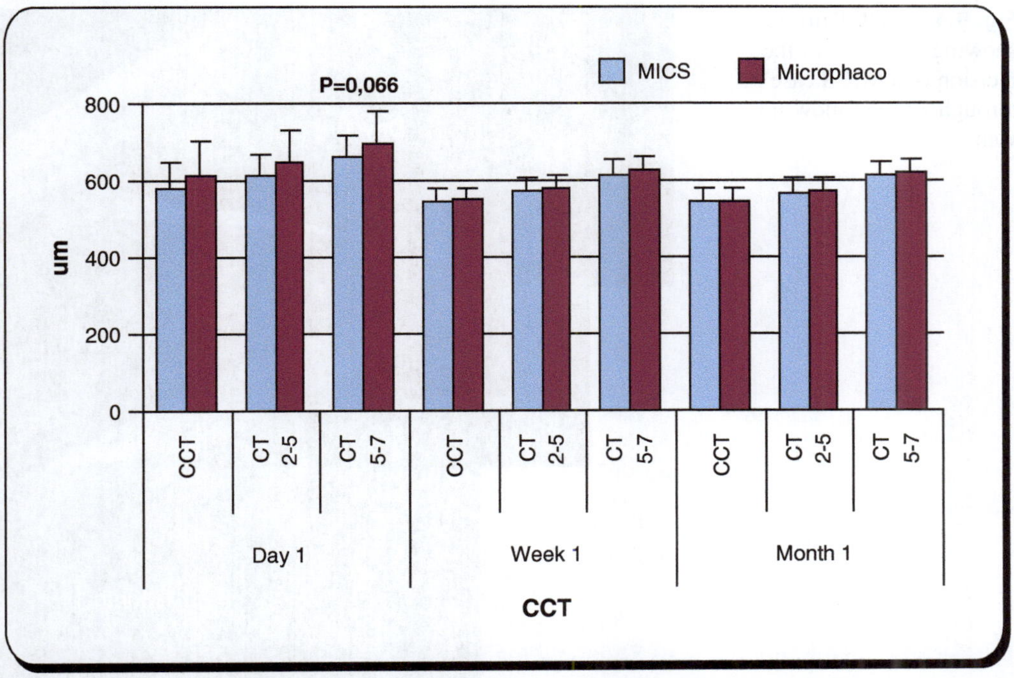

Fig. 9.4.36 OCT measured central corneal thickness and mean thickness in an area of 2–5 and 5–7 mm of the cornea among study groups, day 1, week 1 and month 1 postoperatively (*P* value denotes the only significant difference)

Table 9.4.2 OCT measured descriptive incision data among study groups, day 1, week 1 and month 1 postoperatively

Parameter	Day 1			Week 1			Month 1		
	MICS (%)	Microphaco (%)	*p*	MICS (%)	Microphaco (%)	*p*	MICS (%)	Microphaco (%)	*p*
Epithelial gaping	0.00	0.00		0.00	0.00		0.00	0.00	
Endothelial gaping	64.00	72.00	0.76	76.00	72.7	1.00	0.00	0.00	
DM detachment	60.00	80.00	0.22	32.00	45.5	0.38	0.0	0.00	
Endothelial bullae	8.00	16.00	0.67	12.00	9.1	1.00	0.00	0.00	
No coaptation	3.12 ± 7.61[a]	2.65 ± 5.48[a]	0.46	1.10 ± 2.51[a]	0.59 ± 1.22[a]	0.82	0.00	0.00	

[a]Mean ± SD

present, and at 1 month, there was no misalignment of either the epithelial or endothelial edges, or Descemet's detachments (Fig. 9.4.37).

Quantitative incision data (incision angle and thickness) revealed that corneal thickness at 1 mm temporal to the incision was slightly less in microphaco only on day-1 (0.95 ± 0.14 vs. 0.88 ± 0.13 mm; p = 0.09), (Fig. 9.4.38). Angle of the incision trigonometrically calculated revealed excellent incision quality in both groups with no statistically significant differences (Table 9.4.3, Figs. 9.4.39 and 9.4.40).

9.4.6.3 Topographic and Aberrometric Outcomes

At 1 month postsurgery, corneal topography maps revealed that the postoperative corneal powers didn't differ (44.12 ± 2.26 D vs. 43.96 ± 1.76 D; p = 0.90). Corneal asphericity differs significantly between BMICS and microphaco, with a more prolate topography in the BMICS group (Q 4.5 mm, −0.08 ± 0.39 vs. 0.2 ± 0.72; p = 0.05; Q 8 mm, −0.22 ± 0.45 vs. 0.05 ± 0.49; p = 0.04), (Fig. 9.4.41).

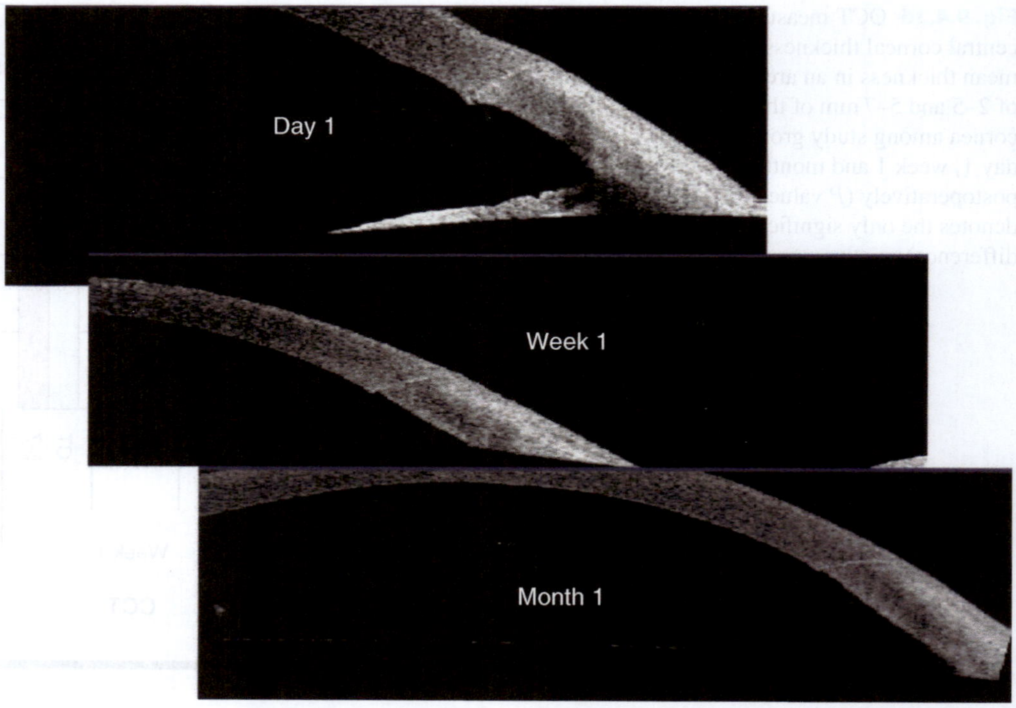

Fig. 9.4.37 OCT images showing evolution of the incision of a MICS case throughout the follow-up visits

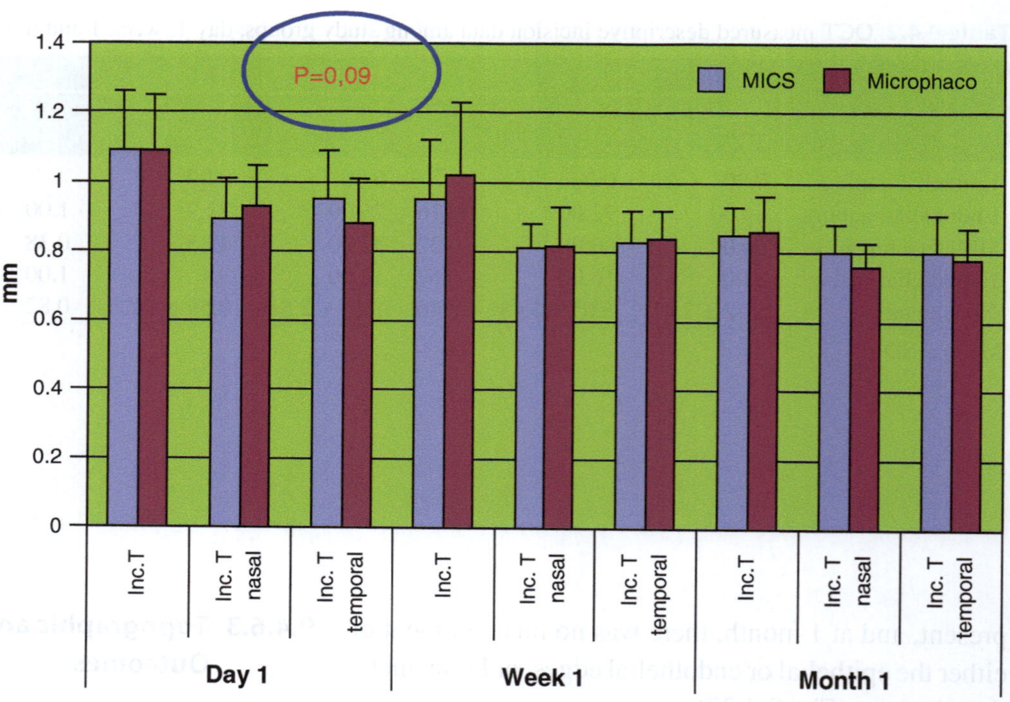

Fig. 9.4.38 OCT measured corneal thickness in the area of the incision and at 1 mm at each side of the incision throughout the follow-up visits

Table 9.4.3 OCT measured incision thickness, central and at 1 mm on either side of the incision and incision angle among study groups, day 1, week 1, and month 1 postoperatively

Parameter	MICS (mean ± SD)	Microphaco (mean ± SD)	*p* value
Central incision thickness (mm)			
Day 1	1.09 ± 0.17	1.09 ± 0.16	0.82
Week 1	0.95 ± 0.17	1.02 ± 0.21	0.16
Month 1	0.85 ± 0.08	0.86 ± 0.1	0.95
Incision thickness 1 mm nasal (mm)			
Day 1	0.89 ± 0.12	0.93 ± 0.12	0.27
Week 1	0.81 ± 0.07	0.82 ± 0.11	0.65
Month 1	0.80 ± 0.08	0.76 ± 0.07	0.11
Incision thickness 1 mm temporal (mm)			
Day 1	0.95 ± 0.14	0.88 ± 0.13	0.09
Week 1	0.83 ± 0.09	0.84 ± 0.08	0.67
Month 1	0.8 ± 0.11	0.78 ± 0.09	0.41
Incision angle (degrees)			
Day 1	42.05 ± 13.23	39.25 ± 9.89	0.4
Week 1	61.81 ± 16.93	42.50 ± 16.67	–
Month 1	46.49 ± 8.98	44.24 ± 10.57	0.37

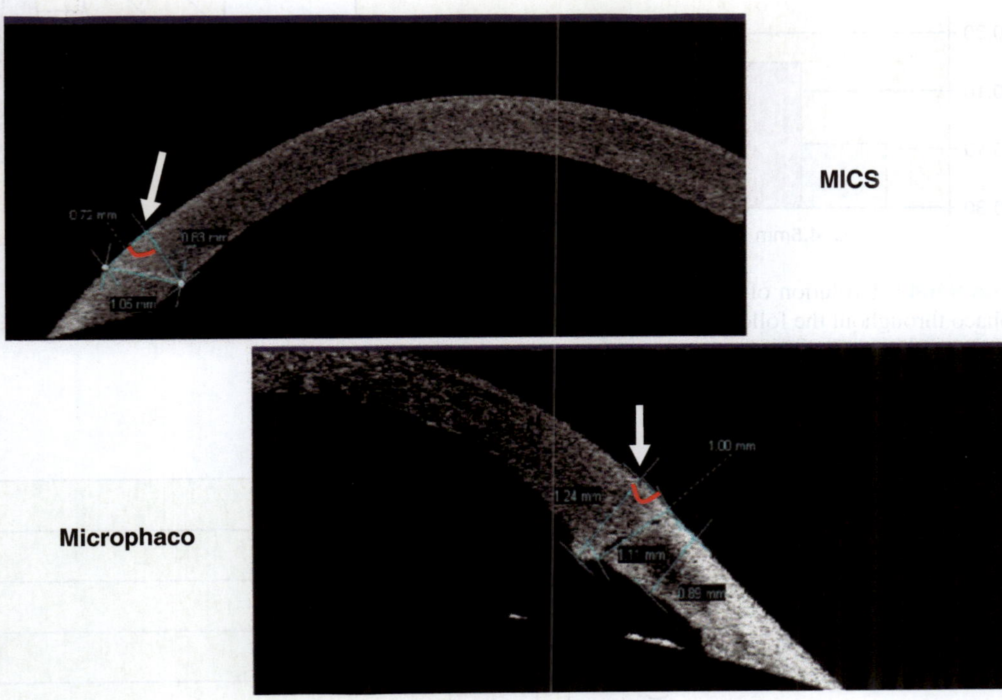

Fig. 9.4.39 OCT images showing angle of the incision MICS vs. microphaco (*white arrows*)

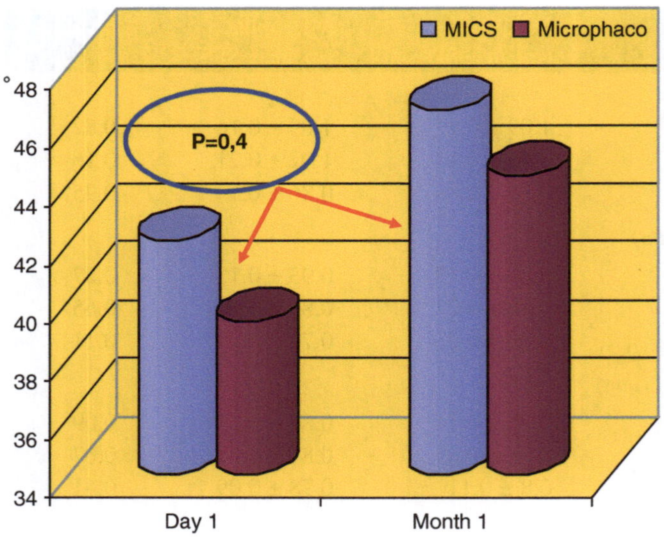

Fig. 9.4.40 Evolution of the angle of the incision MICS vs. microphaco throughout the follow-up visits

Corneal aberrations with the corresponding p values are shown (Fig. 9.4.42) denoting that RMS values for astigmatism and HOA were slightly better in BMICS, $p = 0.06$ and 0.05 respectively. Strehl ratio didn't differ significantly between groups (0.12 ± 0.03 vs. 0.12 ± 0.05; $p = 0.53$).

No statistically significant differences between groups were observed in ocular aberrometry parameters: RMS total (1.97 ± 0.91 vs. $2.35 \pm 1.12\,\mu m$; p = 0.2) and RMS higher-order aberrations (HOA) (0.64 ± 0.22 vs. $0.74 \pm 0.1\,\mu m$; p = 0.1) with good optical quality in both groups (Fig. 9.4.43).

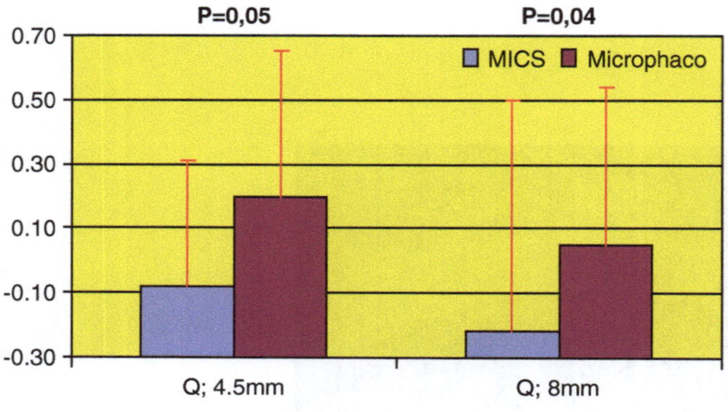

Fig. 9.4.41 Evolution of corneal asphericity MICS vs. microphaco throughout the follow-up visits

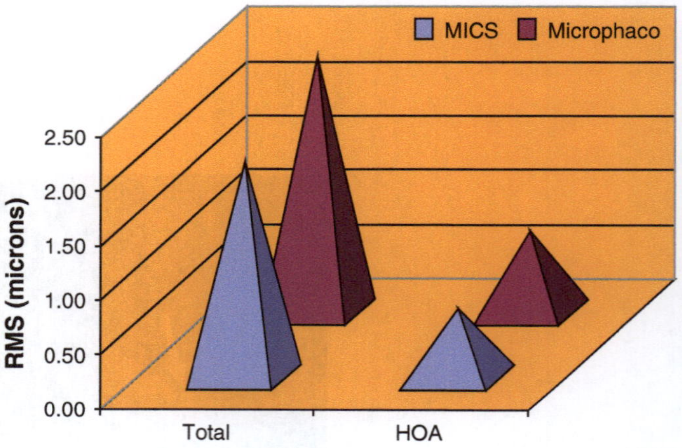

Fig. 9.4.43 Ocular aberrations for both groups

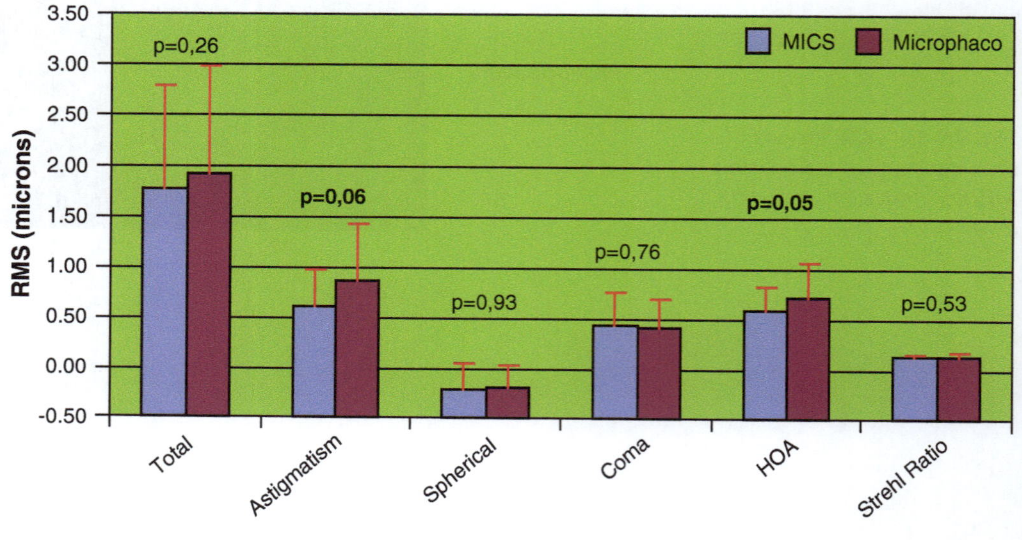

Fig. 9.4.42 Corneal aberrations at 6-mm pupil diameter for both groups with the corresponding *p* values

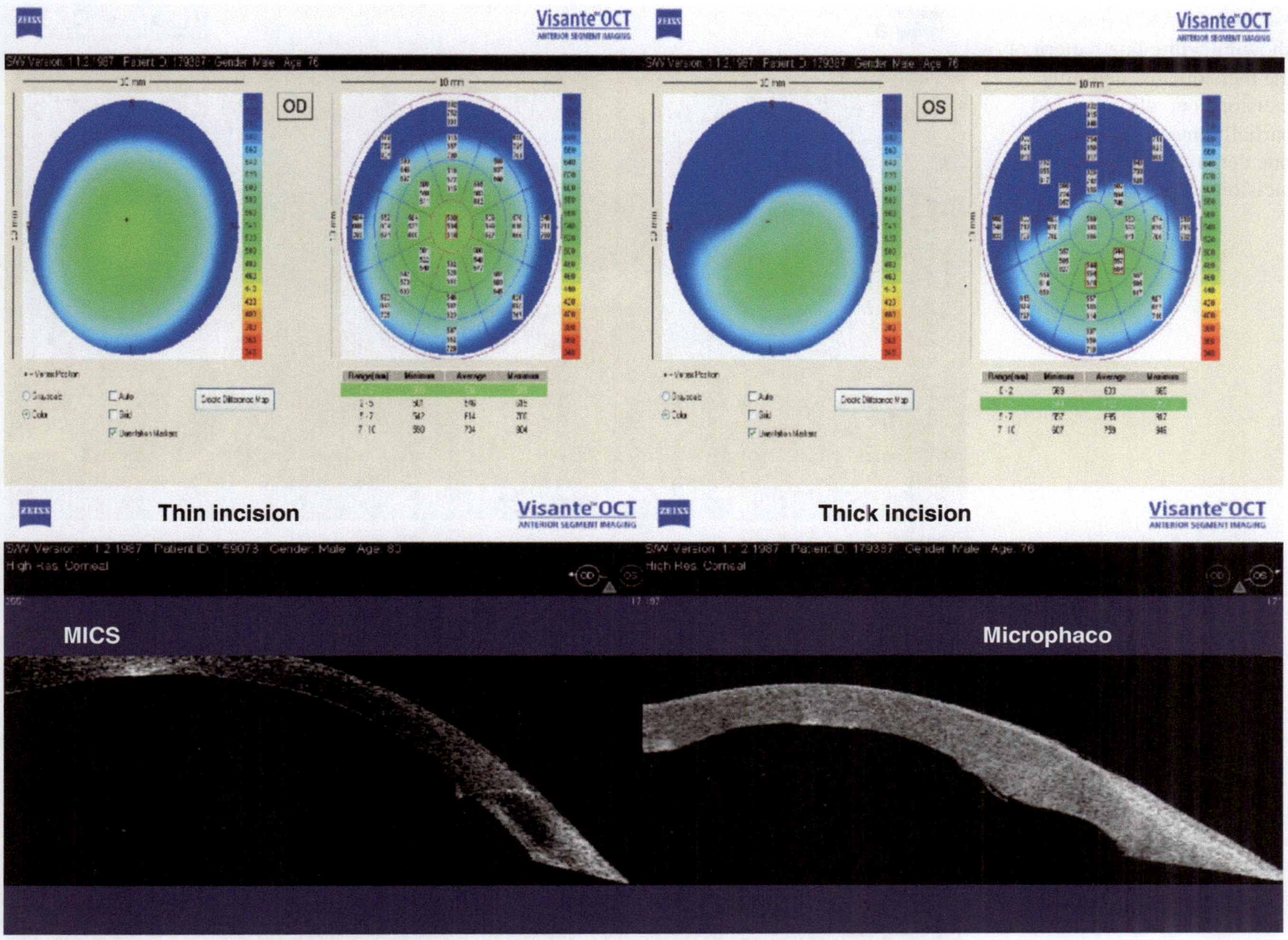

Fig. 9.4.44 An example of a thin incision in a MICS case and a thick incision in a microphaco case, correlation between OCT pachymetric values and OCT imaging assessment

9.4.7 Special Focus on the Role of OCT in the Evaluation of Incision Quality in BMICS

We have to refer that our clinical observations about BMICS incision were subsequently confirmed objectively by OCT assessment parameters (Fig. 9.4.44), confirming the role of OCT as an accurate quantitative tool assessing the incision effect and quality [17].

The importance of OCT as a tool for evaluating tiny incisions results in the fact that it is a noncontact modality and therefore, introduces no artifacts and is more precise than slit-lamp evaluations, (Fig. 9.4.45) [17, 27, 28].

An important parameter of incision quality is the angle of the incision. Our study [21] shows that BMICS provides an incision angle previously described as critical for self-sealability [29], to obtain secure ocular incisions unaffected by the level of IOP, especially among sutureless cataract incisions, which provide a perfectly coapted barrier against the invasion of pathogenic organisms, supported by the fact that we did not have any single case of endophthalmitis in our study [21]. Although variable and sometimes poor incision apposition with fluctuation with IOP has been reported by many authors [27, 29–31], our results were obtained using a large number of eyes, with longer follow-up, compared with others who used either postmortem human globes or animal eyes.

Interestingly, we may encounter a localized subclinical Descemet's membrane detachment. This could be explained by double-cut incisions or by stretching the incisions during IOL insertion [17, 21, 32].

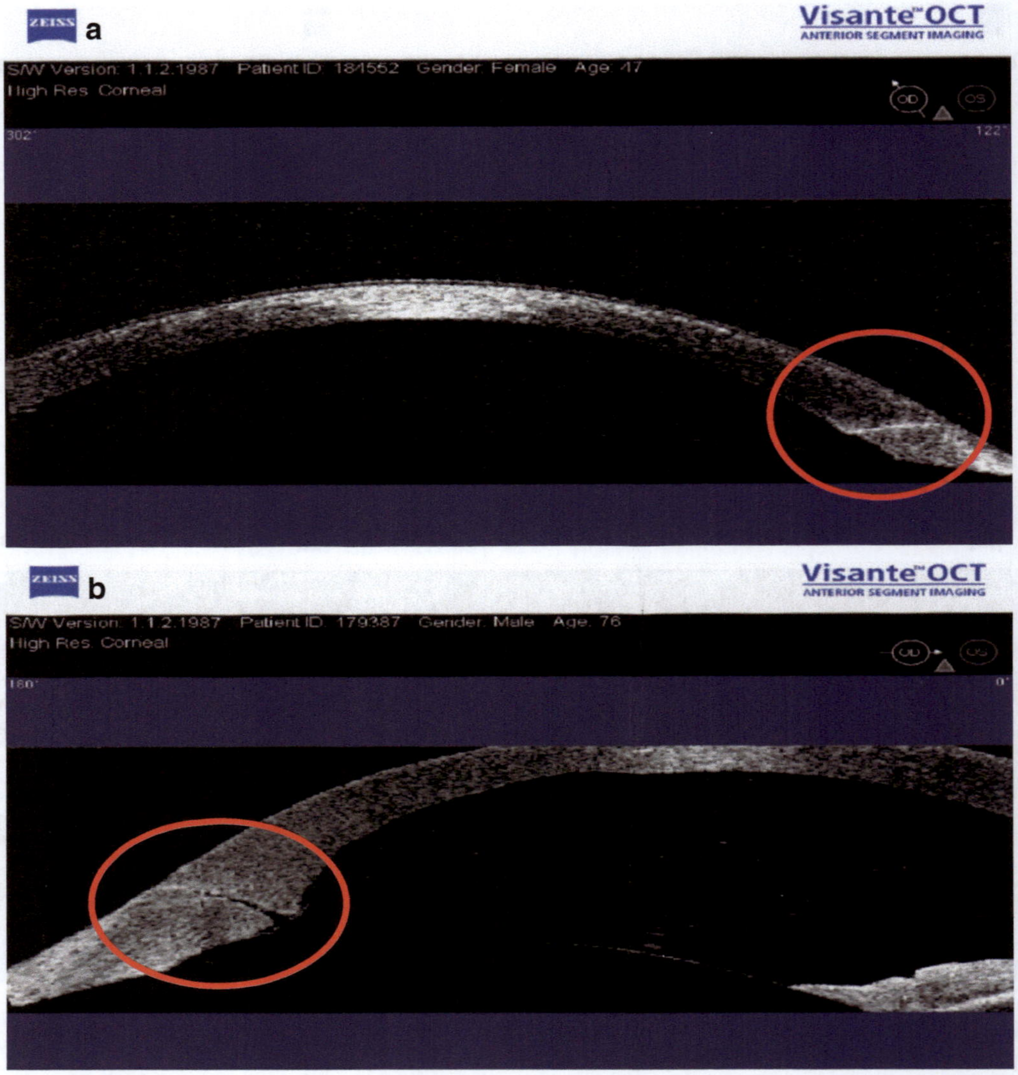

Fig. 9.4.45 OCT images showing white line pattern of the incision area denoting incision coaptation (**a**) and partially interrupted white line denoting some degree of incision gaping (**b**)

9.4.8 Conclusion

Minimizing the incision size can reduce intraoperative corneal trauma and result in more rapid visual recovery, and allow lenticular modalities a more prominent role in refractive surgery.

BMICS provides optically high quality incisions compared with other microincision techniques for lens surgery, with immediate postoperative visual rehabilitation as anticipated by refractive surgery candidates and increasingly by cataract surgery patients.

OCT is a very useful tool in assessing corneal incision quality.

Take Home Pearls

- BMICS provides optically excellent incisions.
- BMICS results in astigmatism neutral incisions.
- BMICS preserves the prolate corneal topography.
- BMICS creates less corneal edema in the short term and less corneal aberrations in the long term.
- OCT is a useful tool in assessing corneal incision quality in BMICS.
- By minimizing incision size in BMICs, we are maximizing outcomes in cataract and refractive lens exchange surgery.

References

1. Alio JL, Rodriguez Prats JL, Galal A, eds. MICS Micro-incision Cataract Surgery. El Dorado, Republic of Panama, Highlights of Ophthalmology, 2004; 1–4
2. Kelman CD (1967) Phaco-emulsification and aspiration. A new technique of cataract removal. A preliminary report. Am J Ophthalmol 64:23–35
3. Alio J.L, Rodriguez-Prats JL, Galal A, et al (2005) Outcomes of microincision cataract surgery versus coaxial phacoemulsification. Ophthalmology 112:1997–2003
4. Alió JL, Klonowski P, El Kady B, et al (2008) MICS (micro-incision cataract surgery). In: Garg A, Fine IH, Alió JL, et al (eds) Mastering the techniques of advanced phaco surgery. Jaypee brothers, New Delhi, pp 121–136
5. Tsuneoka H, Shiba T, Takahashi Y (2001) Feasibility of ultrasound cataract surgery with a 1.4 mm incision. J Cataract Refract Surg 27:934–940
6. Shock JP (1972) Removal of cataracts with ultrasonic fragmentation and continuous irrigation. Trans Pac Coast Otoophthalmol Soc Annu Meet 53:139–144
7. Girard LJ (1978) Ultrasonic fragmentation for cataract extraction and cataract complications. Adv Ophthalmol 37:127–135
8. Shearing SP, Relyea RL, Loaiza A, Shearing RL (1985) Routine phacoemulsification through a one-millimeter non-sutured incision. Cataract 2:6–10
9. Hara T, Hara T (1989) Endocapsular phacoemulsification and aspiration (ECPEA) – recent surgical technique and clinical results. Ophthalmic Surg 20(7):469–475
10. Agarwal A, Agarwal S (1998). No anesthesia cataract surgery. In: Agarwal S (ed) Phacoemulsification, laser cataract surgery, and foldable IOLs.: Jaypee Brothers, New Dehli, pp 144–154
11. Elkady B, Alió J, Ortiz D, et al (2008) Corneal aberrations after microincision cataract surgery. J Cataract Refract Surg 34:40–45
12. Osher RH, Injev VP (2006) Thermal study of bare tips with various system parameters and incision sizes. J Cataract Refract Surg 32:867–872
13. Berdahl JP, DeStafeno JJ, Kim T (2007) Corneal incision architecture and integrity after phacoemulsification: evaluation of coaxial, microincision coaxial, and microincision bimanual techniques. J Cataract Refract Surg 33:510–515
14. Yao K, Tang X, Ye P (2006) Corneal astigmatism, high order aberrations, and optical quality after cataract surgery: micro-incision versus small-incision. J Refract Surg 22: S1079–S1082
15. Jiang Y, Le Q, Yang J, et al (2006) Changes in corneal astigmatism and high order aberrations after clear corneal tunnel phacoemulsification guided by corneal topography. J Refract Surg 22:S1083–S1088
16. Guirao A, Tejedor J, Artal P (2004) Corneal aberrations before and after small-incision cataract surgery. Inves Ophthalmol Vis Sci 45:4312–4319
17. Behrens A, Stark WJ, Pratzer KA, et al (2008) Dynamics of small-incision clear cornea incisions after phacoemulsification surgery using optical coherence tomography in the early postoperative period. J Refract Surg 24:46–49
18. Chee SP, Bacsal K (2005) Endophthalmitis after microincision cataract surgery. J Cataract Refract Surg 31:1834–1835
19. Herretes S, Stark WJ, Pirouzmanesh A, et al (2005) Inflow of ocular surface fluid into the anterior chamber after phacoemulsification through sutureless corneal cataract incisions. Am J Ophthalmol 140:737–740
20. Taban M, Sarayba MA, Ignacio TS, et al (2005) Ingress of India ink into the anterior chamber through sutureless clear corneal cataract incisions. Arch Ophthalmol 123:643–648
21. Elkady B, Piñero D, Alió JL. Corneal incision quality: microincision cataract surgery versus microcoaxial phacoemulsification. J Cataract Refract Surg. 2009; 35(3): 466–74
22. Radhakrishnan S, Rollins AM, Roth JE, et al (2001) Real-time optical coherence tomography of the anterior segment at 1310 nm. Arch Ophthalmol 119:1179–1185
23. Chylack LT Jr, Wolfe JK, Singer DM, et al (1993) The lens opacities classification system III. The Longitudinal Study of Cataract Study Group. Arch Ophthalmol 111:831–836
24. Haripriya A, Aravind S, Vadi K, et al (2006) Bimanual microphaco for posterior polar cataracts. J Cataract Refract Surg 32:914–917
25. Rongé LJ (2004) Step-by-Step Guide to microphaco. EyeNet Magazine >> Catarac-Jan http://development.aao.org/aao/news/eyenet/cataract/cataract_jan_2004.htm
26. Guttman C (2005) Coaxial microphaco considered a significant advance in cataract surgery. Ophthalmol Times 30:1–22
27. McDonnell PJ, Taban M, Sarayba M, et al (2003) Dynamic morphology of clear corneal cataract incisions. Ophthalmology 110:2342–2348
28. Fine IH, Hoffman RS, Packer M (2007) Profile of clear corneal cataract incisions demonstrated by ocular coherence tomography. J Cataract Refract Surg 33:94–97
29. Taban M, Rao B, Reznik J, et al (2004) Dynamic morphology of sutureless cataract incisions–effect of incision angle and location. Surv Ophthalmol Suppl 2:S62–S72
30. Khng C, Packer M, Fine IH, et al (2006) Intraocular pressure during phacoemulsification. J Cataract Refract Surg 32:301–308
31. May W, Castro-Combs J, Camacho W, et al (2008) Analysis of clear corneal incision integrity in an ex vivo model. J Cataract Refract Surg 34:1013–1018
32. Johar SR, Vasavada AR, Praveen MR, et al (2008) Histomorphological and immunofluorescence evaluation of bimanual and coaxial phacoemulsification incisions in rabbits. J Cataract Refract Surg 34:670–676

Index

MIX
Papier aus verantwortungsvollen Quellen
Paper from responsible sources
FSC® C105338

If you have any concerns about our products,
you can contact us on
ProductSafety@springernature.com

In case Publisher is established outside the EU,
the EU authorized representative is:
Springer Nature Customer Service Center GmbH
Europaplatz 3, 69115 Heidelberg, Germany

Printed by Libri Plureos GmbH
in Hamburg, Germany